Serum Free Light Chain Analysis
plus Hevylite

7th Edition
Fully revised for 2015

Disclaimer

Some of the products or applications discussed in this book may not be approved or available in all countries. Please contact info@bindingsite.co.uk for more information.

The content we share is for educational purposes only. Some of the content may involve forward-looking use of The Binding Site Group Ltd's products. Nothing is intended to promote off-label use of any of The Binding Site Group Ltd's products and we strongly recommend that you refer to the applicable product instructions for clarification of intended use. We cannot advise on individual clinical test results as they are contextually dependent on other laboratory test results alongside clinical signs and symptoms. Please contact your physician or local patient group.

Trademark notices

Freelite®, Hevylite®, Combylite®, SPAPLUS® and Optilite® are registered trademarks of The Binding Site Group Ltd (Birmingham, UK) in certain countries.

BN™II, BN ProSpec™ and ADVIA™ are trademarks of Siemens Healthcare Diagnostics Inc.

Other brand or product names may be trademarks of their respective holders.

Published by The Binding Site Group Ltd, 8 Calthorpe Road, Edgbaston, Birmingham B15 1QT, UK

Design and page creation by Grays Associates.

British Library Cataloguing in Publication Data

A catalogue record for this book is available from the British Library.

ISBN 978-0-9932196-0-3

Wikilite.com

A full electronic version of the 7th edition of Serum Free Light Chain Analysis plus Hevylite is available online at www.wikilite.com. The format is similar to that of Wikipedia, with a search facility and hyperlinks between the chapters and to bibliographic information via PubMed™. Wikilite.com is available on a read-only basis. A dedicated team of writers at The Binding Site regularly monitor the literature and add new data, while a chief editor ensures consistency of content and style. In this manner, Wikilite.com is maintained as an up-to-date literature review for all those who are interested in Serum Free Light Chain Analysis plus Hevylite.

Acknowledgement

Binding Site would like to acknowledge the many people who have contributed to the writing and editing of this book, as well as those who have provided data and figures presented within. They include Binding Site staff members (past and present), as well as numerous Clinical and Scientific collaborators. Our grateful thanks go to them all.

Contents

Section 1 - The biology and measurement of immunoglobulins

Section 2 - Practical considerations of Freelite immunoassays

Section 4 - Monoclonal gammopathies

Section 5 - Diseases with monoclonal light chain deposition

Section 6 - Other diseases with monoclonal or increased polyclonal FLCs

Section 7 - Instrumentation and external quality assurance

How remarkable free light chain (FLC) analysis has become! First emerging in 1846 as Bence Jones proteinuria, the analysis lived quietly in the backwaters for 150 years, until 2001 when successful development of a blood test reignited interest. Serum measurement cleared the fog caused by renal tubular resorption of the light chains, so that in a mere dozen years the new assay has stolen the tumour marker limelight: wide ranging applications, high sensitivity for the diagnosis of numerous tumour types with great utility for monitoring patients.

However, its clinical value comes with complexity. It is not just a simple, one dimensional test, such as the measurement of carcinoembryonic antigen: where high levels mean disease and low levels mean normal, but two dimensional; two tests in one - kappa (κ) and lambda (λ). And, their values can be interpreted in various ways. Let me elaborate:

First, since the two tests are used in combination, where each can be high, medium or low, there are nine possible results making interpretation multifaceted. Second, the two results can be analysed in several different ways. Each pair can be; a), divided (κ/λ) to provide a tumour diagnostic ratio; b), used directly to provide an involved FLC (iFLC) or uninvolved (uFLC) monitoring value; c), subtracted to provide a more accurate indicator of production (by correcting for impaired renal function); and d), summated (ΣFLC) to produce a measure of polyclonal B-cell activation. Third, the test can be used for a multitude of different diseases.

The tumours range from the classic monoclonal gammopathies of multiple myeloma, Waldenström's macroglobulinaemia and their ilk to the ten or more B-cell, non-Hodgkin lymphomas and the subsets of B-cell chronic lymphocytic leukaemia. Of the non-tumour diseases, FLCs are a sensitive marker of renal impairment and useful when monitoring a variety of inflammatory diseases ranging from rheumatoid arthritis, Sjögren's syndrome, multiple sclerosis and vasculitides to infections such as hepatitis and HIV; indeed, just about any illness that has an inflammatory component. Dramatically, FLC molecules are the cause of two disorders. Not in the manner of parathyroid hormone initiating bone disease via an effector cell, but the actual causal molecule of the disease in AL amyloidosis and light chain deposition disease. No other tumour marker can claim such wide ranging clinical prominence.

However, κ and λ light chain molecules are complicated: two main types, ten sub-groups, 70 genes plus allotypes and through combinatorial mechanisms, over a million epitopes. How, with all these variations, can they be properly measured? The Freelite® polyclonal, homogeneous immunoassay is a good start; a fine benchmark. Monoclonal antibody assays are and will remain, a problem. Different assays will produce different results depending upon their antibody specificity, resulting in varied normal ranges and varied concentrations for monoclonal light chains; never quite comparable. And they are likely to miss the occasional patient's disease. Perhaps assays that can identify the multitude of molecular structures should be used, such as mass-spectrometry, but that is for the future.

That takes me to Hevylite® – tests that measure intact immunoglobulin heavy chain/light chain pairs. Just as serum FLC κ and λ are more powerful tools when measured separately, so Ig'κ and Ig'λ pairs add to total immunoglobulin analysis. A tumour produced molecule eg. IgGκ, can be more accurately monitored by excluding the non-tumour produced IgGλ; the ratio of IgGκ/IgGλ is a measure of clonality and the non-tumour IgGλ becomes suppressed during tumour growth providing information about tumour staging and prognosis. But these are early days. Hevylite analysis is where FLC analysis was 10 years ago – there is much more to be discovered.

Free light chains deserve their Greek names of kappa and lambda. They add linguistic gravitas to extraordinary molecules. If any clinical tests required a monograph to clarify their utility then this is surely true of serum FLC (and Hevylite) analyses.

AR Bradwell, January 2015

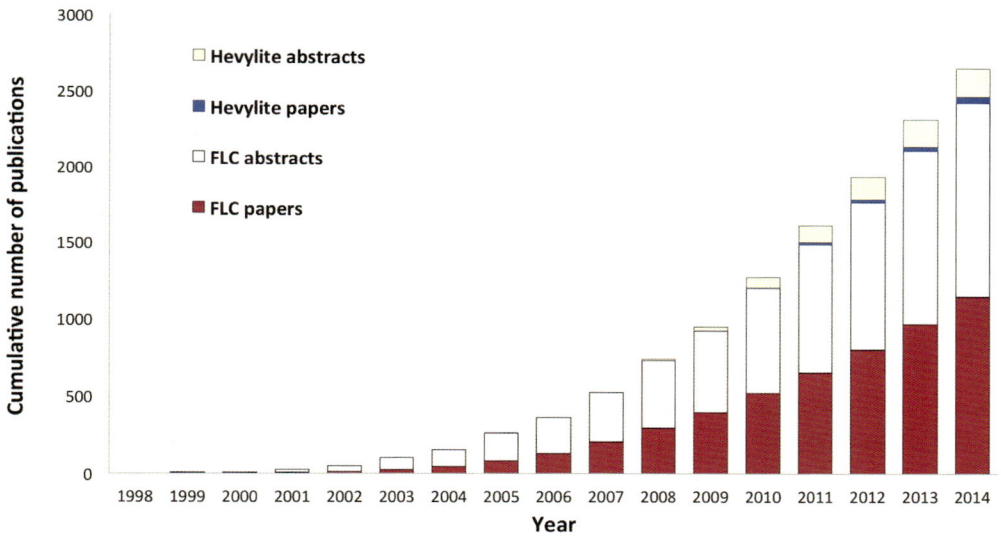

Cumulative number of FLC and Hevylite publications.

The clinical importance of serum free light chain and Hevylite analysis

1.1. Introduction

Multiple myeloma (MM) is a disease with many faces. It usually presents in old age but may occur in youth. Bone pain and fractures are characteristic, but soft tissue involvement by plasmacytomas may also occur. Some patients may die within weeks of presentation, while others "smoulder" for years. Patients may develop renal failure, acute and chronic infections or AL amyloidosis, and many will require stem cell transplantation or intensive chemotherapy. Consequently, many specialists, including haematologists, nephrologists, immunologists, orthopaedic surgeons and chemical pathologists, become involved in disease management. Furthermore, the prevalence of MM is increasing due to a slowly rising incidence and a longer life expectancy *(Section 12.2)*. Other plasma cell dyscrasias encompass a similar, if not greater, diversity of outcomes. Monoclonal gammopathy of undetermined significance (MGUS) can be found in approximately 3% of the (Caucasian) population over the age of 50 years but of this 3%, the vast majority will die of unrelated causes *(Chapter 13)*[2]. By contrast, for patients with plasma cell leukaemia or AL amyloidosis with cardiac involvement, median survival is close to 12 months *(Chapters 22 and 28)*[3,4].

One feature that MM and other plasma cell dyscrasias have in common is the production of monoclonal immunoglobulin proteins that can be detected in the serum, with the exception of a very small percentage of patients whose clonal plasma cells appear to be non-secretory, e.g. in nonsecretory MM *(Chapter 16)*[5] or POEMS syndrome *(Section 34.4)*[6]. The monoclonal protein may be intact immunoglobulin: IgG, IgA, IgM, IgD or (very rarely) IgE *(Figure 1.1)*. Immunoglobulin free light chain (FLC) production frequently accompanies the intact immunoglobulin or it can be found in isolation as in light chain MM (LCMM *(Chapter 15)*; rarely isolated immunoglobulin heavy chain may be produced *(Section 34.3)*. Plasma cell tumours are generally "hidden" within the bone marrow and initially give rise to symptoms that are vague and non-specific. Therefore, the presence of monoclonal proteins in the serum is a significant aid, not only for the diagnosis of these disorders but also their clinical management; indicating the response to treatment and persistence of residual disease. The majority of serum tumour markers (for non-plasma cell cancers) are relatively non-specific: the markers are present in healthy individuals but abnormally high concentrations indicate the possibility that a tumour may be present. By contrast, monoclonal immunoglobulins are highly specific tumour markers, the occurrence of a monoclonal immunoglobulin defines the presence of a clone of cells responsible for its production. However, it should be noted that apart from plasma cells, clones of less mature B-lymphocytes may also produce monoclonal immunoglobulin proteins *(Chapters 31, 32 and 33)* so, in fact, the presence of monoclonal immunoglobulin indicates the existence of a clone of cells of the B-lymphocyte lineage (i.e. a lymphoproliferative disorder).

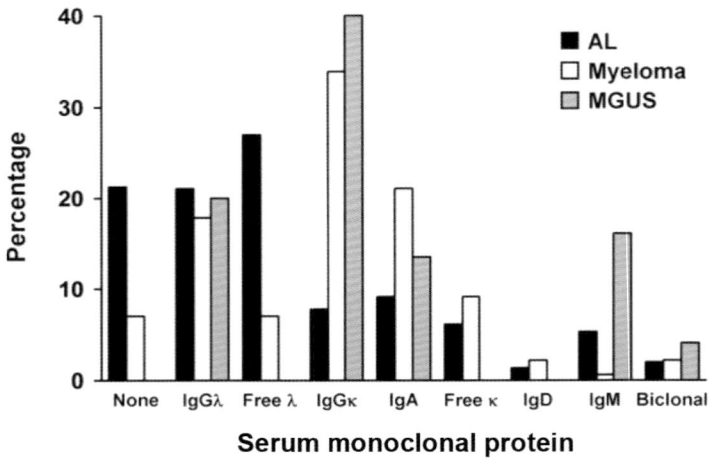

Figure 1.1. Types of serum monoclonal proteins found on immunofixation results.
The percentage of each type of monoclonal protein is shown in samples from patients with monoclonal gammopathy of undetermined significance (MGUS), MM, and AL amyloidosis. (Reproduced with permission from the American Journal of Hematology[1] and John Wiley and Sons).

Monoclonal immunoglobulin proteins (specifically FLCs) have been linked to MM since they were first reported by Dr Henry Bence Jones over 150 years ago *(Chapter 2)*[7,8]. Notwithstanding their substantial history and great utility, measurement of these tumour markers, particularly FLCs, remained problematic for many years. Principally, this was a consequence of attempting to measure FLC concentrations in urine. An important function of the kidneys is to prevent the loss of FLCs and other small protein molecules into the urine. FLCs are rapidly cleared through the renal glomeruli with half-lives of 2 - 6 hours before being metabolised in the proximal tubules of the nephrons with reabsorption of the constituent amino acids. Under normal circumstances, little protein escapes to the urine so serum FLC (sFLC) concentrations have to increase many-fold before absorption mechanisms are overwhelmed *(Chapter 26)*. Hence, urinalysis is an unreliable method for detecting changes in monoclonal FLC production.

An alternative strategy is to measure FLCs in serum. Experimental assays from the 1970s onwards revealed the potential for sFLC measurement, but the assay technology was never sufficiently practical or accurate enough for general use *(Section 2.3)*. Why, therefore, have adequate serum immunoassays not been produced before? It is now apparent that the overriding barrier was the difficulty in developing satisfactory antibodies for use in the assays. To function correctly, these antibodies must not only be of high affinity to allow measurement of low concentrations of sFLCs, but must also be highly specific. Concentrations of sFLCs are several orders of magnitude lower than those of light chains bound to intact immunoglobulins, so even minor antibody cross-reactivity produces unacceptable results. Only recently have suitable antibodies been developed that bind exclusively to the hidden epitopes of FLC molecules *(Chapter 5)*. These antibodies have facilitated the development of Freelite® sFLC assays that are specific, sensitive and quantitative.

Serum concentrations of FLCs are dependent upon the balance between production by plasma cells (and their progenitors) and renal clearance *(Chapter 3)*. When there is increased polyclonal immunoglobulin production and/or renal impairment, both κ and λ FLC concentrations can increase 30-40 fold. However, the relative concentrations of κ to λ (i.e. the κ/λ ratio) remain unchanged, or only slightly increase *(Section 6.3)*. By contrast, tumours produce a monoclonal excess of only one of the light chain types, often with bone marrow suppression of the alternate light chain, so that κ/λ ratios become highly abnormal. Accurate measurement of κ/λ ratios underpins the utility of sFLC immunoassays and provides a numerical indicator of clonality[9]. This same concept is the basis for the immunoglobulin heavy/light chain (Hevylite®, HLC) assays, which have more recently been developed and allow accurate measurement of the different light chain types of intact immunoglobulin, such that κ/λ ratios can be determined (eg. the IgGκ/IgGλ ratio) *(Chapter 9)*. The availability of Freelite assays, after 2001, provoked a "renaissance" of interest in FLC studies and a dramatic rise in publications. Although HLC assays do not provide the same "step change" that sFLC assays did (with the move from urine to serum measurement) they should also stimulate further research, notably through insight into HLC pair suppression (e.g. the suppression of IgGλ by an IgGκ tumour) and the existence of different bone marrow "niches" *(Sections 13.2.2 and 18.4.4)*.

1.2. Overview of established uses

Since the first availability of Freelite, many applications for sFLC analysis have become standard practice and indeed, are now recommended in various guidelines for best practice. All guidelines relevant to sFLC analysis are described in Chapter 25 (MM) and Chapter 28 (AL amyloidosis). The main applications for sFLC analysis are described briefly below. The chapters/sections cited in the text contain more detailed discussions plus references.

The sensitivity of sFLC analysis for identifying low levels of monoclonal FLC production indicates that it has a role in the initial screening for plasma cell dyscrasias. Many studies have been performed adding sFLC tests to the (previously) recommended standard of serum and urine electrophoresis assays and reported that extra patients were identified *(Chapter 23)*. Also the efficacy of different screening panels has been assessed using sera from many hundreds of patients with well-characterised plasma cell disorders. The consensus from these studies has been that sFLC analysis plus serum electrophoresis tests comprise a suitable screening algorithm unless AL amyloidosis is suspected, for which the addition of urine electrophoresis will identify a few rare AL amyloidosis patients who are negative by the serum tests. This protocol was recommended in international guidelines published in 2009[10].

Some of the earliest studies with sFLC assays were performed with sera from LCMM patients. All patients with positive urines were found to have abnormal serum results and it was apparent that sFLC analysis was generally more sensitive for detection of residual disease *(Chapter 15)*. This sensitivity was recognised by the incorporation of a normal sFLC ratio as one of the criteria defining a "stringent complete response" (sCR) in guidelines for response criteria and the uniform reporting of clinical trials *(Section 25.3.5)*[11]. Guidelines from the International Myeloma Working Group in 2009[10] recommended that Freelite assays were used for monitoring any "oligosecretory" LCMM patients whose urinary FLC was <200 mg/24 hours and considered unreliable for accurate measurement.

Approximately 3 - 4% of myeloma patients were routinely classified as having nonsecretory disease until it was demonstrated that up to 70% of these patients were actually producing small amounts of FLC that could be identified by sFLC assays *(Chapter 16)*. sFLC analysis was quickly identified as a significant benefit for these patients as it allows their disease to be monitored without recourse to frequent bone-marrow biopsies and permits them to be included in clinical trials. Guideline recommendations for sFLC use encompassed these patients within the definition of oligosecretory disease[10].

The majority of patients with MM produce monoclonal intact immunoglobulin (i.e. IIMM) which is used for monitoring their responses to treatment. However, more than one publication has reported that up to 96% of these patients also produce monoclonal FLCs, detectable by sFLC analysis *(Section 17.2)*. Interestingly, the serum concentrations of FLCs and intact monoclonal immunoglobulins are not correlated ($R^2 < 0.1$). Monoclonal sFLCs are therefore independent markers of the disease process. This is of potential clinical use particularly when the tumour produces large amounts of FLCs and small amounts of intact monoclonal immunoglobulins. sFLC may be a more sensitive marker of complete response and the designation of sCR is also applied to patients with IIMM[11]. Patients with IIMM may relapse with expression of FLC alone ("FLC escape"). A number of case studies have now been published illustrating how sFLC analysis readily identifies this phenomenon *(Section 18.2)* so it is advisable to include tests for FLC production when monitoring IIMM patients. One particularly interesting aspect of sFLCs is their short half-life in the blood (κ: 2 - 4 hours; λ: 3 - 6 hours). This is approximately 100 - 200 times shorter than the 21 day half-life of IgG molecules. Hence, responses to treatment can be seen much more rapidly if sFLCs are monitored. This also has been identified in a number of clinical studies *(Section 18.3.1)*.

An additional feature of FLC molecules is that, in contrast to intact immunoglobulins, they are frequently nephrotoxic. Indeed, "myeloma kidney", which presents as acute kidney injury (AKI), occurs in up to 10% of MM patients *(Section 27.1)*. If renal recovery is not achieved, the life expectancy of these patients is significantly reduced. The benefit of rapid removal of FLCs from these patients has yet to be proven, but it is clear that early diagnosis and treatment of the underlying tumour is essential *(Section 27.5)* and the International Kidney and Monoclonal Gammopathy Research Group recommended the use of SPE and sFLC analysis to screen for monoclonal disease in all patients presenting with AKI[12].

sFLC assays have made a particular contribution to the diagnosis and management of patients with AL amyloidosis *(Chapter 28)*. This may be unsurprising because it is the FLCs that directly cause the disease whilst the underlying tumours are typically slow-growing and difficult to detect. Characteristically, light chain fibrils form amyloid deposits in various organs and tissues, disrupting their normal function. Concentrations of circulating sFLCs are often insufficient for measurement by serum electrophoretic tests, but sFLC assays provide quantification of the circulating fibril precursors in 75 - 98% of patients *(Section 28.2.1)*. Furthermore, the concentrations of sFLCs and their reduction after treatment have been shown to be prognostic in various studies. sFLC analysis is advocated in both national and international guidelines for management of AL amyloidosis *(Sections 28.3 and 28.6)*[10,13,14,15]. As stated by Dispenzieri et al.[16] from The Mayo Clinic:

"The introduction of the serum immunoglobulin free light chain assay has revolutionized our ability to assess hematological responses in patients with low tumor burden..."

Monoclonal gammopathy of undetermined significance (MGUS) and smouldering myeloma (SMM) are precursor conditions which progress to active disease at rates of approximately 1% and 10% per year, respectively *(Chapters 13 and 14)*. Abnormal sFLC ratios are found in approximately 30% of subjects with MGUS but 80 – 90% of those with SMM. In both conditions, sFLC analysis provides an independent prognostic indication that can help identify those patients who will benefit from more frequent monitoring and those who can be reassured and discharged (low-risk MGUS). Again, these prognostic utilities have been included in guideline recommendations *(Chapter 25)*[17,18].

In summary, sFLC tests fulfill an important role in the detection, monitoring and prognosis of plasma cell dyscrasias; bringing benefits to a multitude of patients. Their inclusion in multiple guidelines for best clinical practice is witness to this role.

1.3. Recent Progress

Prior to the current edition, the last printed version of "Serum free light chain analysis plus Hevylite" was the 6th edition in 2010. What is new in the field of FLC and HLC analysis since that time? The following comprise a small selection from the many publications that have helped to consolidate or extend the field of knowledge *(Figure 1.2)*. More detailed discussions can be found in the relevant chapters and have been referenced in the text.

1.3.1. Monoclonal FLC studies

A recent study monitoring overall survival of MM patients after high dose melphalan and autologous stem cell transplant has substantiated the value of achieving a stringent complete response (sCR). The inclusion of sFLC analysis in the definition of sCR (i.e. requiring the presence of a normal κ/λ sFLC ratio in addition to other criteria) was first introduced into guidelines in response to observational studies which had demonstrated that a proportion of patients achieving a conventional CR still had abnormal sFLC ratios *(Sections 15.2 and 18.2.2)*. In 2013, Kapoor et al.[19] published follow-up data, comparing patients who had achieved a sCR (n=109) with those who had only achieved a conventional CR (n=37) or near CR (n=91). Significantly improved long-term survival was seen for those achieving a sCR (compared to either lesser response), demonstrating the clinical relevance and desirability of attaining this degree of response *(Section 20.3.1)*.

There has been much interest in recent years in the clonal heterogeneity of MM and how the dominant clone(s) may change during the course of a patient's disease, a concept referred to as clonal evolution *(Chapter 19)*. Many of the studies have utilised genetic analysis of the tumour cells but there has also been some interest in identifying how changes in the monoclonal proteins produced can give an insight into clonal evolution. This concept was explored by Brioli et al.[20], who analysed changes in protein production at relapse amongst 520 MM patients. It was found that just over 10% (54 patients) relapsed with light chain escape and had a significantly shorter survival. The authors considered this represented the outgrowth of a more aggressive tumour clone and commented on the importance of using sFLC analysis for monitoring patients with IIMM in order to ensure that light chain escape was not missed *(Section 18.2.1)*.

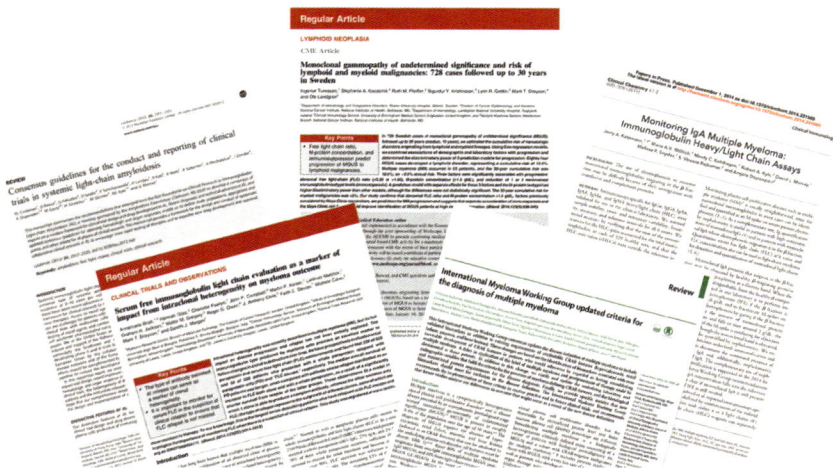

Figure 1.2. A selection of new publications.

The first publication identifying abnormal sFLC ratios as a risk factor for MGUS progression (by Rajkumar and colleagues from the Mayo Clinic in 2005)[21] was, arguably, definitive; not least due to the size of the study population (n=1148) and length of follow-up (median 15 years). Few other research groups would be able to access a comparable study population. However, in 2013, Turesson and colleagues[22] published data from 728 Swedish people with MGUS who had been followed for up to 30 years (median 10 years). They confirmed the previous findings that an abnormal sFLC ratio and high monoclonal protein concentration predicted progression to lymphoid malignancies and differed only in their selection of general immunoparesis as a third risk factor, ahead of the immunoglobulin isotype (IgA and IgM indicating higher risk) *(Chapter 13)*. It now seems unlikely that any future data will challenge the role of abnormal sFLC ratios as a risk factor in MGUS progression.

1.3.2. Polyclonal FLC studies

The previous edition summarised data from many observational studies reporting elevated polyclonal sFLCs in association with various diseases. Subsequently, in 2012, Dispenzieri et al.[23] published data from follow-up of over 15000 people seen at the Mayo Clinic in Rochester, Minnesota, USA. After removal of all subjects with an abnormal sFLC ratio or other evidence of a monoclonal process, there was a significant association between elevated polyclonal sFLC concentrations and early mortality *(Section 35.10)*. These findings have been corroborated in two further, independent, populations by Eisele et al.[24] and Anandram et al.[25]. The risk associated with elevated sFLC was found to be independent of other markers of renal function, inflammation or acute-phase response but the early mortality was attributable to multiple causes, indicating no obvious path for clinical intervention. This remains an area of active research.

1.3.3. HLC studies

HLC assays had only recently been developed when the 6th edition of this book was published. Few HLC studies had been completed and discussion was confined to a separate chapter at the back of the book. In the current edition, HLC data and FLC data are integrated within the same chapters. For example, if your interest is in risk stratification of MGUS, Chapter 13 contains data from both FLC and HLC prognostic studies.

With regard to the potential utility of HLC analysis in the management of MM, there have been several important publications. Bradwell et al.[26] reported that abnormal HLC ratios at presentation were predictive of shorter progression-free survival, predominantly due to the influence (on the ratios) of HLC pair suppression *(Section 20.4)*. A staging system using β_2-microglobulin and extreme HLC ratios was prognostically more accurate than the current International Staging System. Ludwig et al.[27] similarly found that highly abnormal HLC ratios at presentation were associated with shorter survival and that β_2-microglobulin and HLC ratios were independent prognostic markers. When monitoring disease, Ludwig et al. noted that HLC assays could give a quantitative assessment of monoclonal protein when other tests were uninformative and, in some patients, they gave a more sensitive measure of residual disease and an earlier indication of relapse *(Section 18.4)*. Katzmann et al.[28] focused on the problems of monitoring MM patients with β-migrating IgA monoclonal proteins. They concluded that HLC assays were a suitable substitute for the alternative of electrophoresis assays and total IgA quantitation *(Section 11.5)*, a utility similarly highlighted in a clinical case study by Donato et al. *(Section 18.4.1)*[29].

For an investigation of MGUS prognosis, Katzmann and colleagues[30] were able to measure HLC concentrations in archived sera from 999 MGUS patients. HLC pair suppression was found to be an independent risk factor for progression and the authors observed that as suppression was apparent several years before malignant transformation, this had implications for the understanding of myeloma biology *(Chapter 13)*.

1.3.4. New guidelines

New guidelines, pertinent to the use of sFLC analysis, have also been published in recent years *(Chapters 25 and 28)*. The revised British guidelines for management of MM[31] now recommend that sFLC assays are used to assess response in all LCMM patients and in the management of patients with renal failure. In addition, an update to the International Myeloma Working Group criteria for MM diagnosis was published by Rajkumar et al.[32]. This included new definitions of light chain MGUS (identified by an abnormal sFLC ratio) and defined sFLC ratios >100 as a biomarker of malignancy for MM diagnosis. This latter definition is of particular importance because a proportion of patients previously classified as having smouldering MM are now re-defined as having MM, justifying treatment. New guidelines for the conduct and reporting of clinical trials in AL amyloidosis have also been published, including updated definitions of haematological response based upon sFLC analysis[13].

And finally, it is worth noting that the revised British MM guidelines[31] include the first (guideline) mention of HLC analysis: Bird et al. refer to the published data showing that HLC ratios can provide prognostic information for patients both at presentation and post-response.

References

1. Gertz MA. Immunoglobulin light chain amyloidosis: 2014 update on diagnosis, prognosis, and treatment. Am J Hematol 2014;89:1133-40

2. Kyle RA, Therneau TM, Rajkumar SV, Larson DR, Plevak MF, Offord JR et al. Prevalence of monoclonal gammopathy of undetermined significance. N Engl J Med 2006;354:1362-9

3. Kumar SK, Gertz MA, Lacy MQ, Dingli D, Hayman SR, Buadi FK et al. Recent improvements in survival in primary systemic amyloidosis and the importance of an early mortality risk score. Mayo Clin Proc 2011;86:12-8

4. Gonsalves WI, Rajkumar SV, Go RS, Dispenzieri A, Gupta V, Singh PP et al. Trends in survival of patients with primary plasma cell leukemia: a population based analysis. Blood 2014;124:907-12

5. Drayson M, Tang LX, Drew R, Mead GP, Carr-Smith H, Bradwell AR. Serum free light-chain measurements for identifying and monitoring patients with nonsecretory multiple myeloma. Blood 2001;97:2900–2

6. Stankowski-Drengler T, Gertz MA, Katzmann JA, Lacy MQ, Kumar S, Leung N et al. Serum immunoglobulin free light chain measurements and heavy chain isotype usage provide insight into disease biology in patients with POEMS syndrome. Am J Hematol 2010;85:431-4

7. Jones HB. Papers on Chemical Pathology, Lecture III. Lancet 1847;II:88-92

8. Jones HB. On the new substance occurring in the urine of a patient with mollities ossium. Philosophical Transactions of the Royal Society of London. Series B: Biological Sciences 1848;138:55-62

9. Katzmann JA, Clark RJ, Abraham RS, Bryant S, Lymp JF, Bradwell AR, Kyle RA. Serum reference intervals and diagnostic ranges for free kappa and free lambda immunoglobulin light chains: relative sensitivity for detection of monoclonal light chains. Clin Chem 2002;48:1437–44

10. Dispenzieri A, Kyle R, Merlini G, Miguel JS, Ludwig H, Hajek R, et al. International Myeloma Working Group guidelines for serum-free light chain analysis in multiple myeloma and related disorders. Leukemia 2009;23:215-24

11. Rajkumar SV, Harousseau JL, Durie B, Anderson KC, Dimopoulos M, Kyle R et al. Consensus recommendations for the uniform reporting of clinical trials: report of the International Myeloma Workshop Consensus Panel 1. Blood 2011;117:4691-5

12. Hutchison CA, Batuman V, Behrens J, Bridoux F, Sirac C, Dispenzieri A et al. The pathogenesis and diagnosis of acute kidney injury in multiple myeloma. Nat Rev Nephrol 2011;8:43-51

13. Comenzo RL, Reece D, Palladini G, Seldin D, Sanchorawala V, Landau H et al. Consensus guidelines for the conduct and reporting of clinical trials in systemic light-chain (AL) amyloidosis. Leukemia 2012;26:2317-25

14. Wechalekar AD, Gillmore JD, Bird J, Cavenagh J, Hawkins S, Kazmi M et al. Guidelines on the management of AL amyloidosis. Br J Haematol 2015;168:207-18

15. Weber N, Mollee P, Augustson B, Brown R, Catley L, Gibson J et al. Management of systemic light chain (AL) amyloidosis: recommendations of the Myeloma Foundation of Australia Medical and Scientific Advisory Group. Intern Med J 2014 In press

16. Dispenzieri A, Gertz MA, Kyle RA. To the editor: Determining appropriate treatment options for patients with primary systemic amyloidosis. Blood 2004;104:2992-3

17. Kyle RA, Durie BG, Rajkumar SV, Landgren O, Blade J, Merlini G, et al. Monoclonal gammopathy of undetermined significance (MGUS) and smoldering (asymptomatic) multiple myeloma: IMWG consensus perspectives risk factors for progression and guidelines for monitoring and management. Leukemia 2010;24:1121-7

18. Bird J, Behrens J, Westin J, Turesson I, Drayson M, Beetham R, et al. UK Myeloma Forum (UKMF) and Nordic Myeloma Study Group (NMSG): guidelines for the investigation of newly detected M-proteins and the management of monoclonal gammopathy of undetermined significance (MGUS). Br J Haematol 2009;147:22-42

19. Kapoor P, Kumar SK, Dispenzieri A, Lacy MQ, Buadi F, Dingli D et al. Importance of achieving stringent complete response after autologous stem-cell transplantation in multiple myeloma. J Clin Oncol 2013;31:4529-35

20. Brioli A, Giles H, Pawlyn C, Campbell J, Kaiser M, Melchor L et al. Serum free light chain evaluation as a marker for the impact of intra-clonal heterogeneity on the progression and treatment resistance in multiple myeloma. Blood 2014;123:3414-9

21. Rajkumar SV, Kyle RA, Therneau TM, Melton LJ, 3rd, Bradwell AR, Clark RJ, et al. Serum free light chain ratio is an independent risk factor for progression in monoclonal gammopathy of undetermined significance. Blood 2005;106:812–7

22. Turesson I, Kovalchik SA, Pfeiffer RM, Kristinsson SY, Goldin LR, Drayson MT, Landgren O. Monoclonal gammopathy of undetermined significance and risk of lymphoid and myeloid malignancies: 728 cases followed up to 30 years in Sweden. Blood 2014;123:338-45

23. Dispenzieri A, Katzmann JA, Kyle RA, Larson DR, Therneau TM, Colby CL et al. Use of nonclonal serum immunoglobulin free light chains to predict overall survival in the general population. Mayo Clin Proc 2012;87:517-23

24. Eisele L, Durig J, Huttman A, Duhrsen U, Fuhrer A, Kieruzel S et al. Polyclonal free light chain elevation and mortality in the German Heinz Nixdorf Recall Study. Blood 2010;116:3903a

25. Anandram S, Assi LK, Lovatt T, Parkes J, Taylor J, MacWhannell A et al. Elevated, combined serum free light chain levels and increased mortality: a 5-year follow-up, UK study. J Clin Pathol 2012;65:1036-42

26. Bradwell A, Harding S, Fourrier N, Mathiot C, Attal M, Moreau P et al. Prognostic utility of intact immunoglobulin Ig'kappa/Ig'lambda ratios in multiple myeloma patients. Leukemia 2013;27:202-7

27. Ludwig H, Milosavljevic D, Zojer N, Faint JM, Bradwell AR, Hubl W, Harding SJ. Immunoglobulin heavy/light chain ratios improve paraprotein detection and monitoring, identify residual disease and correlate with survival in multiple myeloma patients. Leukemia 2013;27:213-9

28. Katzmann JA, Willrich MA, Kohlhagen MC, Kyle RA, Murray DL, Snyder MR et al. Monitoring IgA multiple myeloma: immunoglobulin heavy/light chain assays. Clin Chem 2014 *In Press*

29. Donato LJ, Zeldenrust SR, Murray DL, Katzmann JA. A 71-year-old woman with multiple myeloma status after stem cell transplantation. Clin Chem 2011;57:1645-8

30. Katzmann JA, Clark R, Kyle RA, Larson DR, Therneau TM, Melton LJ, III et al. Suppression of uninvolved immunoglobulins defined by heavy/light-chain pair suppression is a risk factor for progression of MGUS. Leukemia 2013;27:208-12

31. Bird J, Owen R, D'Sa S, Snowden J, Ashcroft J, Yong K et al. Guidelines for the diagnosis and management of multiple myeloma 2014. BCSH guideline 2014. *Published online (www.bcshguidelines.com)*

32. Rajkumar SV, Dimopolous MA, Palumbo A, Blade J, Merlini G, Mateos MV et al. International Myeloma Working Group updated criteria for the diagnosis of multiple myeloma. Lancet Oncology 2014;15:e538-e548

A brief history of diagnostic tests for myeloma: Bence Jones protein and beyond

Summary:

- Dr William MacIntyre was the first person to characterise the precipitate in the urine from a patient with multiple myeloma, and his findings were reported by Henry Bence Jones in a Lancet article in 1847.
- Korngold and Lapiri characterised two types of Bence Jones protein (subsequently designated κ and λ in tribute to them).
- Tiselius reported how serum globulins can be separated into alpha, beta and gamma fractions using moving boundary electrophoresis.
- Waldenström described the key concept of monoclonal vs. polyclonal gammopathy.

2.1. The identification of Bence Jones protein

Although immunoglobulin free light chains (FLCs) are synonymous with Bence Jones proteins, history might have been more generous to others involved in their discovery[1,2,3,4,5].

On Friday, October 30th 1845, the 53-year-old Dr William MacIntyre, physician to the Western General Dispensary, St. Marylebone, London, left his rooms in Harley Street. He had been called to see Mr Thomas Alexander McBean, a 45-year-old, highly respectable grocer, who had severe bone pain and fractures. He had been under the care of his general practitioner, Dr Thomas Watson, for several months. Upon examination of the patient, William MacIntyre noted the presence of oedema. Considering the possibility of nephrosis, he tested the urine for albumin. To his consternation, the albuminous protein precipitate found on warming the urine, uncharacteristically, redissolved when heated to 75°C.

Both Dr MacIntyre and Dr Watson then sent urine samples to the chemical pathologist at St. George's Hospital. A note accompanying the urine sent by Dr Watson read as follows:

"Dear Dr Bence Jones,
The tube contains urine of very high specific gravity. When boiled it becomes highly opaque. On the addition of nitric acid, it effervesces, assumes a reddish hue, and becomes quite clear; but as it cools assumes the consistence and appearance which you see. Heat reliquifies it. What is it?"

Over the next 2 months, the patient deteriorated, became emaciated, weak, and was racked with pain. He eventually died on January 1st 1846, in full possession of his mental faculties. Dr MacIntyre subsequently published the post-mortem examination and the description of the peculiar urine in 1850[6].

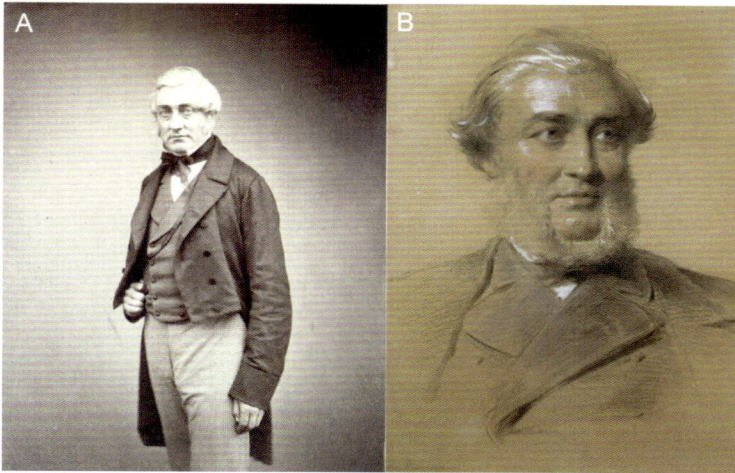

Figure 2.1. Henry Bence Jones. (A) Albumen print by Maull and Polyblank c.1850s (B) Charcoal and chalk on paper by George Richmond 1865. (Reproduced with permission from The Royal Institution, London, UK and Bridgeman Images).

Unfortunately for him, Henry Bence Jones[7,8] *(Figure 2.1)* had already described the patient's urinary findings in two, single-author articles, one of which was published in The Lancet, in 1847. He considered the protein to be an *"hydrated deutoxide of albumen"*. He wisely commented:

"I need hardly remark on the importance of seeking for this oxide of albumen in other cases of mollities ossium".

Bence Jones's reputation was assured, while the contributions of his colleagues were consigned to the footnotes of history.

For all the apparent injustice to his colleague, William MacIntyre, Henry Bence Jones achieved much else in his career. He published over 40 papers and became rich and famous based on his clinical practice, lecturing and original observations, and was elected to fellowship of The Royal Society at the tender age of 33. Florence Nightingale once described him as "the best chemical doctor in London." Surprisingly, there was no mention of Bence Jones protein in his obituary and the eponym (and the hyphen in his name) was not used until after his death[2].

By 1909, over 40 cases of Bence Jones proteinuria had been reported[9], and the protein was thought to originate in bone marrow plasma cells that were first identified by Waldeyer in 1875. In 1922, Bayne-Jones and Wilson characterised two types of Bence Jones protein by observing precipitation reactions using antisera made by immunising rabbits with the urine of several patients. The proteins were classified as group I and group II types. However, it was not until 1956 that Korngold and Lapiri, using the Ouchterlony technique, showed that antisera raised against the different groups also reacted with myeloma proteins. As a tribute to their observations the two types of Bence Jones protein were designated kappa and lambda (κ and λ). Edelman and Gally, in 1962, subsequently showed that FLCs prepared from IgG monoclonal proteins were the same as Bence Jones protein. It had taken 117 years from the original observation for the function of Bence Jones protein to be finally determined.

2.2. The identification of serum monoclonal proteins

In parallel with the clinical and scientific observations of the role of Bence Jones protein, electrophoretic techniques for protein separation were evolving and eventually entered clinical laboratories. Perlzweig et al.[10] were the first to report hyperproteinaemia in MM in 1928. Shortly after in 1930, Tiselius reported the homogeneity of certain serum globulins using a technique he devised, termed moving boundary electrophoresis[11]. In this technique, proteins moved through a U-shaped electrophoretic cell and the detection system was based on the refraction of light by proteins as they moved through the tube. Tiselius found that there was a difference in the refractive index of light at boundary interfaces between major protein fractions, and in 1937 he described how serum globulins could be separated into alpha, beta and gamma components[12]. In 1939, Tiselius and Kabat[13] demonstrated antibody activity in the gamma globulin fraction. Moving boundary electrophoresis became commercially available, but was very labour-intensive and the technique was limited in its ability to detect subtle abnormalities[14]. Using this technique, in 1939, Longsworth et al.[15] recognised tall, narrow-based, "church spire" peaks in the sera of patients with multiple myeloma (MM). Electrophoresis was subsequently improved by using filter paper as a support, which allowed the separation of protein into discrete zones that could be visualised with dyes[16]. The method was further improved using cellulose acetate and agarose gels in the 1950s and 1960s, and subsequently automated using capillary zone electrophoresis in the 1990s *(Chapter 4)*[14]. Finally, immunofixation electrophoresis was first introduced in 1964 by Wilson et al.[17] and became established in the 1980s[18].

Jan Waldenström[17], in a seminal lecture series in 1961, was the first to describe the key concept of monoclonal vs. polyclonal gammopathy. Importantly, he distinguished monoclonal proteins (characterised by a narrow band of gammaglobulin on electrophoresis, often associated with MM or macroglobulinaemia) from hypergammaglobulinaemia (characterised by a broad band, and regarded as a polyclonal increase in proteins, that was associated with an inflammatory or reactive process).

2.3. FLC assays

Clear identification of κ and λ molecules became possible with the use of antibodies specific for each type of protein. Immunodiffusion was initially used[19], followed by immunoelectrophoresis in 1953[20], radial immunodiffusion and ultimately nephelometry and turbidimetry. The first successful attempt to measure FLCs in serum was in 1975. Size-separation column chromatography[21,22,23] was used to isolate them from intact immunoglobulins, prior to analysis. Although the results were accurate and showed the potential use of serum analyses, these assays were clearly impractical for routine use. However, serum immunoassays for Bence Jones protein (serum FLCs; sFLCs) remained unattainable because the antibodies could not distinguish between sFLCs and the overwhelming amounts of light chains bound in intact immunoglobulin molecules.

Subsequent assays focussed on the use of antibodies directed against "hidden" epitopes on FLC molecules. These are located at the interface between the light and heavy chains of intact immunoglobulins and become detectable when the FLCs are unbound. Radioimmunoassays and enzyme immunoassays using polyclonal antisera against FLCs were used to analyse urine samples, but specificity remained inadequate for serum measurements[24,25] and variations in FLC polymerisation caused measurement errors[26,27].

The use of monoclonal antibodies was an obvious approach to improving specificity, but satisfactory reagents were difficult to develop and their use was initially restricted to radio-immunoassays and enzyme immunoassays[28,29,30,31]. Early attempts to develop turbidimetric[32,33] and latex-enhanced nephelometric assays[34] using polyclonal antibodies could not detect normal sFLC concentrations, and cross-reactions with intact immunoglobulins were unacceptable. In 2001, immunoassays based on polyclonal antibodies were finally developed that could measure FLCs at normal serum concentrations[35]. Their utility was quickly made apparent when monoclonal FLCs were detected in the sera of most patients classified as having nonsecretory MM *(Chapter 16)*[36]. Furthermore, as described in The Lancet, all of 224 patients with light chain MM who had Bence Jones proteinuria also had elevated sFLC concentrations *(Chapter 15)*[37]. The serum tests were also better at detecting residual disease than urinalysis *(Chapter 24)*.

These results and many others, heralded the widespread use of sFLC immunoassays, and the incorporation of Freelite® assays into International Myeloma Working Group guidelines *(Chapter 25)*.

2.4. Immunoglobulin heavy/light chain assays

One of the great diagnostic benefits of sFLC analysis is the κ/λ ratio. This is because: 1) it provides a quantitative assessment of clonality; 2) the clinical ranges are enhanced due to immunosuppression of the non-tumour FLCs; and 3) there is automatic compensation for variable metabolism *(Section 3.5)*. These same advantages can be exploited for intact immunoglobulins if the different light chain types are measured (eg. to produce a ratio of IgGκ/IgGλ). Raising polyclonal antibodies specific for the unique, junctional epitopes, spanning the heavy and light chain immunoglobulin constant regions, is a significant challenge but reagents have now been developed for the 3 main immunoglobulins (i.e. IgGκ, IgGλ, IgAκ, IgAλ, IgMκ and IgMλ) *(Chapter 9)*[35]. Turbidimetric/nephelometric immunoglobulin heavy/light chain (HLC) assays were made available for general use in 2009 – 2010 with the trade name of Hevylite®.

HLC assays typically have a greater clinical sensitivity than SPE (for monoclonal immunoglobulin) and can exceed that of IFE in some instances *(Section 18.4)*. In addition, the assays can be particularly helpful for monitoring patients with IgA myeloma if their monoclonal immunoglobulin co-migrates with other proteins in the β-region of SPE gels[38]. Preliminary studies have also indicated that suppression of the uninvolved HLC-pair (e.g. IgGλ in an IgGκ patient) may be more informative than assessment of general immunoparesis and HLC analysis has provided prognostic information in both monoclonal gammopathy of undetermined significance and MM *(Chapters 13 and 20)*. It is too early to judge how valuable HLC assays may be in the management of myeloma and related disorders but, in an editorial, Keren described Hevylite assays as "an important addition to our armamentarium for detecting and quantifying monoclonal proteins"[14].

Test Questions

1. Who was the first person to observe "Bence Jones proteinuria"?
2. Why are the two immunoglobulin light chain types termed kappa and lambda?

References

1. Clamp JR. Some aspects of the first recorded case of multiple myeloma. Lancet 1967;2:1354-6

2. Rosenfeld L. Henry Bence Jones (1813-1873): the best "chemical doctor" in London. Clin Chem 1987;33:1687–92

3. Kyle RA. Multiple myeloma: an odyssey of discovery. Br J Haematol 2000;111:1035–44

4. Kyle RA. Henry Bence Jones - physician, chemist, scientist and biographer: a man for all seasons. Br J Haematol 2001;115:13–8

5. Hajdu SI. A note from history: the first biochemical test for detection of cancer. Ann Clin Lab Sci 2006;36:222–3

6. MacIntyre W. Case of mollities and fragilitas ossium, accompanied with urine strongly charged with animal matter. Med Chir Tran 1850;33:211–232

7. Jones HB. Papers on Chemical Pathology, Lecture III. Lancet 1847;II:88-92

8. Jones HB. On the new substance occurring in the urine of a patient with mollities ossium. Philosophical Transactions of the Royal Society of London. Series B: Biological Sciences 1848;138:55-62

9. Parkes Weber F, Ledingham JCG. A note on the histology of a case of Myelomatosis (Multiple Myeloma) with Bence-Jones protein in the urine (Myelopathic Albumosuria). Proc R Soc Med 1909;2(Pathol Sect):193–206

10. Perlzweig WA, Delrue G, Geschicter C. Hyperproteinemia associated with multiple myelomas: report of an unusual case. JAMA 1928;90:755-7

11. Kyle RA, Rajkumar SV. Multiple myeloma. Blood 2008;111:2962-72

12. Tiselius A. A new apparatus for electrophoretic analysis of colloidal mixtures. Trans Faraday Soc 1937;33:524

13. Tiselius A, Kabat EA. Electrophoretic study of immune sera and purified antibody preparation. J Exp Med 1939;69:119-31

14. Keren DF. Protein electrophoresis in clinical diagnosis. Arnold (Hodder Headline), 2003

15. Longsworth LG, Shedlovsky T, Macinnes DA. Electrophoretic patterns of normal and pathological human blood serum and plasma. J Exp Med 1939;70:399-413

16. Kunkel H, Tiselius A. Electrophoresis of proteins on filter paper. J Gen Physiol 1951;35:89-118

17. Waldenström J. Studies on conditions associated with disturbed gamma globulin formation (gammopathies). Harvey Lect 1961;56:211-31

18. Whicher JT, Hawkins L, Higginson J. Clinical applications of immunofixation: a more sensitive technique for the detection of Bence Jones protein. J Clin Pathol 1980;33:779–80

19. Ouchterlony O. Antigen-antibody reactions in gels. IV. Types of reactions in coordinated systems of diffusion. Acta Pathol Microbiol Scand 1953;32:230–40

20. Grabar P, Williams CA. [Method permitting the combined study of the electrophoretic and the immunochemical properties of protein mixtures; application to blood serum. Biochim Biophys Acta 1953;10:193–4

21. Sölling K. Free light chains of immunoglobulins in normal serum and urine determined by radioimmunoassay. Scand J Clin Lab Invest 1975;35:407–12

22. Sölling K. Polymeric forms of free light chains in serum from normal individuals and from patients with renal diseases. Scand J Clin Lab Invest 1976;36:447–52

23. Cole PW, Durie BG, Salmon SE. Immunoquantitation of free light chain immunoglobulins: applications in multiple myeloma. J Immunol Methods 1978;19:341–9

24. Robinson EL, Gowland E, Ward ID, Scarffe JH. Radioimmunoassay of free light chains of immunoglobulins in urine. Clin Chem 1982;28:2254–8

25. Brouwer J, Otting-van de Ruit M, Busking-van der Lely H. Estimation of free light chains of immunoglobulins by enzyme immunoassay. Clin Chim Acta 1985;150:267–74

26. Sölling K. Free light chains of immunoglobulins. Scand J Clin Lab Invest Suppl 1981;157:1–83

27. Heino J, Rajamaki A, Irjala K. Turbidimetric measurement of Bence-Jones proteins using antibodies against free light chains of immunoglobulins. An artifact caused by different polymeric forms of light chains. Scand J Clin Lab Invest 1984;44:173–6

28. Ling NR, Lowe J, Hardie D, Evans S, Jefferis R. Detection of free kappa chains in human serum and urine using pairs of monoclonal antibodies reacting with C kappa epitopes not available on whole immunoglobulins. Clin Exp Immunol 1983;52:234–40

29. Axiak SM, Krishnamoorthy L, Guinan J, Raison RL. Quantitation of free kappa light chains in serum and urine using a monoclonal antibody based inhibition enzyme-linked immunoassay. J Immunol Methods 1987;99:141–7

30. Nelson M, Brown RD, Gibson J, Joshua DE. Measurement of free kappa and lambda chains in serum and the significance of their ratio in patients with multiple myeloma. Br J Haematol 1992;81:223–30

31. Abe M, Goto T, Kosaka M, Wolfenbarger D, Weiss DT, Solomon A. Differences in kappa to lambda (kappa:lambda) ratios of serum and urinary free light chains. Clin Exp Immunol 1998;111:457–62

32. Hemmingsen L, Skaarup P. The 24-hour excretion of plasma proteins in the urine of apparently healthy subjects. Scand J Clin Lab Invest 1975;35:347–53

33. Tillyer CR, Iqbal J, Raymond J, Gore M, McIlwain TJ. Immunoturbidimetric assay for estimating free light chains of immunoglobulins in urine and serum. J Clin Pathol 1991;44:466–71

34. Wakasugi K, Suzuki H, Imai A, Konishi S, Kishioka H. Immunoglobulin free light chain assay using latex agglutination. Int J Clin Lab Res 1995;25:211–5

35. Bradwell AR, Carr-Smith HD, Mead GP, Tang LX, Showell PJ, Drayson MT, Drew R. Highly sensitive, automated immunoassay for immunoglobulin free light chains in serum and urine. Clin Chem 2001;47:673–80

36. Drayson M, Tang LX, Drew R, Mead GP, Carr-Smith H, Bradwell AR. Serum free light-chain measurements for identifying and monitoring patients with nonsecretory multiple myeloma. Blood 2001;97:2900–2

37. Bradwell AR, Carr-Smith HD, Mead GP, Harvey TC, Drayson MT. Serum test for assessment of patients with Bence Jones myeloma. Lancet 2003;361:489–91

38. Katzmann JA, Willrich MA, Kohlhagen MC, Kyle RA, Murray DL, Snyder MR et al. Monitoring IgA Multiple Myeloma: Immunoglobulin Heavy/Light Chain Assays. Clin Chem 2014. *In press*

The biology of immunoglobulins

Summary:
- Immunoglobulin light and heavy chains contain variable and constant domains.
- The structural diversity of immunoglobulin antigen-binding sites arises from genetic recombination and somatic hypermutation of genes corresponding to the light and heavy chain variable region domains.
- Further diversity of κ and λ light chain constant domains arises from isotypic and allotypic variation.
- FLCs are secreted by plasma cells.
- sFLCs have a half-life of a few hours due to rapid renal clearance.
- Serum IgG has a prolonged and variable half-life due to FcRn recycling.

3.1. Immunoglobulin structure

Antibody (immunoglobulin) molecules are composed of two identical heavy chains and two identical light chains. Heavy chains are each paired with a single light chain via a disulphide bridge and non-covalent interactions to form a heavy-light chain pair (or half-molecule). Two heavy-light chain pairs are linked by disulphide bonds in the so-called 'hinge region' to form a Y-shaped structure that is arranged symmetrically about a two-fold axis *(Figure 3.1)*.

Immunoglobulin heavy and light chains each have constant and variable regions. A pair of heavy and light chain variable regions together forms the antigen-binding site. The variable regions exhibit enormous structural diversity, particularly of antigen-binding contacts, allowing the recognition of a huge variety of antigens.

Antibody heavy and light chains are composed of homologous structural units known as 'immunoglobulin domains'. Each domain is approximately 110 amino acids long and is constructed from a series of antiparallel β-strands connected to form two β-pleated sheets. The sheets are covalently linked by an intrachain disulphide bridge and each domain adopts a roughly barrel-shaped structure characteristic of an immunoglobulin fold[1,2].

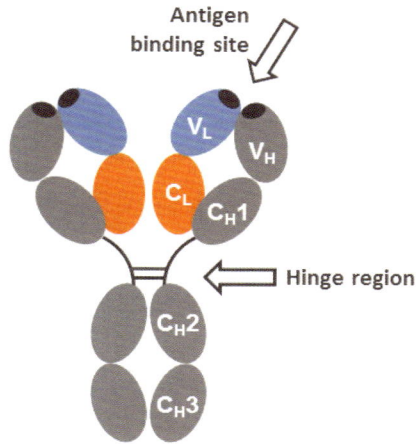

Figure 3.1. An immunoglobulin molecule showing light and heavy chain constant and variable region domains. *V_L: light chain variable domain; C_L: light chain constant domain; V_H: heavy chain variable domain; C_H1 - C_H3: heavy chain constant domains 1 - 3.*

The light chain tertiary structure consists of two immunoglobulin domains joined by a loop to form a single variable region and single constant region *(Figure 3.2)*. In humans, light chains are encoded by two different gene loci, resulting in the serologically distinguishable light chain types, κ and λ. Immunoglobulin molecules are assembled in plasma cells with exclusively κ or λ light chain types, never both.

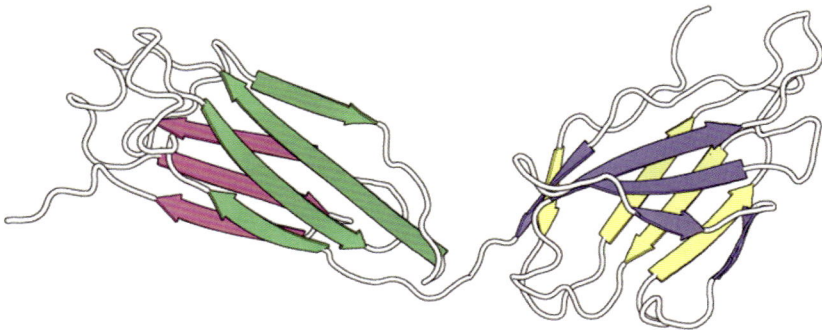

Figure 3.2. A FLC molecule showing the constant region (left) and variable region (right). *Each colour represents a β-pleated sheet.*

Similar to light chains, the heavy chain contains one variable domain corresponding to a single variable region. By contrast, the number of heavy chain constant domains (comprising the constant region) varies between immunoglobulin classes, of which there are five: IgG, IgA, IgM, IgD and IgE. Human IgG and IgA can be further divided into closely related subclasses IgG1, 2, 3 and 4, IgA1 and 2. These classes and subclasses are encoded by separate heavy chain constant genes (γ1-4, α1-2, μ, δ and ε, respectively). The constant regions of the heavy chain mediate most of the biological functions of antibodies by interacting with other effector molecules and immune cells. The majority of secreted antibodies are monomeric, although several immunoglobulin subtypes form oligomers, such as IgA and IgM *(Figure 3.3)*.

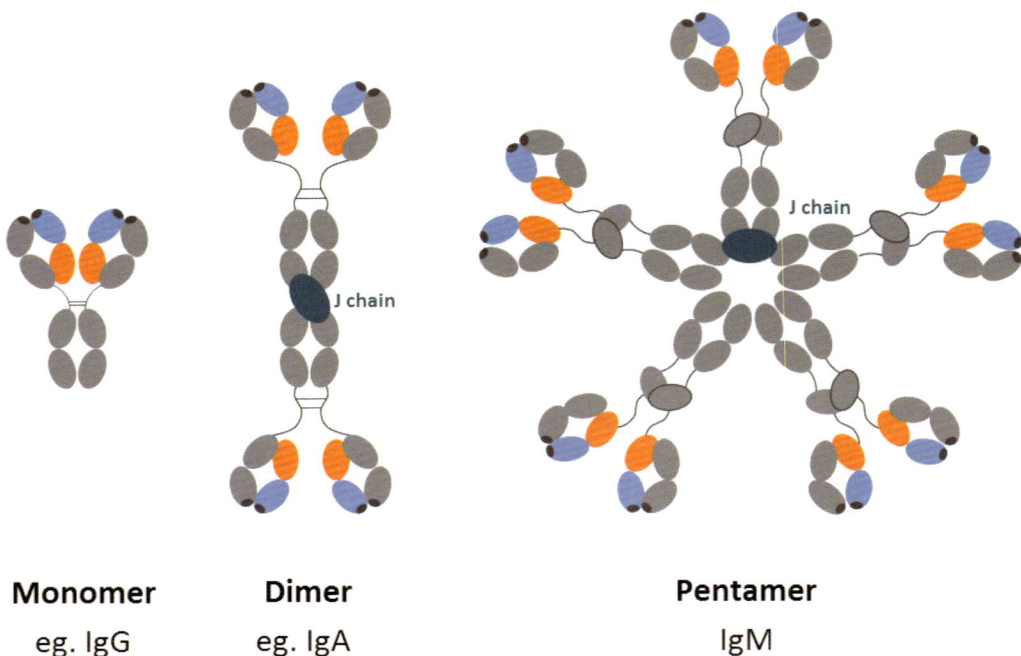

Monomer

eg. IgG

Dimer

eg. IgA

Pentamer

IgM

Figure 3.3. Different forms of secreted antibodies.

In B-cells, the heavy chains, κ light chains and λ light chains are each encoded by independent chromosomal loci containing multiple copies of analogous gene segments. The gene segments within each locus are rearranged stochastically by somatic recombination and RNA processing mechanisms, ultimately resulting in the expression of functional immunoglobulin proteins. The light chain variable domain is constructed from variable (V) and joining (J) gene segments, whilst the constant domain is encoded by a separate constant (C) gene segment *(Figure 3.4)*. The heavy chain variable domain is constructed from three gene segments: V, D (diversity) and J.

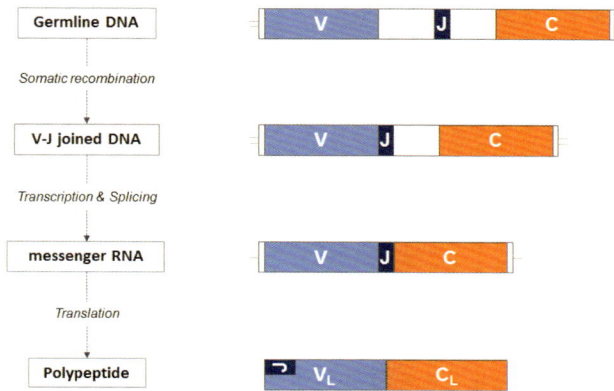

Figure 3.4. Construction of a light chain.

3.2. Immunoglobulin diversity

In humans it is calculated that there are at least 10^{11} unique antibody structural variants possible which allows for the recognition of a vast number of different antigens[3]. Such diversity is generated in four main ways:

Firstly, different combinations of gene segments are used in the rearrangement of heavy and light chain genes during early B-cell development. κ light chains are constructed from one of approximately 40 functional V_κ gene segments, one of 5 J_κ gene segments and a single C_κ gene. λ light chains are constructed from one of approximately 30 V_λ gene segments, and one of four (or more) pairs of functional J_λ gene segments and C_λ genes *(Figure 3.5)*[3]. The heavy chain variable region is formed from one of around 60 V_H, one of 30 D_H, and one of six J_H gene segments[3]. This combinational diversity accounts for a substantial amount of variable region diversity. Secondly, diversity arises from the addition or removal of nucleotides at the junctions between V (D) and J gene segments during recombination. A third source of diversity arises from the many different combinations of heavy and light chains, and finally, somatic hypermutation introduces point mutations in the variable region genes of light and heavy chains in mature activated B-cells[3].

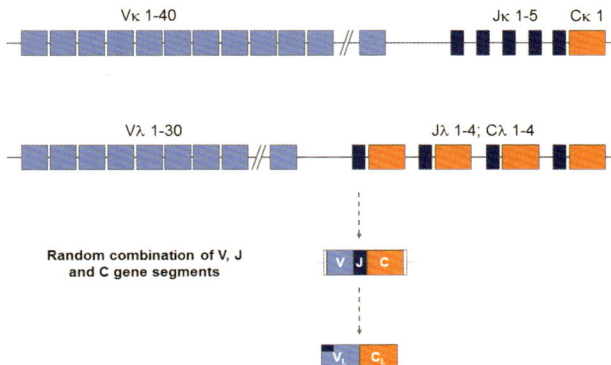

Figure 3.5. Organisation of light chain genes

In light chains, variations are also found in a region of the variable domain corresponding to the first 23 amino acids of the first framework region (a region not associated with antigen binding). Using monoclonal antibodies, four κ (V_κ I - V_κ IV) and six λ subgroups (V_λ I - V_λ VI) have been identified[4] *(Figure 3.6A)*. The specific subgroup structures influence the potential of free light chains (FLCs) to polymerise. For example, AL amyloidosis is associated with V_λ VI, and light chain deposition disease (LCDD) with V_κ I and V_κ IV.

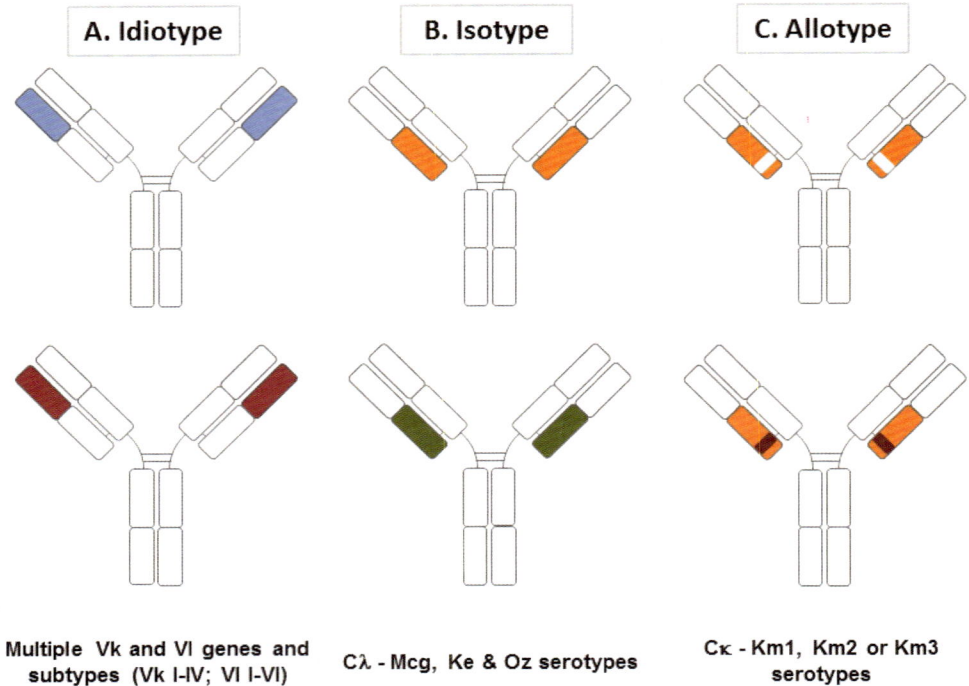

A. Idiotype	B. Isotype	C. Allotype
Multiple Vk and Vl genes and subtypes (Vk I-IV; Vl I-VI)	Cλ - Mcg, Ke & Oz serotypes	Cκ - Km1, Km2 or Km3 serotypes

Figure 3.6. Idiotypic, isotypic and allotypic variation of light chains.

3.3. Isotypic and allotypic variation of light chain constant domains

In addition to genetic recombination and somatic hypermutation of the variable domains, further heterogeneity of light chains arises from isotypic and allotypic variation of the constant domains *(Figure 3.6B and C)*. The human genome contains a variable number of λ constant genes, giving rise to multiple λ chain isotypes, which can be distinguished serologically by the expression of Mcg, Kern and Oz markers. Additionally, the genome contains a single κ constant gene for which three serologically-defined allotypes have been identified, designated Km1, Km2 and Km3[5]. These allotypes define three Km alleles, which differ in two amino acids, as presented in Table 3.1. There is no evidence that these constant region variants affect FLC measurements using Freelite® assays, which are based on polyclonal antisera *(Chapter 5)*.

Km allele	Amino acids
Km1	Val(153) Leu(191)
Km1,2	Ala(153) Leu(191)
Km3	Ala(153) Val(191)

Table 3.1. Amino acid substitutions in κ light chain constant domains.

3.4. Immunoglobulin and FLC production

Immunoglobulins and FLCs are produced by B-cells. During their development the earliest immunoglobulin polypeptide to be produced is the μ heavy chain, in the pre-B-cell. Immature and mature B-cells produce either κ or λ light chains, which associate with μ heavy chains to form membrane-bound IgM. Upon activation, mature B-cells differentiate into plasma cells, which secrete immunoglobulin into the serum. Activation may also stimulate plasma cells to switch the heavy chain constant domain, and hence the class of antibody produced, for example, IgM to IgG. Approximately 40% more light chains than heavy chains are synthesised[6], and this excess of FLCs is thought to favour accurate assemblty of intact immunoglobulin molecules. Light chains which remain unbound from their heavy chain partner are secreted into the blood as FLCs. Secretion of FLCs is highest from plasma cells, with twice as many producing κ-chains than λ-chains. κ FLCs are normally monomeric, while λ FLCs tend to be dimeric, joined by disulphide bonds; however, higher polymeric forms of both FLCs may occur *(Figure 3.7)*. Tumours associated with the different stages of B-cell maturation may secrete monoclonal FLCs and/or monoclonal intact immunoglobulins into the serum *(Figure 3.8)*.

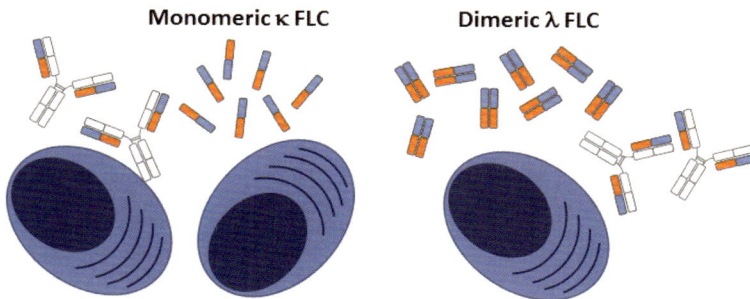

Monomeric κ FLC   **Dimeric λ FLC**

Figure 3.7. Diagrammatic representation of plasma cells producing intact immunoglobulins with monomeric κ and dimeric λ FLC molecules.
There are approximately twice as many κ FLC-producing plasma cells as λ FLC-producing plasma cells.

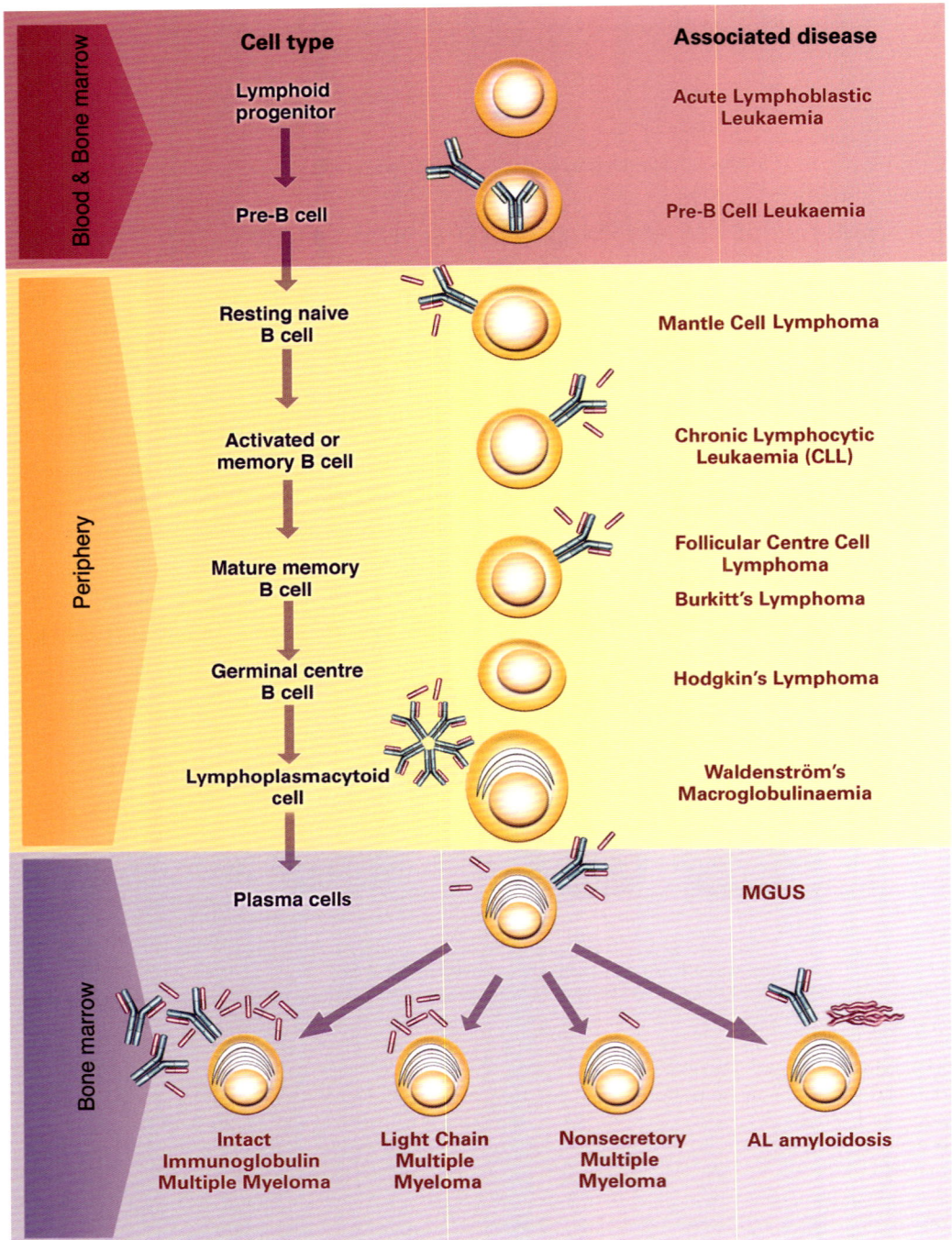

Figure 3.8. Development of the B-cell lineage and associated diseases.

In normal individuals, approximately 500 mg of FLCs are produced each day from bone marrow and lymph node cells[4,6]. The molecules enter the blood and are rapidly partitioned between the intravascular and extravascular compartments. The normal plasma cell content of the bone marrow is about 1%, whereas in multiple myeloma (MM) this can rise to over 90%. In chronic infections and autoimmmune diseases the bone marrow may contain 5 - 10% plasma cells, and may be associated with hypergammaglobulinaemia and corresponding increases in polyclonal serum FLC (sFLC) concentrations. Identification of monoclonal plasma cells in the bone marrow by histology or flow cytometry is an essential part of MM diagnosis, and is frequently based on identifying intracellular κ and λ light chains by direct immunofluorescence techniques *(Figure 3.9)*.

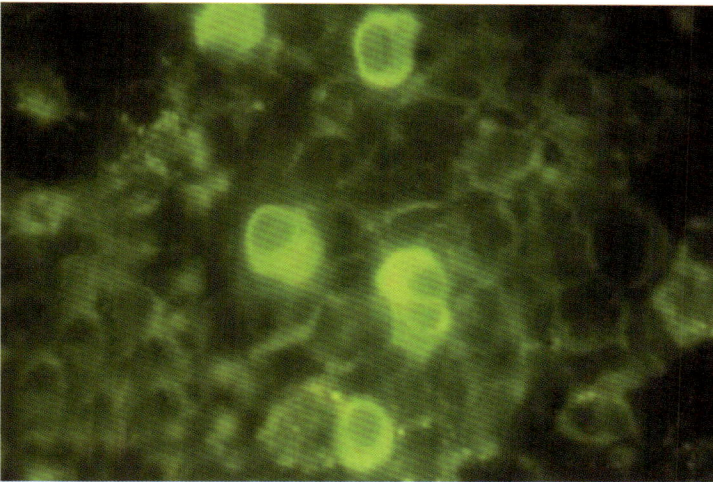

Figure 3.9.
Immunohistochemical staining of κ-producing bone marrow plasma cells from a patient with MM using fluorescein-conjugated, anti-κ antiserum. Five plasma cells can be seen.

3.5. Clearance and metabolism

Serum concentrations of FLCs and intact immunoglobulins reflect the balance between their production and clearance rates. An understanding of immunoglobulin clearance mechanisms in both normal and pathological conditions is important when considering the utility of sFLCs and intact immunoglobulins as tumour markers in monoclonal gammopathies.

3.5.1. Half-life of sFLCs

sFLCs are rapidly cleared and metabolised by the kidneys. At around 25 kDa in size, monomeric FLCs, characteristically κ, are cleared in 2 - 4 hours at 40% of the glomerular filtration rate. Dimeric FLCs of around 50 kDa, typically λ, are cleared in 3 - 6 hours at 20% of the glomerular filtration rate *(Figure 3.10)*, while larger polymers are cleared more slowly[6,7]. In contrast, IgG has a half-life of approximately 21 days with minimal renal clearance *(Section 5.3)*. Although κ FLC production rates are estimated to be twice that of λ, their faster removal ensures that actual serum concentrations are approximately 50% lower *(Chapter 5)*. The half-life of FLCs is dependent upon kidney function, so that FLC removal may be prolonged to 2 - 3 days in MM patients with complete renal failure[4,6,7,8]. In patients with chronic kidney disease (CKD), κ and λ sFLC concentrations increase due to reduced renal clearance[9]. When renal clearance is reduced, a greater proportion of sFLC are removed through pinocytosis by cells of the reticuloendothelial system[10]. This mechanism removes κ and λ sFLC at the same rate so the relative FLC concentrations change to reflect more closely the higher rate of κ production and there are minor increases in the κ/λ sFLC ratio[9].

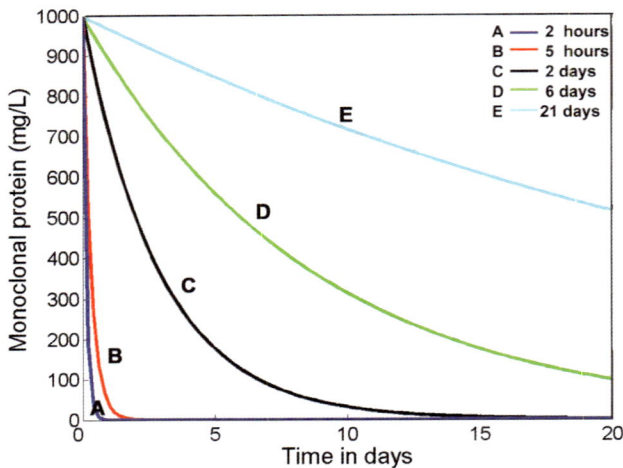

Figure 3.10. Calculated serum half-life curves for different immunoglobulin molecules.
(A) monomeric κ sFLCs; (B) dimeric λ sFLCs; (C) monomeric κ sFLCs with renal failure; (D) IgA and (E) IgG. (Courtesy of N. Evans and M. Chappell).

3.5.2. Renal clearance of FLCs

Figure 3.11 shows the glomerular filtration and metabolism of FLCs within a kidney nephron. Each nephron contains a glomerulus with basement membrane fenestrations, which allow filtration of serum molecules into the proximal tubules. Pore sizes are variable, with restricted filtration of molecules that are greater than 20 kDa in size, and a molecular weight cut-off of around 60 kDa. Protein molecules that pass through the glomerular pores are bound by the multi-ligand megalin and cubulin receptors on proximal tubule epithelium; these are then absorbed unchanged, degraded in the proximal tubular cells into their constituent amino acids, or excreted as fragments[12]. This megalin/cubulin absorption pathway is designed to prevent loss of large amounts of proteins and peptides into urine. It is very efficient and can process between 10 and 30 g of small molecular weight proteins daily. Therefore, the 500 mg of FLCs produced each day by the normal lymphoid system are filtered by the glomeruli and completely processed in the proximal tubules[8,13,14].

In normal individuals, between 1 and 10 mg of FLCs are excreted per day into the urine. Their exact origin is unclear, but they probably enter the urine via the mucosal surfaces of the distal part of the nephrons and the urethra, alongside secretory IgA. This secretion is part of the mucosal defence system that prevents infectious agents entering the body.

Because of the huge metabolic capacity of the proximal tubule, the amount of FLCs in urine (even when production is considerably increased in a patient with MM), is more dependent upon renal function than synthesis by the tumour. As a consequence, serum and urine FLC concentrations may differ during the evolution of light chain MM (LCMM) *(Figure 3.12)*. From low initial starting concentrations, sFLCs increase steadily with growing tumour mass, while concentrations in the urine show little change until the proximal tubular metabolism is exceeded and overflow proteinuria develops. Hence, early disease and oligo-secretory disease are not identified from urine tests. Subsequently, urine FLCs rise rapidly as overflow occurs, to reach a maximum. Concentrations then decrease as renal impairment occurs, and are low in complete renal failure. By contrast, sFLC levels increase as renal impairment develops due to the lengthening half-life of FLCs that are no longer cleared by the kidneys. Because of the biphasic urine curve, decreasing concentrations may indicate response to treatment or deterioration of renal function. Urine measurements are therefore unreliable during disease monitoring. Serum levels, however, rise or fall in correct relationship to worsening or improving disease status. The merits of serum over urine testing are further discussed in Chapter 24.

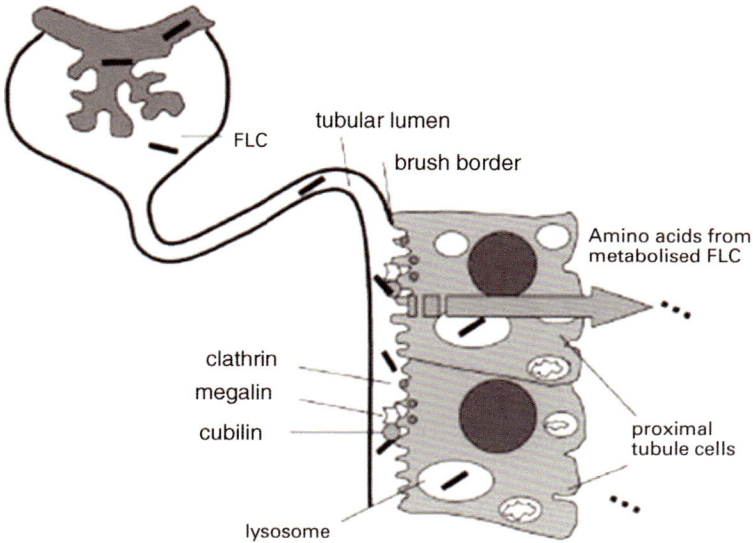

Figure 3.11. Filtration and metabolism of FLCs. *FLCs are filtered through the glomerulus and pass into the proximal tubule, where they are endocytosed via the megalin/cubulin receptor system. Within the proximal tubular cells they are degraded in lysosomes.* (Reprinted by permission from Macmillan Publishers Ltd: Leukemia[11], copyright 2008).

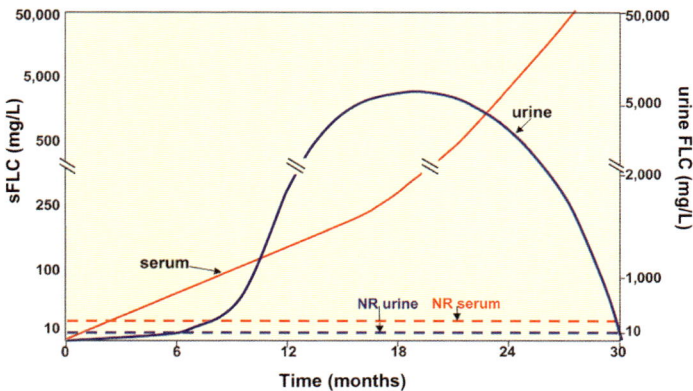

Figure 3.12. Changes in serum and urine free light chain concentrations during the evolution of a hypothetical patient with light chain multiple myeloma. *NR: Normal range.*

3.5.3. Half-life of IgG, IgA and IgM

Under normal circumstances, most serum proteins that are too large for renal filtration (> around 60 kDa) are removed by pinocytosis, a process that occurs in all nucleated cells as they obtain their essential nutrients from plasma. This accounts for the half-life of IgA and IgM, which is constant at around 5 - 6 days. By contrast, IgG has a concentration-dependent half-life of approximately 21 days due to recycling by FcRn receptors[16,17,18,15]. These receptors have a structure similar to Class I MHC molecules with a heavy chain of three domains and a single domain light chain comprising β_2-microglobulin *(Figure 3.13)*. FcRn receptors are functional in most nucleated cells, including renal podocytes, which may account for the presence of IgG in the urine at high serum concentrations *(Chapter 24)*[18,19,20,21,22,23,24]. These are the same receptors that transport IgG from the pregnant mother to the developing foetus in the last trimester of pregnancy.

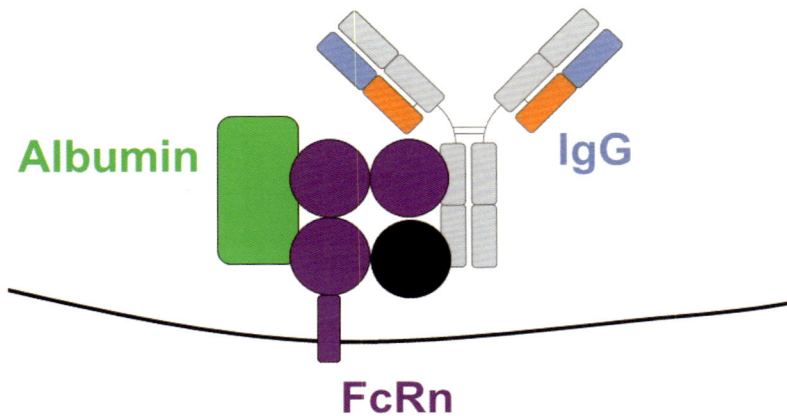

Figure 3.13. Diagram of FcRn structure showing binding of IgG and albumin molecules.
Albumin and IgG are bound non-competitively.

The heterodimeric FcRn molecules protect both IgG and albumin from acid digestion in lysosomes, recycling them back to the cell surface *(Figure 3.14)*. Interestingly, IgG and albumin molecules do not compete for the same sites on the receptor, although the exact mechanism and sites of binding are unknown. In the absence of functioning FcRn receptors, as in patients with familial hypercatabolic hypoproteinaemia (a disease associated with a genetic deficiency of β_2-microglobulin), the half-lives of IgG and albumin are only 3 days. Such patients have hypogammaglobulinaemia, not from failure of production, but simply from excessive catabolism.

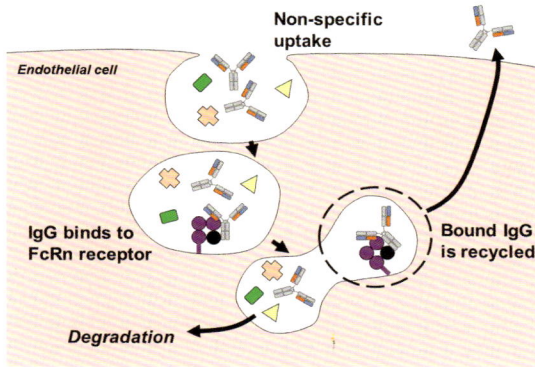

Figure 3.14. Recycling of IgG molecules by FcRn receptors.

At high IgG concentrations, the FcRn recycling system can reach saturation and the half-life of IgG falls as there are insufficient FcRn receptors to protect all IgG molecules *(Figure 3.15)*. Hence, a patient presenting with, for example, a monoclonal IgG of 90 g/L is producing far more than 3 times the amount of IgG than a patient presenting with 30 g/L of IgG. In contrast, at low IgG concentrations, when FcRn receptor protection is maximal, the IgG half-life extends to several months. Serum IgG concentrations may therefore be an unreliable indicator of tumour production rates in patients with IgG MM *(Chapter 18)*.

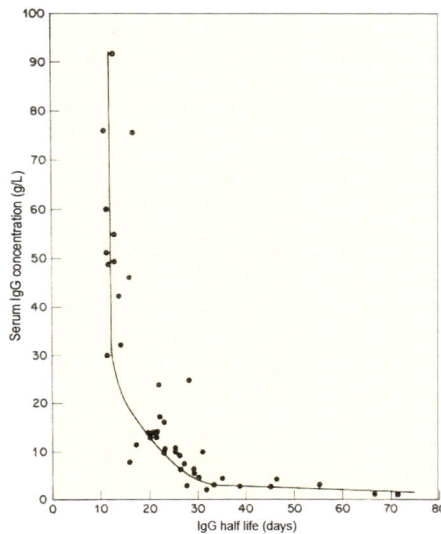

Figure 3.15. The relationship between IgG half-life and serum IgG concentration[15]. (Copyright © 1969 Karger Publishers, Basel, Switzerland).

Test Questions

1. What accounts for immunoglobulin light chain heterogeneity?
2. What are the normal serum half-lives of IgG and FLCs?
3. Do urine FLC concentrations always increase alongside rising sFLC concentrations?
4. Why does the IgG half-life vary with concentration?

Answers

1. Light chain heterogeneity arises from genetic recombination, isotypic, allotypic and idiotypic variation and somatic hypermutation of the variable regions after antigen exposure *(Sections 3.1 and 3.2)*.

2. IgG is approximately 21 days and FLCs 2 - 6 hours *(Section 3.4)*.

3. No. If there is significant renal impairment, urine FLC excretion falls *(Section 3.4)*.

4. FcRn receptors saturate at high IgG concentrations so the half-life shortens *(Section 3.4)*. At low IgG concentrations, the half-life lengthens because FcRn receptor recycling is maximal *(Section 3.4)*.

References

1. Edmundson AB, Ely KR, Abola EE, Schiffer M, Panagiotopoulos N, Deutsch HF. Conformational isomerism, rotational allomerism, and divergent evolution in immunoglobulin light chains. Fed Proc 1976;35:2119-23

2. Epp O, Lattman EE, Schiffer M, Huber R, Palm W. The molecular structure of a dimer composed of the variable portions of the Bence-Jones protein REI refined at 2.0-A resolution. Biochemistry 1975;14:4943-52

3. Janeway CA, Jr., Travers P, Walport M. The generation of diversity in immunoglobulins. Immunobiology: the immune system in health and disease. New York: Garland Science, 2001

4. Solomon A. Light chains of human immunoglobulins. Methods Enzymol 1985;116:101-21

5. Jefferis R, Lefranc MP. Human immunoglobulin allotypes: possible implications for immunogenicity. MAbs 2009;1:332-8

6. Waldmann TA, Strober W, Mogielnicki RP. The renal handling of low molecular weight proteins. II. Disorders of serum protein catabolism in patients with tubular proteinuria, the nephrotic syndrome, or uremia. J Clin Invest 1972;51:2162-74

7. Miettinen TA, Kekki M. Effect of impaired hepatic and renal function on[131]I Bence Jones protein catabolism in human subjects. Clin Chim Acta 1967;18:395-407

8. Wochner RD, Strober W, Waldmann TA. The role of the kidney in the catabolism of Bence Jones proteins and immunoglobulin fragments. J Exp Med 1967;126:207-21

9. Hutchison CA, Harding S, Hewins P, Mead GP, Townsend J, Bradwell AR, Cockwell P. Quantitative assessment of serum and urinary polyclonal free light chains in patients with chronic kidney disease. Clin J Am Soc Nephrol 2008;3:1684-90

10. Hutchison CA, Basnayake K, Cockwell P. Serum free light chain assessment in monoclonal gammopathy and kidney disease. Nat Rev Nephrol 2009;5:621-8

11. Dimopoulos MA, Kastritis E, Rosinol L, Blade J, Ludwig H. Pathogenesis and treatment of renal failure in multiple myeloma. Leukemia 2008;22:1485-93

12. Christensen EI, Birn H, Storm T, Weyer K, Nielsen R. Endocytic receptors in the renal proximal tubule. Physiology (Bethesda) 2012;27:223-36

13. Abraham GN, Waterhouse C. Evidence for defective immunoglobulin metabolism in severe renal insufficiency. Am J Med Sci 1974;268:227-33

14. Maack T, Johnson V, Kau ST, Figueiredo J, Sigulem D. Renal filtration, transport, and metabolism of low-molecular-weight proteins: a review. Kidney Int 1979;16:251-70

15. Waldmann TA, Strober W. Metabolism of immunoglobulins. Prog Allergy 1969;13:1-110

16. Kim J, Hayton WL, Robinson JM, Anderson CL. Kinetics of FcRn-mediated recycling of IgG and albumin in human: pathophysiology and therapeutic implications using a simplified mechanism-based model. Clin Immunol 2007;122:146-55

17. Akilesh S, Christianson GJ, Roopenian DC, Shaw AS. Neonatal FcR expression in bone marrow-derived cells functions to protect serum IgG from catabolism. J Immunol 2007;179:4580-8

18. Anderson CL, Chaudhury C, Kim J, Bronson CL, Wani MA, Mohanty S. Perspective - FcRn transports albumin: relevance to immunology and medicine. Trends Immunol 2006;27:343-8

19. Tryggvason K, Wartiovaara J. How does the kidney filter plasma? Physiology (Bethesda) 2005;20:96-101

20. Haymann JP, Levraud JP, Bouet S, Kappes V, Hagege J, Nguyen G et al. Characterization and localization of the neonatal Fc receptor in adult human kidney. J Am Soc Nephrol 2000;11:632-9

21. Kobayashi N, Suzuki Y, Tsuge T, Okumura K, Ra C, Tomino Y. FcRn-mediated transcytosis of immunoglobulin G in human renal proximal tubular epithelial cells. Am J Physiol Renal Physiol 2002;282:F358-F365

22. Chaudhury C, Mehnaz S, Robinson JM, Hayton WL, Pearl DK, Roopenian DC, Anderson CL. The major histocompatibility complex-related Fc receptor for IgG (FcRn) binds albumin and prolongs its lifespan. J Exp Med 2003;197:315-22

23. Akilesh S, Huber TB, Wu H, Wang G, Hartleben B, Kopp JB et al. Podocytes use FcRn to clear IgG from the glomerular basement membrane. Proc Natl Acad Sci U S A 2008;105:967-72

24. Roopenian DC, Christianson GJ, Sproule TJ, Brown AC, Akilesh S, Jung N et al. The MHC class I-like IgG receptor controls perinatal IgG transport, IgG homeostasis, and fate of IgG-Fc-coupled drugs. J Immunol 2003;170:3528-33

Laboratory techniques for monoclonal immunoglobulin measurement

Summary:

- Serum protein electrophoresis detects the majority of monoclonal intact immunoglobulins, but is considerably less sensitive than sFLC analysis for identifying monoclonal FLCs.

- Capillary zone electrophoresis offers a more automated alternative to serum protein electrophoresis, and is increasingly being used by laboratories with a large workload.

- Once identified, monoclonal proteins are typed using immunofixation electrophoresis or immunosubtraction.

- Monoclonal intact immunoglobulins that co-migrate with other serum protein peaks on serum electrophoresis may be more accurately quantifed using total immunoglobulin or Hevylite® immunoassays.

- There are wide variations in laboratory protocols for urine protein electrophoresis.

4.1. Introduction

The detection of monoclonal intact immunoglobulins and/or free light chains (FLCs) forms part of the diagnostic criteria for many plasma cell disorders, although the requirement for the presence of a monoclonal protein is no longer mandatory for the diagnosis of multiple myeloma (MM) (*Section 25.2*). The same tests, which are used diagnostically, are frequently employed for monitoring disease and defining the response to treatment *(Chapter 25)*[1,2,3,4,5,6]. This chapter provides an overview of the methodology and analytical sensitivity of routine laboratory methods used to identify and quantify monoclonal immunoglobulins.

4.2. Detection and quantification of serum monoclonal proteins

4.2.1. Serum protein electrophoresis

Serum protein electrophoresis (SPE) is performed in agarose gels, resulting in the separation of serum proteins according to their size and charge and producing two major fractions: albumin and globulins. Albumin is the most abundant serum protein and forms a dense band close to the anode. The globulin fraction is subdivided into five regions, each containing several serum proteins. These are α1, α2, β1, β2 and γ, with the γ region being closest to the cathode *(Figure 4.1)*.

After proteins have been separated, they are fixed in the gel with an acid fixative and generally stained with Coomassie Brilliant Blue or Amido Black. Stained gels may be examined by eye and are often scanned with a densitometer to produce an electrophoretogram. This is a digital interpretation of the stained gel and is similar in appearance to electrophoretograms generated by capillary zone electrophoresis *(CZE; Figure 4.2)*. Monoclonal proteins may appear as a peak in any region on the electrophoretogram. Other features suggestive of a monoclonal gammopathy may be detected by SPE e.g. hypogammaglobulinaemia (identified by reduced staining in the γ region). If a monoclonal gammopathy is suspected, further investigation is warranted, including serum immunofixation electrophoresis *(sIFE; Section 4.3.1)*[7,8].

Serum monoclonal proteins are typed by sIFE *(or immunosubtraction; Section 4.3)*, while the concentration of each band is determined by scanning densitometry of the SPE gel in combination with serum total protein measurements.

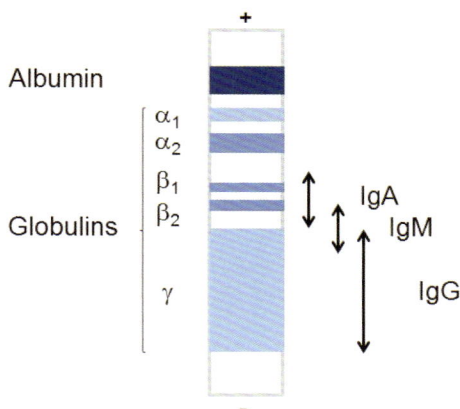

Figure 4.1. Schematic of serum protein electrophoresis. *The approximate position of polyclonal immunoglobulins in normal serum and the anode (+) and cathode (-) are indicated.*

4.2.2. Capillary zone electrophoresis

CZE offers an alternative to agarose gel electrophoresis for the detection and quantification of serum proteins. Protein separation is performed in a liquid buffer system running through narrow-bore capillaries made of fused silica. The separated proteins pass an ultraviolet detector that measures absorbance at 200 to 215 nm to determine the protein concentration.

Electrophoretograms generated by CZE are similar in appearance to those produced by SPE, and can be used for monoclonal protein quantitation (in combination with serum total protein measurements) *(Figure 4.2)*. Katzmann and colleagues[10] reported a good correlation between monoclonal protein concentration obtained by CZE and SPE for values <20 g/L, but above 20 g/L, values for CZE tended to be greater.

The main advantage of CZE over SPE is that it is an automated technique with faster throughput. In addition, most[10,11,12], but not all[13] reports conclude that capillary-based methods have slightly higher sensitivity than agarose gel-based electrophoresis *(Table 4.1)*. The superior sensitivity of CZE over SPE has been shown to identify additional cases of monoclonal serum free light chains (sFLCs) and small monoclonal protein peaks in either the β-region or on a polyclonal background[10,11,12].

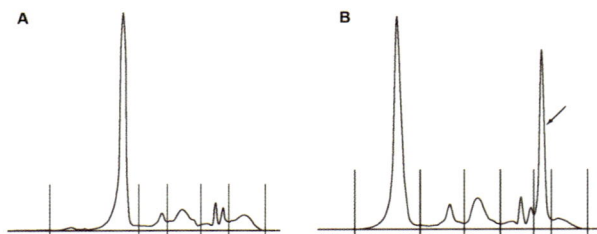

Figure 4.2. Capillary zone electrophoresis. (A) *Normal serum.* **(B)** *Monoclonal protein peak in γ-region, indicated by an arrow. (These figures were originally published in[9], reproduced with permission from Taylor & Francis Group).*

Method	Analytical sensitivity
SPE	~0.5 g/L
sIFE	0.1 g/L
UPE	20 mg/L
uIFE	3 - 5 mg/L
CZE	0.25 g/L
Total κ and λ	~4 g/L
sFLC	0.25 - 3 mg/L*

Table 4.1. Detection limits for various methods used to detect monoclonal immunoglobulins. *Based on manufacturers' information and published studies[7,14,15]. UPE: urine protein electrophoresis. * This is the analytical sensitivity of FLC measurement and not the limit for detection of monoclonal FLC, which is dependent upon the presence of an abnormal κ/λ sFLC ratio.*

4.2.3. Diagnostic sensitivity of SPE and CZE compared with other laboratory techniques

The analytical sensitivity of SPE, CZE and other routine laboratory tests for monoclonal immunoglobulin detection is summarised in Table 4.1. In practice, the detection limit of electrophoretic techniques is dependent on a number of factors including: 1) the position of the monoclonal protein; 2) the level of polyclonal background immunoglobulins (in the γ-region); and 3) the width of the monoclonal protein peak[14]. Not all monoclonal proteins can be accurately quantified by SPE due to co-migration or dye saturation issues (Section 17.4).

When the diagnostic sensitivity of CZE and SPE is compared with that of sIFE, both methods fail to detect a small percentage of monoclonal proteins (Table 4.2). A high proportion of these samples are monoclonal IgA, IgM or sFLCs[13]. Such monoclonal proteins represent a diagnostic challenge as they may be small and co-migrate with other serum protein peaks, making detection and accurate quantification challenging (Section 17.4). In some cases, an abnormal κ/λ sFLC ratio may prompt sIFE to be performed, and reveal the presence of a hidden monoclonal intact immunoglobulin (Section 23.3)[16]. The diagnostic specificity of SPE and CZE are similar, although the reported values are variable between different studies (Table 4.2).

Study	SPE		CZE	
	Diagnostic sensitivity (%)	Diagnostic specificity (%)	Diagnostic sensitivity (%)	Diagnostic specificity (%)
Bossuyt 1998[17]	86.0	Not reported	93.0	Not reported
Katzmann 1998[10]	90.7	98.9	94.9	98.6
Poisson 2012[11]	89.9	75.4	97.4 (or 92.3)*	57.6 (or 72.2)*
Yang 2007[13]	90.0	100	81	100

Table 4.2. Comparison of the diagnostic sensitivity of SPE and CZE to detect monoclonal proteins identified by sIFE.
* Values refer to Sebia CAPILLARYS™2 (or Helena V8™) instruments.

4.2.4. sFLC analysis

Freelite® sFLC assays are quantitative, latex-enhanced immunoassays that are performed on routine nephelometric or turbidimetric instruments (Chapters 5 and 37). Of all the methods used to detect monoclonal immunoglobulins, sFLC analysis has the highest analytical sensitivity for identifying monoclonal sFLCs (Table 4.1)[18,19,20].

The high clinical sensitivity of sFLC assays is dependent upon assessing the individual sFLC concentrations and the κ/λ sFLC ratio. Tumour suppression of the normal plasma cells in the bone marrow reduces the concentration of polyclonal uninvolved sFLCs, and thereby enhances the sensitivity of the κ/λ ratio.

Katzmann et al.[21] concluded that a combination of sFLC and SPE provided a simple and efficient initial diagnostic screen for the high-tumour-burden monoclonal gammopathies such as MM, Waldenström's macroglobulinaemia (WM) and smouldering MM (SMM) (Chapter 23). International guidelines recommend that sFLC analysis in combination with SPE and sIFE is sufficient to screen for all pathological monoclonal plasmaproliferative disorders other than AL amyloidosis, which requires IFE of a 24-hour urine sample in addition to the serum tests (Chapters 25 and 28).

4.2.5. Hevylite immunoassays

Immunoglobulin heavy/light chain (Hevylite®, HLC) assays separately quantify the different light chain types of each immunoglobulin isotype (i.e. IgGκ, IgGλ, IgAκ, IgAλ, IgMκ and IgMλ, *Chapter 9*). HLC assays are performed on routine nephelometric or turbidimetric instruments *(Chapters 9 and 38)*. The molecules are assessed in pairs to produce HLC ratios (e.g. IgGκ/IgGλ) in the same manner as κ/λ sFLC ratios. HLC assays provide an alternative tool to aid in the management of diseases associated with monoclonal intact immunoglobulins, including monoclonal gammopathy of undetermined significance (MGUS), SMM and intact immunoglobulin multiple myeloma (IIMM) *(Chapters 13, 14, and 18)*.

HLC assays may overcome many of the known limitations of serum electrophoresis (including co-migration and dye saturation) and are less labour-intensive and less subjective. The sensitivity of the HLC ratio to detect monoclonal intact immunoglobulins is dependent upon the concentration of both the involved and uninvolved immunoglobulin HLC. In a study of 999 patients with MGUS, IgA and IgM HLC assays were generally as sensitive as SPE, whereas IgG HLC assays did not identify a monoclonal immunoglobulin in almost half of patients, presumably due to the lack of polyclonal uninvolved HLC suppression[10]. By contrast, Katzmann et al.[22] demonstrated that whilst IgG HLC assays had a similar sensitivity to SPE for the detection of IgG monoclonal proteins in sera from IgG MM patients (n=155, *Table 4.3)*, the sensitivity of IgA HLC assays was greater than SPE and comparable to that of IFE for IgA monoclonal proteins in IgA MM patient sera (n=149, *Table 4.4)*. The authors concluded that IgA HLC assays can substitute for the combination of SPE, IFE and total IgA quantification for monitoring β-migrating IgA monoclonal proteins.

Serum sample	n	Abnormal SPE*	Abnormal IgGκ/IgGλ HLC ratio
Presentation	32	31 (97%)	30 (94%)
Post-treatment	123	104 (85%)	106 (86%)
All	155	135 (87%)	136 (88%)

Table 4.3. SPE and HLC ratio abnormalities in IgG MM[22]. Data are n (%); * Monoclonal protein band or small, fuzzy band.

Serum sample	n	SPE monoclonal protein quantified	Abnormal IgAκ/IgAλ HLC ratio	Positive IFE	Total IgA >upper limit of normal*
Presentation	30	23 (78%)	29 (97%)	30 (100%)	26 (87%)
Post-treatment	119	18 (15%)	54 (45%)	56 (50%)[‡]	48 (40%)
All	149	41 (28%)	83 (56%)	86 (61%)[†]	74 (50%)

Table 4.4. SPE, HLC, IFE and total IgA abnormalities in IgA MM[10]. Data are n (%); * >3.56 g/L; ‡ n=111; † n=141.

Laboratory techniques for monoclonal
immunoglobulin measurement

4.3. Typing of serum monoclonal proteins

4.3.1. Immunofixation electrophoresis

For sIFE, a patient's serum is applied to several lanes of an agarose gel, and after electrophoresis, specific antisera are overlaid on individual lanes of the gel. These antisera are typically against IgG, IgA, IgM, κ and λ, although other specificities may be useful for identifying unusual bands (e.g. IgD, IgE or fibrinogen). A lane fixed with acid (which fixes all proteins) is also included for comparison. Following removal of the antisera, gels are washed and stained with Coomassie Brilliant Blue or Amido Black *(Figure 4.3)*. Although IFE is non-quantitative (due to the presence of the precipitating antibody, which also absorbs dye), it is considered the "gold standard" method to confirm the presence of a monoclonal protein and to distinguish its heavy and light chain type[23].

IFE is approximately 10-fold more sensitive than SPE, and is included in MM guidelines in the definition of a stringent complete response *(Chapter 25)*[6]. It should be noted that judging whether there is or is not a discrete (monoclonal) protein band present after IFE can be subjective, and this may lead to discordance in the response category assigned by different operators *(Section 18.4.3)*[24].

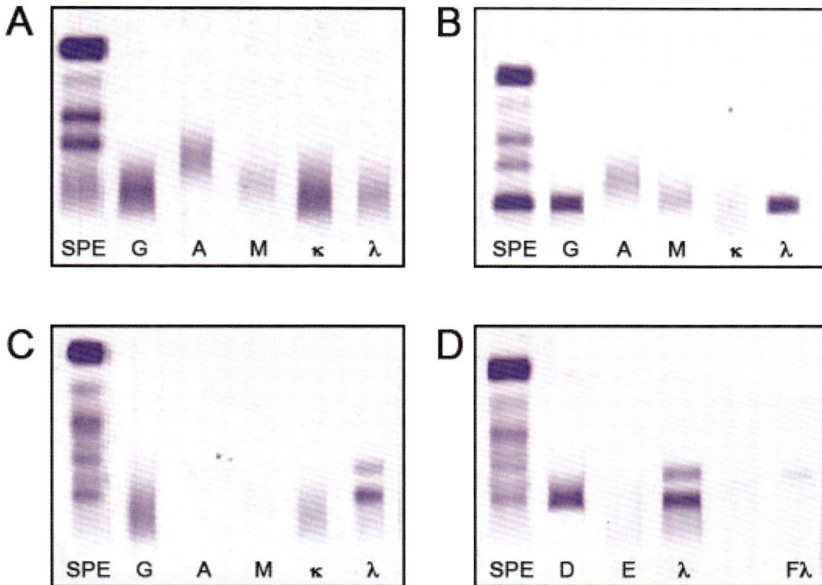

Figure 4.3. Serum immunofixation electrophoresis. (A) Normal serum. (B) Monoclonal IgGλ intact immunoglobulin. (C,D) Monoclonal IgDλ intact immunoglobulin with λ FLCs. Fλ: anti-free λ antisera. (Courtesy of Me Musset Hôpital Pitié-Salpétrière – Paris, France).

4.3.2. Immunosubtraction

Immunosubtraction can be used in place of IFE for typing the majority of monoclonal protein bands, but it is less sensitive[23]. In this technique, antibodies against IgG, IgA, IgM, κ or λ (bound to solid phase beads) are incubated with serum aliquots, then CZE is performed to determine which reagent(s) remove an electrophoretic abnormality *(Figure 4.4)*.

This procedure works well with samples producing discrete monoclonal protein spikes and is easier to perform than sIFE[10]. However, IFE may still be required as a complementary method to determine the monoclonal protein type in a number of situations[10,11,17]. These include detection/typing of: 1) monoclonal sFLCs of the same type as the characterised monoclonal intact immunoglobulin; 2) multiple monoclonal proteins, e.g. biclonal gammopathies or oligoclonal banding; 3) "hidden" monoclonal proteins, e.g. small (<3 g/L) IgA or IgM monoclonal proteins that co-migrate with other serum proteins in the β-region; and 4) IgD and IgE monoclonal proteins.

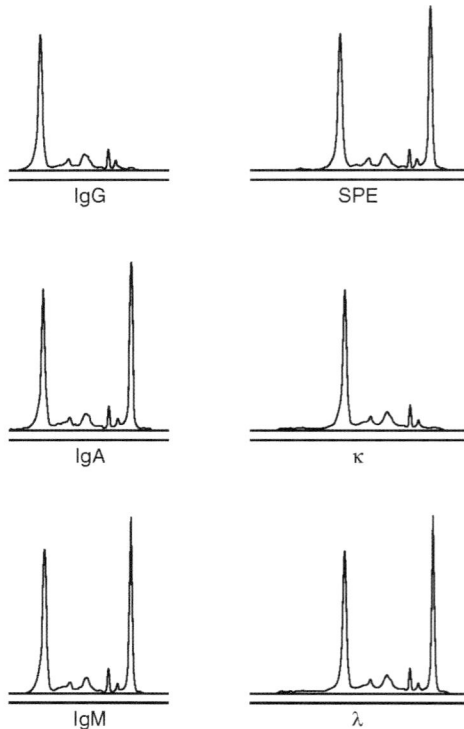

Figure 4.4. IgGκ immunosubtraction example. *The monoclonal protein peak is removed with addition of anti-IgG and -κ antibodies. (This figure was originally published in[9], reproduced with permission from Taylor & Francis Group).*

4.4. Other serum assays

4.4.1. Total immunoglobulin assays

Once a monoclonal protein has been identified in a serum sample, it is recommended that total immunoglobulins (IgG, IgA and IgM) are also measured by nephelometric/turbidimetric methods[23]. Whilst it is preferred that monoclonal proteins are monitored by densitometric quantification, in cases where small monoclonal proteins are obscured by other serum proteins (e.g. transferrin), nephelometric measurements may be more accurate[7,23]. However, total nephelometric measurements cannot discriminate between monoclonal and polyclonal immunoglobulins, which may limit their usefulness as the serum concentration approaches the normal range[25]. In their study of 149 patients with IgA MM, Katzmann et al.[22] showed that total IgA assays are less sensitive than IgA Hevylite assays for detection of monoclonal IgA in diagnostic and post-treatment samples (Table 4.4).

It is important that densitometric and nephelometric methods are not used interchangeably as they do not always yield the same result[7,23]. For example, nephelometry may overestimate high concentrations of monoclonal IgM, and will also overestimate monoclonal protein concentrations if samples contain significant levels of polyclonal immunoglobulin. Electrophoresis may underestimate high concentrations of IgG (possibly due to dye saturation, Section 17.5).

4.4.2. Total κ/λ assays

Nephelometric total light chain assays measure the concentration of all intact immunoglobulin and FLCs of a particular light chain type (e.g. total κ assays measure IgGκ + IgAκ + IgMκ + IgDκ + IgEκ + κ sFLCs). Results are expressed as a κ/λ ratio and are used by some laboratories as a screen for monoclonal gammopathy. However, it is an insensitive approach. The presence of background polyclonal immunoglobulins prevents the detection of monoclonal proteins smaller than around 4 g/L[15].

The sensitivity of sFLC assays and total κ and λ assays were compared in a study by Marien et al.[26]. Sixteen serum samples from patients with light chain MM (LCMM) were investigated. Total κ and λ concentrations were measured using Beckman-Coulter reagents on the IMMAGE® nephelometer and sFLC concentrations were measured by Freelite assays from The Binding Site. All samples were abnormal by sFLC assays (Figure 4.5). This compared with only five of the 16 samples by total κ and λ assays, and one λ patient was mistyped as κ. Other studies have confirmed that total light chain assays are less sensitive than sFLC analysis for the diagnosis of LCMM, nonsecretory MM (NSMM) and AL amyloidosis[27,28,29]. Thus, the benefits of the total κ/λ assays are limited, and they are not recommended by international guidelines (Chapter 25)[30.]

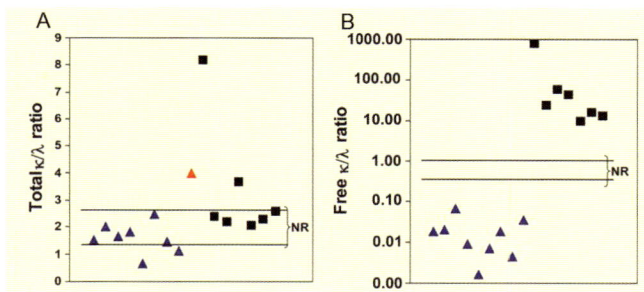

Figure 4.5. Comparison of (A) total serum light chains and (B) sFLC κ/λ ratios for identifying patients with κ and λ LCMM. κ patients: black squares; λ patients: blue triangles. The red triangle is a mistyped sample. Normal range limits are shown.

4.5. Detection and quantification of urine monoclonal proteins

4.5.1. Urine protein electrophoresis

Urine protein electrophoresis (UPE) and urine immunofixation (uIFE) use essentially the same gels and equipment as SPE and sIFE. UPE produces a heterogeneous range of patterns depending on the presence and relative concentrations of proteins including albumin, glomerular and tubular proteins, monoclonal FLCs (urinary Bence Jones protein, uBJP) and polyclonal FLCs *(Figure 4.6)*[7].

There are wide variations in laboratory protocols for UPE. These include the use of 24-hour vs. random urine collections, with or without urine concentration, and with or without correction for creatinine excretion[31]. Difficulties associated with 24-hour urine collections are further discussed in Section 24.3. Whilst some guidelines recommend that urine aliquots from 24-hour collections are concentrated (up to 100-fold) prior to electrophoresis[23], many laboratories routinely use neat random urine samples for analysis.

The concentration of uBJP is calculated using scanning densitometry in combination with total protein measurements. With optimal conditions, UPE can detect monoclonal FLCs at <20 mg/L, although most laboratories claim a detection limit in the region of 40 - 50 mg/L. In practice, high concentrations of background proteins and "ladder banding" caused by polyclonal FLCs prevent attainment of the ideal sensitivity. In addition, false positive UPE results may be produced by a variety of proteins including β_2-microglobulin, and lysozyme[9]. Therefore, the visual interpretation of electrophoretic gels presents many challenges, even to experienced users. As with SPE, the presence of any suspicious band after UPE requires IFE to determine the identity of the protein. Compared with SPE, UPE produces many more "false-positive" bands which are found not to be monoclonal FLC or immunoglobulin after performing uIFE[9].

Urine electrophoresis is required for all patients if a diagnosis of MM is established[23]. However, some patients with plasma cell dyscrasias produce only small amounts of monoclonal FLCs, so little, if any, passes the absorptive surface of the renal proximal tubules *(Chapter 3)*. As a result, these patients may have undetectable levels of FLCs in the urine, and sFLC immunoassays are usually preferable *(Chapter 24)*. It is important to note that small amounts of monoclonal FLCs have occasionally been identified in the urine of some AL amyloidosis patients with normal sFLC ratios. This is further discussed in Section 7.6.1.

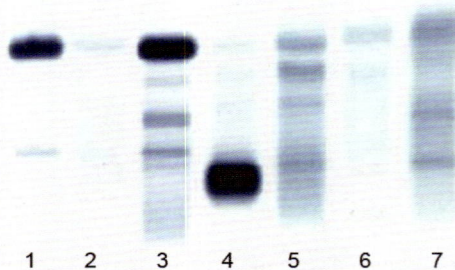

Figure 4.6. UPE examples. (1) Slight glomerular proteinuria; (2) albumin only; (3) normal serum control; (4) probable monoclonal protein (uIFE identifies λ FLC); (5) tubular proteinuria (uIFE negative); (6) slight tubular proteinurea (uIFE identifies IgGκ plus κ FLC); (7) query monoclonal protein (uIFE shows κ banding, no monoclonal protein detected).

4.5.2. Urine capillary zone electrophoresis

The analysis of urine proteins by CZE is more challenging than serum analysis because urine contains electrolytes, organic acids and other metabolites that can interfere with the technique. To prevent this interference, urine samples need to be pre-treated by filtration, dialysis or precipitation[32] and for this reason, the routine use of urine CZE is limited.

4.5.3. Urine FLC assays

FLC immunoassays can be used on urine samples as an alternative to urine electrophoretic tests. However, urinary FLC immunoassays do not solve any of the practical problems of urine collection or overcome the influence of the renal threshold for passage of FLCs into the urine. Indeed, the broad normal range for the κ/λ FLC ratio in urine (*Section 6.4*) ensures that uIFE is usually more sensitive for the detection of monoclonal FLC. For this reason, international guidelines do not recommend the measurement of urine FLC levels *(Chapter 25)*[23]. This is further discussed in Chapter 24, which brings together all the arguments for the use of serum rather than urine for the measurement of FLCs.

Test Questions

1. What assays are available to monitor patients with small monoclonal immunoglobulins that co-migrate with other serum proteins?

2. What UPE artefact can be associated with the presence of polyclonal FLCs in urine?

References

1. Durie BG, Harousseau JL, Miguel JS, Blade J, Barlogie B, Anderson K et al. International uniform response criteria for multiple myeloma. Leukemia 2006;20:1467-73

2. Gertz MA, Merlini G. Definition of organ involvement and response to treatment in AL amyloidosis: an updated consensus opinion. Amyloid 2010;17:CP-Ba

3. Kyle RA, Rajkumar SV. Criteria for diagnosis, staging, risk stratification and response assessment of multiple myeloma. Leukemia 2009;23:3-9

4. Palladini G, Dispenzieri A, Gertz MA, Wechalekar A, Hawkins P, Schonland SO et al. Validation of the criteria of response to treatment in AL amyloidosis. Blood 2010;116:1364a

5. Palladini G, Dispenzieri A, Gertz MA, Kumar S, Wechalekar A, Hawkins PN et al. New criteria for response to treatment in immunoglobulin light chain amyloidosis based on free light chain measurement and cardiac biomarkers: impact on survival outcomes. J Clin Oncol 2012;30:4541-9

6. Rajkumar SV, Harousseau JL, Durie B, Anderson KC, Dimopoulos M, Kyle R et al. Consensus recommendations for the uniform reporting of clinical trials: report of the International Myeloma Workshop Consensus Panel 1. Blood 2011;117:4691-5

7. Tate J, Caldwell G, Daly J, Gillis D, Jenkins M, Jovanovich S et al. Recommendations for standardized reporting of protein electrophoresis in Australia and New Zealand. Ann Clin Biochem 2012;49:242-56

8. Lakshminarayanan R, Li Y, Janatpour K, Beckett L, Jialal I. Detection by immunofixation of M proteins in hypogammaglobulinemic patients with normal serum protein electrophoresis results. Am J Clin Pathol 2007;127:746-51

9. Keren DF. Protein electrophoresis in clinical diagnosis. Arnold (Hodder Headline), 2003

10. Katzmann JA, Clark R, Sanders E, Landers JP, Kyle RA. Prospective study of serum protein capillary zone electrophoresis and immunotyping of monoclonal proteins by immunosubtraction. Am J Clin Pathol 1998;110:503-9

11. Poisson J, Fedoriw Y, Henderson MP, Hainsworth S, Tucker K, Uddin Z, McCudden CR. Performance evaluation of the Helena V8 capillary electrophoresis system. Clin Biochem 2012;45:697-9

12. McCudden CR, Mathews SP, Hainsworth SA, Chapman JF, Hammett-Stabler CA, Willis MS, Grenache DG. Performance comparison of capillary and agarose gel electrophoresis for the identification and characterization of monoclonal immunoglobulins. Am J Clin Pathol 2008;129:451-8

13. Yang Z, Harrison K, Park YA, Chaffin CH, Thigpen B, Easley PL et al. Performance of the Sebia CAPILLARYS 2 for detection and immunotyping of serum monoclonal paraproteins. Am J Clin Pathol 2007;128:293-9

14. Bradwell AR, Harding SJ, Fourrier NJ, Wallis GL, Drayson MT, Carr-Smith HD, Mead GP. Assessment of monoclonal gammopathies by nephelometric measurement of individual immunoglobulin kappa/lambda ratios. Clin Chem 2009;55:1646-55

15. Laine ST, Soppi ET, Morsky PJ. Critical evaluation of the serum kappa/lambda light-chain ratio in the detection of M proteins. Clin Chim Acta 1992;207:143-9

16. Robson EJD, Taylor J, Beardsmore C, Basu S, Mead G, Lovatt T. Utility of serum free light chain analysis when screening for lymphoproliferative disorders. Lab Med 2009;40:325-9

17. Bossuyt X, Schiettekatte G, Bogaerts A, Blanckaert N. Serum protein electrophoresis by CZE 2000 clinical capillary electrophoresis system. Clin Chem 1998;44:749-59

18. Bradwell AR, Carr-Smith HD, Mead GP, Harvey TC, Drayson MT. Serum test for assessment of patients with Bence Jones myeloma. Lancet 2003;361:489-91

19. Drayson M, Tang LX, Drew R, Mead GP, Carr-Smith H, Bradwell AR. Serum free light-chain measurements for identifying and monitoring patients with nonsecretory multiple myeloma. Blood 2001;97:2900-2

Development and validation of Freelite immunoassays

Summary:

- Freelite® assays use sheep polyclonal antisera directed against the hidden epitopes of FLC molecules located at the interface between the light and heavy chains of immunoglobulins.
- Batch-to-batch consistency of Freelite reagents is maintained using a rolling pool of polyclonal antisera.
- Freelite assays are validated according to protocols set out by the Clinical and Laboratory Standards Institute, including precision, linearity, interference and stability.

5.1. Assay overview

Freelite κ and λ serum free light chain (sFLC) assays use polyclonal antisera directed against the "hidden" epitopes of FLC molecules that are located at the interface between the light and heavy chains of intact immunoglobulins *(Figure 5.1)*. These epitopes are only accessible when light chain molecules are not associated with the immunoglobulin heavy chain. κ and λ FLCs are measured in pairs to produce κ/λ sFLC ratios, or calculate the difference between the involved and uninvolved sFLC concentrations *(Section 7.2.2)*. Polyclonal antibodies raised in sheep provide the most attractive method of recognising the highly polymorphic FLC molecules *(Chapter 3)*. Latex enhancement increases the sensitivity of Freelite assays, to a few mg/L, and the assays are performed by turbidimetry or nephelometry on a number of automated laboratory instruments *(Chapter 37)*.

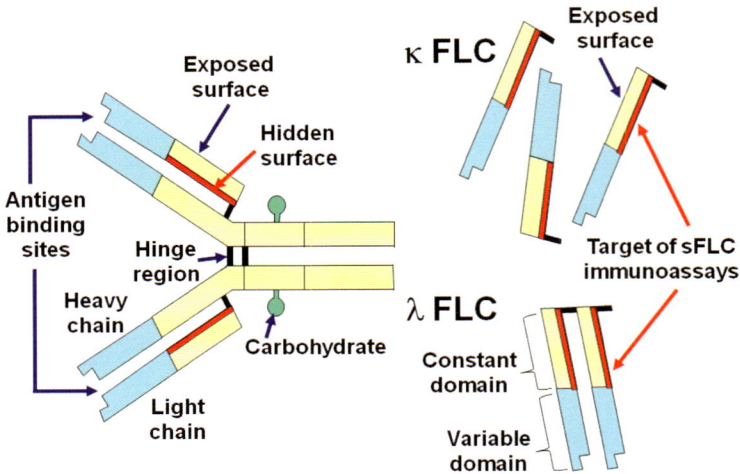

Figure 5.1. An antibody molecule showing the immunoglobulin heavy and light chain structure, together with free κ and λ FLC epitopes.

5.2. Polyclonal antisera versus monoclonal antibodies

It is essential that FLC immunoassays utilise antibodies that have high specificity and affinity. Early FLC immunoassays, from other groups, used polyclonal antisera but good specificity was difficult to obtain *(Chapter 2)*. Monoclonal antibodies seemed to be the obvious solution to the problem. However, considerable effort failed to produce antibodies that reliably recognised a full range of monoclonal FLCs *(Chapter 3)*. Similar findings have been reported for other monoclonal antibody-based FLC immunoassays and are discussed further in Chapter 8.

In contrast, an assay based on polyclonal antisera can recognise a wide variety of FLC epitopes, including the diverse range of pathological monoclonal FLCs produced by patients with monoclonal gammopathies. Therefore, research focussed on optimising polyclonal FLC antisera to ensure the reliable detection of the huge variety of monoclonal FLCs. The following description is an outline of the successful procedures involved in the development of Freelite sFLC assays. In summary, sheep were immunised with κ or λ molecules that had been purified from urine samples containing Bence Jones proteins. The resultant antisera were adsorbed against purified IgG, IgA and monoclonal proteins and then affinity purified against mixtures of the respective FLCs that had been immobilised onto Sepharose. Antisera requiring further adsorption, as judged by the tests described below, were recycled through the adsorption and testing procedures, resulting in antisera highly specific for FLCs and deemed satisfactory for assay use.

5.3. Antisera specificity testing

Specificity is the most important aspect of the immunoassays and was evaluated using several techniques.

5.3.1. Immunoelectrophoresis

Polyclonal antiserum was purified until it showed no cross-reactions by immunoelectrophoresis with the alternate FLC and intact immunoglobulin molecules *(Figure 5.2)*.

5.3.2. Western blot analysis

Western blot analysis is a sensitive technique used to assess the reactivity of the antisera against immunoglobulin fragments and FLC polymers. The results showed that both κ and λ FLC antisera reacted strongly, with two closely migrating bands at 25 - 30 kDa, and weakly with several larger and smaller molecular weight fragments. Similar staining patterns were observed using monoclonal antibodies. The FLC antisera were readily able to detect monomers and dimers of both κ and λ molecules *(Figure 5.3)*.

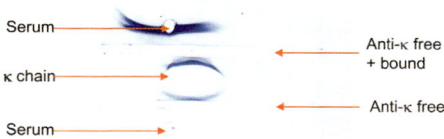

Figure 5.2. Immunoelectrophoresis showing the specificity of κ FLC antisera. The anti κ FLC antibody shows no cross reaction to proteins in normal human serum, including intact immunoglobulins (bottom well). Good anti-κ FLC activity is demonstrated by the presence of the arc against the purified κ chains (Serum = normal human serum, κ chain = purified κ light chains).

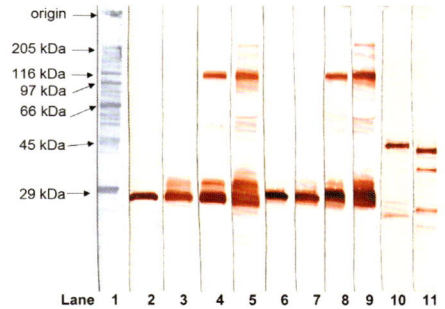

Figure 5.3. Western blots showing the specificity of polyclonal FLC antisera compared with monoclonal antibodies, and the reaction of polyclonal antisera against FLC monomers and dimers; all separated by non-reducing sodium dodecyl sulfate-polyacrylamide gel electrophoresis. Lane 1: molecular weight markers; Lanes 2 and 3: urine containing κ FLCs; and Lanes 4 and 5: normal serum. Even lanes probed with mono- and odd lanes probed with polyclonal anti-κ. Lanes 6 and 7: urine containing λ FLCs; and Lanes 8 and 9: normal serum. Even lanes probed with mono- and odd lanes probed with polyclonal anti- λ. Lanes 10 and 11: polyclonal FLC antisera (κ and λ, respectively) reacting with monomers and dimers of κ and λ.

5.3.3. Haemagglutination assays

Haemagglutination assays are far more sensitive than immunoelectrophoresis, and provide better assessment of specificity. Sheep red blood cells were sensitised with individual FLCs and purified IgG, IgA and IgM, and tested against the FLC antisera. The results showed that κ and λ FLC antibodies reacted with the appropriately labelled cells at >1:16,000 dilution and at <1:2 against cells coated with the alternate FLCs or intact immunoglobulins *(Figure 5.4)*.

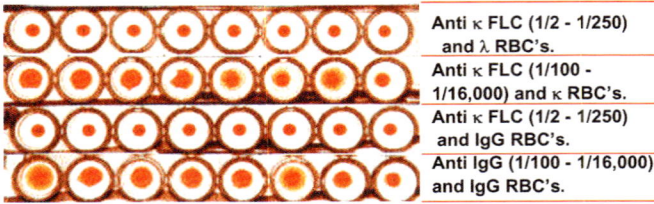

	Anti κ FLC (1/2 - 1/250) and λ RBC's.
	Anti κ FLC (1/100 - 1/16,000) and κ RBC's.
	Anti κ FLC (1/2 - 1/250) and IgG RBC's.
	Anti IgG (1/100 - 1/16,000) and IgG RBC's.

Figure 5.4. Haemagglutination assays showing the specificity of κ FLC antisera against red blood cells coated with purified FLCs and IgG.

5.3.4. Nephelometry

Latex-conjugated FLC antisera were tested for specificity by nephelometry. Potentially interfering substances were added to serum containing known concentrations of FLCs and the changes in values indicated the effect on the assays (*Figure 5.5*). Nephelometric assays demonstrated that FLC antisera had minimal reactivity with light chains on intact immunoglobulins and other potentially interfering substances (0.2 - 0.01%). These values are within the purity specification for FLC contamination in the tested interfering materials.

There have been no published independent specificity analyses of the nephelometric Freelite latex reagents. Nakano et al.[1] reported an evaluation but, in error, only tested FLC antisera that were manufactured for immunofixation electrophoresis (IFE), where specificity requirements are less demanding.

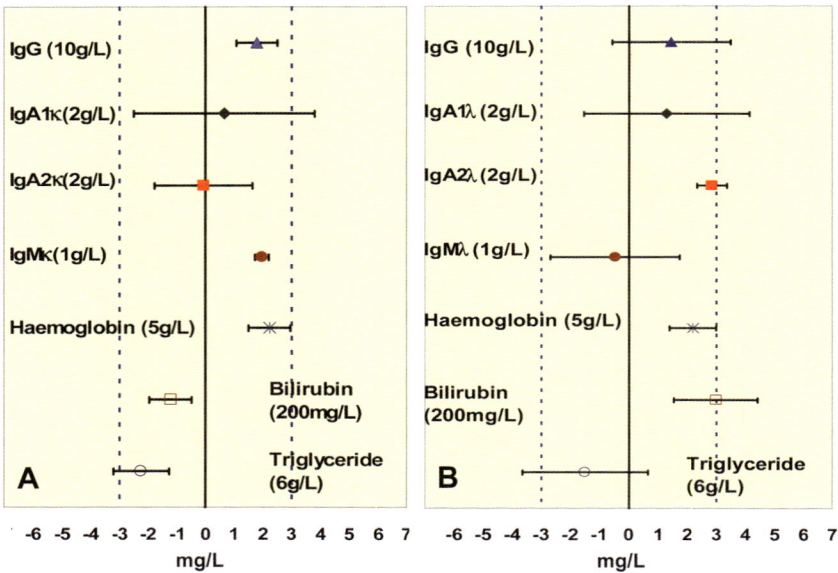

Figure 5.5. Specificity of (A) κ and (B) λ FLC antisera assessed by interference with the results of typical nephelometric assays upon the addition of various substances. Mean and 95% confidence limits for each added substance are shown.

5.4. Accuracy and standardisation

Assay accuracy is defined as the degree of closeness of achieved results relative to their actual (true) values. Unfortunately, international standards do not exist for FLC measurements, so there are no reference points from which to assess the accuracy of results. In order to ensure accuracy in Freelite immunoassays, a suitable basis for standardisation and calibration was required. It was considered that polyclonal FLCs should be used in order to minimise any potential problems that might arise from the use of unique monoclonal proteins.

The production of assay calibrators was achieved in the following manner: 1) production and accurate quantification of pure polyclonal, primary κ and λ FLC standards; 2) production of secondary internal reference standards; and 3) production of calibration materials for use in the FLC kits (calibrated to the internal reference) (Figure 5.6).

Each primary standard was found to be greater than 99% pure by silver-stained sodium dodecyl sulfate polyacrylamide gel electrophoresis (SDS-PAGE), whilst the alternate FLC was not detected by haemagglutination-inhibition and dot blot assays. The amino acid content of each primary standard was then determined in order to produce an accurate estimation of the protein content. Secondary standards were initially prepared from pools of different monoclonal κ and λ proteins. These were not considered ideal for use as working calibrators, so additional polyclonal standards were prepared from a pool of sera that contained elevated polyclonal sFLCs. These standards are known as κ or λ Internal Reference standards. The primary standards were used to assign κ and λ FLC concentrations to the Internal Reference standards by nephelometry. Each stage of the value transfer was completed at three dilutions and repeated three times. The final FLC values for the Internal Reference standards were 46.0 mg/L and 71.4 mg/L for κ and λ sFLCs, respectively. These values were used for all subsequent laboratory and clinical studies and used to assign values to kit calibrators and controls.

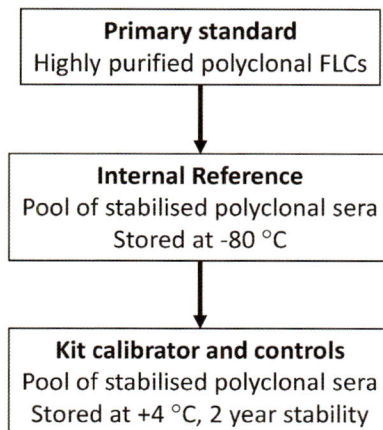

```
┌─────────────────────────────────────┐
│          Primary standard           │
│   Highly purified polyclonal FLCs   │
└─────────────────────────────────────┘
                   │
                   ▼
┌─────────────────────────────────────┐
│          Internal Reference         │
│   Pool of stabilised polyclonal sera│
│           Stored at -80 °C          │
└─────────────────────────────────────┘
                   │
                   ▼
┌─────────────────────────────────────┐
│       Kit calibrator and controls   │
│   Pool of stabilised polyclonal sera│
│   Stored at +4 °C, 2 year stability │
└─────────────────────────────────────┘
```

*Figure 5.6. Flow chart for the production
of standards for FLC assays.*

The measuring ranges of Freelite nephelometric/turbidimetric assays are dependent upon two factors: the slope of the respective calibration curve and the portion selected for the assay. The latter should be chosen to allow the maximum number of normal and abnormal clinical samples to be measured at the initial sample dilution. Typical analytical ranges (at the standard dilution) on the Binding Site SPAPLUS® for κ and λ sFLCs are 4.0 - 180 mg/L and 4.5 - 165 mg/L, respectively (*Figure 5.7*). Samples containing higher concentrations require further dilution. Calibration curves are validated by the measurement of high and low control samples. It is also recommended that all laboratories take part in external quality assurance schemes, to allow comparison of performance and results among different test sites (*Chapter 39*).

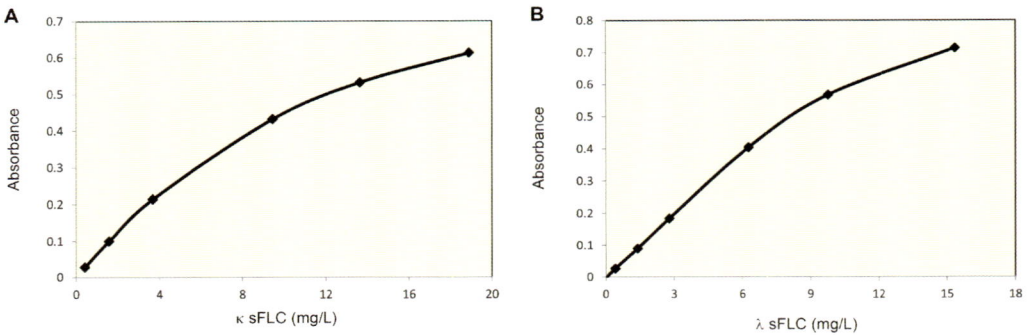

Figure 5.7. Calibration curves for (A) κ, and (B) λ FLC assays on the Binding Site SPAPLUS.

5.5. Maintaining batch-to-batch consistency of polyclonal antisera-based latex reagents

Maintaining batch-to-batch consistency is essential, as sFLC assays may be used for monitoring individual patients over many years. The key component of any nephelometric or turbidimetric immunoassay is the polyclonal antisera. Therefore, it is essential to minimise any change in the composition of the antisera over time.

In order to ensure consistency between production batches of polyclonal antisera, a virtual "rolling pool" of antisera has been established. This pool consists of a list of pre-approved antisera (*Section 5.3* explains how suitable antisera are identified). During the manufacture of a batch of reagent, an equal portion of each approved antiserum from the list is mixed. As individual antiserum volumes vary, stocks become exhausted at different times. When this occurs, the antiserum is replenished with a new pre-approved antiserum. The pool of polyclonal antisera used in the manufacture of Freelite assays will always contain at least 90% of the same constituent antisera as the previous batch of reagent. The use of rolling pools of antisera during FLC assay manufacture has minimised batch-to-batch variation whilst ensuring a full range of FLC epitopes are recognised[2].

Once a pool of suitable polyclonal antisera has been created, the sheep antibodies are attached to latex particles (in order to enhance their performance in nephelometric and turbidimetric immunoassays).

5.6. Overview of Freelite assay validation

During the development of Freelite assays there is a rigorous validation process to ensure that the assays perform correctly and provide the correct diagnostic information. The validation protocols follow those set out by the Clinical and Laboratory Standards Institute, and are outlined in *Table 5.1*.

Validation	Comments	Validation protocol
Precision	At multiple levels across the measuring range	Within run, between analyser, between batch, and total precision
Analytical sensitivity	At the lower end of the measuring range	Limit of detection, limit of quantitation, and limit of blank
Linearity	Across the measuring range	Disease state sera
Interference	By the most common assay interferents	Haemoglobin, bilirubin, lipid, relevant drugs etc.
Stability	Of kit to determine kit expiry	Real time
	Of open reagents	On board
	Of reagents that are removed from the analyser and refrigerated when not in use	Open vial
	Of kits that are heated or frozen to mimic worst case conditions during shipment to customers	Extremes of temperature
Comparison to predicate device	Using a range of samples relevant to the utility of the assay	Healthy blood donors and disease state sera
Confirmation of normal reference range	Quoted by the manufacturer	Healthy blood donor sera

Table 5.1. Summary of Freelite assay validation protocols.

5.7. Overview of Freelite kit manufacture

The manufacture of Freelite assays follows established validated protocols. Each batch of reagents undergoes rigorous testing to ensure the quality of the kit components *(Figure 5.8)*. Once the latex and supplementary reagent has been manufactured, the precision and linearity of the assay is tested. Next, a value is assigned to the kit calibrators using the Internal Reference standard. This is achieved using 100 separate assays and 10 separate calibration curves. Values are assigned to control samples using similar protocols.

For each new batch of antisera, specificity is controlled by comparing sFLC results for panels of samples with results from previous batches. The panel samples include normal sera and patient sera containing polyclonal or monoclonal sFLCs (typically from multiple myeloma patients). The results are compared using Passing-Bablok analysis and are considered acceptable when they fall within a defined set of criteria. Typical batch-to-batch comparison data is shown in Figure 5.9.

Analytical comparisons are also made using a large number of normal sera. A typical evaluation of a panel of 90 normal samples on the Binding Site SPAPLUS produced the following results: mean $\kappa = 8.86$ mg/L (range 4.32 - 20.6 mg/L), mean $\lambda = 11.85$ mg/L (range 3.77 - 28.77 mg/L). Freelite normal ranges are further discussed in Chapter 6. Once a final pre-packaging test is complete, the kit is packaged ready for release.

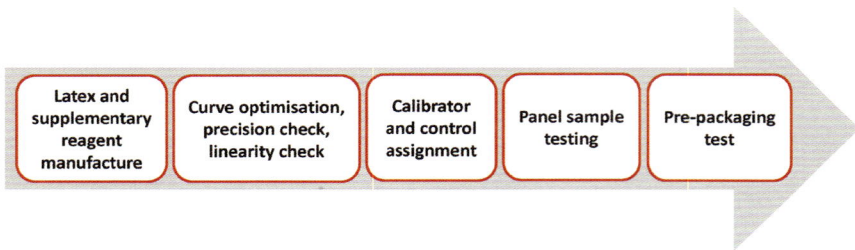

Figure 5.8. Overview of Freelite kit manufacture.

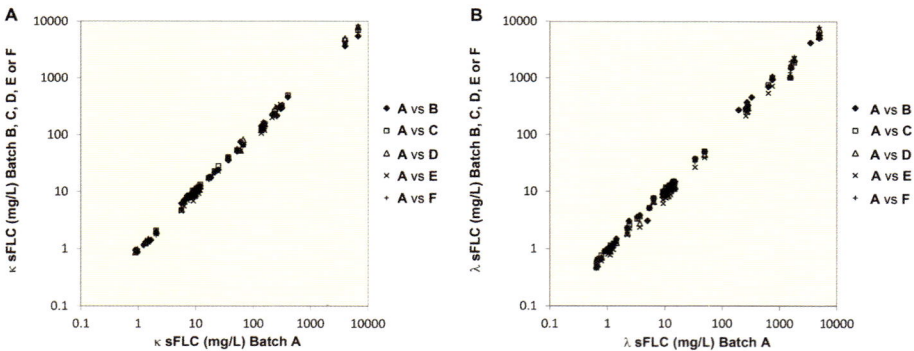

Figure 5.9. Batch-to-batch analysis for the Freelite κ and λ assays. (A) Six κ batches; and (B) six λ batches were compared using an in-house quality control panel. In each analysis, values obtained from a predicate batch (A) were compared with values from five separate batches (B to F).

5.8. Immunoassay development on different platforms

Freelite assays were initially developed for the Siemens BN™II nephelometer, and following their successful launch in the year 2000, the range of platforms has expanded and the assays are currently available on a total of 10 different instruments. Developing Freelite assays across different platforms poses a challenge as each instrument has unique features (summarised in *Table 5.2*). These include differences in the optical detection systems and the methods for reagent and sample handling. Therefore, assays developed for each platform may vary slightly in terms of sensitivity, measuring range, precision and antigen excess detection. However, there is good agreement between the sFLC results obtained with the different instruments. An example of κ and λ sFLC results obtained for BNII and SPAPLUS instruments is shown in Figure 5.10.

System feature	Examples
Sampling	Cuvettes (disposable/semi-disposable/non-disposable), cuvette cleaning method, probes/pipettes
System liquids	Wash solutions, sample diluent, tubing and pumps
Reagent storage	Compartments and carousels, temperature control (refrigerated/non-refrigerated)
Sample dilution	Automatic on-board/manual off-line
Detection system	Light source, light detector (nephelometric/turbidimetric)
Channels	Open/closed
Software and parameters	Sample flags, automatic antigen excess detection
Integration	Tracked system/stand-alone, laboratory information system integration

Table 5.2. Features that may vary between different analytical platforms.

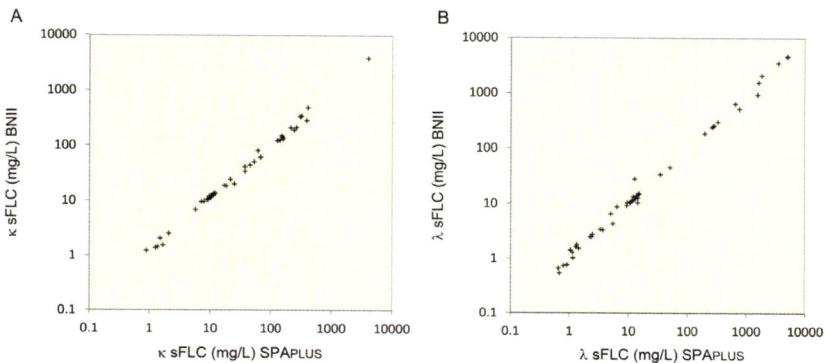

Figure 5.10. Comparison of (A) κ and (B) λ results on the Binding Site SPAPLUS and Siemens BNII.

Test Questions

1. How are Freelite assays routinely standardised?

Answers

1. As no international standards exist for FLC measurements, Freelite assays are standardised against κ and λ internal reference materials, which, in turn, are calibrated to highly purified primary standards *(Section 5.4)*.

References

1. Nakano T, Nagata A. ELISAs for free human immunoglobulin light chains in serum: improvement of assay specificity by using two specific antibodies in a sandwich detection method. J Immunol Methods 2004;293:183–9

2. Matters DJ, Showell PJ, Harding SJ, Carr-Smith HD, Smith LJ. Inter-batch variation and within batch precision of The Binding Site Freelite light chain assays. Clin Chem 2013;59:A-253a

Freelite reference intervals

Summary:

- sFLC concentrations and κ/λ ratios are maintained within narrow limits in normal individuals.
- Ethnicity appears to have minimal influence on sFLC normal ranges.
- sFLC concentrations increase substantially and κ/λ sFLC ratios increase slightly with decreasing renal function. Use of a modified renal reference interval for the ratio increases the diagnostic specificity for detecting monoclonal FLC production in patients with renal impairment.
- FLC concentrations in serum are less variable than in urine.

6.1. Freelite serum reference intervals

The most substantial study of serum free light chain (sFLC) concentrations in normal individuals using Freelite® was published by Katzmann et al.[1]. Serum samples were obtained from 127 healthy blood donors (21 - 62 years) and 155 older, normal individuals (51 - 90 years). The κ and λ sFLC concentrations for the 282 serum samples are plotted in Figure 6.1 and the normal range data is summarised in Table 6.1. The 95% reference ranges for κ and λ sFLC concentrations and κ/λ sFLC ratio were 3.3 - 19.4 mg/L, 5.7 - 26.3 mg/L and 0.3 - 1.2, respectively. It was proposed that the 100% reference range for the ratio (0.26 - 1.65) should be used diagnostically, in order to minimise the number of false-positive results when screening for monoclonal FLC production. This 100% diagnostic range has now been generally adopted and is incorporated into guidelines *(Chapter 25)*. The utility of Freelite sFLC measurements for identifying FLC monoclonal gammopathies is discussed in Chapter 23.

Normal adult serum	Mean	Median	95% reference range	100% diagnostic range
κ sFLC	8.4 mg/L	7.3 mg/L	3.3 - 19.4	
λ sFLC	13.4 mg/L	12.7 mg/L	5.7 - 26.3	
κ/λ sFLC ratio	0.63	0.59	0.3 - 1.2	0.26 - 1.65

Table 6.1. Mean/median values and ranges for FLC concentrations and κ/λ sFLC ratios in the sera of 282 normal individuals[1].

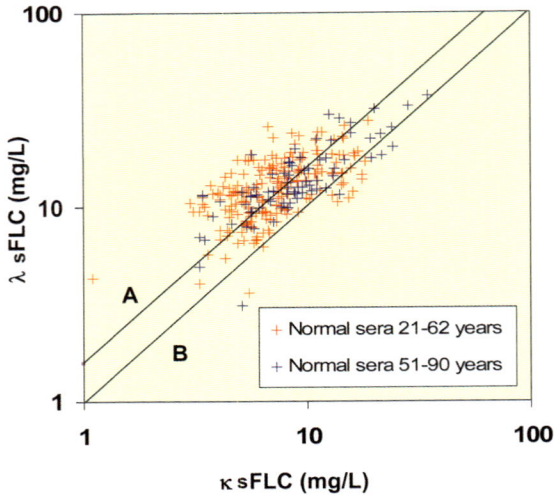

Figure 6.1. κ and λ FLC concentrations in 282 normal sera plotted on a logarithmic scale. *In general λ sFLC concentrations are higher than κ in normal individuals. A: Axis at the normal κ/λ sFLC ratio of 0.6, and B: axis at a κ/λ ratio of 1.00. (Courtesy of J.A. Katzmann).*

Katzmann et al. observed that κ sFLC concentrations tended to be lower than λ, giving a median κ/λ sFLC ratio of 0.59. This is because sFLC levels are dependent upon the balance between production and clearance. There are approximately twice as many plasma cells producing κ FLC as there are producing λ FLC. However, as κ molecules are normally monomeric (25 kDa), their renal clearance is faster than λ molecules, which tend to be dimeric (50 kDa). Consequently the serum half-life of κ FLCs is shorter than λ, and κ FLCs accumulate less in serum leading to lower concentrations of κ sFLC in normal individuals *(Chapter 3)*.

In elderly people there was a trend towards higher sFLC concentrations *(Figure 6.2 a,b and Table 6.2)*[1]. The same trend was observed for the renal function marker, cystatin C, which was measured in the same samples *(Figure 6.2d)*. When the results were expressed as sFLC κ/λ ratio or a ratio of sFLC concentration/cystatin C concentration, the effect of age was eliminated or reduced *(Figure 6.2 c,e,f)*. This indicates that the higher sFLC values seen in older people can be largely explained by small reductions in glomerular filtration rate (GFR)[1]. Whilst several other groups have similarly observed no significant age-related differences in the sFLC ratio[2,3], others have reported an increase in the κ/λ sFLC ratio reference range in elderly populations, prompting the suggestion that age-dependent reference ranges should be considered[4,5].

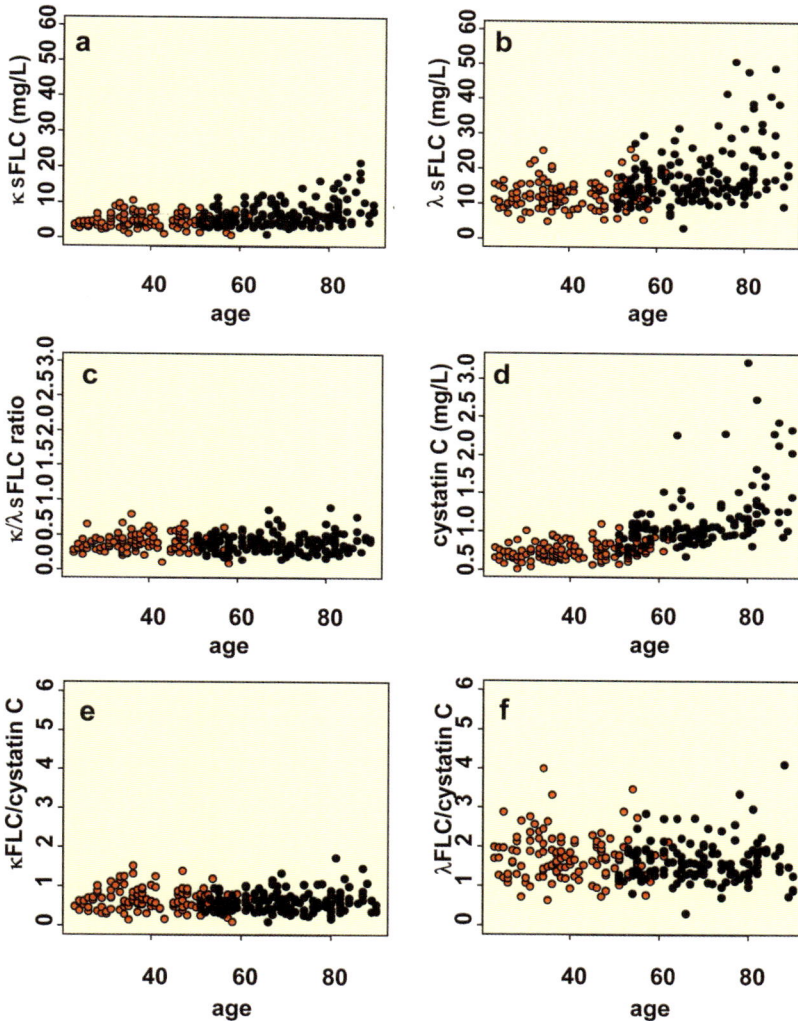

Figure 6.2. (a) κ sFLC concentration, (b) λ sFLC concentration and (c) κ/λ sFLC ratios versus age (years) in 282 normal serum samples together with (d) cystatin C results in the same patients. sFLC/cystatin C ratios (e) and (f) show no change with age, confirming renal deterioration as the cause of increased sFLC levels in elderly individuals. (red = fresh sera, black = frozen sera). (Courtesy of J. A. Katzmann).

Age (years)	κ sFLC (mg/L)	λ sFLC (mg/L)	κ/λ sFLC ratio
20 – 29	6.3	12.4	0.49
30 – 39	7.2	13.6	0.55
40 – 49	7.5	12.8	0.58
50 – 59	6.4	11.3	0.59
60 – 69	6.9	11.8	0.70
70 – 79	8.0	11.9	0.65
80 – 90	9.1	15.1	0.64

Table 6.2. Median values for sFLCs and κ/λ ratios in different age groups[1].

The normal ranges published by Katzmann et al. were very similar to those previously reported by Bradwell et al., who observed a mean κ/λ sFLC ratio of 0.6 and a 95% reference range of 0.35 - 1.0[6]. Slightly lower κ and λ sFLC concentrations (95% reference ranges of 4.2 - 13.1 mg/L and 9.2 - 22.7 mg/L, respectively) observed in the Bradwell study may be attributed to a younger study population (17 - 71 years).

6.1.1. Ethnic influences

The Freelite normal ranges published by Katzmann et al.[1] were established in an American, predominantly white, population. Known ethnic differences in the normal ranges of total immunoglobulins *(Chapter 10)* have prompted a number of laboratories to determine normal sFLC ranges for their local populations.

European research groups have reported Freelite reference ranges for normal individuals that are comparable to Katzmann et al.[7,8]. Similarly, sFLC concentrations in a small South African cohort including Black (57/113), mixed-race (44/113) and Caucasian (12/113) subjects were not significantly different, both for the local population as a whole, and for the Black and mixed-race populations independently[9]. In a Han Chinese population of 326 subjects, although a narrower κ/λ sFLC ratio normal range was observed (0.32 - 1.52), this local range and the Katzmann range (0.26 - 1.65) provided the same diagnostic sensitivity and specificity for multiple myeloma (MM) (area under ROC curve 0.99 in both cases)[10].

6.2 Borderline Freelite results

All laboratory tests can produce borderline results, which should be considered in their clinical context and alongside other laboratory test results. Borderline κ/λ sFLC ratios may be attributed to a variety of causes. Increases in FLC concentrations and borderline elevated ratios due to renal impairment in the absence of monoclonal gammopathy are well documented[11,12,13]. For such patients, the use of a renal reference interval for the κ/λ sFLC ratio may reduce the number of false-positive results *(Section 6.3)*.

Borderline high κ/λ sFLC ratios have also been reported in conditions associated with polyclonal inflammatory responses, such as infections, inflammation and autoimmune diseases[12,14,15]. In an audit reported by Marshall et al., 4.9% (47/955) of individuals tested had a borderline abnormal κ/λ sFLC ratio (between 1.67 and 3.2) with no known plasma cell disorder[12]. In the majority of cases this could be attributed to renal impairment or an inflammatory process. The authors commented that borderline low sFLC ratios were infrequently associated with renal impairment or inflammatory states, and that such borderline low ratios should prompt further investigation.

In addition to renal impairment and inflammatory conditions, borderline abnormal Freelite results may occur in a variety of monoclonal diseases encompassing intact immunoglobulin MM, many lymphomas and leukaemias *(Chapters 31 and 33)*, AL amyloidosis *(Chapter 28)* and monoclonal gammopathy of undetermined significance (MGUS) *(Chapter 13)*. It is now recognised that the probability of a malignant plasma cell disorder increases in relation to the degree of abnormality of the κ/λ sFLC ratio *(Section 7.2.4)*.

6.3 Freelite renal reference intervals

Severe renal impairment changes the dynamics of FLC clearance. As GFR reduces, the clearance of FLCs decreases and becomes more dependent upon the reticulo-endothelial system, which shows no size preference and clears both κ and λ FLCs at the same rate. Therefore, as renal impairment increases, the serum half-life of κ FLCs approaches that of λ FLCs and their serum levels become more influenced by their underlying production rates. Consequently, the increase in the concentration of κ sFLCs is greater than λ sFLCs, and in a minority of patients the κ/λ ratio can increase above the normal reference interval in the absence of monoclonal gammopathy. This was demonstrated in a study using Freelite on serum samples from 688 patients with chronic kidney disease (CKD) and no evidence of monoclonal gammopathy[11]. As both κ and λ sFLC concentrations increased in patients with deteriorating renal function, their relative amounts changed slightly *(Figure 6.3A)*. As a consequence, with increasing CKD stage, the median sFLC ratios were found to increase progressively from 0.6 to 1.1, with a 100% range of 0.37 - 3.10 *(Figure 6.3B)*. Therefore, a κ/λ sFLC reference interval of 0.37 - 3.10, termed the "renal reference interval", was proposed for patients with renal impairment[16].

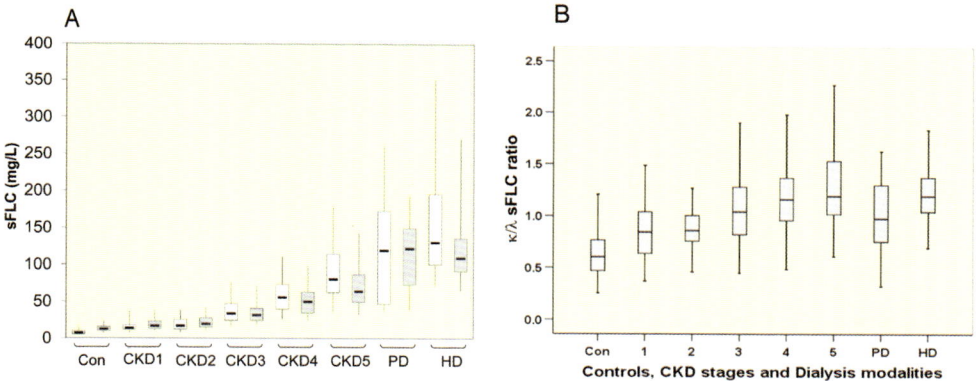

Figure 6.3. (A) κ (white) and λ (grey) sFLC concentrations and (B) κ/λ sFLC ratio in CKD stages 1 – 5 plus patients on peritoneal dialysis (PD), haemodialysis (HD) and controls (Con). Data presented as box plots (1st – 3rd inter-quartile ranges, central line is median value) with whiskers (5th – 95th percentile values). *(Courtesy of Colin Hutchison).*

The diagnostic accuracy of the Freelite renal reference range was assessed in an unselected group of 142 patients who presented with dialysis-dependent acute kidney injury (AKI) of unknown cause[16]. All 41 patients with MM had abnormal κ/λ sFLC ratios by both the published reference range and renal reference range (*Figure 6.4*). Receiver operating characteristic (ROC) analysis showed that application of the renal reference range for the ratio increased the specificity from 93% to 98% with no loss of sensitivity. The diagnostic utility of the κ/λ sFLC renal reference range was further demonstrated by Park et al.[13]. A combination of sFLC analysis (using the renal reference interval) in combination with SPE, was the optimal screening algorithm for detecting MM in patients with renal impairment (*Section 23.3.1, Table 23.4*).

In conclusion, use of the Freelite renal reference interval in routine clinical practice may lead to increased diagnostic accuracy for the diagnosis of monoclonal gammopathy. For patients with CKD, a κ/λ sFLC ratio of 1.66 - 3.1 is likely to be caused by the change in FLC clearance and further investigation is only warranted if there is a significant clinical suspicion of monoclonal gammopathy.

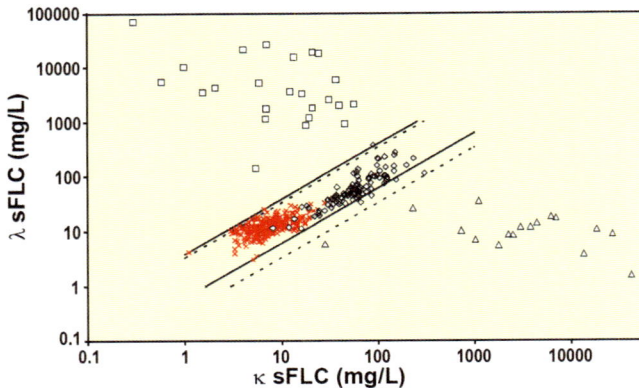

Figure 6.4. sFLCs in 142 patients presenting with dialysis-dependent, acute renal failure. 41 patients with κ (triangles) and λ (squares) MM are distinct from blood donors (red crosses: p<0.001) and from patients with acute renal failure from other causes (diamonds: p<0.001). Solid lines indicate the κ/λ sFLC normal reference interval (0.26 - 1.65); broken lines indicate the κ/λ sFLC renal reference interval (0.37 - 3.10). (Reproduced from[16] with permission from BioMed Central).

6.4 Freelite urine reference intervals

Bradwell et al.[6] measured κ and λ concentrations in early morning urine samples from 66 normal individuals using Freelite immunoassays (*Figure 6.5 and Table 6.3*). When compared to sFLC data from the same study, the range of urine FLC concentrations was much wider than for serum, and κ/λ urine FLC ratios were more variable. Presumably, this reflects differences in renal handling, urine dilution and mucosal secretion of FLCs between individuals.

A wide range of normal urine FLC concentrations was similarly observed by Snyder et al.[17], who established a 95% reference range for the urine Freelite ratio of 1 - 19 using 91 healthy adult donors. The authors attributed the relatively poor diagnostic sensitivity of the urine FLC assay (80%) to the wide reference ranges and a high background of polyclonal FLC in the urine. It is important to note that international guidelines do not recommend the use of urinary FLC immunoassays[18]. Arguments in favour of serum over urine FLC assays are further discussed in Chapter 24.

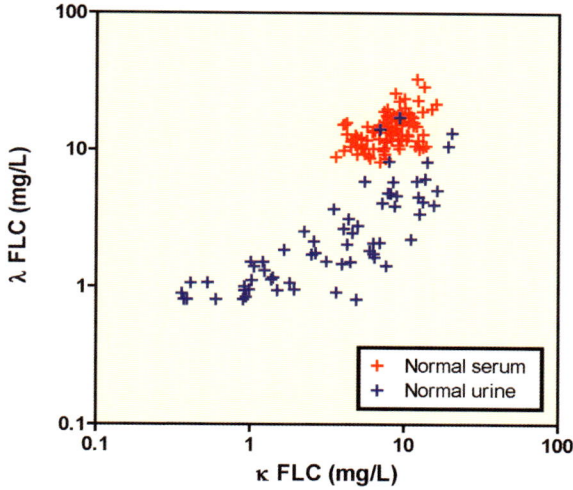

Figure 6.5. Comparison of FLC measurements in serum and early morning urine samples from healthy individuals. (Courtesy of J.A. Katzmann).

Normal adult urine	Mean	95% reference range
κ FLC	5.4 mg/L (± 4.95)	0.39 - 15.1 mg/L
λ FLC	3.17 mg/L (± 3.3)	0.81 - 10.1 mg/L
κ/λ ratio	1.85	0.46 - 4.0

Table 6.3. Mean values (± standard deviation) and ranges for FLC concentrations and κ/λ ratios in early morning urine samples from 66 normal individuals[6].

Test Questions

1. Why is the normal κ/λ ratio inverted in serum compared with urine?
2. Why do κ/λ sFLC ratios increase slightly in patients with severe renal impairment?

Answers

1. Because the smaller monomeric κ molecules are cleared faster by the kidneys and enter the urine more readily than dimeric λ molecules (*Section 6.1*).

2. Because FLC removal in renal impairment becomes dependent upon the reticuloendothelial system which removes κ and λ FLC at the same rate. Serum levels begin to reflect production rates and κ concentrations therefore increase relative to λ (*Section 6.3 and Chapter 3*).

References

1. Katzmann JA, Clark RJ, Abraham RS, Bryant S, Lymp JF, Bradwell AR, Kyle RA. Serum reference intervals and diagnostic ranges for free kappa and free lambda immunoglobulin light chains: relative sensitivity for detection of monoclonal light chains. Clin Chem 2002;48:1437–44

2. Altinier S, Seguso M, Zaninotto M, Varagnolo M, Adami F, Angeli P, Plebani M. Serum free light chain reference values: a critical approach. Clin Biochem 2013;7-8:691-3

3. Abadie JM, Bankson DD. Assessment of serum free light chain assays for plasma cell disorder screening in a Veterans Affairs population. Ann Clin Lab Sci 2006;36:157-62

4. Hernandez JM, Muñoz H, Jimenez Cobaleda MJ, Queizan JA, Latorre M, de la Hoz B et al. Normal ranges and reference intervals of serum free light chains values are higher in elderly people: study in a Spanish urban population. Haematologica 2011;96:0863a

5. Machalkova K, Vavrova J, Maisnar V, Radocha J, Tichy M. Age dependancy of reference values of immunoglobulin heavy/light chain pairs and free light chains serum levels. Clinical Lymphoma, Myeloma & Leukaemia 2013;13:P-418a

6. Bradwell AR, Carr-Smith HD, Mead GP, Tang LX, Showell PJ, Drayson MT, Drew R. Highly sensitive, automated immunoassay for immunoglobulin free light chains in serum and urine. Clin Chem 2001;47:673-80

7. Hernandez JM, Jimenez-Cobaleda MJ, Muñoz H, Caro R, Qiueizan JA, Latorre M et al. Normal ranges and reference intervals of serum free light chains concentrations in a Spanish urban population. Hematology Reports 2010;2:A9a.

8. Callis M, Garcia L, Gironella M, Rodrigo MJ, Garcia E, Castella D. Serum free light chain reference intervals. A study of 133 blood donors. Haematologica 2008;93:1332a.

9. Zemlin AE, Rensburg MA, Ipp H, Germishuys JJ, Erasmus RT. Verification of serum reference intervals for free light chains in a local South African population. J Clin Pathol 2013;66:992-5

10. Liang YF, Chen WM, Wang QT, Zhai YH, Yang YJ, Liu JY et al. Establishment and validation of serum free light chain reference intervals in an ethnic Chinese population. Clin Lab 2014;60:193-8

11. Hutchison CA, Harding S, Hewins P, Mead GP, Townsend J, Bradwell AR, Cockwell P. Quantitative assessment of serum and urinary polyclonal free light chains in patients with chronic kidney disease. Clin J Am Soc Nephrol 2008;3:1684-90

12. Marshall G, Tate J, Mollee P. Borderline high serum free light chain k/l ratios are seen not only in dialysis patients but also in non-dialysis-dependent renal impairment and inflammatory states. Am J Clin Pathol 2009;132:309

13. Park JW, Kim YK, Bae EH, Ma SK, Kim SW. Combined analysis using extended renal reference range of serum free light chain ratio and serum protein electrophoresis improves the diagnostic accuracy of multiple myeloma in renal insufficiency. Clin Biochem 2012;45:740-4

14. Hill PG, Forsyth JM, Rai B, Mayne S. Serum free light chains: an alternative to the urine Bence Jones proteins screening test for monoclonal gammopathies. Clin Chem 2006;52:1743-8

15. Abadie JM, van Hoeven KH, Wells JM. Are renal reference intervals required when screening for plasma cell disorders with serum free light chains and serum protein electrophoresis? Am J Clin Pathol 2009;131:166-71

16. Hutchison CA, Plant T, Drayson M, Cockwell P, Kountouri M, Basnayake K et al. Serum free light chain measurement aids the diagnosis of myeloma in patients with severe renal failure. BMC Nephrol 2008;9:11

17. Snyder MR, Clark R, Bryant SC, Katzmann JA. Quantification of urinary light chains. Clin Chem 2008;54:1744-6

18. Dispenzieri A, Kyle R, Merlini G, Miguel JS, Ludwig H, Hajek R et al. International Myeloma Working Group guidelines for serum-free light chain analysis in multiple myeloma and related disorders. Leukemia 2009;23:215-24

Implementation and interpretation of Freelite immunoassays

Summary:
- FLCs are stable in serum stored at 2 - 8 °C for up to 21 days.
- Freelite® assays available on some instruments include prozone parameters for antigen excess detection.
- FLC polymerisation leads to over-estimation of antigen concentrations determined by immunoassay.
- Freelite non-linearity may occur in some samples due to non-specific interference (matrix effects) or the inherent variability of monoclonal FLCs.

7.1. Implementation of Freelite assays

Freelite serum free light chain (sFLC) assays are polyclonal antisera-based immunoassays, and can be performed on a number of automated laboratory instruments. κ and λ sFLCs are measured separately, then results can be expressed as a κ/λ sFLC ratio, or when there is monoclonal production of a FLC, as the difference (dFLC) between the involved (iFLC) and uninvolved (uFLC) concentrations. This chapter discusses both the practical aspects of implementation of Freelite assays (including choice of instrument, sample types and biological variation) and interpretation of results.

7.1.1 Choice of instrument

Freelite immunoassays are available for the majority of nephelometric and turbidimetric laboratory instruments *(Chapter 37)*. Between-platform agreement of sFLC results is good *(Section 5.8)*. Factors that may influence a laboratory's choice of instrument include features of the sFLC assays on a particular platform (assay time, prozone parameters etc.), as well as those related to general laboratory organisation (workload, complete testing menu offered, existing platforms already present etc.). It is recommended that all laboratories performing sFLC assays participate in external quality assurance (EQA) schemes. These are further discussed in Chapter 39.

7.1.2 Reporting units

It is important to ensure that sFLC concentrations are reported in consistent units. In the UK the preferred reporting units are mg/L. Within the USA, results may be either in mg/L or mg/dL.

7.1.3 Choice of sample

All Freelite sFLC assays are validated for the quantification of κ or λ FLCs in serum or urine. In addition, Freelite assays are also available for the measurement of FLCs in cerebrospinal fluid *(Chapter 36)*.

In general, samples that are haemolysed, lipaemic, or with highly elevated bilirubin should be avoided. The maximum concentration of interfering substance that can be reliably assessed is stated in the product insert. An example of interference testing of κ and λ sFLC assays is shown for the Binding Site SPAPLUS® in Table 7.1.

Interfering substance	Concentration	Deviation from target value	
		κ sFLC	λ sFLCs
Haemoglobin	3 g/L	2.1%	-1.6%
Intralipid	0.3%	-9.1%	-3.0%
Bilirubin	300 mg/L	-5.0%	-2.4%

Table 7.1. Freelite assay interference for κ and λ Freelite assays on the Binding Site SPAPLUS. Interference was tested using a control serum containing ≤10 mg/L sFLCs, tested at the minimum sample dilution (1/1).

7.1.4 Sample and reagent stability

An in-house study was conducted to assess the stability of FLCs in unpreserved serum samples (n=30) stored at 2 to 8°C for up to 7 weeks. For each sample, κ and λ sFLCs were measured at regular intervals. After 3 weeks there was a significant drop in the κ sFLC concentrations *(Figure 7.1A)*. Therefore, it is recommended that samples are stored for a maximum of 21 days at 2 to 8 °C prior to analysis.

A second study assessed the stability of FLCs in unpreserved serum samples stored at -20°C. At each time point, an aliquot was defrosted and κ and λ sFLCs were measured. There was no deterioration in κ or λ sFLC concentrations over 7 months *(Figure 7.2)*. Therefore, for long term storage of serum samples prior to sFLC analysis, it is recommended that samples are stored frozen at ≤-20°C.

Stability of the Freelite reagent is also an important issue. "Open-vial stability" refers to the shelf-life of the antisera after their first use. This is a minimum of 40 days for the SPAPLUS, but for other instruments the open vial stability may vary due to differences in instrument storage conditions *(Chapter 37)*.

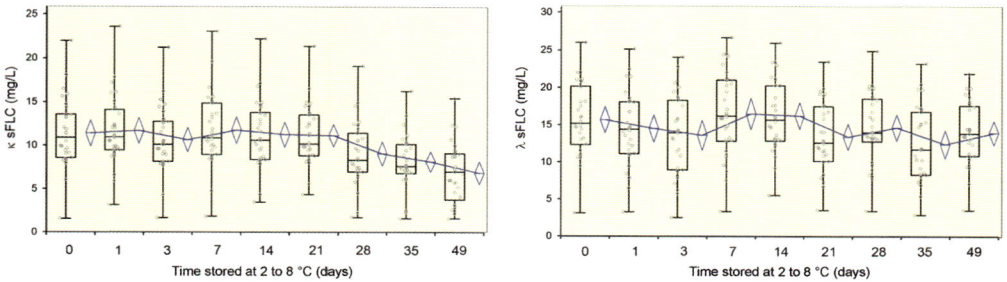

Figure 7.1. Stability of (A) κ and (B) λ sFLCs stored at 4 °C. *Data presented as box plots (interquartile range, central line is median value) with whiskers (5th - 95th percentile values). Blue diamonds represent the mean value (central line) and the limits of the 95% confidence interval (tips of diamond above and below the mean). Mean values are connected by a blue line.*

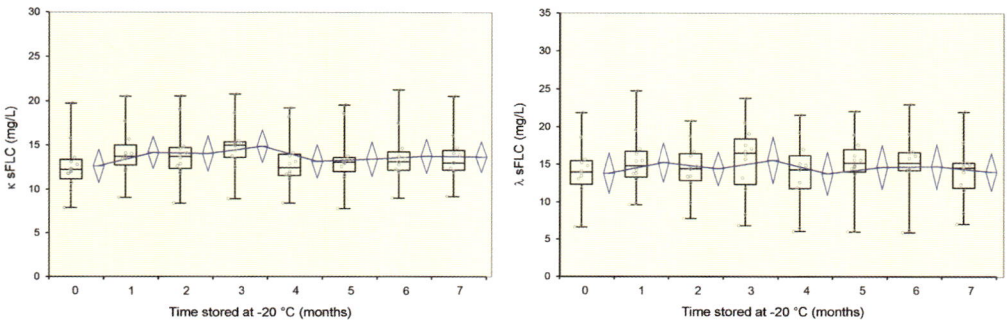

Figure 7.2. Stability of (A) κ and (B) λ sFLCs stored at -20 °C. *Data presented as box plots (interquartile range, central line is median value) with whiskers (5th - 95th percentile values). Blue diamonds represent the mean value (central line) and the limits of the 95% confidence interval (tips of diamond above and below the mean). Mean values are connected by a blue line.*

7.1.5 Changing batch of reagent or instrument

Great effort is made during Freelite assay manufacture to maintain batch-to-batch consistency *(Section 5.5)*. Moving from one batch to the next should not present the laboratory with any issues. However, it is recommended that identical internal quality control samples are measured with both the new batch and the existing batch to confirm consistency, before moving entirely over to the new batch. Correlation of Freelite sFLC measurements obtained using different platforms is good *(Section 5.8)*. However, before a laboratory changes platform, it is recommended that they compare the results obtained using the new and existing platforms as part of their validation protocol.

7.2. Interpretation of Freelite assays

As with any laboratory test, Freelite results should be interpreted alongside a patient's clinical details and other laboratory tests including serum electrophoresis and renal function. When serial monitoring data is available, results should be compared with previous measurements to check they are consistent and to identify trends.

7.2.1. Normal reference intervals

Normal reference intervals for κ sFLCs, λ sFLCs and the κ/λ sFLC ratio were published by Katzmann et al.[1]. These ranges have been locally validated and widely adopted by many centres and are further discussed in Chapter 6. For patients with renal impairment, application of a modified renal reference interval may increase the specificity of the κ/λ sFLC ratio for detecting monoclonal FLC production *(Section 6.3)*.

7.2.2 Terminology

For each sample, both κ and λ sFLCs should always be measured, and the κ/λ sFLC ratio calculated. Some centres (especially those taking part in clinical trials) may also wish to calculate the difference (dFLC) between the involved (iFLC) and uninvolved (uFLC) sFLCs. Definitions of other common terms/abbreviations are summarised in Table 7.2.

Term	Definition	Comment	For a κ FLC tumour
iFLC	Involved FLC	The FLC type that is produced by the tumour	κ
uFLC	Uninvolved FLC	The FLC type that is the alternate light chain type to the iFLC (not to be confused with urine FLCs)	λ
κ/λ sFLC ratio	κ/λ	A ratio of the concentration of κ to λ sFLCs	κ/λ
dFLC	iFLC - uFLC	The difference in the concentration between the iFLC and uFLC	κ - λ
ΣFLC	Summated FLC	The sum of κ and λ sFLC concentrations, determined by two separate assays	κ + λ

Table 7.2. Summary of FLC terminology

International Myeloma Working Group (IMWG) guidelines for sFLC analysis in multiple myeloma (MM) and related disorders recommend that the κ/λ sFLC ratio is calculated as part of the standard investigative workup of patients with suspected MM *(Chapter 25)*[2]. The ratio is also important when documenting a stringent complete response *(Chapter 25)*.

For serial measurements, either the iFLC or the dFLC is recommended[2]. There are two principal reasons for this: 1) when the concentration of uFLCs is very low, due to immunosuppression, this may lead to analytical variation in the values measured and fluctuations in the κ/λ sFLC ratio which do not represent any change in the tumour; and 2) using dFLC can remove some of the variation see in iFLC values due to changes in renal function.

7.2.3 The FLC dot plot

In some cases it may be helpful to plot an individual patient's result (or an entire cohort of patients' results) on a FLC dot plot *(Figure 7.3)*. This is a graph displaying κ sFLC concentrations (x-axis) against λ sFLC concentrations (y-axis), both on logarithmic scales. The limits of the normal reference interval for the κ/λ sFLC ratio are represented by two diagonal parallel lines. Each patient is represented by a single point. If the κ/λ sFLC ratio is normal, the result will fall within the parallel lines. For monoclonal κ or λ sFLCs, the result will lie below or above the lines, respectively.

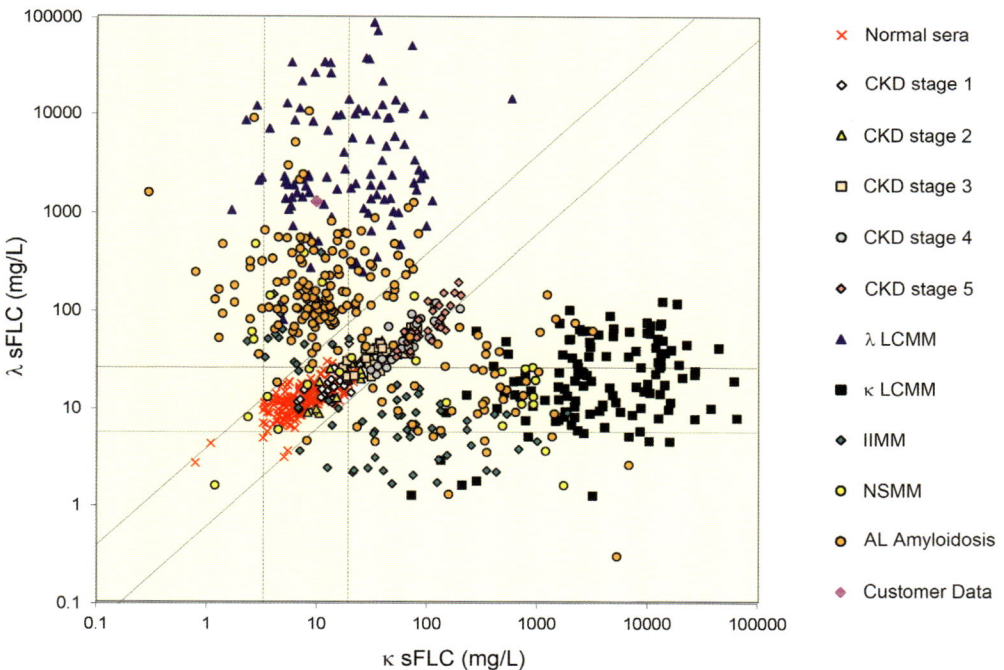

Figure 7.3. The Freelite dot plot. *CKD: chronic kidney disease; LCMM: light chain MM; IIMM: intact immunoglobulin MM; NSMM: nonsecretory MM.*

7.2.4 Result interpretation

Abnormally high concentrations of κ and λ sFLCs may result from a number of clinical situations including immune stimulation, reduced renal clearance, or monoclonal plasma cell proliferative disorders[2]. Patients with either polyclonal hypergammaglobulinemia or renal impairment often have elevated κ and λ sFLCs due to increased synthesis *(Chapter 35)* or reduced renal clearance *(Chapter 26)*, respectively. For patients with renal impairment, use of a renal reference interval for the κ/λ sFLC ratio may reduce the number of false-positive results *(Section 6.3)*.

A significantly abnormal κ/λ sFLC ratio would only be expected to be due to a plasmaproliferative or lymphoproliferative disorder that secretes monoclonal FLCs and disturbs the normal balance between κ and λ secretion. Use of likelihood ratios when interpreting κ/λ sFLC ratios may improve clinical interpretation of sFLC results for the diagnosis of malignant plasma cell disorders[3].

7.2.5 sFLCs and intact immunoglobulins are independent tumour markers

An abnormal κ/λ sFLC ratio is not always present in patients with monoclonal intact immunoglobulins, as sFLCs and intact immunoglobulins are independent tumour markers *(Section 17.2)*. For example, an abnormal sFLC ratio is present in around 89% of intact immunoglobulin MM (IIMM) patients, 80% of smouldering MM patients and 33% of monoclonal gammopathy of undetermined significance (MGUS) patients *(Chapters 17, 14, and 13, respectively)*.

7.2.6 Biological variation

Biological variation studies define the physiological fluctuation of analyte concentrations in a biological fluid around its homeostatic set point[4]. Knowledge of the biological variation of FLCs in serum is useful when interpreting monitoring data for individual patients. Braga et al.[5] studied the biological variation of sFLC measurements in 21 healthy volunteers (12 women and 9 men), measured at the same time on the same day, every 2 weeks over the course of 2 months. λ sFLC concentrations were significantly higher in men than women ($p<0.01$), whereas no difference was found for κ sFLC concentrations. Intra-individual variances of κ or λ FLCs were similar (8.1% and 7.0%, respectively), and were not different between men and women. By contrast, the inter-individual variance of λ sFLCs was higher than that of κ sFLCs (27.5% vs. 14.1%, respectively), and was higher for men than women (33.0% vs. 22.6%, respectively). The reference change value (RCV) defines the minimum significant difference ($p<0.05$) between two consecutive measurements in the same individual. In this study the RCV for κ and λ sFLCs was similar: 22.6% and 19.6%, respectively. Similar findings were reported by Hansen et al.[6].

Katzmann et al.[7] studied the long-term biological variation of monoclonal FLCs in 158 patients with clinically stable monoclonal gammopathy. For each patient, at least three serial samples were obtained within a 5 year period. During the study, each patient received no treatment, had no change in clinical diagnosis, and had a <5 g/L change in serum monoclonal immunoglobulin quantification by protein electrophoresis. A total of 52/158 patients had measurable monoclonal sFLCs (defined as iFLC ≥100 mg/L with an abnormal κ/λ sFLC ratio). The total coefficient of variation (CV) for iFLC measurements was 28.4%, which was almost entirely attributable to biological variation (CV=27.8%) and, to a lesser extent, due to inter-assay analytical variation (CV=5.8%). The variation in iFLC was more comparable to that of monoclonal protein quantification by urine protein electrophoresis (Total CV=35.8%) than serum protein electrophoresis (Total CV=8.1%). This is likely to reflect the short serum half-life of FLCs compared with intact immunoglobulins *(Chapter 3)*. The RCV for monoclonal sFLCs was 54.5%. This value is significantly higher than that reported by other smaller studies[5,6], and may reflect differences in the length of patient follow-up (5 years vs. less than a week). Several authors now recommend that biological variation data should be taken into account to update the definitions of sFLC response criteria *(Chapter 25)*[6,7].

7.3. Non-linearity

Sample non-linearity can be defined as a sample that when measured at different dilutions gives a substantially different result. Two examples are shown in Table 7.3. Sample A is an example of a non-linear sample, while sample B shows a linear response (i.e. further dilution [1/100] gives a value close to that obtained at the initial dilution [1/10]).

Non-linear sample	Dilution	Result (mg/L)
Sample A	1/10	50
	1/100	100

Linear sample	Dilution	Result (mg/L)
Sample B	1/10	50
	1/100	60

Table 7.3. Examples of non-linear and linear sample behaviour.

Sample non-linearity should not be confused with assay linearity; if an assay is non-linear all samples will give substantially different results when measured at different dilutions. Assessment of Freelite assay linearity forms an important part of immunoassay development and validation (Section 5.6).

As with all immunoassays, FLC assays are potentially prone to sample non-linearity. Pretorius et al.[8] concluded that non-linearity of FLC assays was a property of the individual sample, and not a method-specific phenomenon. Sample specific non-linearity may occur in some samples when measured with Freelite FLC assays due to: 1) non-specific interference (matrix effects); or 2) the inherent structural diversity of monoclonal FLCs (Chapter 3).

7.3.1 Managing non-linearity

Binding Site recommend following the sample dilution protocol as shown in each product insert and reporting the first plausible result only. The use of non-standard sample dilutions, or skipping dilutions should be avoided. Examples of non-linear samples are shown in Table 7.4 and 7.5.

	Dilution	Result (mg/L)
Sample A	1/100	**95.3**
	1/2000	202

	Dilution	Result (mg/L)
Sample B	1/100	**145**
	1/2000	467

Table 7.4. Examples of non-linear κ Freelite results using a Siemens BN™ II analyser. The first plausible result should be reported (values in bold).

	Dilution	Result (mg/L)
Sample A	1/10	>165
	1/100	>1650
	1/1000	**790**

Table 7.5. Example of non-linear λ Freelite results using a Binding Site SPAPLUS analyser. The first plausible result should be reported (value in bold).

It is important to note that Freelite results should not be interpreted in isolation and other laboratory findings and clinical symptoms should be considered when evaluating the status of the patient. In addition, the results from two consecutive measurements should be assessed when interpreting disease response[9].

7.4. Antigen excess

Antigen excess occurs when an antigen is present in such high levels that it interferes with antigen-antibody crosslinking, resulting in the formation of smaller immune complexes *(Figure 7.4)*. This causes immunoassays to underestimate high concentrations of protein. sFLC concentrations can range from <1 mg/L to >10,000 mg/L. This is a greater range than almost any other serum protein test. Consequently, a small proportion of samples may be underestimated because of antigen excess. Monoclonal sFLCs produced by different patients can exhibit considerably different points of equivalence (the concentrations above which the assay is in antigen excess). It is therefore not possible to predict the concentration at which Freelite antigen excess may occur – it could be 300, 3000 or 30,000 mg/L for different patients. It is important to note that for the majority of patients, their samples will never demonstrate Freelite antigen excess.

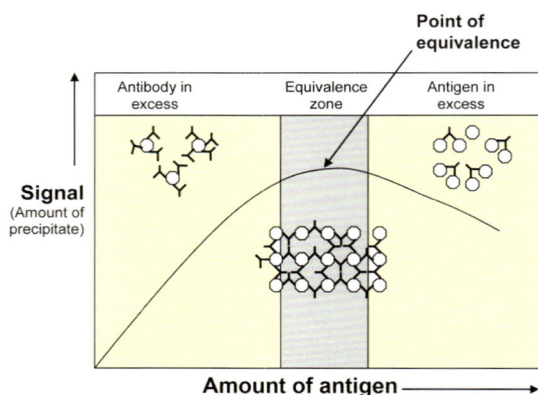

Figure 7.4. Diagram illustrating the mechanism of antigen excess. The light scattering signal falls in antigen excess because of smaller immune complexes.

Assessment of antigen excess forms an important part of immunoassay development and validation *(Section 5.6)*. Freelite sFLC assays available on some instruments include prozone parameters *(Chapter 37)*. For example, the Binding Site SPAPLUS instrument monitors the initial reaction kinetics of each sample at three separate time intervals *(Figure 7.5)* and compares the results with reaction limits set by the manufacturer through testing of an extensive myeloma library. Samples detected as being in antigen excess are automatically flagged by the instrument and retested at a higher sample dilution. A very small proportion of samples in antigen excess have normal reaction kinetics so will not prompt the flag. Such undetected antigen excess is a rare event but cannot be excluded. Therefore, it is recommended that the following statement accompanies all FLC results "Undetected antigen excess is a rare event but cannot be excluded. If these free light chain results do not agree with other clinical or laboratory findings, or if the sample is from a patient that has previously demonstrated antigen excess, the result must be checked by retesting at a higher dilution".

Freelite sFLC assays available on other instruments, such as the Siemens BNII, do not include automatic antigen excess checks. On these instruments, samples should be tested for antigen excess following advice given in the product insert. Section 7.4.2 has further information on distinguishing antigen excess from sample non-linearity.

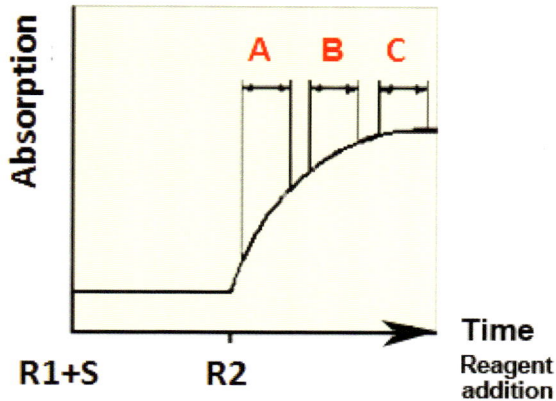

Figure 7.5. Prozone parameters on the SPAPLUS monitor the change in scatter
signal at three different time intervals (labelled A, B, C). R1: reagent 1;
S: sample; R2: reagent 2.

7.4.1 Incidence of antigen excess

Several studies have evaluated the incidence of antigen excess in large numbers of consecutive patients. Murata et al.[10] studied 7,538 serum samples over a 4-month period using 1:100 and 1:400 sample dilutions on a Siemens BNII. There were nine samples with κ antigen excess but no samples with λ antigen excess giving an incidence of 1/840 (0.12%). Importantly, all the antigen excess samples had elevated FLC concentrations or abnormal κ/λ ratios at the initial dilution of 1:100 so they would not have been classified as normal. Bosmann et al.[11] studied the incidence of antigen excess in 91 patients. Samples from two patients (2.2%) exhibited antigen excess: one, a patient with λ FLC-monoclonal gammopathy of undetermined significance *(Chapter 13)* and the other, a κ FLC patient with a known IgAκ monoclonal gammopathy. The authors concluded that the interpretation of FLC measurements is facilitated in many cases, when combined with electrophoresis results and clinical information.

Vercammen et al.[12] studied 865 patients using 1:100 and 1:2000 sample dilutions on a Siemens BNII. Antigen excess was defined as a greater than 4-fold difference between the results obtained at the two dilutions. A total of 5.4% (44/811) and 1.2% (9/773) of κ and λ samples exhibited antigen excess respectively. It is unclear why the incidence of antigen excess reported in this study is much higher than that reported by others[10,11]. The authors highlight the importance of selecting the correct dilution for reporting results, and state that if the result at the 1:2000 dilution is greater than 4 times the result obtained at the 1:100 dilution, then the 1:2000 result should be reported; if the result at the 1:2000 dilution is less than 4 times the result obtained at the 1:100 dilution, then the 1:100 result should be reported. This approach improves the consistency of reporting FLC values and is discussed further in Section 7.4.2 below.

7.4.2 Distinguishing between non-linearity and antigen excess

To check for antigen excess, Binding Site recommend performing an antigen excess check dilution in addition to the initial sample dilution, as described in the relevant product insert *(Table 7.6)*. Such a protocol minimises reagent usage and ensures consistency.

Instrument	Initial dilution for κ and λ Freelite assays	Antigen excess check dilution for κ and λ Freelite assays
Binding Site SPAPLUS	1/10	1/1000*
Siemens BNII/ProSpec™	1/100	1/2000

Table 7.6. Antigen excess check dilutions on Binding Site SPAPLUS and Siemens instruments. *This is the overall dilution: 1/10 initial dilution + 1/100 manual dilution*

Distinguishing between non-linearity and antigen excess is important because with non-linearity the lower result should be reported, whereas with antigen excess the higher result should be reported. The Binding Site recommends that when the result obtained at the antigen excess check dilution is more than 4-fold greater than the result obtained at the initial sample dilution, this sample should be considered to be in antigen excess. In this case the result obtained at the higher dilution should be reported. On the other hand, if the result from the antigen excess check dilution is less than 4-fold greater than that from the initial dilution, the sample should be considered non-linear and the value at the initial dilution should be reported. Examples of the use of this guidance to distinguish between antigen excess and non-linearity are shown in Table 7.7.

Sample 1	Dilution	Result (mg/L)
	1/100	**95.3**
	1/2000	202
Dilution results ratio*		2.1
Non-linear		

Sample 2	Dilution	Result (mg/L)
	1/100	**145**
	1/2000	467
Dilution results ratio*		3.2
Non-linear		

Sample 3	Dilution	Result (mg/L)
	1/100	78.1
	1/2000	**4310**
Dilution results ratio*		55
Antigen excess		

Table 7.7. Examples of κ FLC non-linearity and antigen excess on a Siemens BNII. *Results from antigen excess check dilution (1/2000) divided by those from the initial dilution (1/100). The results in bold should be reported.*

7.5. Polymerisation

FLC molecules are usually monomers or dimers, but higher polymeric forms frequently occur[13,14,15,16,17]. These act as multi-antigenic targets in immunoprecipitation assays, accelerating the formation of aggregates and leading to over-estimation of antigen concentrations *(Figure 7.6)*. This occurs in some patients with nonsecretory multiple myeloma (NSMM) who have undetectable concentrations of sFLCs by IFE but can have high concentrations by nephelometry *(Chapter 16)*.

In order to determine the effect of polymerisation on Freelite quantification, FLC monomers, dimers and polymers were purified from myeloma sera and concentrations compared with total protein measurements. It was apparent that purified dimers were over-estimated by 1.5-fold and higher polymers by 1.5- to 3.5-fold[18]. In a study by Émond et al.[15] greater than 7-fold over-estimation was observed in two samples (when compared with CZE) in association with polymers of up to 200 kDa.

An additional factor to consider is that SPE tests can underestimate FLC concentrations. Variable polymerisation may cause smearing of monoclonal bands on the gels so that only a proportion of the monoclonal protein is measured[18]. FLCs also take up less protein stain than albumin so their concentration is underestimated by scanning densitometry. It is likely that a combination of these factors causes the disparities between nephelometry and electrophoresis that are seen with the sera of some patients.

Whatever the explanation for the unexpectedly high results for samples containing polymerised sFLCs, it is important to note: 1) never try to disrupt polymers, treat as a normal sample; and 2) sFLC polymers are consistently produced so sFLC results provide valuable monitoring information and should be reported. In a patient with high sFLC results, if the patient responds to treatment the sFLC concentrations will reduce and the κ/λ sFLC ratio will eventually normalise in patients who achieve a stringent complete response *(Chapter 25)*.

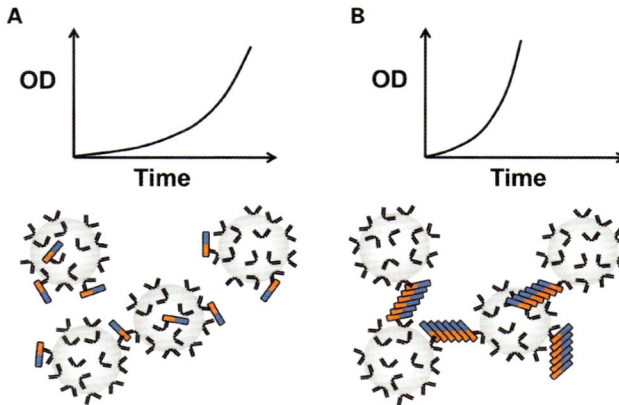

Figure 7.6. Diagram illustrating how FLC polymerisation affects reaction kinetics (A) Monomeric FLC molecules, normal reaction kinetics. (B) FLC polymers, enhanced crosslinking, faster reaction kinetics.

7.6. Discrepant results

When comparing serum and urine FLC results (e.g. serum Freelite results vs. urine electrophoresis) it is essential to ensure that the samples are from the same time point. If there is a significant time delay between the collection of serum and urine samples, even a few days, any observed difference may simply reflect response to treatment or disease progression because of the short serum half-life of FLCs *(Chapter 3)*.

7.6.1 Monoclonal FLCs in urine, normal sFLCs

FLC analysis is generally more sensitive than urine electrophoresis for indicating the presence of monoclonal FLCs. However, this advantage is dependent upon efficient renal reabsorption of FLCs *(Section 3.4)*. Small amounts of monoclonal FLCs have occasionally been identified in the urine of patients with normal sFLC ratios.

In a prospective screening study by Beetham et al.[19] monoclonal proteins were detected in 105 (22%) patients, 34 of whom had urinary Bence Jones protein (monoclonal FLCs). Of these 34 patients, eight had normal sFLC κ/λ ratios; however, seven were found to be positive for intact monoclonal immunoglobulins by SPE/sIFE and the remaining patient was considered to have a urine-only MGUS (<50 mg/L) of no apparent clinical consequence. These results support the findings of other studies, which recommend that SPE/sIFE and sFLC analysis can replace urine studies when screening for monoclonal gammopathy *(Chapter 23)*. However, Beetham expressed some disquiet as to why monoclonal FLCs were present in urine when sFLC κ/λ ratios were normal[19]. There is more than one mechanism whereby this may occur. One theory, proposed by Holding et al.[20] suggests that false positive results could be generated by the catabolism of intact immunoglobulins in urine. Although this theory remains unproven, it is known that renal podocytes express Fc receptors, which facilitate clearance of IgG that has traversed the glomerular filtration barrier into the urine *(Section 3.5.3)*[21], with subsequent separation of FLCs from intact IgG molecules.

A small proportion of AL patients may have trace amounts of urinary BJP but a normal sFLC ratio. Mead et al.[18] compared sFLC and urine IFE results in a cohort of 219 AL amyloidosis patients attending clinics at the National Amyloidosis Centre, London. Of these patients, 56 had abnormal sFLC ratios and monoclonal FLC detected in the urine; 52 had abnormal sFLC ratios but urine that was negative by IFE, and 16 had small monoclonal bands detected by uIFE but sFLC ratios within the normal range. Of this latter group, 12/16 had nephrotic-range proteinuria (>3 g/day), so saturation of protein reabsorption mehanisms by albumin and other proteins would explain the increased passage of FLCs into their urine *(Chapter 3)*. Serum levels, in contrast, may not be raised sufficiently to produce abnormal κ/λ ratios. For the other 4/16 patients, other mechanisms must have been responsible. All four of these patients had sFLC ratios biased towards the tumour light chain (0.30, 0.34 and 0.49 for λ patients and 1.61 for the κ patient).

In a separate study by Palladini et al.[22] five of 115 (4%) AL amyloidosis patients had monoclonal bands detectable by uIFE but sFLC ratios within the normal range. Interestingly these five patients were all λ-type AL patients. This may reflect the higher proportion of λ AL patients with nephrotic-range proteinuria compared with κ patients[23.]

7.6.2. Monoclonal FLCs detectable by sIFE but undetectable by sFLC immunoassay

On very rare occasions, sFLCs may be undetectable by immunoassay but detectable in the serum by IFE. In such cases, further investigation is always warranted. Possible explanations include: 1) antigen excess *(Section 7.4)*; and 2) failure of the sFLC immunoassay to recognise a particular patient's FLC epitopes. This is highly unlikely. There has been only one reported case in light chain MM, in 2004[24], where κ sFLCs were underestimated during a period of follow-up. The authors supplied Binding Site with urine from the patient, and purified FLCs were incorporated in the antigen pool used to produce subsequent batches of Freelite antisera[25].

7.6.3. No monoclonal proteins detectable by any routine laboratory method

For a small proportion of AL amyloidosis patients, no monoclonal FLCs are detected by any routine laboratory methods. In a large screening study by Katzmann et al., 11 of 581 (2%) AL patients were normal by sFLC analysis, sIFE and uIFE *(Chapter 23)*[26]. Three possible explanations include: 1) some FLC molecules may have a high affinity for the amyloid deposits, resulting in circulating FLCs being rapidly removed; 2) in a similar manner, patients with extensive amyloid deposits might have a huge capacity for FLC removal. Any newly synthesised molecules would be cleared rapidly by a combination of binding to the amyloid mass and glomerular filtration, thereby preventing the accumulation of FLCs in serum; or 3) the amyloid is due to the deposition of a different protein[27].

7.7. Biclonal gammopathies

Approximately 1 - 2% of patients with MM have biclonal gammopathies. When the light chain types differ (as occurs in around half of all biclonal cases), so that the patient has both κ and λ monoclonal sFLCs, κ/λ ratios can be normal[22]. Since it is likely that both FLC concentrations would be elevated, and in different amounts, the clinician would usually be alerted to an abnormality *(Figure 7.7)*[28]. The issue can be resolved by testing the sample using IFE and identifying two monoclonal bands of different FLC types. Renal function should also be determined to assess the degree of polyclonal elevation of sFLCs that might be attributed to reduced glomerular clearance.

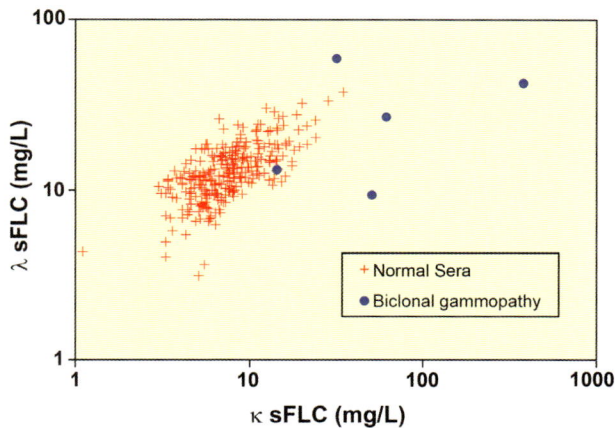

Figure 7.7. sFLC concentrations in 5 patients with biclonal gammopathies. (Courtesy of I. Ramasamy).

Test Questions

1. What is the maximum time that samples for sFLC analysis should be stored at 2-8 ℃?

2. What should users confirm before moving from one lot of sFLC kit to another?

3. What causes sample non-linearity?

4. How can non-linearity be distinguished from antigen excess?

Answers

1. 21 days *(Section 7.1.4)*.

2. That internal quality control samples give consistent results with both the new and existing batches of reagent *(Section 7.1.5)*.

3. Non-specific interference (matrix effects) or the inherent variability of monoclonal FLCs *(Section 7.3)*.

4. Perform an antigen excess check dilution (in addition to the initial sample dilution, as described in the product insert). If the result obtained at the antigen excess dilution is more than 4-fold greater than the result obtained at the initial sample dilution, the sample should be considered to be in antigen excess *(Section 7.4.2)*.

References

1. Katzmann JA, Clark RJ, Abraham RS, Bryant S, Lymp JF, Bradwell AR, Kyle RA. Serum reference intervals and diagnostic ranges for free kappa and free lambda immunoglobulin light chains: relative sensitivity for detection of monoclonal light chains. Clin Chem 2002;48:1437-44

2. Dispenzieri A, Kyle R, Merlini G, Miguel JS, Ludwig H, Hajek R et al. International Myeloma Working Group guidelines for serum-free light chain analysis in multiple myeloma and related disorders. Leukemia 2009;23:215-24

3. Vermeersch P, Vercammen M, Holvoet A, Broeck IV, Delforge M, Bossuyt X. Use of interval-specific likelihood ratios improves clinical interpretation of serum FLC results for the diagnosis of malignant plasma cell disorders. Clin Chim Acta 2009;410:54-8

4. Fraser CG, Harris EK. Generation and application of data on biological variation in clinical chemistry. Crit Rev Clin Lab Sci 1989;27:409-37

5. Braga F, Infusino I, Dolci A, Panteghini M. Biologic variation of immunoglobulin free light chains in serum. Biochimica Clinica 2013;37:376-82

6. Hansen CT, Munster AM, Nielsen L, Pedersen P, Abildgaard N. Clinical and preclinical validation of the serum free light chain assay: identification of the critical difference for optimized clinical use. Eur J Haematol 2012;89:458-68

7. Katzmann JA, Snyder MR, Rajkumar SV, Kyle RA, Therneau TM, Benson JT, Dispenzieri A. Long-term biologic variation of serum protein electrophoresis M-spike, urine M-spike, and monoclonal serum free light chain quantification: implications for monitoring monoclonal gammopathies. Clin Chem 2011;57:1687-92

8. Pretorius CJ, Klingberg S, Tate J, Wilgen U, Ungerer JP. Evaluation of the N Latex FLC free light chain assay on the Siemens BN analyser: precision, agreement, linearity and variation between reagent lots. Ann Clin Biochem 2012;49:450-5

9. Rajkumar SV, Harousseau JL, Durie B, Anderson KC, Dimopoulos M, Kyle R et al. Consensus recommendations for the uniform reporting of clinical trials: report of the International Myeloma Workshop Consensus Panel 1. Blood 2011;117:4691-5

10. Murata K, Clark RJ, Lockington KS, Tostrud LJ, Greipp PR, Katzmann JA. Sharply increased serum free light-chain concentrations after treatment for multiple myeloma. Clin Chem 2010;56:16-8

11. Bosmann M, Kossler J, Stolz H, Walter U, Knop S, Steigerwald U. Detection of serum free light chains: the problem with antigen excess. Clin Chem Lab Med 2010;48:1419-22

12. Vercammen M, Meirlaen P, Broodtaerts L, Broek IV, Bossuyt X. Effect of sample dilution on serum free light chain concentration by immunonephelometric assay. Clin Chim Acta 2011;412:1798-804

13. Abraham RS, Charlesworth MC, Owen BA, Benson LM, Katzmann JA, Reeder CB, Kyle RA. Trimolecular complexes of lambda light chain dimers in serum of a patient with multiple myeloma. Clin Chem 2002;48:1805-11

14. Berggard I, Peterson PA. Polymeric forms of free normal kappa and lambda chains of human immunoglobulin. J Biol Chem 1969;244:4299-307

15. Émond JP, Harding S, Lemieux B. Aggregation of serum free light chains (FLC) causes overestimation of FLC nephelometric results as compared to serum protein electrophoresis (SPE) while preserving clinical usefulness. Blood 2007;110:4767a

16. Heino J, Rajamaki A, Irjala K. Turbidimetric measurement of Bence-Jones proteins using antibodies against free light chains of immunoglobulins. An artifact caused by different polymeric forms of light chains. Scand J Clin Lab Invest 1984;44:173-6

17. Solling K, Solling J, Lanng Nielsen J. Polymeric Bence Jones proteins in serum in myeloma patients with renal insufficiency. Acta Med Scand 1984;216:495-502

18. Mead GP, Stubbs PD, Carr-Smith HD, Drew R, Drayson MT, Bradwell AR. Nephelometric measurement of serum free light chains in nonsecretory myeloma. Clin Chem 2002;48:70a

19. Beetham R, Wassell J, Wallage MJ, Whiteway AJ, James JA. Can serum free light chains replace urine electrophoresis in the detection of monoclonal gammopathies? Ann Clin Biochem 2007;44:516-22

20. Holding S, Spradbery D, Hoole R, Wilmot R, Shields ML, Levoguer AM, Dore PC. Use of serum free light chain analysis and urine protein electrophoresis for detection of monoclonal gammopathies. Clin Chem Lab Med 2011;49:83-8

21. Sarav M, Wang Y, Hack BK, Chang A, Jensen M, Bao L, Quigg RJ. Renal FcRn reclaims albumin but facilitates elimination of IgG. J Am Soc Nephrol 2009;20:1941-52

22. Palladini G, Russo P, Bosoni T, Verga L, Sarais G, Lavatelli F et al. Identification of amyloidogenic light chains requires the combination of serum-free light chain assay with immunofixation of serum and urine. Clin Chem 2009;55:499-504

23. Kumar S, Dispenzieri A, Katzmann JA, Larson DR, Colby CL, Lacy MQ et al. Serum immunoglobulin free light chain measurement in AL amyloidosis: prognostic value and correlations with clinical features. Blood 2010;116:5126-9

24. Tate JR, Mollee P, Dimeski G, Carter AC, Gill D. Analytical performance of serum free light-chain assay during monitoring of patients with monoclonal light-chain diseases. Clin Chim Acta 2007;376:30-6

25. Robson E, Mead G, Carr-Smith H, Bradwell A. In reply to Tate et al Clin Chim Acta 2007;376:30-6. Clin Chim Acta 2007;380:247

26. Katzmann JA, Kyle RA, Benson J, Larson DR, Snyder MR, Lust JA et al. Screening panels for detection of monoclonal gammopathies. Clin Chem 2009;55:1517-22

27. Lachmann HJ, Booth DR, Booth SE, Bybee A, Gilbertson JA, Gillmore JD et al. Misdiagnosis of hereditary amyloidosis as AL (primary) amyloidosis. N Engl J Med 2002;346:1786-91

28. Ramasamy I. Serum free light chain analysis in B-cell dyscrasias. Ann Clin Lab Sci 2007;37:291-4

Other free light chain immunoassays

Summary:

- Freelite® FLC assays utilise sheep polyclonal antisera, and are validated for use with serum, urine and CSF.

- FLC assays from other manufacturers are typically restricted to a different range of sample types.

- Many other FLC assays utilise monoclonal antibodies, which may not recognise all FLC polymorphisms.

- Freelite assays have been used as the "gold standard" reference calibrators for other FLC assays, although, in practice, values frequently show poor correlation.

- Freelite is the only FLC assay recommended by name by the International Myeloma Working Group. Guidelines that are based on Freelite data cannot be applied to N Latex FLC assays.

8.1. Introduction

Clinical studies involving the use of free light chain (FLC) immunoassays have been published in scientific journals since the 1960s. A variety of assay formats have been described including radioimmunoassay, enzyme immunoassay (EIA), radial immunodiffusion, turbidimetry and nephelometry; and some have been claimed to be specific for the measurement of FLCs in serum[1.] However, it is only since Freelite FLC assays (Binding Site, UK) became commercially available that serum FLC (sFLC) measurement has come to be an integral part of routine clinical practice for the diagnosis and management of monoclonal gammopathies. Indeed, sFLC analysis is now included in various national and international guidelines *(Chapter 25)*. In some countries, products intended for measurement of FLCs are commercially available from other manufacturers. This chapter provides an overview of the assays available, discusses the relative merits of monoclonal versus polyclonal antisera and presents data from the various published comparison studies.

8.2. Overview of commercial FLC assays

A summary of the main commercial FLC assays that are currently being marketed is shown in Table 8.1.

Freelite assays are latex-enhanced immunoassays that utilise sheep polyclonal antisera. They are the only FLC assays that are recommended by name in International Myeloma Working Group (IMWG) guidelines *(Section 8.5.4)*. By contrast, each of the other commercial FLC assays has features that may limit their usefulness. New Scientific Company (NSC), from Italy, manufactures FLC assays that are intended for use with urine/CSF. However, to our knowledge, there are no peer-reviewed publications containing data of NSC assay performance. The Biovendor FLC assays are enzyme-linked immunosorbent assays (ELISAs). Whilst this assay format can achieve high sensitivity, they are intended for research use only. Serascience manufactures lateral flow FLC immunoassays, but there are currently no published studies describing their use in clinical practice. Siemens N Latex FLC assays are latex-enhanced nephelometric assays[2]. Similar to Freelite sFLC assays, the assays are rapid and have good analytical sensitivity. However, a critical difference between N Latex FLC and Freelite assays is the choice of antisera. Siemens N Latex FLC assays utilise mouse monoclonal antibodies and this can lead to problems when measuring sFLCs; this is further discussed below.

Supplier	Assay	Antisera	Method	Instrumentation	Specimen types	Intended use	Regulatory approval
Binding Site	Freelite	Polyclonal	Latex-enhanced immunoassay	Nephelometry, turbidimetry	Serum, urine, CSF	Diagnosis and monitoring of MG	CE-marked FDA approved
New Scientific Company	Free light chains kit	Polyclonal	Antisera-based immunoassay	Nephelometry, turbidimetry	Urine, CSF	Diagnosis and monitoring of MG	CE-marked
Biovendor	Human immunoglobulin free light chains κ and λ ELISA	Monoclonal	Sandwich ELISA	Microplate reader	Serum, plasma, urine	Research only	None
Serascience	Seralite™ (dual kappa and lambda test)	Monoclonal	Lateral flow immunoassay	Test strip reader	Blood, serum, urine	Diagnosis and monitoring of MG	CE-marked
Siemens	N Latex FLC	Monoclonal	Latex-enhanced immunoassay	Nephelometry, turbidimetry	Serum, plasma, urine	Diagnosis and monitoring of MG	CE-marked

Table 8.1. A summary of commercial FLC immunoassays. MG: monoclonal gammopathy; ELISA: enzyme-linked immunosorbent assay; CSF: cerebrospinal fluid.

8.3. Monoclonal vs. polyclonal antisera

Historically, polyclonal antisera raised in rabbits or sheep have been used in most FLC assays and only a minority have utilised mouse monoclonal antibodies[1]. This is probably a reflection of the difficulty of producing monoclonal antibodies which are specific for free but not bound light chains, but also recognise all the variations of shape which different monoclonal FLCs can exhibit *(Chapter 3)*.

8.3.1. Monoclonal antibody production

To produce monoclonal antibodies, individual B-cells are isolated from immunised animals and fused with an immortal (myeloma) cell line to produce hybridoma cells. The hybridoma cells are similarly immortal and hopefully, produce antibodies with the desired specificity. Multiple mouse immunisations and subsequent hybridoma screening are frequently required before clones are identified that produce a suitable monoclonal antibody. Appropriate clones are then propagated in large quantities and the monoclonal antibody is purified from the culture supernatant *(Figure 8.1A)*.

Monoclonal antibodies recognise a single epitope *(Figure 8.2A)*, and are particularly suited as primary antibodies in ELISA assays, or in competitive immunoassays measuring drugs, hormones or other analytes, in which the antigenic target has a defined structure with minimal variation.

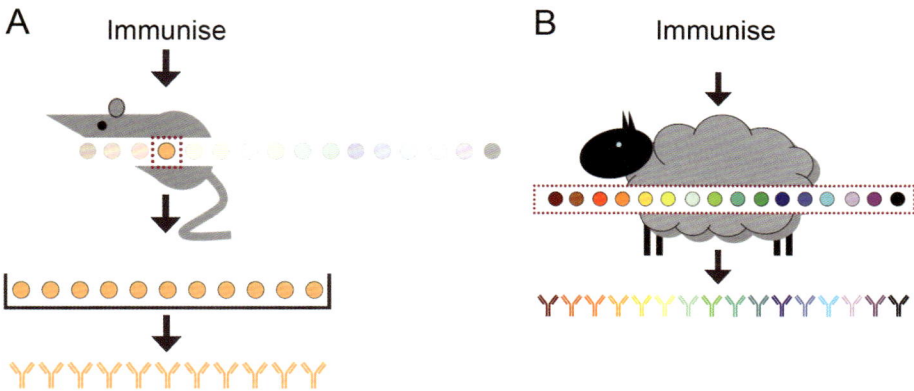

Figure 8.1. Production of monoclonal and polyclonal antisera. (A) Following immunisation, multiple B-cells are activated to produce antibodies. An individual B-cell clone is selected to propagate in vitro which secretes monoclonal antibody. *(B)* Following immunisation, multiple B-cells are activated to produce antibodies, resulting in polyclonal antisera.

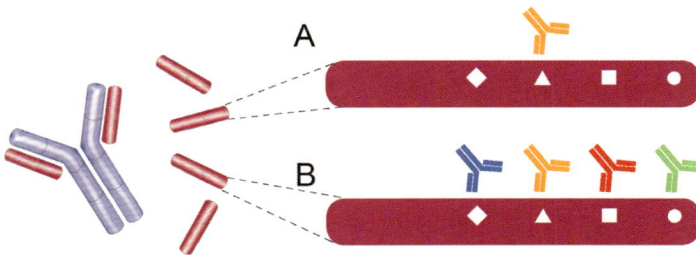

Figure 8.2. FLC epitope(s) recognised by (A) monoclonal or (B) polyclonal antisera.

8.3.2. Polyclonal antisera production

To produce polyclonal antisera, animals (typically rabbits or sheep) are immunised with a particular antigen (e.g. FLCs). As a result, multiple B-cells are activated to multiply, differentiate and produce antibodies, which each target a specific epitope on the antigen *(Figure 8.1B)*. As a result, serum collected from the immunised animal contains polyclonal antibodies that collectively, will demonstrate a range of different specificities and epitope affinities *(Figure 8.2B)*. For Freelite assays, the repertoire of polyclonal antibodies is further increased through blending a large array of polyclonal antisera that have been raised in different sheep and against a wide variety of different monoclonal FLCs *(Chapter 5)*. Prior to use in the assays, the polyclonal sheep antibodies are purified by positive- and negative-affinity chromatography against a diverse range of FLCs and intact immunoglobulins. This is necessary to produce the high-specificity, high-titre and high-affinity antibodies that are required for Freelite sFLC assays.

8.3.3. Requirements for anti-FLC antibodies for use in FLC immunoassays

Regardless of whether an anti-FLC antibody is monoclonal or polyclonal in nature, it should have a number of features for optimum performance in tubidimetric/nephelometric FLC immunoassays. These are summarised in Table 8.2.

Desired feature	Monoclonal antibody	Binding Site polyclonal antisera
Specificity	+++ or 0*	+++
Affinity/avidity	+++	+++
Immune complex formation	+[#] Small soluble complexes	+++ Large insoluble complexes
Recognition of all polymorphic FLCs?	No	Yes

Table 8.2. A summary of desired features of a FLC immunoassay, and the characteristics of monoclonal and polyclonal antisera.
Whilst monoclonal antibodies are highly specific for a given epitope, if this epitope is distorted, hidden or absent, they will not recognise the protein. [#]As a single monoclonal antibody is unable to form large immune complexes (unless the target antigen has repeated epitopes), a mixture of monoclonal antibodies is required in turbidimetric/nephelometric assays. However, it is difficult to create a mixture of monoclonal antibodies with balanced reactivity against a broad range of FLC molecules.

For any FLC assay, the antibodies used must be highly specific as FLC assays are required to discriminate "free" from "bound" light chains (in intact immunoglobulins), which may be 1000-fold more abundant in serum. Even minor cross reactivity with intact immunoglobulins can cause significant overestimation, and should be avoided. The antibodies must also be of high affinity, to produce FLC immunoassays that are suitably sensitive. In order to maximise light scattering in turbidimetric/nephelometric assays, the antibodies must form large immune complexes. Analytical sensitivity can be enhanced using latex-conjugated antibodies. Polyclonal antibodies are ideally suited for latex-enhanced turbidimetric/nephelometric assays due to their ability to cross-link via the recognition of different epitopes on an antigen. In contrast, large immune complexes cannot be formed with a single monoclonal antibody, unless the relevant epitope is repeated on the antigen. To overcome this limitation, more than one monoclonal antibody can be used; both N Latex FLC κ and λ assays use two monoclonal antibodies[3]. However, it can be difficult to produce multiple antibodies that provide balanced reactivity against the full range of FLC molecules.

Immunoglobulins and FLC molecules are highly polymorphic *(Chapter 3)*. Therefore, an important feature of a FLC assay must be the ability to recognise all the various forms of FLC molecules with comparable affinity. This is necessary to ensure that the assay is not only effective for diagnosing all patients, but is also quantitatively consistent, allowing comparisons of protein production between patients. All routine assays for the quantification of total immunoglobulins (IgG, IgA and IgM) use polyclonal antisera and the issues discussed above suggest that polyclonal antibodies would be the best choice for measuring polymorphic FLCs.

8.4. Analytical performance of N Latex FLC and Freelite assays

The FLC assays most frequently used as an alternative to Freelite are the Siemens N Latex FLC assays. These assays have been used in a number of evaluation and comparison studies, and are described below.

8.4.1. Calibration

An international reference material is not available for FLCs, therefore, master standards for the N Latex FLC assays were calibrated against the Freelite assays[2]. However, the absolute values returned by the two assays do not compare well. This is discussed further in Section 8.5.3.

8.4.2. Precision

As the measuring ranges of Freelite and N Latex FLC assays are different, samples used in precision studies must be suitably selected to ensure a fair comparison. This was illustrated in a precision study by Pretorius et al.[4] in which the samples with the lowest concentrations were well within the standard N Latex FLC measuring range (above the second calibrator point), but at or below the standard Freelite measuring range. Unsurprisingly, the total %CV of the lowest sample for the Freelite assays was >20%, but <7% for N Latex FLC *(Figure 8.3)*.

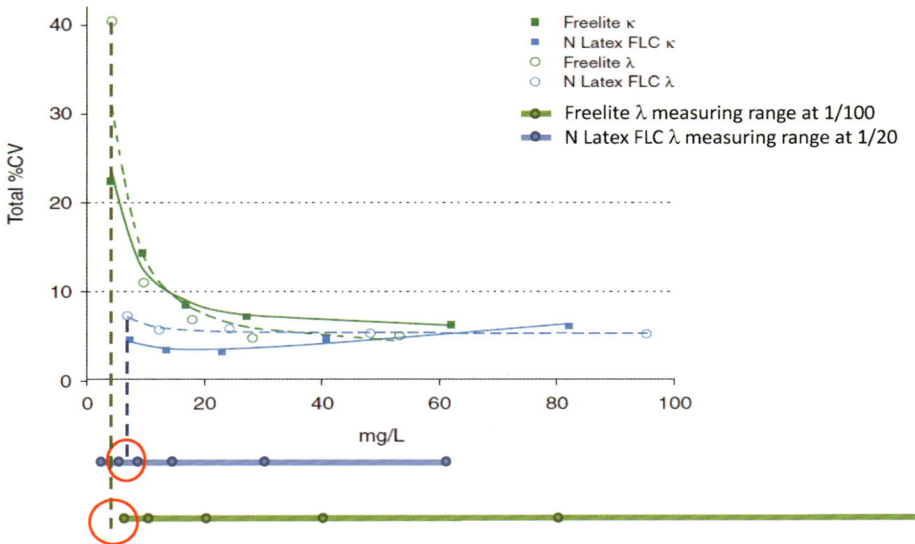

Figure 8.3. Precision of Freelite and N Latex FLC assays. *Thick lines below the axis represent Freelite and N Latex FLC measuring ranges at the standard dilution, individual standard values are indicated (filled circles). (Reproduced by permission of SAGE Publications Ltd., London, Los Angeles, New Delhi, Singapore and Washington DC, from[4] [©Pretorius, 2012]).*

A better-designed precision study by Lock et al.[5] used samples that either fell within the reference range or were moderately elevated by both FLC assays. The authors concluded that the within-batch and between-batch precision of both Freelite and N Latex FLC assays was acceptable (Table 8.3). A report by Sharrod-Cole et al.[6] reached similar conclusions. Maintaining batch-to-batch consistency is an essential requirement for any FLC assay, which may be used to monitor patients over the course of many years. Freelite polyclonal antisera are produced using standardised manufacturing procedures that include careful blending to achieve balanced, reproducible recognition of FLC molecules, with good between-batch consistency. This is further discussed in Section 5.5.

	Assay	Precision fluid	Freelite (%CV)	N Latex FLC (%CV)
Within-batch precision	κ sFLC	Normal	9.8	2.2
	λ sFLC	Normal	7.6	1.8
Between-batch precision	κ sFLC	Normal	7.1	5.1
		Elevated	5.8	6.4
	λ sFLC	Normal	7.0	3.6
		Elevated	6.4	5.6

Table 8.3. Precision of Freelite and N Latex FLC assays[5]. Reproducibility data based on 10 replicates, except N Latex FLC between-batch which was based on 3 replicates.

A theoretical advantage of monoclonal over polyclonal antibodies is reduced variation between reagent lots. Pretorius et al.[4] assessed variance between two N Latex FLC reagent lots, calibrated with the same material. Whilst the κ N Latex FLC assay demonstrated negligible bias (-1.7%), the λ N Latex FLC assay demonstrated significant bias (-5.4%). For both κ and λ N Latex FLC assays the difference in values for a number of samples was >20% (Figure 8.4). This included one notable extreme value which showed a >80% difference in λ sFLC concentration between reagent lots (Figure 8.4B). This indicates that use of monoclonal antibodies does not eliminate between-batch variation.

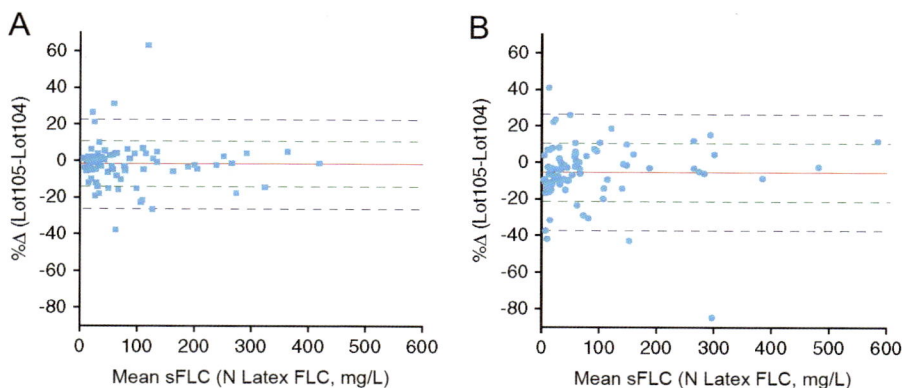

Figure 8.4. *Bland-Altman plots comparing patient results for two batches of N Latex FLC reagent. (A) κ sFLC, (B) λ sFLC. The variance predicted from precision is indicated by the shaded area. (Reproduced by permission of SAGE Publications Ltd., London, Los Angeles, New Delhi, Singapore and Washington DC, from[4] (©Pretorius, 2012]).*

8.4.3. Linearity

Occasional sample non-linearity (i.e. when a sample measured at different dilutions gives a substantially different result) occurs with most immunoassays. Examples of sample non-linearity with Freelite assays are described and discussed in Section 7.3. Pretorius et al.[4] reported that sample non-linearity occurred in approximately half of all monoclonal and polyclonal samples, with both Freelite and N Latex FLC assays. The authors concluded that non-linearity of FLC assays is a property of the individual sample and not a method-specific phenomenon. Freelite assays undergo validation during development (based on protocols defined by the Clinical and Laboratory Standards Institute) to ensure that the assays are linear *(Section 5.6)*.

8.4.4. Antigen excess

Antigen excess causes immunoassays to underestimate high concentrations of protein *(Section 7.4)*. Freelite antigen excess checks can be performed on all platforms, and are carried out in one of two ways: 1) automatic prozone parameters, e.g. Binding Site SPAPLUS® and Optilite®; or 2) a sample dilution protocol detailed in the product insert, e.g. Siemens BN™II. Freelite antigen excess is further discussed in Section 7.4.

The Siemens N Latex FLC assays include antigen excess detection parameters based on a pre-reaction protocol. For the pre-reaction, a small volume of sample is initially added, followed by the rest of the sample for the primary reaction. If the signal at the end of the pre-reaction is above a certain threshold value, the instrument automatically performs a higher dilution. te Velthuis et al.[2] described the initial validation of N Latex FLC antigen excess parameters. In that study, over 2,000 serum samples were screened to identify the two with the highest concentration of κ or λ sFLCs: 23,000 and 57,000 mg/L, respectively. Serial dilutions of these two high samples failed to demonstrate antigen excess. However, this protocol does not provide a good assessment of antigen excess susceptibility because 1) only two samples were tested; and 2) they were chosen in a manner that was most likely to select samples not subject to antigen excess.

Jacobs et al.[7] compared the results from Freelite and N Latex FLC assays for 46 samples containing polyclonal or monoclonal sFLCs and using multiple sample dilutions. For monoclonal κ FLCs measured by Freelite or N Latex FLC, the discrepancies of concentrations between different dilutions were sometimes large. In addition, λ sFLC concentrations were underestimated at higher concentrations by both methods. However, this study failed to give a clear definition of non-linearity or antigen excess and the incidence of neither phenomenon was reported.

Two further studies compared the incidence of antigen excess and gross non-linearity for Freelite and Siemens N Latex FLC assays by testing samples at higher sample dilutions, on the BNII[8,9]. Harding et al.[9] reported that κ sFLC antigen excess was observed in 3/91 (3%) samples by Freelite and 4/91 (4%) by N Latex FLC; all cases of Freelite antigen excess were correctly identified using the manufacturer's dilution protocol. λ sFLC antigen excess was not observed with Freelite assays, in keeping with previous reports that suggest that these λ assays are less prone to antigen excess than κ assays (Section 7.4.1). In contrast, 3/91 (3%) of samples showed λ sFLC antigen excess with the N Latex FLC assay. Burden et al.[8] reported that a proportion of samples measured with κ or λ N Latex FLC assays gave results that were 5-9 times greater at the higher sample dilution compared with the result at the initial dilution (Table 8.4); this is indicative of antigen excess despite the fact that the assays should have automatic protection from antigen excess issues.

N Latex FLC		Freelite		N Latex FLC		Freelite	
Dilution	κ FLC (mg/L)	Dilution	κ FLC (mg/L)	Dilution	λ FLC (mg/L)	Dilution	λ FLC (mg/L)
1:100	7	1:100	>171	1:20	4	1:100	>155
1:400	NR	1:400	>684	1:100	61	1:400	>620
1:2000	289	1:2000	617	1:400	158	1:2000	1020

Table 8.4. sFLC concentrations measured by N Latex FLC and Freelite assays at several sample dilutions[8]. NR: not reported.

Therefore, it should be noted that: 1) both Freelite and N Latex FLC assays show antigen excess in a small number of samples; 2) antigen excess parameters utilised in the N-Latex assays do not prevent all samples from exhibiting antigen excess; and 3) discrepant results between the two assays could be due to antigen excess. This third point is discussed further in Section 8.5.6.

8.5. Clinical performance of N Latex FLC and Freelite assays

8.5.1. Normal reference intervals

Published reference intervals for Freelite and N Latex FLC assays are similar *(Table 8.5)*[2,10]. Freelite assay standardisation and normal ranges are further discussed in Chapters 5 and 6, respectively.

		κ sFLC (mg/L)	λ sFLC (mg/L)	κ/λ sFLC ratio
Freelite	95% reference interval	**3.3 - 19.4**	**5.7 - 26.3**	0.3 - 1.2
	Diagnostic range			**0.26 - 1.65**
N Latex FLC	95% reference interval	**6.7 - 22.4**	**8.3 - 27.0**	0.50 - 1.27
	Diagnostic range			**0.31 - 1.56**

Table 8.5. A comparison of reference intervals for Freelite and N Latex FLC assays. Figures in bold indicate the limits for result interpretation. The diagnostic range includes 100% of the reference population.

8.5.2. Renal reference interval

Patients with renal impairment but no evidence of monoclonal gammopathy may have κ/λ sFLC ratios (measured by Freelite) which are slightly above the normal range[11,12,13]. The reason is that as renal clearance of sFLCs declines, the sFLC concentrations increase to more closely reflect the production rates, which are higher for κ than λ FLCs. Consequently, a modified renal reference range for the Freelite κ/λ sFLC ratio (0.37 – 3.10) has been proposed[14]. Use of the renal reference range when screening for monoclonal gammopathy in patients with renal impairment may increase specificity and is further discussed in Section 6.3.

Jacobs et al.[15] studied the effect of renal impairment on N Latex FLC concentrations in 284 patients with chronic kidney disease (CKD, stage 1-5). κ and λ FLC concentrations increased through each CKD stage. However, whilst κ N Latex FLC assays gave similar results to Freelite, the increase in λ FLC concentrations in the CKD5/dialysis groups was significantly greater for the N Latex FLC assays *(Figures 8.5, 8.6A and 8.6B)*. As a result, none of the patients with CKD had a κ/λ sFLC ratio exceeding the N Latex FLC reference interval and, in fact, the ratio was significantly lower in the CKD5/dialysis group compared to healthy controls (p<0.0001; *Figure 8.6C*).

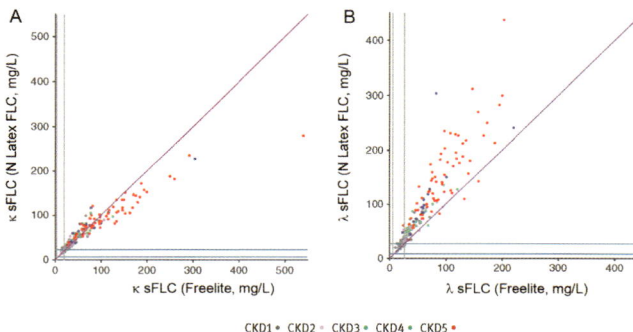

CKD1 • CKD2 • CKD3 • CKD4 • CKD5 •

Figure 8.5. Comparison of sFLC results for Freelite and N Latex FLC assays in patients with renal impairment. (A) κ sFLC (B) λ sFLC. Purple line is y=x. (Courtesy of J. F. M. Jacobs).

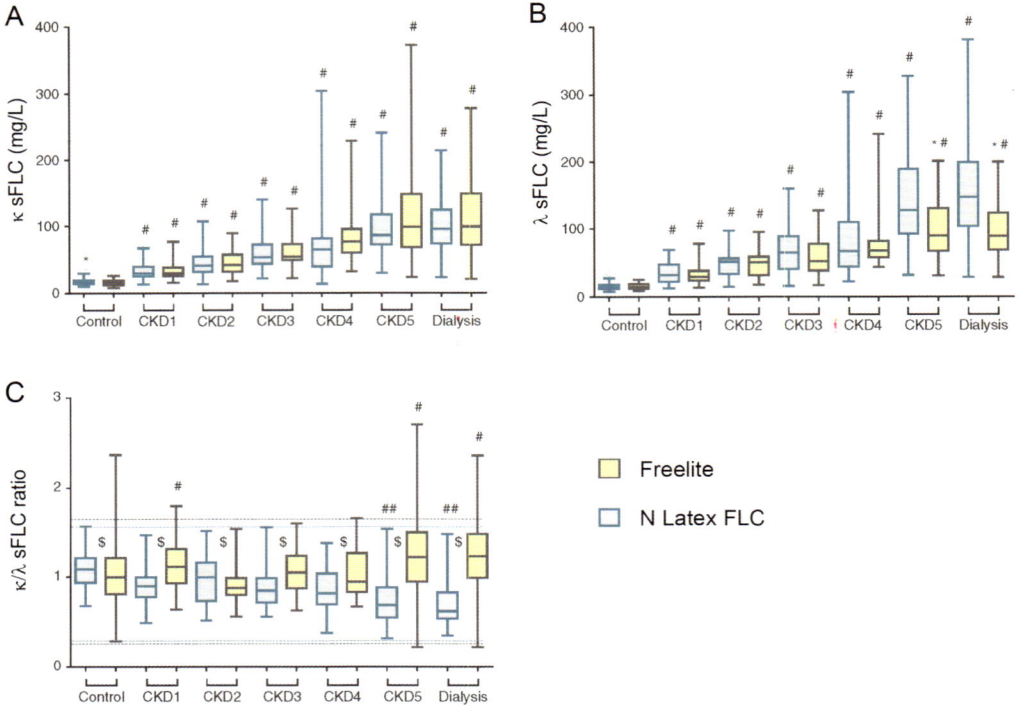

Figure 8.6. Box and whiskers plots comparing Freelite and N Latex FLC results for (A) κ sFLC, (B) λ sFLC, and (C) κ/λ sFLC ratio in patients with renal impairment. *Boxes: 2.5 – 97.5 percentile ranges; bars: min – max values; dotted lines in (C): min – max of normal reference intervals; #: significant increase from control group; ##: significant decrease from control group; *: significant difference between Freelite and N Latex FLC assays (λ sFLC). $: significant difference between Freelite and N Latex assays. (Courtesy of J. F. M. Jacobs).*

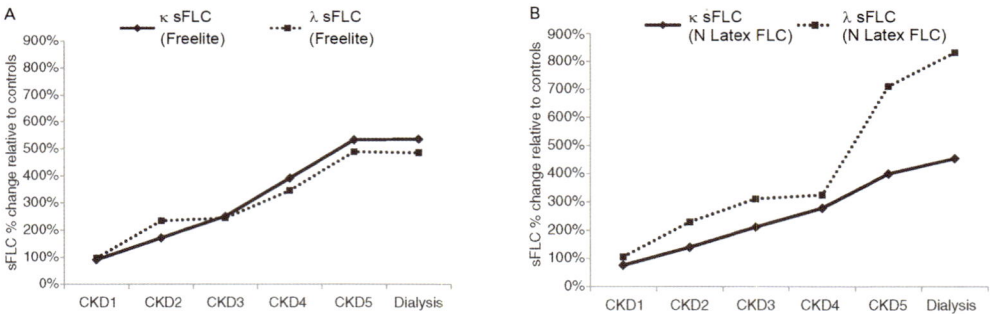

Figure 8.7. Percentage change in sFLC results in patients with renal impairment compared to controls. (A) *Freelite and* (B) *N Latex FLC. (Courtesy of O. Berlanga).*

Berlanga et al.[16] re-analysed the data reported by Jacobs et al., and plotted the percentage increase in sFLC levels relative to controls for both assays *(Figure 8.7)*. Freelite measured a progressive elevation of κ over λ FLC with worsening renal function, which resulted in some patients having an abnormal κ/λ sFLC ratio. By contrast, N Latex FLC assays indicated an approximately equal increase of both FLCs throughout CKD1-4, but a sharp increase in λ FLC levels in the fifth group, that comprised both CKD5 and dialysis patients. One potential explanation for this anomaly was provided by Tate et al.[17] who compared sFLC concentrations in serum samples pre- and post-high flux haemodialysis with Freelite and N Latex FLC assays. Pre-dialysis λ sFLC concentrations were much higher as measured by the N Latex FLCs assays than Freelite, but post-haemodialysis, a larger reduction in λ sFLCs was indicated by the N Latex FLC assays *(Table 8.6)*. This resulted in similar post-dialysis λ sFLC concentrations as measured by both assays. The authors proposed that a positively interfering substance may have been present in pre-dialysis samples that affected the λ N Latex FLC assay (causing an over-read) more than the Freelite assays. If this interfering substance was of low molecular weight and was removed by haemodialysis, this would explain the greater fall in λ FLC concentrations indicated by the N Latex FLC assays. Further investigations are now required to try and identify the putative interfering substance and test this hypothesis.

	N Latex FLC			Freelite		
	κ (mg/L)	λ (mg/L)	κ/λ (range)	κ (mg/L)	λ (mg/L)	κ/λ (range)
Pre-haemodialysis (n=29)	196	243	0.48 - 1.35	195	166	0.79 - 2.38
Post-haemodialysis (n=11)	118	146		110	145	

Table 8.6. Comparison of Freelite and N Latex FLC sFLC concentrations in patients with dialyisis-dependent chronic kidney disease[17]. Mean concentrations of sFLCs are reported for patients pre- and post-high-flux haemodialysis.

8.5.3. Comparison studies

A number of studies have compared the absolute values returned by the Freelite and N Latex FLC assays[2,4,5,15,18,19,20,21]. All have reached similar conclusions: the two assays do not compare well and are not interchangeable. For example, a well-designed study by Lock et al.[5] compared quantitative results of Freelite and N Latex FLC assay for 327 serum samples submitted for analysis to four routine diagnostic laboratories in the UK; a total of 79% were from patients with known monoclonal gammopathies. Comparing the results produced by the two assays, standard linear regression gave r^2 values of 0.86 and 0.71 for κ and λ sFLCs, respectively. This level of agreement is well below the requirements of the Clinical Laboratory Standards Institute (which requires an $r^2 \geq 0.95$ to establish that two assays are equivalent)[22]. Bland-Altman plots identified 17/327 (5.2%) samples that had the most discrepant results *(Figure 8.8)*. This included 14 patients whose sera contained clonal FLC that were "poorly detected" by the N Latex FLC but not the Freelite assays[5]. Of most concern was the fact that 2 of the 14 patients had LCMM (prior to treatment) but their N Latex FLC assay results indicated normal sFLC ratios while their Freelite assay results were clearly abnormal *(Table 8.8)*. These 2 patients and other examples of missed diagnoses are discussed further in section 8.5.6 below. Whilst some comparison studies have been limited to small numbers of patients with monoclonal gammopathy[17] or a lack of clinical information[3], all have reported a similar poor concordance of Freelite and N Latex FLC assay results. This lack of agreement can be clinically important and is discussed further in Section 8.5 below.

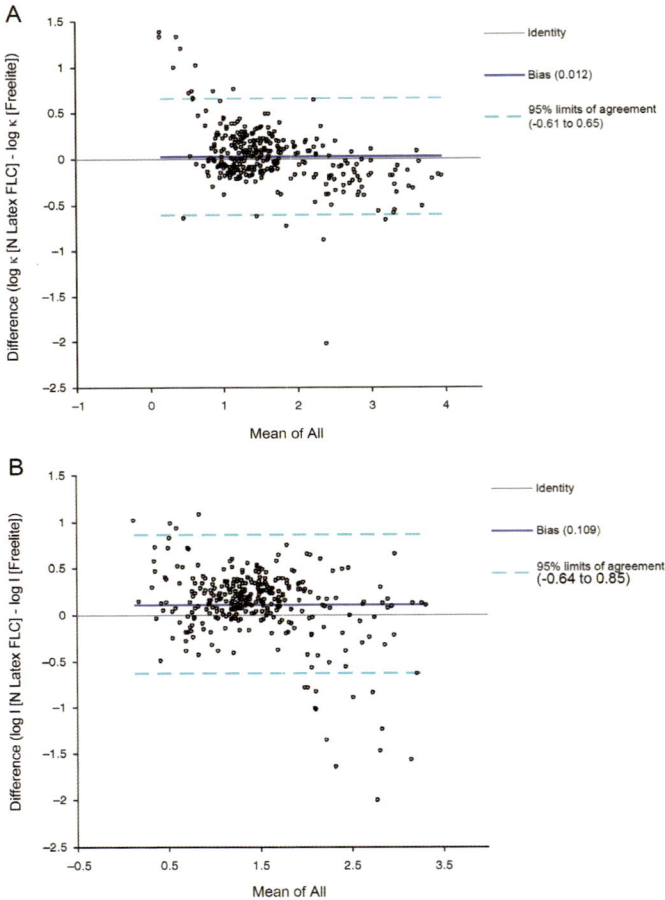

Figure 8.8. Bland-Altman plots comparing results for Freelite and N Latex sFLC assays. (A) κ sFLC, (B) λ sFLC. (Reproduced by permission of SAGE Publications Ltd., London, Los Angeles, New Delhi, Singapore and Washington DC, from[5] [©Lock, 2013]).

8.5.4. Compliance with guidelines

Freelite assays are the only FLC assays recommended by name in International Myeloma Working Group guidelines and an involved/uninvolved Freelite sFLC ratio ≥100 is designated as a biomarker of malignancy *(Chapter 25)*[23,24]. Guidelines and response criteria that are based on Freelite data should not be applied on the basis of N Latex FLC results because of the poor concordance between the absolute values[25,26,27]. A summary of clinical definitions that are based upon quantitative Freelite results are shown in Table 8.7.

Popat et al.[26] compared the assessment of response indicated by N Latex and Freelite FLC assays for 42 MM patients who had been treated after relapse. The response criteria used were those defined by Rajkumar et al.[32]. A total of 17/42 patients had measurable disease by both assays and 11 by neither; one patient was evaluable by N Latex FLC only but 13 had measurable disease by Freelite only. For the 17 patients with measurable disease by both assays, there was poor agreement in the assigned response to treatment *(Figure 8.9, weighted Kappa 0.75)*.

Guideline	Definition	sFLC concentration
AL amyloidosis [28,29,30]	Measurable disease	dFLC >50 mg/L
	VGPR	dFLC <40 mg/L
MM [31,32,24]	Measurable disease	100 mg/L

Table 8.7. A summary of international guidelines based on quantitative Freelite results. *VGPR: very good partial response; dFLC: the difference between involved and uninvolved sFLC concentrations.*

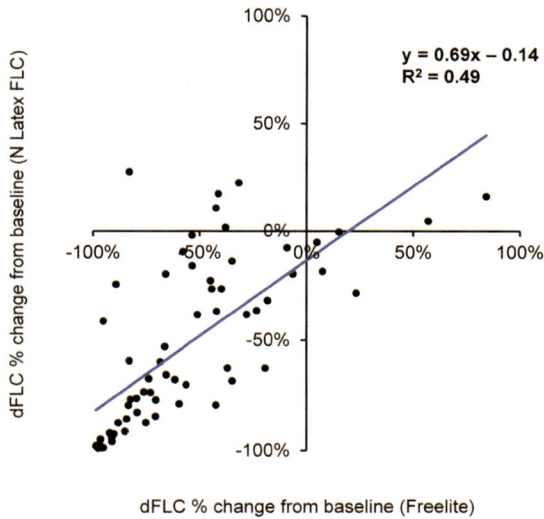

dFLC % change from baseline (Freelite)

Figure 8.9. Correlation between Freelite and N Latex sFLC results for 17 MM patients with measurable disease. *(Results are expressed as the percentage change in dFLC (difference between involved and uninvolved FLC concentrations). Blue line: line of best fit. (Courtesy of R. Popat).*

87

8.5.5. Diagnostic performance in LCMM

In a total of five studies published to date, which incorporated approximately 50 LCMM patients, the Siemens N Latex FLC assays failed to detect abnormalities in 6 λ LCMM and 1 κ LCMM patients *(Table 8.8)*[4,5,18,33,34.] By comparison, the same five studies reported that all of these LCMM patients were correctly identified by the Freelite assays. The best described cohorts of confirmed cases of LCMM were included in the studies by Schneider and Hoedemakers[18,34] in which 3/26 of confirmed LCMM cases were not detected by the N Latex FLC assays. In contrast, an abnormal Freelite κ/λ sFLC ratio has been detected in all of 692 LCMM patients at diagnosis *(Chapter 15)*. The recommendation that sFLC analysis plus serum electrophoresis constitutes a suitable primary screening protocol for monoclonal gammopathies[35,23] should, arguably, only be applied to FLC analysis with Freelite assays and not N Latex FLC or any other FLC assays, which are not validated in this context.

Study	Total no. of LCMM patients	Missed LCMM	N Latex FLC			Freelite		
			κ FLC mg/L	λ FLC mg/L	κ/λ ratio	κ FLC mg/L	λ FLC mg/L	κ/λ ratio
Lock 2013[5]	n.s (189 MM)	λ LCMM	19.5	59.7	0.33 Normal	4.66	6070	<0.01 Abnormal
		λ LCMM	12.8	40.2	0.32 Normal	7.9	422	0.02 Abnormal
Hoedemakers 2011[18]	3 κ LCMM 6 λ LCMM	λ LCMM	n.s	n.s	n.s. Normal	n.s	n.s	n.s Abnormal
Schneider 2013[34]	17 LCMM	λ LCMM	n.s	n.s	0.8 Normal	n.s	n.s	0.02 Abnormal
		κ LCMM	n.s	n.s	0.8 Normal	n.s	n.s	1.89 Abnormal
Cavalcanti 2013[33]	1 λ LCMM	λ LCMM	16.5	23.0	0.71 Normal	9.14	818.8	0.01 Abnormal
Pretorius 2012[4]	n.s	λ LCMM	29	84	0.35 Normal	18	464	0.04 Abnormal

Table 8.8. Summary of missed cases of LCMM by N Latex FLC assays. Patients were categorised as misclassified if the N Latex FLC assays reported a normal κ/λ ratio (n.s.=not stated).

8.5.6. Rationale for the diagnoses of LCMM missed by N Latex FLC assays

The clinical studies discussed above have provided a number of examples where patients known to have LCMM have had normal N Latex FLC results but abnormal results with Freelite assays. There are two reasons why FLC assays may fail to identify the presence of monoclonal sFLCs: 1) antigen excess *(Section 8.4.4)*, or 2) complete non-reaction, in which the monoclonal antibodies fail to recognise a particular FLC clone.

Pretorius et al.[4] performed a comparison of Freelite and N Latex FLC results for 116 samples sent to the laboratory for routine FLC analysis (after exclusion of samples with Freelite <50 mg/L), and investigated any samples that were highly discordant. For 6/116 (5.2%) samples, N Latex FLC assays gave markedly higher κ results *(Figure 8.10A)*. When these six samples were further diluted and retested using Freelite assays, the results significantly increased, consistent with antigen excess in the Freelite assays. In contrast, 4/116 samples (3.4%) had markedly higher λ Freelite results *(Figure 8.10B)*. Further dilution did not increase the N Latex FLC λ results for these samples. These four patients included one with confirmed λ LCMM for whom the κ/λ sFLC ratio was normal by N Latex FLC assays, but abnormal by Freelite *(Table 8.8)*.

It is noteworthy that the majority of diagnoses that were missed by the N Latex FLC assays were of λ type. Whilst the κ constant domain is typically encoded by a single C gene segment, the λ constant domain is encoded by one of a number of C gene segments *(Section 3.3)*. It is probable that the monoclonal antibody-based assays fail to detect all polymorphic forms of FLCs, particularly λ FLCs that are more genetically diverse.

A further patient with λ LCMM that was not diagnosed by the N Latex FLC assays is presented as a clinical case study below. In this example, serum immunofixation confirmed the presence of monoclonal FLCs that were detected by the Freelite sFLC assays, but not the monoclonal antibody-based N Latex FLC assays.

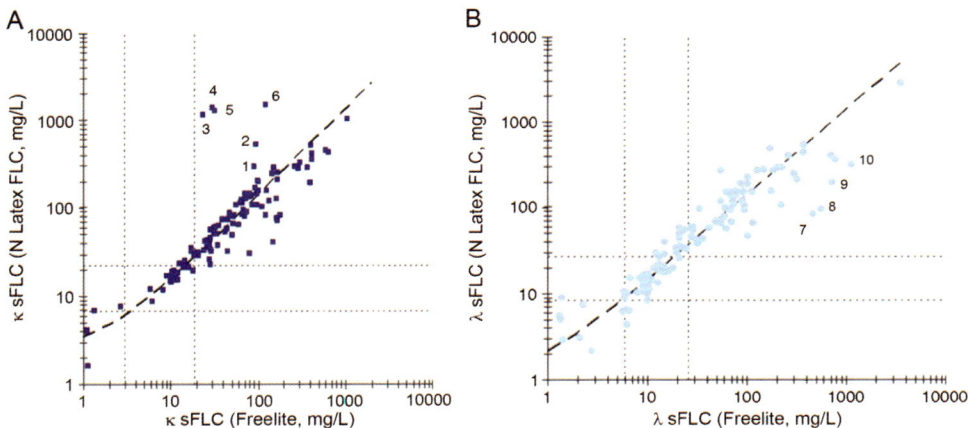

***Figure 8.10. Scatter plot comparing Freelite and N Latex sFLC results. (A)** κ sFLC. Six samples with markedly elevated N Latex FLC results are indicated (1 – 6). **(B)** λ sFLC. Four samples with markedly elevated Freelite results are indicated (7 – 10). Further dilution did not increase the N Latex FLC λ results. Dotted lines: normal reference intervals. (Reproduced by permission of SAGE Publications Ltd., London, Los Angeles, New Delhi, Singapore and Washington DC, from[4] [©Pretorius, 2012]).*

Clinical case history

A patient with λ LCMM identified by Freelite but not N Latex FLC assays[33]

A 47-year-old woman was admitted to the Istituto Nazionale Tumori, Naples, with bone pain. An X-ray of her pelvis revealed osteolytic lesions, and a serum protein electrophoresis (SPE) was ordered but this revealed no obvious monoclonal protein. Subsequently, sFLC analysis was performed using both Freelite and N Latex FLC assays. Whilst the Freelite assay identified monoclonal λ sFLCs, the N Latex FLC assay results were normal *(Table 8.9)*. High-resolution agarose electrophoresis of serum and urine samples identified a monoclonal protein band *(Figure 8.11A)*, which was typed by immunofixation electrophoresis (IFE) as monoclonal λ FLCs (in the absence of intact immunoglobulins including IgD/IgE; *Figures 8.11B and C*. A bone-marrow biopsy confirmed the diagnosis of λ LCMM. The patient was admitted to the Hematology-Oncology Unit, and one month after the start of therapy, serum and urine IFE became negative and the Freelite sFLC assay values returned to normal.

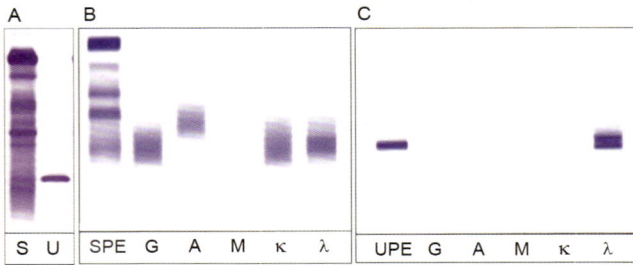

Figure 8.11. Serum and urine electrophoresis. (A) *High-resolution agarose electrophoresis of serum and urine samples.* (B) *Serum IFE* (C) *Urine IFE. (Reproduced with permission from Bioclinical Clinica[33]).*

	Freelite		N Latex FLC	
	Results	Reference interval	Results	Reference interval
κ sFLC (mg/L)	9.1	3.3 - 19.4	16.4	6.7 - 22.4
λ sFLC (mg/L)	818.8	5.7 - 26.3	23.0	8.3 - 27.0
κ/λ sFLC ratio	0.01	0.26 - 1.65	0.71	0.31 - 1.56

Table 8.9. Freelite and N Latex FLC patient results and reference intervals.

8.5.7. Diagnostic performance in cast nephropathy

The International Kidney and Monoclonal Gammopathy Research Group (IKMGRG) recommend the use of SPE and sFLC analysis to screen for monoclonal disease in patients presenting with acute kidney injury *(Chapter 27)*[36]. The IKMGRG suggest that if the concentration of monoclonal FLCs is ≥500 mg/L in patients with acute kidney injury (AKI), a diagnosis of tubular interstitial pathology is likely, and the most common renal lesion in such cases is cast nephropathy[22]. For such patients, further haematological work-up and prompt treatment, to reduce FLC production, is essential.

In the only study performed to date using the Siemens N Latex FLC assays in the context of AKI, the authors concluded that the IKMGRG recommendations could not be carried out satisfactorily[37]. In this study, five of the 28 patients (18%) with AKI secondary to MM were misclassified by the N Latex FLC assays. For one patient, the N Latex FLC assay reported a λ FLC concentration of 1 mg/L, whereas a value of 1810 mg/L was reported by the Freelite assay. Once again, this suggests that the pathogenic monoclonal λ FLC clone was not recognised by the monoclonal antibody-based assay.

8.5.8. Diagnostic performance in AL amyloidosis

The largest study that has compared the performance of N Latex FLC and Freelite assays in AL amyloidosis was published by Palladini et al.[38] This included 426 patients with newly-diagnosed AL amyloidosis from two specialist centres (Pavia, n=353; and Limoges, n=73). A poor agreement of quantitative results between the two methods was observed but the diagnostic sensitivity of the Freelite (82%) and N-latex (84%) assays was similar, and both improved to 98% in combination with serum and urine immunofixation. During follow-up, the dFLC concentration by either method was of prognostic significance, although the optimal cut off values varied according to the method (>50% dFLC decrease by Freelite; >33% dFLC decrease by N Latex FLC). The authors concluded that although the two assays have similar diagnostic and prognostic performance, the assays are not interchangeable and follow-up should be performed with a single method. Similar findings were reported by two further studies which included patients with AL amyloidosis[20,39]. Due to the different quantitative changes recorded by the two assay systems, new response criteria would need to be derived and validated for the N Latex FLC assays if they are to be used in routine clinical practice.

8.6. Conclusion

It is reasonable to assume that any assay calibrated against another assay should produce similar quantitative results. However, it has been shown that this is not the case for the N Latex FLC and Freelite assays, and it cannot be assumed that N Latex FLC assays will have the same clinical utility or give compliance with current guidelines *(Chapter 25)*. Of particular concern is the number of clinically confirmed diagnoses of LCMM that have been missed by the N Latex FLC assays. This is most likely due to the failure of the monoclonal antibodies to recognise the full repertoire of polymorphic monoclonal FLCs.

Test Questions

1. Can an individual monoclonal antibody directed against FLC epitopes be used to produce a turbidimetric/nephelometric FLC immunoassay?

2. Are κ/λ sFLC ratios, measured with N Latex FLC assays, found to be higher in patients with severe renal impairment (CKD5)?

3. Are international guidelines applicable to N Latex FLC assays?

1. No. Lack of cross linking between the antibody and FLC antigen fails to produce the large immune complexes that are required to scatter light *(Section 8.3.3)*.

2. No. In fact λ sFLC concentrations measured by N Latex FLC assays are relatively higher in CKD5, resulting in a κ/λ sFLC ratio that is significantly lower than healthy controls. It has been suggested this may be an analytical artefact due to a low molecular weight interfering substance *(Section 8.5.2)*.

3. No. Absolute values reported by N Latex FLC and Freelite sFLC assays do not compare well *(Section 8.5.3)*, and N Latex FLC assays fail to identify monoclonal sFLCs in cases of LCMM that are detected by Freelite assays *(Section 8.5.5)*. Therefore, it cannot be assumed that international guidelines (that are based on quantitative Freelite data) are applicable to the monoclonal antibody-based assays *(Section 8.5.4 and Chapter 25)*.

References

1. Nakano T, Miyazaki S, Takahashi H, Matsumori A, Maruyama T, Komoda T, Nagata A. Immunochemical quantification of free immunoglobulin light chains from an analytical perspective. Clin Chem Lab Med 2006;44:522-32

2. te Velthuis H, Knop I, Stam P, van den Broek M, Bos HK, Hol S et al. N Latex FLC - new monoclonal high-performance assays for the determination of free light chain kappa and lambda. Clin Chem Lab Med 2011;49:1323-32

3. Wagner C, Gentzer W, te Velthuis H. Add consistency to monoclonal gammopathy testing: N Latex FLC kappa and lambda assays. Siemens Healthcare Diagnostics 2012;A91DX-120143-XC1-4A00

4. Pretorius CJ, Klingberg S, Tate J, Wilgen U, Ungerer JP. Evaluation of the N Latex FLC free light chain assay on the Siemens BN analyser: precision, agreement, linearity and variation between reagent lots. Ann Clin Biochem 2012;49:450-5

5. Lock R, Saleem R, Roberts E, Wallage M, Pesce T, Rowbottom A et al. A multicentre study comparing two methods for serum free light chain analysis. Ann Clin Biochem 2013;50:255-61

6. Sharrod-Cole H, Matters D, Showell P, Harding S. Serum free light chain assessments: Comparison of precision and linearity. Biochmica Clinica 2013;37:T390a

7. Jacobs JF, Hoedemakers RM, Teunissen E, van der Molen RG, te Velthuis H. Effect of sample dilution on two free light chain nephelometric assays. Clin Chim Acta 2012;413:1708-9

8. Burden JM, Matters DJ, Carr-Smith HD, Young P, Harding SJ. Comparison of Freelite and N Latex FLC utilising diagnostically relevant samples. Clin Chem 2012;58:C44a

9. Harding SJ, Popat R, Berlanga O, Sharrod H, Cavenagh J, Oakervee H. Comparison of the analytical performance of polyclonal and monoclonal antibody based FLC assays in refractory multiple myeloma patients. Clinical Chemistry 2013;59:A22a

10. Katzmann JA, Clark RJ, Abraham RS, Bryant S, Lymp JF, Bradwell AR, Kyle RA. Serum reference intervals and diagnostic ranges for free kappa and free lambda immunoglobulin light chains: relative sensitivity for detection of monoclonal light chains. Clin Chem 2002;48:1437-44

11. Hutchison CA, Harding S, Hewins P, Mead GP, Townsend J, Bradwell AR, Cockwell P. Quantitative assessment of serum and urinary polyclonal free light chains in patients with chronic kidney disease. Clin J Am Soc Nephrol 2008;3:1684-90

12. Marshall G, Tate J, Mollee P. Borderline high serum free light chain k/l ratios are seen not only in dialysis patients but also in non-dialysis-dependent renal impairment and inflammatory states. Am J Clin Pathol 2009;132:309

13. Park JW, Kim YK, Bae EH, Ma SK, Kim SW. Combined analysis using extended renal reference range of serum free light chain ratio and serum protein electrophoresis improves the diagnostic accuracy of multiple myeloma in renal insufficiency. Clin Biochem 2012;45:740-4

14. Hutchison CA, Plant T, Drayson M, Cockwell P, Kountouri M, Basnayake K et al. Serum free light chain measurement aids the diagnosis of myeloma in patients with severe renal failure. BMC Nephrol 2008;9:11

15. Jacobs JF, Hoedemakers RM, Teunissen E, te Velthuis H. N Latex FLC serum free light-chain assays in patients with renal impairment. Clin Chem Lab Med 2014;52:853-9

16. Berlanga O, Carr-Smith H, Harding S. Response to Jacobs: N Latex FLC serum free light-chain assays in patients with renal impairment. Clin Chem Lab Med 2014;52:e243-e245

17. Tate J, Bazeley S, Klingberg S, Pretorius CJ, Hawley C, Mollee P. Comparison of the Freelite and N Latex serum free light chain (FLC) assays in chronic kidney disease. Clin Biochem Rev 2012;33:P53a

18. Hoedemakers RM, Pruijt JF, Hol S, Teunissen E, Martens H, Stam P et al. Clinical comparison of new monoclonal antibody-based nephelometric assays for free light chain kappa and lambda to polyclonal antibody-based assays and immunofixation electrophoresis. Clin Chem Lab Med 2011;50:489-95

19. Jurkeviciene J, Gogeliene L, Vitkus D. Comparison of two immunoassays for free light chain kappa and lambda: established (Freelite) and incoming (Siemens). Clinical Chemistry and Laboratory Medicine 2014;52:0691a

20. Mollee P, Tate J, Pretorius CJ. Evaluation of the N Latex free light chain assay in the diagnosis and monitoring of AL amyloidosis. Clin Chem Lab Med 2013;2303-10

21. HS, Kim HS, Shin KS, Song W, Kim HJ, Kim HS, Park MJ. Clinical comparisons of two free light chain assays to immunofixation electrophoresis for deteecting monoclonal gammopathy. BioMed Research International 2014 In press

22. Clinical and Laboratory Standards Institute. EP09-A3. Measurement procedure comparison and bias estimation using patient samples; approved guideline - Third Edition. 2013

23. Dispenzieri A, Kyle R, Merlini G, Miguel JS, Ludwig H, Hajek R et al. International Myeloma Working Group guidelines for serum-free light chain analysis in multiple myeloma and related disorders. Leukemia 2009;23:215-24

24. Rajkumar SV, Dimopolous MA, Palumbo A, Blade J, Merlini G, Mateos MV et al. International Myeloma Working Group updated criteria for the diagnosis of multiple myeloma. Lancet Oncology 2014;15:e538-e548

25. Palladini G, Jaccard A, Milani P, Lavergne D, Foli A, Bender S et al. Comparison of the N-latex and Freelite assays for serum free light chain: clinical performance in AL amyloidosis. Presented at XIV International Symposium on Amyloidosis 2014;OP-35a

26. Popat R, Berlanga O, Cavenagh J, Oakervee H, Williams C, Harding S, Cook M. Polyclonal and monoclonal antibody based FLC assays provide discrepant information for monitoring relapsed multiple myeloma patients. Clinical Chemistry and Laboratory Medicine 2014;52:0680a

27. Weber N, Mollee P, Augustson B, Brown R, Catley L, Gibson J et al. Management of systemic light chain (AL) amyloidosis: recommendations of the Myeloma Foundation of Australia Medical and Scientific Advisory Group. Intern Med J 2014 In press

28. Gertz MA, Merlini G. Definition of organ involvement and response to treatment in AL amyloidosis: an updated consensus opinion. Amyloid 2010;17:CP-Ba

29. Palladini G, Dispenzieri A, Gertz MA, Wechalekar A, Hawkins P, Schonland SO et al. Validation of the criteria of response to treatment in AL amyloidosis. Blood 2010;116:1364a

30. Palladini G, Dispenzieri A, Gertz MA, Kumar S, Wechalekar A, Hawkins PN et al. New criteria for response to treatment in immunoglobulin light chain amyloidosis based on free light chain measurement and cardiac biomarkers: impact on survival outcomes. J Clin Oncol 2012;30:4541-9

31. Kyle RA, Rajkumar SV. Criteria for diagnosis, staging, risk stratification and response assessment of multiple myeloma. Leukemia 2009;23:3-9

32. Rajkumar SV, Harousseau JL, Durie B, Anderson KC, Dimopoulos M, Kyle R et al. Consensus recommendations for the uniform reporting of clinical trials: report of the International Myeloma Workshop Consensus Panel 1. Blood 2011;117:4691-5

33. Cavalcanti E, Barchiesi V, Cuomo M, Di Paola F, Morabito F, Cavalcanti S. A particular case of lambda chain multiple myeloma. Biochimica Clinica 2013;37:428-30

34. Schneider N, Wynckel A, Kolb B, Sablon E, Gillery P, Maquart FX. [Comparative analysis of immunoglobulin free light chains quantification by Freelite (The Binding Site) and N Latex FLC (Siemens) methods]. Ann Biol Clin (Paris) 2013;71:13-9

35. Dimopoulos M, Kyle R, Fermand JP, Rajkumar SV, San MJ, Chanan-Khan A et al. Consensus recommendations for standard investigative workup: report of the International Myeloma Workshop Consensus Panel 3. Blood 2011;117:4701-5

36. Hutchison CA, Batuman V, Behrens J, Bridoux F, Sirac C, Dispenzieri A et al. The pathogenesis and diagnosis of acute kidney injury in multiple myeloma. Nat Rev Nephrol 2011;8:43-51

37. Hutchison CA, Cockwell P, Cook M. Diagnostic accuracy of monoclonal antibody based serum immunoglobulin free light chain immunoassays in myeloma cast nephropathy. BMC Clin Pathol 2012;12:12

38. Palladini G, Hegenbart U, Milani P, Kimmich C, Foli A, Ho AD et al. A staging system for renal outcome and early markers of renal response to chemotherapy in AL amyloidosis. Blood 2014;124:2325-32

39. Mahmood S, Wassef N, Sachchithanantham S, Rannigan L, Taylor W, Lane T et al. Comparison of Freelite and N Latex serum free light chain assays and predicting survival. Haematologica 2013;98:P787a

Development and validation of Hevylite immunoassays

Hevylite® assays:

- Are based on polyclonal antisera raised in sheep.
- Are standardised using International standards for total IgG, IgA and IgM.
- Undergo rigorous testing during assay manufacture to ensure the quality of the kit components.

9.1. Assay overview

Intact immunoglobulin molecules contain unique junctional epitopes across the heavy chain and light chain constant regions that are the target of immunoglobulin heavy/light chain assays (Hevylite, HLC) *(Figure 9.1)*[1]. HLC assays quantify the different light chain types of each immunoglobulin class, i.e. IgGκ, IgGλ, IgAκ, IgAλ, IgMκ and IgMλ *(Figure 9.2)*. These molecules are measured in pairs, e.g. IgGκ/IgGλ, to produce ratios in the same manner as serum free light chain (sFLC) κ/λ ratios.

As with Freelite® sFLC immunoassays, polyclonal antibodies raised in sheep provide the most attractive method of recognising polymorphic immunoglobulin molecules. There are theoretically four HLC epitope regions per immunoglobulin molecule - one on each side of each heavy/light chain contact region. Multiple HLC epitopes enable immune complexes to form readily, allowing homogeneous immunoassays to be produced that are suitable for turbidimeters and nephelometers. Latex enhancement is not necessary for IgG and IgA HLC assays, but is required for IgM assays.

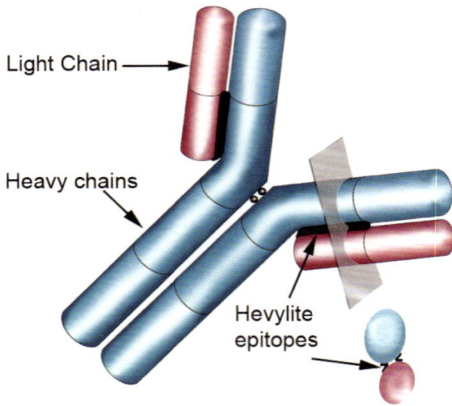

Figure 9.1. Target epitopes (in black) for HLC antibodies are on the constant regions (CH1 and CL) between the heavy and light chains of immunoglobulin molecules.

Light Chain

Heavy chains

Hevylite epitopes

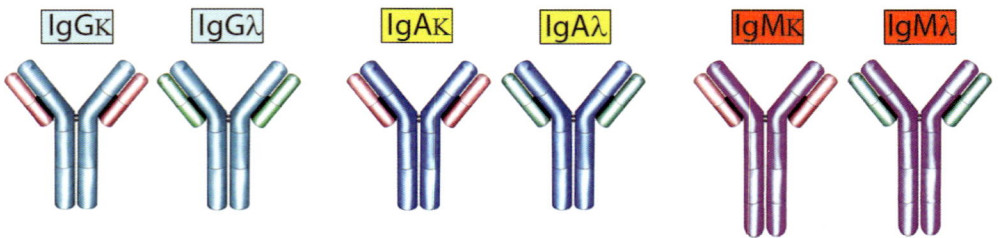

Figure 9.2. Heavy/light chain pairs of IgG, IgA and IgM molecules showing the target epitopes for HLC immunoassays in black.

9.2. Polyclonal antisera production

To produce polyclonal antisera for HLC assays, sheep are immunised using individual monoclonal immunoglobulins of a single class and light chain type (e.g. IgGκ)[1]. Sheep are simultaneously tolerised with: 1) monoclonal immunoglobulins of the same class but opposite light chain type (i.e. IgGλ); 2) monoclonal immunoglobulins of different classes but the same light chain type (i.e. IgAκ); and, 3) monoclonal free light chains (FLCs) of the same light chain type (i.e. κ FLC). Antigens for immunisation and tolerisation are purified from the serum or urine of patients with monoclonal gammopathies. Antigen purity is assessed using silver-stained sodium dodecyl sulfate polyacrylamide gel electrophoresis (SDS-PAGE) and Western blot analysis.

9.3. Antisera specificity testing

Inevitably, one of the most demanding aspects of HLC assay production is to ensure specificity. A panel of antigens is used to test specificity; this panel includes sera containing monoclonal immunoglobulins of each class, subclass, and light chain type.

Initial immunisation and tolerisation procedures result in antisera that are strongly reactive against each HLC molecule, with a degree of cross-reaction with other immunoglobulin specificities. Cross-reacting antisera are recycled through affinity adsorption columns until specificity is satisfactory. Antisera with subclass bias are purified against immobilized monoclonal immunoglobulins of other subclass types. Antisera are considered specific when they react in a balanced manner with the appropriate panel of immunoglobulins, and no cross-reactivity occurs with other molecules, including FLCs. The final purified reagents are produced using positive affinity chromatography against the target HLC immunoglobulin. Antisera specificity is the most important aspect of the HLC immunoassays, and is evaluated using several techniques, described below.

To test specificity by radial immunodiffusion (RID), HLC antisera are immobilised in an agarose gel and a panel of antigens are applied to wells cut into the gel. The diameters of the resulting immunoprecipitates are used to determine specificity.

Neat or latex-conjugated HLC antisera are tested for specificity by turbidimetry/nephelometry. Known concentrations of purified potential interfering substances are added to a normal serum containing concentrations of immunoglobulins within the reference interval for each assay. Results for IgG and IgA HLC assays are shown in Figure 9.3. Overall, the specificity assessments show that HLC antisera have minimal reactivity with intact immunoglobulins of the alternate light chain type or class. HLC antisera also have no significant reactivity with FLCs or other potentially interfering substances.

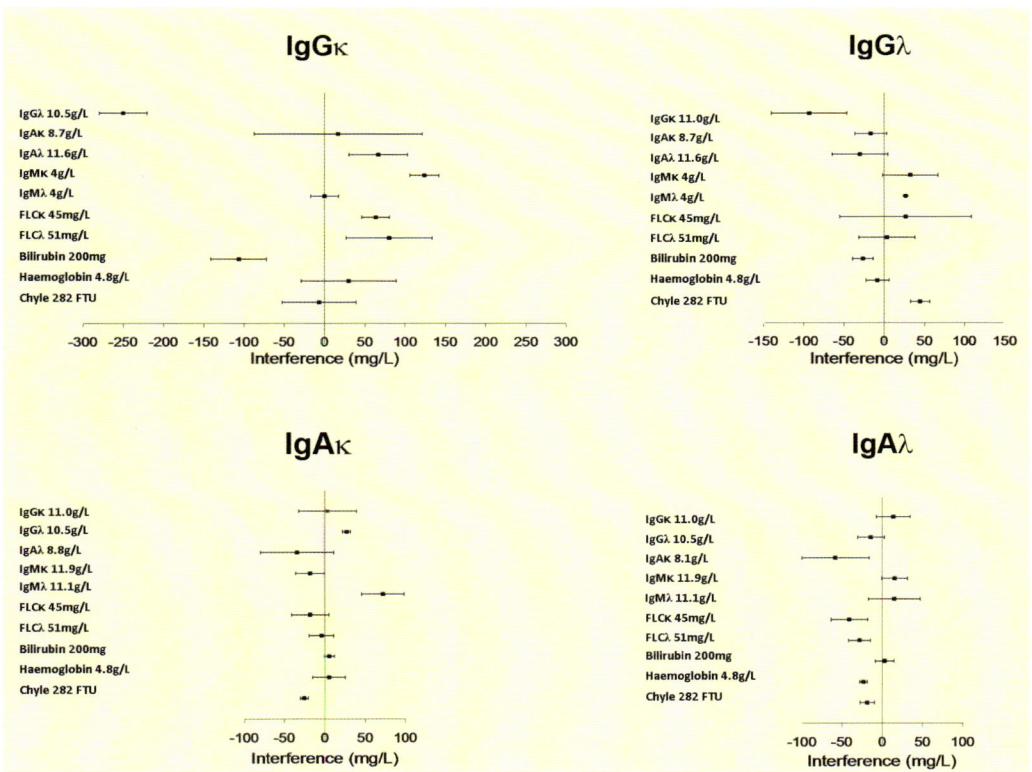

Figure 9.3. Interference data for IgG and IgA HLC assays. *Data points are the mean values of 3 analyses with 95% confidence intervals shown as bars. Changes in the measured Ig concentrations upon the addition of potentially interfering substances are shown. Concentration of added substances (× normal median serum values) were as follows: IgGκ 11.0 g/L (×1.5); IgGλ 10.5 g/L (×2.5); IgAκ 8.7 g/L (×7); IgAλ 11.6 g/L (×13), IgMκ 4 g/L (×6); IgMλ 4 g/L (×8), FLCκ 45 mg/L (×6); FLCλ 51 mg/L (×4); Chyle 282 formazin turbidity units (FTU) (×25); haemoglobin 4.8 g/L (×100); bilirubin 200 mg/L (×30). (Republished with permission of Clinical Chemistry[1]; permission conveyed through Copyright Clearance Center, Inc).*

9.4. Accuracy and standardisation

Assay accuracy is defined as the degree of closeness of achieved results relative to their actual (true) values. International standards exist for total IgG, IgA and IgM (CRM 470 and DA470k)[2,3]. Therefore, these standards were used to assign values to HLC assay reference materials to ensure accurate results. An overview of the process of calibrator assignment for HLC assays is described below, using the IgA assays as an example.

9.4.1. Primary standards and internal reference standards

For IgA HLC assays, polyclonal IgA was purified from pooled normal human sera by ammonium-sulfate precipitation, anion-exchange chromatography, and immunoaffinity chromatography. Low-level contamination with alternate classes of immunoglobulins was removed by immunoaffinity adsorption and/or protein G affinity chromatography. Fractionation of κ from λ light chain forms was achieved using both protein L and anti–light chain immunoaffinity matrices.

Purified IgAκ and IgAλ were >99% pure by silver-stained SDS-PAGE, *(Figure 9.4)* and light chain specific as indicated by enzyme immunoassays and Western blot analysis *(Figures 9.5 and 9.6)*. Contamination with other immunoglobulin and light chain types was <0.5% by enzyme immunoassay. Finally, the total protein concentration of the primary standards (determined using the bicinchoninic acid method) and CRM 470 plus DA470k were used to assign IgAκ and IgAλ values to the IgA HLC internal reference standard *(Figure 9.7)*. Similar methods were used for the calibration of the IgG and IgM HLC assays.

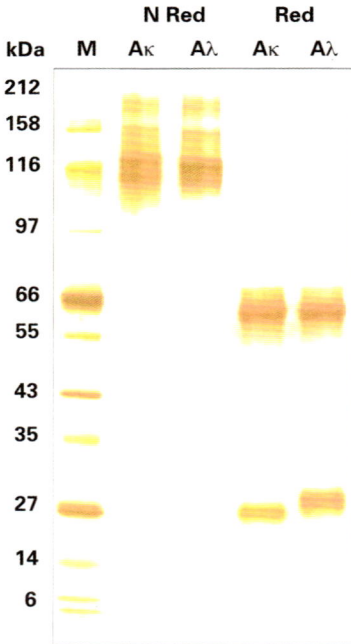

Figure 9.4. Analysis of pure polyclonal IgAκ and IgAλ preparations by silver stain. Each lane contains 1 µg of purified protein. N Red: non-reduced; Red: reduced.

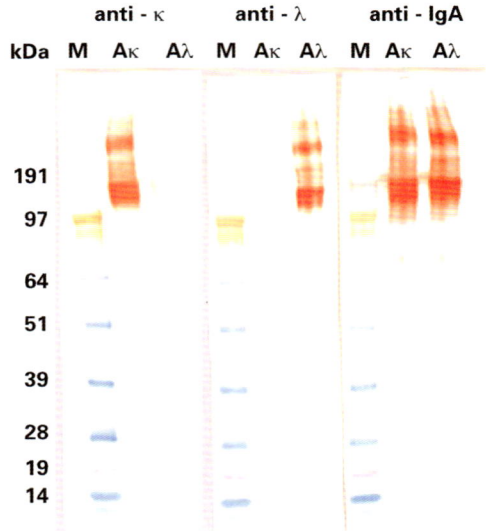

Figure 9.5. Analysis of pure polyclonal IgAκ and IgAλ preparations by Western blot analysis. SDS-PAGE was performed using 0.5 µg of non-reduced protein per lane and immunostained for κ, λ, and IgA as indicated.

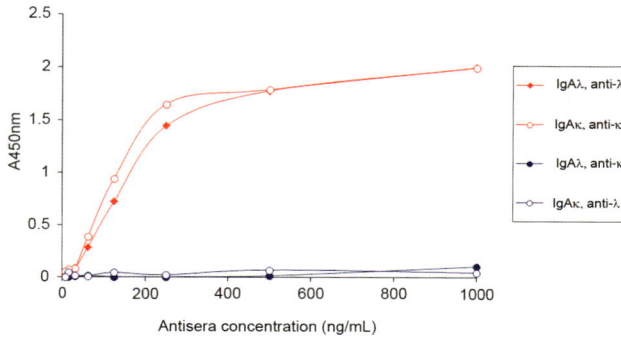

Figure 9.6. Analysis of the light chain composition of pure polyclonal IgAκ and IgAλ by enzyme immunoassays.
Light chain antisera (anti-κ or -λ) was titrated against pure IgAκ and IgAλ.

9.4.2. Kit calibrators and controls

HLC kit calibrators are prepared from pooled normal human sera, and kit controls from human sera containing high concentrations of polyclonal immunoglobulins. Values are assigned to kit calibrators using the internal reference materials *(Figure 9.7)*. This is achieved by turbidimetry/nephelometry over five calibration curves, with the internal reference material assayed at four different dilutions with values across the curve range.

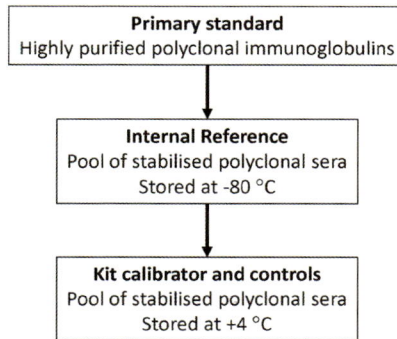

Figure 9.7. Flow chart for the production of standards for HLC assays.

9.4.3. Calibration curves

The measuring ranges of HLC assays are dependent upon two factors: the slope of the respective calibration curve and the portion selected for the assay. The latter should be chosen to allow the maximum number of normal and abnormal clinical samples to be measured at the initial sample dilution.

Typical analytical ranges (at the standard dilution) on the Binding Site SPAPLUS® are shown in Table 9.1, and typical calibration curves are shown in Figure 9.8. Samples containing higher concentrations require further dilution. Samples containing lower concentrations can be re-assayed at a lower dilution (or neat on the SPAPLUS).

Calibration curves are validated by the measurement of high and low control samples. It is also recommended that all laboratories take part in external quality assurance schemes, to allow comparison of performance and results among different test sites *(Chapter 39)*.

Specificity	Dilution	Approximate measuring range (g/L)
IgGκ	1/20	1.9 – 40.0
IgGλ	1/20	0.92 – 29.5
IgAκ	1/10	0.18 – 11.2
IgAλ	1/10	0.16 – 10.4
IgMκ	1/10	0.20 – 5.00
IgMλ	1/10	0.18 – 4.50

Table 9.1. Measuring ranges for HLC assays on the Binding Site SPAPLUS.

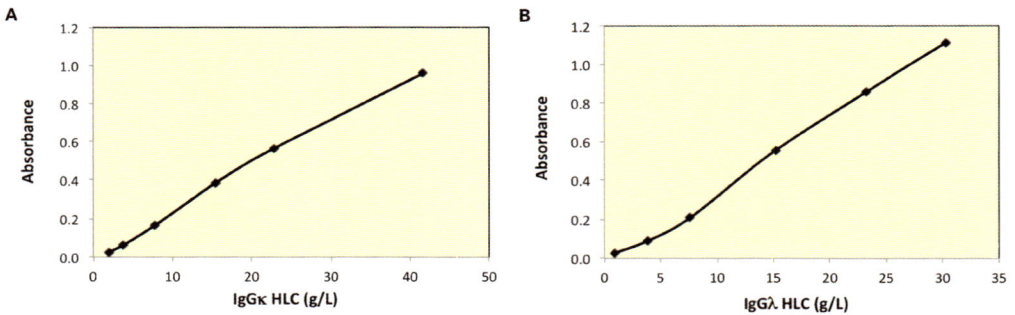

Figure 9.8. Calibration curves for (A) IgGκ and (B) IgGλ HLC assays on the Binding Site SPAPLUS.

9.4.4. Correlation with total immunoglobulin measurements

During validation, a detailed comparison study is performed for each assay: summated concentrations of HLC immunoglobulin pairs (e.g. IgAκ + IgAλ) are compared with total immunoglobulin measurements (e.g. IgA) as a test of assay accuracy. All specificities demonstrate a high degree of correlation, and the results are summarised in each product insert. An example is shown in *(Figure 9.9)*.

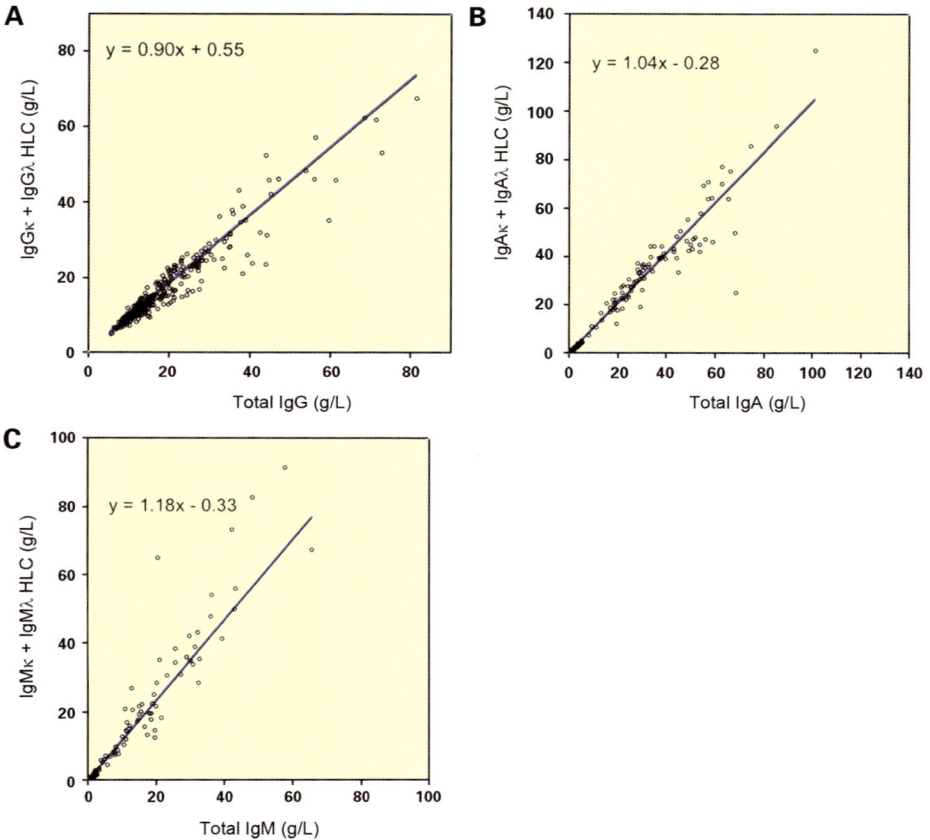

Figure 9.9. Comparison of summated (A) IgG; (B) IgA; and (C) IgM HLC to total immunoglobulin concentrations by Passing-Bablok analysis. IgG HLC: 143 normal sera and 216 IgG MM patient sera (121 IgGκ and 95 IgGλ); IgA HLC: 138 normal sera and 94 IgA MM patient sera (58 IgAκ and 36 IgAλ); IgM HLC: 110 normal sera and 78 sera from patients with IgM monoclonal gammopathies.

9.5. Maintaining batch-to-batch consistency of polyclonal antisera-based reagents

Maintaining batch-to-batch consistency is essential as HLC assays may be used for monitoring individual patients over many years. The key component of any turbidimetric or nephelometric immunoassay is the polyclonal antisera. Therefore, it is essential to minimise any change in the specificity and performance of the antisera over time.

In order to ensure consistency between batches of polyclonal antisera, a virtual "rolling pool" of antisera has been established. This pool consists of a list of pre-approved antisera (*Section 9.3* explains how suitable antisera are identified). During the manufacture of a batch of reagent, an equal portion of each approved antiserum from the list is mixed. As individual antiserum volumes vary, stocks become exhausted at different times. When this occurs, the antiserum is replenished with a new pre-approved antiserum. The pool of polyclonal antisera used in the manufacture of HLC assays always contains at least 90% of the same constituent antisera as the previous batch of reagent. The use of rolling pools of antisera during HLC assay manufacture has minimised batch-to-batch variation whilst ensuring a full range of HLC epitopes are recognised. Batch-to-batch variation is further discussed in Section 9.7. For IgM HLC assays, once a pool of suitable polyclonal antisera is made, sheep antibodies are attached to latex particles (in order to enhance their performance in nephelometric and turbidimetric immunoassays).

9.6. Overview of Hevylite assay validation

During the development and production of Hevylite assays there is a rigorous validation process to ensure that the assays perform correctly and provide the correct diagnostic information. The validation protocols used follow those set out by the Clinical and Laboratory Standards Institute (CLSI), and are outlined in Section 5.6. These include assessment of assay precision, sensitivity, linearity, stability, comparison to predicate devices (serum protein electrophoresis and serum immunofixation electrophoresis) and confirmation of the normal reference range.

9.7. Overview of Hevylite kit manufacture

The manufacture of Hevylite assays follows established, validated protocols, and each batch of reagents undergoes rigorous testing to ensure the quality of the kits *(Figure 9.10)*.

Once all the raw materials for a kit have been manufactured the curve performance and antigen excess capacity of the reagents are evaluated. Values are then assigned to the kit calibrator(s) and controls using the internal reference standard.

Specificity is evaluated by testing panel samples. HLC results for each new batch of antisera are compared with assigned values and results from previous batches. The panel samples include normal sera and patient sera containing polyclonal or monoclonal immunoglobulins (typically from patients with multiple myeloma or Waldenström's macroglobulinaemia). The results are compared using Passing-Bablok analysis and are considered acceptable when they fall within a defined set of criteria. Typical batch-to-batch comparison data on the Binding Site SPAPLUS is shown in Figure 9.11.

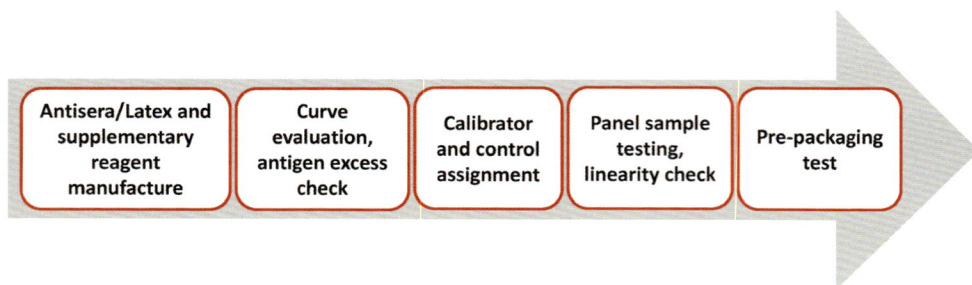

Figure 9.10. Overview of Hevylite kit manufacture.

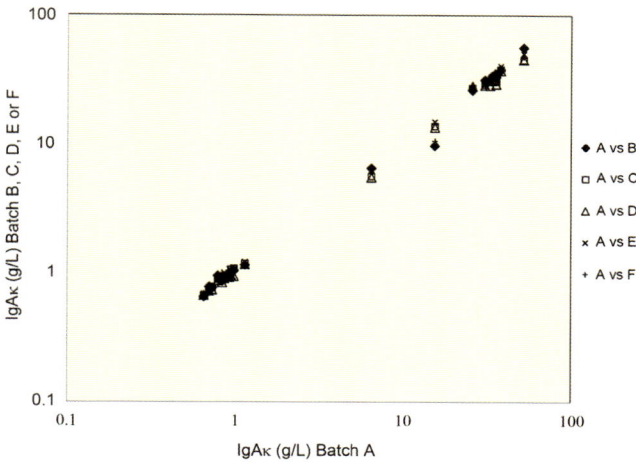

Figure 9.11. Batch-to-batch analysis for IgAκ HLC. *Six IgAκ batches were compared using an in-house quality control panel. In each analysis, values obtained from a predicate batch (A) were compared with values from five separate batches (B to F).*

Assay calibration and kit performance are also controlled by analysing large numbers of normal sera. The results are compared with the normal ranges defined in the product insert *(Chapter 10)*. The results are also summated and compared with the relevant total immunoglobulin assay by Passing-Bablok analysis. The linearity of the kit is evaluated by assaying dilutions of a polyclonal fluid, then once a final pre-packaging test is complete, the kit is packaged, ready for release.

9.8. Immunoassay development on different platforms

IgG, IgA and IgM Hevylite assays were initially launched in 2009/2010, and are available on the Binding Site SPAPLUS and Siemens BN™II instruments. Hevylite assays for the Binding Site Optilite® instrument are also in development. A summary of the features of Hevylite IgM assays is shown in Table 9.2. A full description of Binding Site instruments is present in Chapter 37. A general discussion of Hevylite assay implementation and interpretation is in Chapter 11.

	The Binding Site SPAPLUS		Siemens BNII	
	IgMκ	**IgMλ**	**IgMκ**	**IgMλ**
Sensitivity (g/L) [Dilution]	0.020 [1/1]	0.018 [1/1]	0.010 [1/5]	0.009 [1/5]
Precision (within run, %CV)	1.5 - 2.4%	1.7 - 2.0%	2.8 - 5.6%	1.7 - 4.2%
Precision (between run, %CV)	1.3 - 4.9%	0.5 - 5.4%	2.7 - 4.8%	1.1 - 9.3%
Prozone parameters	Yes	Yes	Yes	Yes
Analytical time (min)	15	15	12	12
Higher dilutions	1 Automatic then off-line	1 Automatic then off-line	Automatic	Automatic

Table 9.2. Comparison of features for IgM HLC assays on the BNII and SPAPLUS.

Test Questions

1. How is the specificity of HLC antisera tested?

2. How are internal reference preparations for HLC assays standardised?

Answers

1. Using a panel of antigens (including monoclonal immunoglobulins of each class, subclass, and light chain type) using RID and turbidimetric/nephelometric techniques *(Section 9.3)*.

2. Using international serum protein reference materials (CRM470 and DA 470k; *Section 9.4)*.

References

1. Bradwell AR, Harding SJ, Fourrier NJ, Wallis GL, Drayson MT, Carr-Smith HD, Mead GP. Assessment of monoclonal gammopathies by nephelometric measurement of individual immunoglobulin kappa/lambda ratios. Clin Chem 2009;55:1646-55

2. Zegers I, Keller T, Schreiber W, Sheldon J, Albertini R, Blirup-Jensen S et al. Characterisation of the new serum protein reference material ERM-DA470k/IFCC: value assignment by immunoassay. Clin Chem 2010;56:1880-8

3. Whicher JT, Ritchie RF, Johnson AM, Baudner S, Bienvenu J, Blirup-Jensen S et al. New international reference preparation for proteins in human serum (RPPHS). Clin Chem 1994;40:934-8

Hevylite reference intervals

Summary:

- Total IgG, IgA and IgM concentrations are standardised using international reference preparations (CRM 470 and DA470k).

- Initial publications of Hevylite® reference intervals were based on prototype Hevylite reagents. Subsequently, reference intervals were published using the fully validated commercial assays.

- Users are recommended to either establish their own local Hevylite reference intervals or validate an existing reference interval.

10.1. Introduction

Total immunoglobulin concentrations in normal individuals are influenced by a number of factors including age, gender and ethnic background[1,2]. In general, immunoglobulin levels are lower when young and increase into adulthood. The exception is IgG in newborn infants: placental transfer of IgG results in high neonatal serum concentrations (near adult levels) that persist for several months after birth.

Significant ethnic differences in immunoglobulin concentrations have been observed. Black Africans have higher levels of IgG and IgM but similar levels of IgA compared with Caucasian populations[3]. Gender may also influence immunoglobulin concentrations and significant differences in IgM reference intervals for males and females have been reported[4].

10.2. Standardisation of immunoglobulin assays

In the early 1970s there were a number of initiatives to standardise immunoglobulin measurements at national levels. This was followed, in 1992, by the release of "Certified Reference Material 470" (CRM 470) by the College of American Pathologists and The Bureau Communitaire de Référence. CRM 470 was prepared from serum collected from several hundred healthy donors in five European cities, which was pooled and processed to produce approximately 40,000 vials, each containing 1 mL of lyophilised serum. After value assignments by reference laboratories in Europe and the USA, this material was accepted as the international standard for 15 commonly measured plasma proteins, including IgG, IgA and IgM[5,6].

By 2008, stocks of CRM 470 were becoming exhausted and the Institute for Reference Materials and Measurements in collaboration with The International Federation of Clinical Chemistry, oversaw an initiative to replace CRM 470 with a new, similar protein reference preparation (DA470k)[7]. Most proteins that had been standardised with CRM 470 were transferred to DA470k, including IgG, IgA and IgM.

10.3. Hevylite standardisation

As DA470k does not have assigned values for the individual light chain types of each immunoglobulin class (that are the targets of the HLC assays), it cannot be used to directly assign values to individual HLC assay calibrators. However, the sum of concentrations measured by pairs of HLC reagents (e.g. IgGκ + IgGλ) should equate to the assigned value for the corresponding total immunoglobulin (i.e. IgG). The calibration of the Hevylite assays is therefore based on this summation, and is further discussed in Section 9.4. It follows that for a particular immunoglobulin class, when the Ig′κ and Ig′λ HLC reference intervals are combined, the range of values should be equivalent to the reference interval for the corresponding total immunoglobulin.

10.4. Hevylite reference intervals

10.4.1. Binding Site Hevylite reference intervals

The first reference intervals for Hevylite assays were established in the Binding Site laboratories with prototype Hevylite reagents on the Siemens BN™II instrument, using different collections of normal serum samples. The results were published in a number of abstracts (Tables 10.1, 10.2 and 10.3)[8,9,10]. In each case, there was a good correlation between the sum of concentrations measured by pairs of HLC reagents and the relevant total immunoglobulin assay (regression coefficient ranged from 0.9 to 0.997)[8,9,10]. A publication by Bradwell et al.[11] followed, which contained HLC reference intervals that were based on a different set of normal samples, but again using prototype reagents. Summation of Ig′κ and Ig′λ HLC results for normal sera produced a good agreement with total immunoglobulin measurements for each HLC specificity.

Shortly after the publication by Bradwell et al.[11], finalised and fully validated HLC reagents became commercially available as CE-marked diagnostic tests for use on the Binding Site SPAPLUS® (a turbidimeter) and the Siemens BNII (a nephelometer) (Chapter 38). Each product insert contains reference intervals determined using the finalised HLC reagents, as well as a comparison of the concentrations determined by summated Ig′κ and Ig′λ HLC compared to total immunoglobulin assays for a range of normal and disease state sera; all showing good agreement. Examples are shown in Figure 9.9.

A summary of the results of these various reference range studies is shown in Tables 10.1, 10.2 and 10.3. From these results, it can be seen that, although there are differences between the various reference intervals for each of the Hevylite parameters, the variations are small. These are likely to reflect sampling variations (when different sets of samples are evaluated) and the use of different instruments which utilise alternative optical detection technologies, namely nephelometry and turbidimetry.

A study using enzyme-linked immunosorbent assays (ELISAs) to measure Ig′κ/Ig′λ ratios (for IgG, IgA and IgM isotypes) in pooled normal sera reported median values that are similar to those obtained with the Hevylite assays[15]. This lends further support to the validity of the IgG HLC ratios determined by Hevylite assays.

Publication	IgGκ (g/L)	IgGλ (g/L)	IgGκ/IgGλ (95% RI)	IgGκ/IgGλ (99% RI)
Harding et al. 2009[10]	3.92 - 12.16	2.28 - 6.05	1.13 - 3.27	
Bradwell et al. 2009[11]	4.23 - 12.18	2.37 - 5.91	1.26 - 3.20	
IgG HLC product inserts: SPAPLUS	3.84 - 12.07	1.91 - 6.74	1.12 - 3.21	
IgG HLC product inserts: BNII	4.03 - 9.78	1.97 - 5.71	0.98 - 2.75	
Katzmann et al. 2013[12]	4.34 - 10.80	1.77 - 5.31	1.30 - 3.70	
Katzmann et al. 2014[13]	4.34 - 10.80	1.77 - 5.31	1.17 - 3.61	1.06 - 4.46

Table 10.1. IgG Hevylite published reference intervals.

Publication	IgAκ (g/L)	IgAλ (g/L)	IgAκ/IgAλ (95% RI)	IgAκ/IgAλ (99% RI)
Bradwell et al. 2008[8]	0.34 - 2.33	0.19 - 2.06	0.67 - 3.12	
Harding et al. 2009[9]	0.51 - 2.48	0.43 - 1.74	0.79 - 2.17	
Bradwell et al. 2009[11]	0.43 - 2.36	0.40 - 1.73	0.58 - 2.52	
IgA HLC product insert: SPAPLUS	0.57 - 2.08	0.44 - 2.04	0.78 - 1.94	
IgA HLC product insert: BNII	0.48 - 2.82	0.36 - 1.98	0.80 - 2.04	
Katzmann et al. 2013[12]	0.53 - 2.62	0.38 - 1.81	0.70 - 2.20	
Katzmann et al. 2014[13]	0.53 - 2.62	0.38 - 1.81	0.70 - 2.21	0.53 - 2.52

Table 10.2. IgA Hevylite published reference intervals.

Publication	IgMκ (g/L)	IgMλ (g/L)	IgMκ/IgMλ (95% RI)	IgMκ/IgMλ (99% RI)
Bradwell et al. 2009[8]	0.33 - 1.54	0.20 - 1.10	0.81 - 2.52	
IgM HLC product insert: SPAPLUS	0.19 - 1.63	0.12 - 1.01	1.18 - 2.74	
IgM HLC product insert: BNII	0.29 - 1.82	0.17 - 0.94	0.96 - 2.30	
Guitarte et al. 2012[14]: SPAPLUS	0.32 - 1.83	0.10 - 0.84	1.38 - 3.54	
Guitarte et al. 2012[14]: BNII	0.26 - 1.53	0.14 - 0.80	1.17 - 2.44	
Katzmann et al. 2013[12]	0.22 - 1.43	0.10 - 0.94	1.00 - 2.40	
Katzmann et al. 2014[13]	0.22 - 1.61	0.10 - 0.94	0.93 - 2.79	0.79 - 4.61

Table 10.3. IgM Hevylite published reference intervals.

10.4.2. Other Hevylite reference intervals

Subsequent to the release of the CE-marked HLC kits, there have been a number of studies in which the reference intervals for the Hevylite assays have been reported. Guirtarte et al.[14] measured IgM HLC in blood donor sera on both the BNII and SPAPLUS instruments, and concluded that reference intervals on each instrument were similar, and comparable to the intervals in the product inserts. Katzmann et al.[12] published reference intervals for all Hevylite specificities on the BNII, and commented that the reference ranges were similar to those previously published by Bradwell et al.[11]. Katzmann et al. report similar reference intervals in their most recent publication[13]. Here they defined both 95% and 99% reference intervals for the IgG, IgA and IgM HLC ratios, and used the 99% intervals to determine clonality. The results from these studies are summarised in Tables 10.1, 10.2 and 10.3.

10.5. Choice of reference interval

Binding Site recommends that users either establish their own local HLC reference intervals, or validate an existing reference interval. The interpretation of HLC assays is further discussed in Chapter 11.

It is notable that the reference intervals for the HLC ratio for each immunoglobulin specificity are consistently different, suggesting that each immunoglobulin isotype makes use of a different repertoire of light chains. Thus, the median value for the IgGκ/IgGλ ratio is 2.0 compared with IgAκ/IgAλ and IgMκ/IgMλ ratios of 1.4 and 1.6, respectively[11].

There are no published studies that investigate the influence of age, gender and ethnic background on HLC concentrations or ratios. Hevylite concentrations in other biological fluids, such as urine and CSF have yet to be studied. Clearly, in any fluid, the sum of the concentrations of each Hevylite pair should equal the total immunoglobulin levels but the ratio of Ig'κ to Ig'λ may differ from that found in serum.

Test Questions

1. What evidence suggests that each immunoglobulin isotype makes use of a different repertoire of light chains?

1. The reference intervals for the HLC ratio for each HLC specificity is different (Section 10.5).

Answers

References

1. Jolliff CR, Cost KM, Stivrins PC, Grossman PP, Nolte CR, Franco SM et al. Reference intervals for serum IgG, IgA, IgM, C3, and C4 as determined by rate nephelometry. Clin Chem 1982;28:126-8

2. Becker W. Variations of immunoglobulins in disease. J Clin Pathol Suppl (Assoc Clin Pathol) 1975;6:92-101

3. Riches PG, Quakyi IA, Gibbs MR, Addison AE. Normal serum immunoglobulin and albumin levels in adult Ghanaians compared with levels in adults in Europe. Trop Geogr Med 1980;32:151-7

4. Rhodes K, Markham RL, Maxwell PM, Monk-Jones ME. Immunoglobulins and the X-chromosome. Br Med J 1969;3:439-41

5. Baudner S, Bienvenu J, Blirup-Jensen S, Carlstrom A, Johnson AM, Milford Ward A. The certification of a matrix reference material for immunochemical measurement of 14 human serum proteins CRM 470. BCR/92/92. Brussels,Belgium: Community Bureau of References (BCR) of the Commission of the European Communities. 1992

6. Whicher JT, Ritchie RF, Johnson AM, Baudner S, Bienvenu J, Blirup-Jensen S et al. New international reference preparation for proteins in human serum (RPPHS). Clin Chem 1994;40:934-8

7. Zegers I, Keller T, Schreiber W, Sheldon J, Albertini R, Blirup-Jensen S et al. Characterisation of the new serum protein reference material ERM-DA470k/IFCC: value assignment by immunoassay. Clin Chem 2010;56:1880-8

8. Bradwell AR, Harding S, Fourrier N, Harris J, Sharp K, Hobbs J et al. Separate nephelometric immunoassays for IgA kappa and IgA lambda for the assessment of patients with multiple myeloma (MM). Clin Chem 2008;54:C116a

9. Harding S, Harris J, Fourrier N, Drayson M, Mead G, Bradwell AR. Quantification of IgA kappa and IgA lambda in human serum using nephelometric assays. Clin Chem Lab Med 2009;47:M-B077a

10. Harding S, Sharp K, Fourrier N, Margetts C, Mead G, Bradwell AR. Nephelometric immunoassays for IgGκ and IgGλ for the assessment of multiple myeloma patients. Clin Chem 2009;55:C23a

11. Bradwell AR, Harding SJ, Fourrier NJ, Wallis GL, Drayson MT, Carr-Smith HD, Mead GP. Assessment of monoclonal gammopathies by nephelometric measurement of individual immunoglobulin kappa/lambda ratios. Clin Chem 2009;55:1646-55

12. Katzmann JA, Clark R, Kyle RA, Larson DR, Therneau TM, Melton LJ, III et al. Suppression of uninvolved immunoglobulins defined by heavy/light-chain pair suppression is a risk factor for progression of MGUS. Leukemia 2013;27:208-12

13. Katzmann JA, Willrich MA, Kohlhagen MC, Kyle RA, Murray DL, Snyder MR et al. Monitoring IgA multiple myeloma: immunoglobulin heavy/light chain assays. Clin Chem 2014 *In press*

14. Guitarte CB, Jiminez J, Campos ML, de Carvalho NB, De Larramendi CH. Specific immunoglobulin heavy/light chain pairs: IgM normal ranges in two different platforms. Clin Chem 2012;58:C-62a

15. Haraldsson A, Kock-Jansen MJ, Jaminon M, van Eck-Arts PB, de Boo T, Weemaes CM, Bakkeren JA. Determination of kappa and lambda light chains in serum immunoglobulins G, A and M. Ann Clin Biochem 1991;28:461-6

Implementation and interpretation of Hevylite immunoassays

Summary:

- Hevylite® assays are validated for the quantification of immunoglobulins in human serum.

- Hevylite results should be interpreted alongside a patient's clinical details and other laboratory tests including serum electrophoresis and total immunoglobulin measurements.

- Summated Hevylite values for a particular immunoglobulin class (Ig′κ + Ig′λ) should equate to the corresponding total immunoglobulin value.

11.1. Implementation of Hevylite assays

IgG, IgA and IgM Hevylite (HLC) assays are polyclonal antisera-based immunoassays, and can be performed on automated laboratory turbidimeters/nephelometers. For each immunoglobulin class, the Ig'κ and Ig'λ (e.g. IgGκ and IgGλ) are measured separately, then results can be expressed as an Ig'κ/Ig'λ HLC ratio (e.g. IgGκ/IgGλ), or as the difference between the involved (iHLC) and uninvolved (uHLC) HLC concentrations (dHLC), in a similar manner to Freelite® serum free light chain (sFLC) assays.

This chapter discusses both the practical aspects of implementing Hevylite assays (including choice of instrument, sample types and biological variation) and interpretation of results.

11.1.1. Choice of instrument

Hevylite immunoassays are available for the Binding Site SPAPLUS® and Siemens BN™II instruments (Chapter 38). Factors that may influence a laboratory's choice of instrument include assay time, workload, complete testing menu offered and existing platforms etc.

It is recommended that all laboratories performing Hevylite assays participate in external quality assurance (EQA) schemes. These are discussed in Chapter 39.

11.1.2. Reporting units

It is important to ensure that IgG, IgA and IgM HLC concentrations are reported in consistent units. In the UK the preferred reporting units are g/L. Within the USA, results may be either in g/L or g/dL.

11.1.3. Choice of sample

IgG, IgA and IgM Hevylite assays are validated for the quantification of immunoglobulins in human serum. Hevylite assays are not validated for use with any other sample types.

Samples that are grossly haemolysed, lipaemic, or with highly elevated billirubin may impact upon the performance of the assay. The maximum concentration of interfering substances that do not cause significant assay interference is stated in the product insert. An example of interference testing for IgGκ and IgGλ HLC assays is shown for the Binding Site SPAPLUS in Table 11.1.

Interfering substance	Concentrations	Deviation from target value	
		IgGκ HLC	IgGλ HLC
Haemoglobin	4.56 g/L	-1.3%	2.2%
Chyle	1540 formazin turbidity units	1.6%	3.8%
Bilirubin	200 mg/L	-2.0%	-1.6%

Table 11.1. Interference testing for IgGκ and IgGλ HLC assays on the Binding Site SPAPLUS. Interference was tested using a control serum containing 0.71 g/L of IgGκ or 0.74 g/L of IgGλ, tested at the minimum sample dilution (1/1).

11.1.4. Sample and reagent stability

An in-house study was conducted to assess the stability of HLC measurements in unpreserved serum samples (n=10) stored first at 22 °C for 2 days, then at 2 - 8 °C for 28 days (in order to mimic shipping followed by refrigerated storage)[1]. For each sample, IgGκ, IgGλ, IgAκ, IgAλ, IgMκ and IgMλ HLCs were measured in triplicate on the day of collection and at regular intervals during storage. There was no significant change observed in HLC values over 28 days (Table 11.2). However, the HLC product inserts recommend that samples are stored for a maximum of 21 days at 2 to 8 °C prior to analysis, to match the guidance in the Freelite product inserts (as sFLCs may be measured in the same sample; Section 7.1.4).

Specificity	Mean concentration at collection (g/L)	Change in concentration at day 28 (% difference from collection value)	
		Mean	Range of values
IgAκ	1.316	4.3	+1 to +5
IgAλ	1.212	1.6	0 to +5
IgGκ	8.400	2.6	0 to +6
IgGλ	3.643	-2.8	-7 to 0
IgMκ	0.503	-1	0 to -11
IgMλ	0.378	-7	-2 to -12

Table 11.2. HLC concentrations in unpreserved sera measured after storage at 2 - 8 °C.

A second in-house study assessed the stability of HLCs in unpreserved serum samples (n=10) stored at 22 °C for 2 days, and then at -20 °C for 28 days[1]. For each sample, IgGκ, IgGλ, IgAκ, IgAλ, IgMκ and IgMλ HLC were measured in triplicate on the day of collection and after 0 and 28 days storage at -20 °C. There was no significant change in HLC values over the time course (Table 11.3, similar to the reported stability of FLCs; Section 7.1.4). Therefore, for long term storage of serum samples prior to HLC analysis, it is recommended that samples are stored frozen at ≤-20 °C.

Specificity	Mean concentration at collection (g/L)	Change in concentration at day 28 (% difference from collection value)
		Mean
IgAκ	1.31	4.0%
IgAλ	1.21	0.8%
IgGκ	8.40	0.4%
IgGλ	3.64	-2.7%
IgMκ	0.50	-5%
IgMλ	0.38	-3%

Table 11.3. Change in HLC values measured after storage of unpreserved sera at -20 °C.

Katzmann et al.[2] studied the stability of all six HLC specificities in 10 serum samples. Sample aliquots were assayed after storage for 7 days at room temperature, storage for 7 days at 4 °C or after 3 freeze/thaw cycles. The observed percentage change in HLC values was minimal *(Table 11.4)*, and the authors concluded that the stability was acceptable for routine use in a clinical laboratory.

Storage	Mean change in HLC concentration from day 0	Maximum decrease in HLC concentration from day 0
7 days at room temperature	-2.5%	4.7%
7 days at 4 °C	-2.2%	4.9%
3 freeze/thaw cycles	-3.4%	6.7%

Table 11.4. Change in HLC values measured after storage of sera under different conditions[2].

Stability of the Hevylite reagents is also an important issue. "Open-vial stability" refers to the shelf-life of the reagents after their first use. Open-vial stability of 3 months has been validated for all HLC specificities.

11.1.5. Changing batch of reagent or instrument

During Hevylite assay manufacture batch-to-batch consistency is maintained *(Section 9.7)*, so that changing from one batch to the next should not present the laboratory with any issues. However, it is still recommended that identical internal quality control samples are measured with both the new batch and the existing batch to confirm consistency. Similar checks should be employed when changing instruments.

11.2. Interpretation of Hevylite assays

As with any laboratory test, Hevylite results should be interpreted alongside a patient's clinical details and other laboratory tests. When serial monitoring data is available, results should be compared with previous measurements to check they are consistent and to identify trends.

11.2.1. Normal reference intervals

A number of published normal reference intervals are available for Hevylite assays. These are discussed further in Chapter 10. Users are recommended to either establish their own local ranges or validate an existing reference interval.

11.2.2. Terminology

For a particular Hevylite specificity, both Ig'κ and Ig'λ HLC should always be measured, and the Ig'κ/Ig'λ HLC ratio calculated. Definitions of commonly used terms are given in Table 11.5. For serial measurements, either the iHLC or the HLC ratio may be used[2,3], with a recent report suggesting dHLC may provide some additional utility[4]. When an abnormal HLC ratio is present, and the concentration of the uninvolved HLC-pair is below the normal reference interval, this is termed "HLC-pair suppression".

Term	Definition	Comment	For an IgGκ MM tumour...
iHLC	Involved HLC	The HLC type that is produced by the tumour, as determined by Hevylite (only applicable if an abnormal HLC ratio is present).	IgGκ
uHLC	Uninvolved HLC	For a particular immunoglobulin class, the HLC type that is the alternate light chain to the iHLC (only applicable if an abnormal HLC ratio is present).	IgGλ
Ig'κ/Ig'λ ratio or HLC ratio	IgGκ	A ratio of the concentration of Ig'κ to Ig'λ HLC.	IgGκ/IgGλ
dHLC	iHLC - uHLC	The difference in concentration between the iHLC and uHLC.	IgGκ - IgGλ

Table 11.5. Summary of HLC terminology.

11.2.3. Result interpretation

A raised concentration of one HLC type, with an abnormal HLC ratio is indicative of monoclonal immunoglobulin production. Renal impairment is not known to influence HLC results, since intact immunoglobulin molecules are not cleared by the kidney *(Chapter 3)*.

11.2.4. The HLC dot plot

In some cases it may be helpful to plot an individual patient's result (or an entire cohort of patients' results) on a HLC dot plot *(Figure 11.1)*. This is a graph displaying Ig'κ HLC concentrations (x-axis) against Ig'λ HLC concentrations (y-axis), both on logarithmic scales. The limits of the normal reference interval for the Ig'κ/Ig'λ HLC ratio are represented by two parallel lines. Each patient result is represented by a single point. If the Ig'κ/Ig'λ HLC ratio is normal, the result will fall within the normal reference interval. A result that lies outside the normal reference interval is consistent with the presence of a monoclonal intact immunoglobulin.

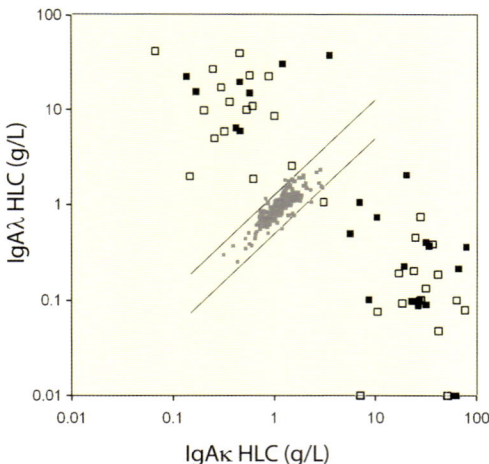

Figure 11.1. HLC dot plot showing results for 56 patients with IgA MM. Solid squares: patients with monoclonal IgA that could be quantified by SPE; open squares: patients with anodal migration of their monoclonal IgA, which made accurate quantification impossible. (Reprinted by permission from Macmillan Publishers Ltd: Leukemia[5], copyright 2013)

11.2.5. Freelite and Hevylite are independent tumour markers

Intact immunoglobulins (and therefore Hevylite measurements) and FLCs are independent tumour markers. For example, a plot of IgGκ HLC vs. κ sFLC concentrations for 170 IgGκ MM patients showed no correlation between the two parameters *(Figure 11.2)*. This important point is discussed further in Section 17.2.

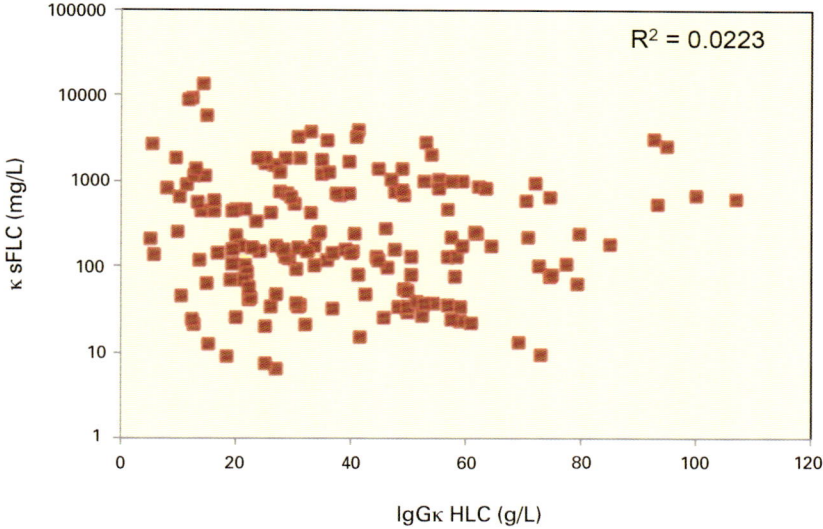

Figure 11.2. A plot of serum IgGκ concentrations vs. κ sFLC concentrations for 170 patients with MM producing monoclonal IgGκ.

11.2.6. Biological variation

Knowledge of the biological variation of HLC in serum is useful when interpreting monitoring data for individual patients. There is currently only limited information on the biological variation of HLC measurements in healthy subjects. Finlay et al.[6] studied the biological variation of IgG and IgA HLC in 15 healthy blood donors. Samples were collected on the same day of the week, every 2 weeks for 6 weeks. The laboratory's analytical performance (CV_A) for all methods was acceptable, ranging from 3.4 to 9.4% *(Table 11.6)*. For all HLC specificities, the within-subject variation (CV_I) was less than the within group variation (CV_G) *(Table 11.6)*.

Analyte	n	Mean (g/L)	CV_A (%)	CV_I (%)	CV_G (%)	RCV (%)
IgGκ	15	6.0	9.4	12.3	24.9	41
IgGλ	15	3.6	3.4	5.9	16.3	28
IgAκ	15	1.1	5.3	7.2	33.3	30
IgAλ	15	1.0	3.8	8.0	35.8	32

Table 11.6. Biological variation of IgG and IgA HLC[5]. CV_A: analytical variation; CV_I: within-subject variation; CV_G: within-group variation; RCV: reference change value.

The reference change value (RCV) defines the minimum difference between two consecutive measurements from the same individual, which can be considered significant ($p<0.05$). In this study the RCV for all analytes was similar, with values of around 30 to 40%. This is similar to the RCV for monoclonal protein measurements determined by SPE, in patients with stable monoclonal gammopathy[7].

11.3. Non-linearity

Sample non-linearity can be defined as a sample that when measured at different dilutions gives a substantially different result *(Section 7.3)*. Sample non-linearity should not be confused with assay non-linearity; if an assay is non-linear all samples will give substantially different results when measured at different dilutions. Assessment of Hevylite assay linearity formed an important part of immunoassay development and validation *(Sections 9.5 and 9.6)*.

As with all immunoassays, Hevylite assays may be prone to occasional sample non-linearity. Sample-specific non-linearity may occur in some samples when measured with Hevylite assays due to: 1) non-specific interference (matrix effects); or 2) the inherent structural variability of monoclonal immunoglobulins *(Chapter 3)*.

11.3.1. Managing non-linearity

Binding Site recommend following the sample dilution protocol as shown in each product insert and reporting the first plausible result only. The use of non-standard sample dilutions, or skipping dilutions should be avoided. Examples of non-linear samples are shown in Table 11.7.

Dilution	IgAκ HLC (g/L)	IgAλ HLC (g/L)
1/100	>11.3	>10.4
1/400	**21.4**	**8.0**
1/2000	19.1	11.2

Table 11.7. Examples of non-linear IgA Hevylite results using a Siemens BNII analyser. The first plausible result should be reported (in bold).

11.4. Antigen excess

Antigen excess occurs when an antigen is present at such high concentrations that it interferes with antigen-antibody crosslinking, resulting in the formation of smaller immune complexes *(Figure 7.4)*. This causes immunoassays to underestimate high concentrations of protein.

Serum Hevylite concentrations can range from <0.020 mg/L to >100 g/L. This is a greater range than most other serum proteins. Hevylite IgM assays on the Binding Site SPAPLUS and Siemens BNII instruments include in built prozone parameters *(Chapter 39)*. For example, the Binding Site SPAPLUS instrument monitors the initial reaction kinetics of each sample at three separate time intervals and compares the results with reaction limits set by the manufacturer (through testing an extensive myeloma library; *Figure 7.5*). Samples detected as being in antigen excess are automatically flagged by the instrument and retested at a higher sample dilution. A very small proportion of samples in antigen excess have normal reaction kinetics so will not prompt the flag. Such cases are considered rare, but cannot be excluded. Hevylite IgA and IgG assays do not include automatic antigen excess detection as the upper limit of the measuring range is higher than that of IgM assays. For these assays, any sample giving unexpected results should be retested at a higher dilution to preclude antigen excess.

The antigen excess capacity is routinely tested during Hevylite assay production. For each HLC assay, a panel of samples containing high concentrations of the corresponding monoclonal intact immunoglobulin type is analysed at the minimum sample dilution over three reagent lots. Samples that give a scatter signal less than the signal produced by the top calibrator are judged to be in antigen excess. Samples are then diluted and the analysis repeated to calculate the antigen excess capacity of each assay. This value is typically between 52 and 100 g/L, depending on the specificity.

11.5. Comparison of Hevylite results with other immunoglobulin tests

11.5.1. Comparison of Hevylite and total immunoglobulin measurements

In general, the agreement between summated Hevylite (e.g. IgGκ + IgGλ) and total immunoglobulin assays (e.g. IgG) is good; indeed, comparison of summation data was used to validate the assays during development and summation checks are used as part of the manufacturing quality control *(Sections 9.4.5 and 9.7)*. As part of an evaluation of HLC assays for monitoring MM patients, Katzmann et al.[2] compared total IgA quantification and the IgA iHLC for 149 IgA MM samples. Passing–Bablok linear regression gave a slope of 1.124 (95% CI 1.015–1.194), r = 0.969 *(Figure 11.3A)*. The more a MM tumour suppresses the production of polyclonal immunoglobulin (of the same immunoglobulin class), the closer will be the correspondence between iHLC concentrations with both the total immunoglobulin concentrations and the monoclonal immunoglobulin concentrations, as measured by densitometry of SPE gels.

When a high concentration of polyclonal immunoglobulins is present, Hevylite measurements may be less sensitive than serum electrophoretic techniques for detecting a monoclonal protein (e.g. MGUS; *Chapter 13*). However, an abnormal HLC ratio has been shown to be present in 97 – 100% of patients with IgG or IgA MM at diagnosis *(Section 17.6)*, including patients with oligosecretory disease *(Section 18.4.2)*.

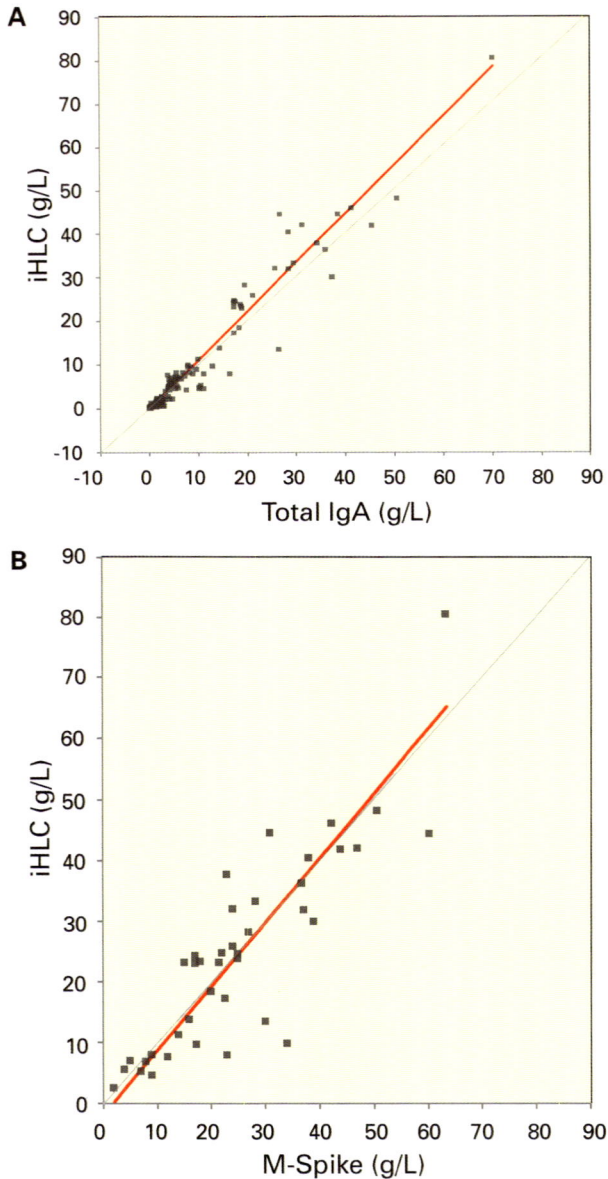

Figure 11.3. (A) A plot of total IgA versus IgA iHLC concentrations for 149 patients with IgA MM. *Passing–Bablok linear regression has a slope of 1.124, r = 0.97.* **(B) A plot of M-spike versus iHLC concentrations for 41 patients with IgA MM.** *Passing–Bablok linear regression has a slope of 1.05, r = 0.87.* *(Republished with permission of Clinical Chemistry[2]; permission conveyed through Copyright Clearance Center, Inc.)*

11.5.2. Comparison of Hevylite and immmunoglobulin measurements by SPE

In an in-house study, the IgG iHLC concentration was compared with the monoclonal concentration, determined by SPE scanning densitometry, for 160 IgG MM patients. In the majority of patients, the concentration determined by the two methods was similar but some samples did show variance *(Figure 11.4)*. Possible explanations for the variance include inaccurate SPE measurements, for example if the monoclonal protein co-migrated with other serum proteins (e.g. transferrin), or dye saturation underestimated the concentration of IgG monoclonal proteins. This is discussed in more detail in Section 17.4.

Katzmann et al.[2] compared the iHLC concentration with the monoclonal protein concentration determined by SPE for 114 IgG and 41 IgA MM serum samples. Each sample had a band present on SPE (M-spike) and a corresponding abnormal HLC ratio. There was a linear correlation between the iHLC concentrations and the M-spike for both IgG and IgA patients *(Figures 11.5 and 11.3B)*. The correlation of iHLC with total IgA *(Figure 11.3A; r=0.97)* was better than SPE M-spike *(Figure 11.3B; r=0.87)*. The authors commented that this was most likely to be due to the difficulty of quantitating β-migrating monoclonal proteins that co-migrate with other serum proteins *(Section 17.4)*. The study also compared the relative changes in the iHLC and serum M-spike concentration for 13 IgG patients for whom diagnostic and four follow-up samples were available. The relative changes of the mean iHLC and mean M-spike were not statistically different *(p>0.75; Figure 11.6)*.

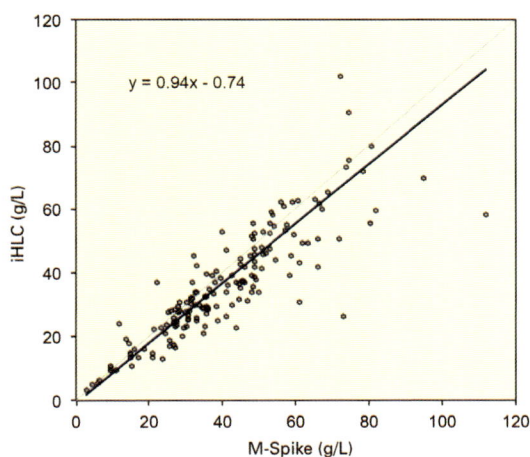

Figure 11.4. A plot of M-spike versus iHLC concentration for 160 IgG MM patients.

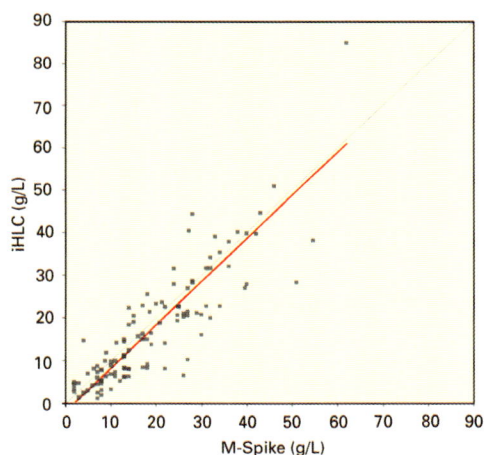

Figure 11.5. A plot of M-spike versus iHLC concentrations for 114 patients with IgG MM, that had both an M-spike and an abnormal IgG HLC ratio. Passing–Bablok linear regression has a slope of 1.02 (95% CI 0.89–1.13), r = 0.87. (Republished with permission of Clinical Chemistry[2]; permission conveyed through Copyright Clearance Center, Inc.)

11.5.3. Comparison of Hevylite and immunofixation electrophoresis

During the follow-up of patients with monoclonal gammopathies, there are occasionally discrepancies between Hevylite and immunofixation results. Two scenarios are discussed below.

1) IFE positive, normal HLC ratio: in IgG patients, recycling of IgG by the FcRn receptor may result in the persistence of small IgG monoclonal proteins in the serum, causing IFE to remain positive long after the tumour has been eradicated and HLC pair suppression has ended *(Section 18.4.5)*. In addition, in a minority of cases, the diagnostic sensitivity of IFE may be superior to that of the HLC ratio. For example, if a small IgG monoclonal protein is present with a large amount of polyclonal IgG[8]. Finally, on rare occasions, Hevylite antigen excess may cause a sample value to be falsely low. If antigen excess is suspected, an additional sample dilution should be performed *(Section 11.4)*.

2) IFE negative, abnormal HLC ratio: in some patients, the HLC ratio may be more sensitive for detecting a monoclonal immunoglobulin than IFE. This is more common for IgA and IgM where there is less polyclonal production so smaller amounts of monoclonal immunoglobulin can produce an abnormal HLC ratio. An abnormal HLC ratio may indicate residual disease in IIMM patients whose electrophoresis results have normalised following therapy *(Section 18.4.3)*.

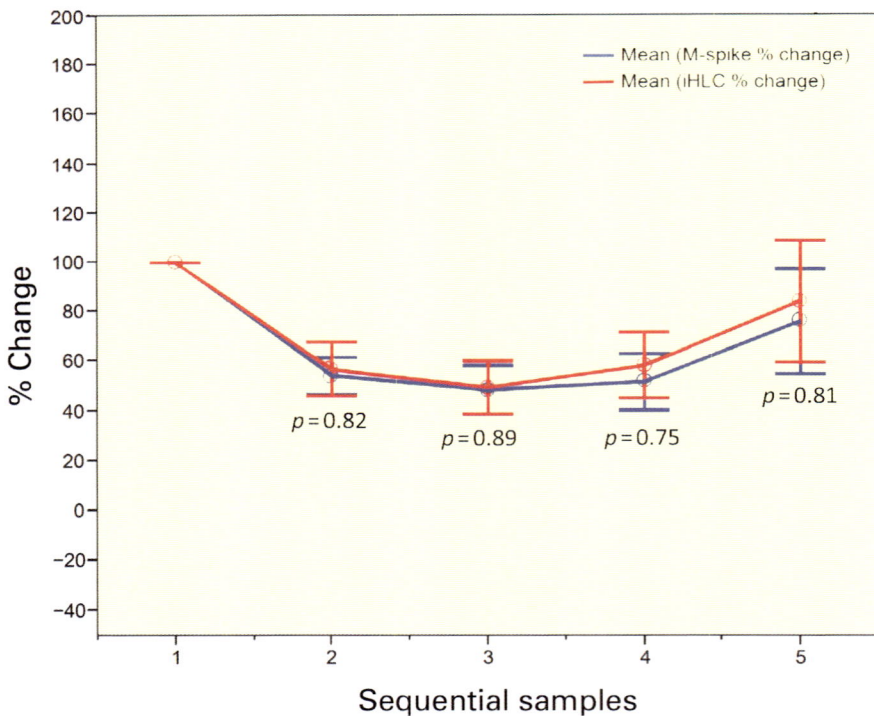

Figure 11.6. Mean M-spike % change and mean iHLC % change for sequential samples from 13 IgG MM patients (with standard error of the mean). Note: Sample 1 = diagnostic sample defined as 100%. Samples 2–5 = post-treatment, follow-up samples. P value derived from unpaired Student t-test. (Republished with permission of Clinical Chemistry[2]; permission conveyed through Copyright Clearance Center, Inc.)

Test Questions

1. When monitoring HLC values in a patient, what percentage change is necessary to be statistically significant (p<0.05)?

Answers

The relative change value (RCV) for HLC measurements has been calculated to be between 30 and 40% (Section 11.2.6).

References

1. Matters D. Stability of free light chains and heavy/light chains in serum samples after an initial shipping period at 22 degrees Celsius. Hematology Reports 2010;2:G73a2.

2. Katzmann JA, Willrich MA, Kohlhagen MC, Kyle RA, Murray DL, Snyder MR et al. Monitoring IgA multiple myeloma: immunoglobulin heavy/light chain assays. Clin Chem 2014 In press

3. Ludwig H, Milosavljevic D, Zojer N, Faint JM, Bradwell AR, Hubl W, Harding SJ. Immunoglobulin heavy/light chain ratios improve paraprotein detection and monitoring, identify residual disease and correlate with survival in multiple myeloma patients. Leukemia 2013;27:213-9

4. Bhutani M, Costello R, Korde N, Manasanch E, Kwok M, Tageja N et al. Serum heavy-light chains (HLC) and free light chains (FLC) as predictors for early CR in newly diagnosed myeloma patients treated with Carfilzomib, Lenalidomide, and Dexamethasone (CRd). Blood 2013;122:762a

5. Finlay JA, Wu AH. Biological variation of immunoglobulin heavy chain-light chain pairs in serum. Clin Chim Acta 2014;25:68-71

6. Katzmann JA, Snyder MR, Rajkumar SV, Kyle RA, Therneau TM, Benson JT, Dispenzieri A. Long-term biologic variation of serum protein electrophoresis M-spike, urine M-spike, and monoclonal serum free light chain quantification: implications for monitoring monoclonal gammopathies. Clin Chem 2011;57:1687-92

7. Katzmann JA, Clark R, Kyle RA, Larson DR, Therneau TM, Melton LJ, III et al. Suppression of uninvolved immunoglobulins defined by heavy/light-chain pair suppression is a risk factor for progression of MGUS. Leukemia 2013;27:208-12

An overview of multiple myeloma and related disorders

12.1. Introduction

The main clinical applications of serum free light chain (sFLC) and immunoglobulin heavy/light chain (Hevylite®, HLC) measurements are for patients with monoclonal gammopathies. Figure 12.1 shows the associated diseases seen at the Mayo Clinic in 2005[1]. Since these data are from a specialist referral centre, general hospitals will probably see different patterns of disease referral with a higher percentage of multiple myeloma (MM) and monoclonal gammopathy of undetermined significance (MGUS) and fewer AL amyloidosis patients.

This section presents an overview of the use of sFLC and HLC measurements in MM and related disorders; from pre-malignant MGUS and smouldering multiple myeloma (SMM), to the symptomatic disorders MM, plasmacytoma and plasma cell leukaemia.

■MGUS   ■Multiple myeloma
■AL amyloidosis   ■Lymphoproliferative
■Smouldering multiple myeloma   ■Solitary or extramedullary plasmacytoma
■Waldenström's macroglobulinaemia   ■Other

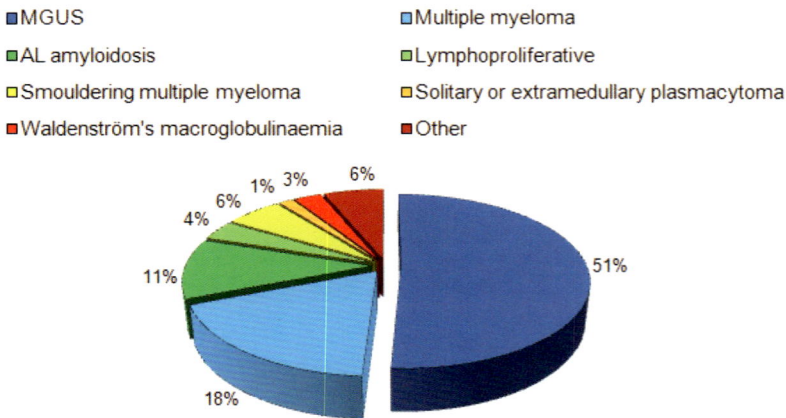

Figure 12.1. Monoclonal gammopathies diagnosed at the Mayo Clinic during 2005.

12.2. Multiple myeloma and related malignant disorders

MM is the second most common form of haematological malignancy after non-Hodgkin lymphoma, and accounts for around 1% of all cancers. In Caucasian populations the annual incidence is approximately 60 per million, and this increases with age[2,3]. The number of new cases diagnosed each year is around 4,800 in the UK and almost 40,000 across Europe[3]. Worldwide, this figure rises to around 114,000, and a large variation in the incidence rates between different populations is observed *(Figure 12.2)*[2]. Furthermore, the incidence is slowly rising. In Europe, the incidence of MM has risen by approximately 10% in the last decade[3]. Survival rates for patients with MM are continually improving as a result of new treatments[4]. For example, 5-year survival in England has increased from around 10% in the early 1970s to >35% in 2005 – 2009 *(Figure 12.3)*[5].

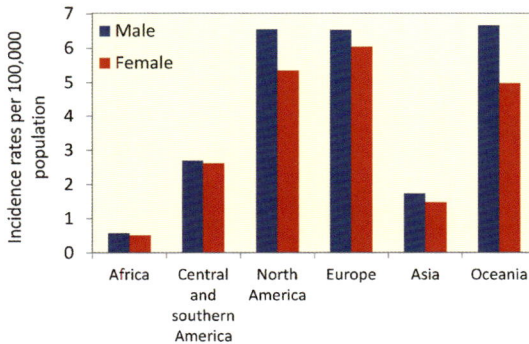

Figure 12.2. Worldwide incidence rates for MM (crude rate/100,000 population)[2].

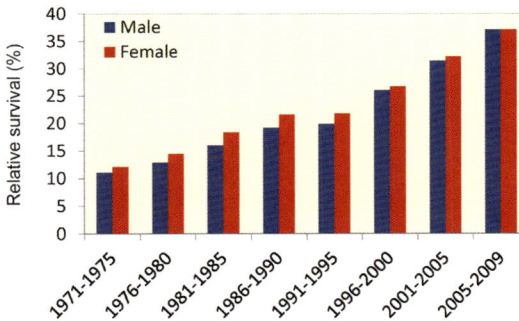

Figure 12.3. Age-standardised five-year myeloma survival rates in England from 1971-2009[5].

According to international guidelines, serum electrophoresis and sFLC analysis constitute an effective screen for monoclonal plasmaproliferative disorders (other than AL amyloidosis, *Chapters 23 and 25*). Until recently, the diagnosis of MM was solely based on the presence of excess monoclonal plasma cells in the bone marrow alongside related organ or tissue impairment (i.e. hypercalcaemia, renal insufficiency, anaemia or bone lesions, *Figure 12.4*). However, guidelines now state that serum markers, including highly abnormal sFLCs (defined as an involved/uninvolved Freelite® sFLC ratio ≥100), can form part of the diagnostic criteria for MM (*Section 25.2*)[6].

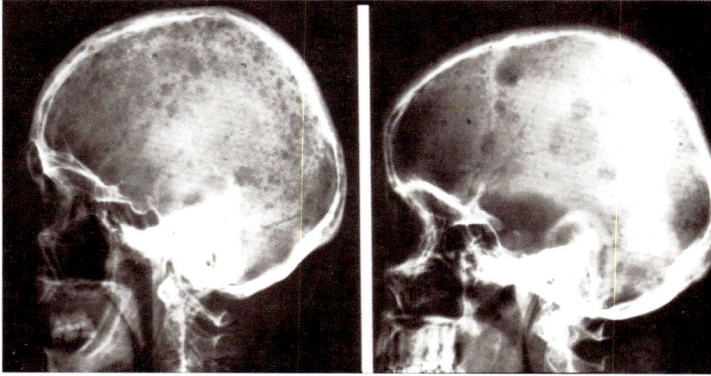

Figure 12.4. Osteolytic lesions in the skulls of 2 patients with MM.

MM patients can be subdivided into secretory and non-secretory types based on the presence or absence of a detectable monoclonal protein, with nonsecretory patients representing only 2% of cases[6]. The majority (85%) of patients with MM secrete an intact immunoglobulin monoclonal protein. The relative frequency of the classes of immunoglobulin secreted by the plasma cell clones reflect the frequencies normally observed in the body. Light chain MM (LCMM) and nonsecretory MM (NSMM) represent a further 13% and 2% of MM patients, respectively. A summary of MM monoclonal protein types is shown in Figure 12.5; this data is from more than 2500 patients entered into the UK Medical Research Council MM trials[7].

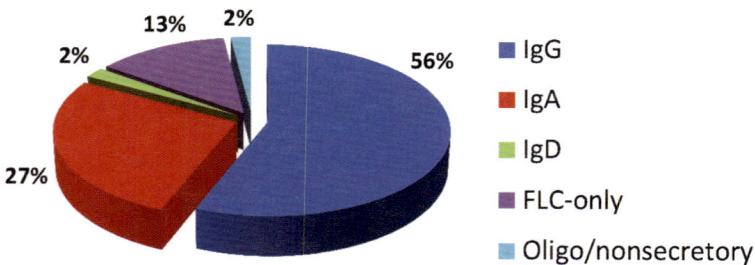

Figure 12.5. Classification of MM based upon monoclonal protein production in 2709 Medical Research Council myeloma trial patients.

Over the past 15 years, there have been publications covering many aspects of sFLC analysis in LCMM (*Chapter 15*), NSMM (*Chapter 16)* and intact immunoglobulin MM (IIMM; *Chapters 17 and 18*). Additionally, clinical applications of sFLC testing have been described in other malignant conditions that are related to MM, including plasmacytoma (*Chapter 21*) and plasma cell leukaemia (*Chapter 22*). These publications, are reviewed in Section 4, addressing the use of sFLCs at initial diagnosis, to monitor treatment response and predict survival. The inclusion of sFLCs for routine monoclonal gammopathy screening and the relative merits of serum versus urine FLC measurements are also discussed (*Chapter 23 and Chapter 24*). It is well established that sFLC measurements provide valuable information in patients with diseases with monoclonal light chain deposition, such as cast nephropathy, AL amyloidosis and light chain deposition disease. These clinical applications are addressed in the succeeding section *(Section 5)*.

Following the introduction of Hevylite assays, there is accumulating evidence showing that HLC analysis provides an additional tool for the management of patients with MM, by giving a quantitative and non-subjective indication of clonality. This evidence is presented in Chapters 17 and 18.

12.3. MGUS and SMM

MGUS is a pre-malignant, asymptomatic plasma cell proliferative disorder that is estimated to affect 3% of the general population aged 50 years or older[8]. Patients with MGUS progress to myeloma or a related malignancy at a rate of around 1% per year[9]. Three distinct types of MGUS can be defined based on the monoclonal protein type: IgM MGUS, non-IgM (IgG or IgA) MGUS, and FLC MGUS (*Table 12.1*)[6]. In general, IgM MGUS is associated with evolution to lymphoplasmacytic tumours such as Waldenström's macroglobulinaemia (WM), whereas non-IgM MGUS is associated with evolution to MM[10].

Monoclonal protein	Pre-malignancy with a low risk of progression (0.3 - 2% per year)	Pre-malignancy with a high risk of progression (5 - 10% per year)	Malignancy
IgG or IgA (non-IgM)	Non-IgM MGUS	SMM	**MM,** Plasmacytoma, NHL, CLL, AL amyloidosis
IgM	IgM MGUS	Smouldering WM	**WM,** IgM MM, NHL, CLL, AL amyloidosis
Light chain	Light chain MGUS	Smouldering LCMM (idiopathic Bence Jones proteinuria)	**LCMM, AL amyloidosis,** NSMM

Table 12.1. Clinical types of MGUS and their evolution into malignant lymphoproliferative disorders[11,12,13,14]. *The most common associated malignancies are highlighted in bold. MGUS: monoclonal gammopathy of undetermined significance; MM: multiple myeloma; SMM: smouldering MM; LCMM: light chain MM; NSMM: nonsecretory MM; WM: Waldenström's macroglobulinaemia; NHL: non-Hodgkin lymphoma; CLL: chronic lymphocytic leukaemia.*

SMM is an intermediate clinical stage between MGUS and MM which carries a higher risk of progression to malignant disease (around 10% per year for the first 5 years)[15]. Recent studies indicate that in the spectrum of disease development from MGUS, through SMM to symptomatic MM, monoclonal FLC production becomes progressively more probable. Approximately one-third of MGUS patients have an abnormal κ/λ sFLC ratio at diagnosis; this increases to around 80% in patients with SMM and 95% in MM.

In both MGUS (*Chapter 13*) and SMM (*Chapter 14)* an abnormal κ/λ sFLC ratio indicates a higher risk of progression to malignancy than a normal ratio[16,17,18,19]. In these patients, sFLC analysis plays an important role in risk stratification and disease management, such that international guidelines recommend that patients with either MGUS or SMM should be risk-stratified at diagnosis to optimise counselling and follow-up (*Chapter 25)*[20]. Whilst the benefits of sFLC analysis in MGUS and SMM risk-stratification are well established, HLC analysis is emerging as a new prognostic tool in these pre-malignant conditions.

12.4. Improving our understanding of disease pathogenesis

Data from measurement of sFLCs and HLCs has made a contribution to our understanding of monoclonal gammopathies. This includes aspects of: 1) clonal heterogeneity; 2) disease evolution, and 3) the bone marrow microenvironment.

Progression from MGUS to MM can involve a complicated branching transformation from benign to malignant clones, resulting in the presence of multiple clones at diagnosis (*Chapter 19)*. Genetic transformations change the clonal composition during the course of disease and these changes may be reflected by changes in monoclonal protein production. Monitoring patients with a combination of HLC and FLC measurements provides information on tumour clones that may evolve over time. One such example is free light chain escape (FLC escape), first characterised in 1969, in which a patient with intact immunoglobulin MM relapsed with an increase in FLCs, but with no associated increase in intact immunoglobulins (*Section 18.2.1)*[21]. The importance of monitoring intact immunoglobulins and FLCs to survey these changes is discussed in Chapters 18 and 19.

More recently, quantitation of uninvolved polyclonal immunoglobulins of the same isotype as the monoclonal immunoglobulin (HLC-pair) has offered insights into tumour biology and the bone marrow microenvironment. Several studies have demonstrated the prognostic value of HLC-pair suppression in MGUS (*Chapter 13*) and MM (*Chapter 20)*.

References

1. Kyle RA, Rajkumar SV. Monoclonal gammopathy of undetermined significance. Br J Haematol 2006;134:573-89

2. International Agency for Research on Cancer. Cancer incidence in five continents, Volume X: ci5.iarc.fr, accessed October 2014

3. Cancer Research UK. Myeloma incidence statistics: http://www.cancerresearchuk.org/cancer-info/cancerstats/types/myeloma/incidence, accessed October 2014

4. Kumar SK, Dispenzieri A, Lacy MQ, Gertz MA, Buadi FK, Pandey S et al. Continued improvement in survival in multiple myeloma: changes in early mortality and outcomes in older patients. Leukemia 2014;28:1122-8

5. Cancer Research UK. Myeloma survival statistics: http://www.cancerresearchuk.org/cancer-info/cancerstats/types/myeloma/survival, accessed October 2014

6. Rajkumar SV, Dimopolous MA, Palumbo A, Blade J, Merlini G, Mateos MV et al. International Myeloma Working Group updated criteria for the diagnosis of multiple myeloma. Lancet Oncology 2014;15:e538-e548

7. Brioli A, Giles H, Pawlyn C, Campbell J, Kaiser M, Melchor L et al. Serum free light chain evaluation as a marker for the impact of intra-clonal heterogeneity on the progression and treatment resistance in multiple myeloma. Blood 2014;123:3414-9

8. Kyle RA, Therneau TM, Rajkumar SV, Larson DR, Plevak MF, Offord JR et al. Prevalence of monoclonal gammopathy of undetermined significance. N Engl J Med 2006;354:1362-9

9. Kyle RA, Therneau TM, Rajkumar SV, Offord JR, Larson DR, Plevak MF, Melton LJ, III. A long-term study of prognosis in monoclonal gammopathy of undetermined significance. N Engl J Med 2002;346:564-9

10. Kyle RA, Therneau TM, Rajkumar SV, Remstein ED, Offord JR, Larson DR et al. Long-term follow-up of IgM monoclonal gammopathy of undetermined significance. Blood 2003;102:3759-64

11. Weiss BM, Abadie J, Verma P, Howard RS, Kuehl WM. A monoclonal gammopathy precedes multiple myeloma in most patients. Blood 2009;113:5418-22

12. Cesana C, Klersy C, Barbarano L, Nosari AM, Crugnola M, Pungolino E et al. Prognostic factors for malignant transformation in monoclonal gammopathy of undetermined significance and smoldering multiple myeloma. J Clin Oncol 2002;20:1625-34

13. Kyle RA, Larson DR, Therneau TM, Dispenzieri A, Melton LJ, Benson JT et al. Clinical course of light-chain smouldering multiple myeloma (idiopathic Bence Jones proteinuria): a retrospective cohort study. Lancet Hematology 2014;1:e28-e36

14. Korde N, Kristinsson SY, Landgren O. Monoclonal gammopathy of undetermined significance (MGUS) and smoldering multiple myeloma (SMM): novel biological insights and development of early treatment strategies. Blood 2011;117:5573-81

15. Kyle RA, Remstein ED, Therneau TM, Dispenzieri A, Kurtin PJ, Hodnefield JM et al. Clinical course and prognosis of smoldering (asymptomatic) multiple myeloma. N Engl J Med 2007;356:2582-90

16. Dispenzieri A, Kyle RA, Katzmann JA, Therneau TM, Larson D, Benson J et al. Immunoglobulin free light chain ratio is an independent risk factor for progression of smoldering (asymptomatic) multiple myeloma. Blood 2008;111:785-9

17. Rajkumar SV, Kyle RA, Therneau TM, Melton LJ, III, Bradwell AR, Clark RJ et al. Serum free light chain ratio is an independent risk factor for progression in monoclonal gammopathy of undetermined significance. Blood 2005;106:812-7

18. Turesson I, Kovalchik SA, Pfeiffer RM, Kristinsson SY, Goldin LR, Drayson MT, Landgren O. Monoclonal gammopathy of undetermined significance and risk of lymphoid and myeloid malignancies: 728 cases followed up to 30 years in Sweden. Blood 2014;123:338-45

19. Watters E, Calder M. MGUS Myeloma UK Infosheet 2013

20. Kyle RA, Durie BG, Rajkumar SV, Landgren O, Blade J, Merlini G et al. Monoclonal gammopathy of undetermined significance (MGUS) and smoldering (asymptomatic) multiple myeloma: IMWG consensus perspectives risk factors for progression and guidelines for monitoring and management. Leukemia 2010;24:1121-7

21. Hobbs JR. Growth rates and responses to treatment in human myelomatosis. Br J Haematol 1969;16:607-17

Monoclonal gammopathy of undetermined significance

Summary:

- Intact immunoglobulin monoclonal gammopathy of undetermined significance (MGUS) accounts for 80% of all MGUS cases, of which approximately one-third have an abnormal sFLC ratio.
- Light chain MGUS accounts for approximately 20% of all MGUS cases and is characterised by an abnormal sFLC ratio and an elevated concentration of the involved FLC.
- sFLCs have been incorporated into an MGUS risk-stratification model, in association with the monoclonal immunoglobulin class and concentration, to guide patient management.
- Hevylite pair suppression is an independent risk factor for progression and improves the standard risk stratification model.

13.1. MGUS definition and frequency

Monoclonal gammopathy of undetermined significance (MGUS) is characterised by the presence of a monoclonal protein in the serum of asymptomatic individuals who do not meet the diagnostic criteria for multiple myeloma (MM), AL amyloidosis, Waldenström's macroglobulinaemia (WM), lymphoproliferative disorders, plasmacytoma or related conditions. Whilst most MGUS patients have a stable condition and remain asymptomatic, a small proportion will progress to MM or a related B-cell or lymphoid cancer. This equates to a 1%-per-year lifelong risk of malignant transformation[1].

MGUS is defined as follows (all criteria must be met): 1) a serum monoclonal protein <30 g/L; 2) clonal bone marrow plasma cells <10%; and 3) the absence of end-organ damage such as hypercalcaemia, renal insufficiency, anaemia, and bone lesions that can be attributed to the plasma cell proliferative disorder. The definition of MGUS should not be confused with the term "monoclonal gammopathy of renal significance" (MGRS), which is used to describe a group of haematological disorders associated with kidney disease that fail to meet the standard definitions for MM or lymphoma *(Chapter 26)*[2].

MGUS is present in approximately 3% of individuals aged 50 or older, and in around 5% of those aged 70 or older[3]; it has a 2-fold higher incidence in African-Americans[4] and is more common in individuals with autoimmune, infectious and inflammatory disorders[5]. Due to the high frequency of MGUS, it typically accounts for between 50 and 65% of all monoclonal proteins detected, although around 80% of individuals will be unaware that they have the condition[6].

Historically, the term MGUS was used only to describe patients with a monoclonal intact immunoglobulin. In a Mayo Clinic study, 70% of monoclonal proteins identified were IgG, 15% IgM, 12% IgA and 3% biclonal[1]. In addition, the term "idiopathic Bence Jones proteinuria" was used to describe the presence of a monoclonal light chain in the urine (>200 mg/24-hour), in the absence of both an intact immunoglobulin monoclonal protein in the serum and end-organ damage attributable to a plasma cell proliferative disorder. Such patients are at high risk for the development of MM or AL amyloidosis, with a cumulative probability of progression of 20% at 5 years[7]. In 2010 a new category termed light chain MGUS was recognised, and this represents the pre-malignant precursor of light chain MM (LCMM) (Section 13.3.2)[8].

13.2. Risk factors for MGUS progression

Whilst the 1% average annual risk of MGUS developing into MM or a related condition is well documented[1], progression among individual MGUS patients is highly variable[9]. Therefore, recognition of risk factors for progression is of clear benefit. Not only does this allow the identification of patients at highest risk, who will benefit most from close monitoring, it also provides reassurance to patients at low risk who do not need to be subjected to further tests. A summary of known risk factors is presented in Table 13.1.

Study	n	Monoclonal protein size	BMPC %	Monoclonal protein type	FLCs	Immunoparesis	Additional risk factors
Blade 1992[10]	128	No	No (n=105)	IgA>IgG, IgM	Unknown	No	
Baldini 1996[11]	335	Yes	Yes	No	Yes (uBJP)	Yes (classical immunoparesis)	
Cesana 2002[12]	1104	No	Yes	No	Yes (uBJP)	Yes (classical immunoparesis)	Increased ESR
Mayo Clinic 2002[1], 2005[13] and 2013[14]	1384	Yes	No (n=160)	IgA, IgM>IgG	No (uBJP) Yes (sFLC ratio)	No (classical immunoparesis) Yes (HLC-pair suppression)	
Rosinol 2007[15]	359	Yes	No (n=228)	IgA>IgG, IgM	Unknown	Unknown	Evolving MGUS
Perez-Persona 2007[16]	407	No	No	No	No (uBJP)	No	% aPC/BMPC DNA aneuploidy
Perez-Persona 2010[17]	311	Unknown	Yes	Unknown	Unknown	Unknown	% aPC/BMPC Evolving MGUS
Turesson 2014[18]	728	Yes	Unknown	No	Yes (sFLC ratio)	Yes (classical immunoparesis)	

Table 13.1. Summary of risk factors for MGUS progression identified by multivariate analysis. Yes: significant risk factor; No: non-significant risk factor; uBJP: urinary Bence Jones protein; aPC: aberrant plasma cells; BMPC: bone marrow plasma cells; HLC: immunoglobulin heavy/light chain (Hevylite); ESR: erythrocyte sedimentation rate.

In the largest study to date, the long-term outcome of 1384 individuals with MGUS was assessed by Kyle et al.[1]. Patients enrolled between 1960 and 1994 were followed up for a median of 15.4 years (range: 0 – 35 years), during which time 115 had progressed to MM or a related condition, a rate of approximately 1% per year. The most important prognostic factor for progression was the initial size of the serum monoclonal protein (>15 g/L). Immunoglobulin class was also important; individuals with monoclonal IgM and IgA, but not IgG, were 5 times more likely to progress.

Cesana et al.[12] reported that at MGUS diagnosis, a bone marrow plasma cell (BMPC) percentage of 6 – 9% carried twice the risk of MGUS progression compared with ≤5% BMPCs. Perez-Persona et al.[16] characterised the phenotype of BMPCs in 407 MGUS patients using multiparametric flow cytometry. Aberrant plasma cells (aPC) were defined by the absence of CD19 and/or CD45, decreased expression of CD38, and overexpression of CD56. Using multivariate analysis, ≥95% aPC/total BMPCs, together with DNA aneuploidy, identified MGUS patients with the highest risk of progression[16].

The presence of urinary Bence Jones protein (uBJP, monoclonal FLCs) was highlighted as risk factor in several, but not all studies (Table 13.1). In part, this may be related to the problems obtaining a urine sample (Chapter 24). For example, in the study of 1384 MGUS patients by Kyle et al.[1], urine data was unavailable for 70% of patients, and the presence of uBJP failed to reach statistical significance. Since the introduction of sFLC assays into routine practice, the κ/λ sFLC ratio has been identified as a more reliable prognostic marker.

13.2.1. Prognostic value of sFLCs in MGUS

Rajkumar et al.[13] measured sFLCs in serum samples from 1148 MGUS patients at diagnosis by using archived (frozen) sera that had been collected from the original Kyle et al. cohort of 1384 MGUS patients[1]. An abnormal κ/λ sFLC ratio (<0.26 or >1.65) was detected in 379 (33%) cases at diagnosis. At a median follow-up of 15 years, malignant progression to MM or a related condition had occurred in 87 (7.6%) patients. The risk of progression in patients with abnormal sFLC κ/λ ratios

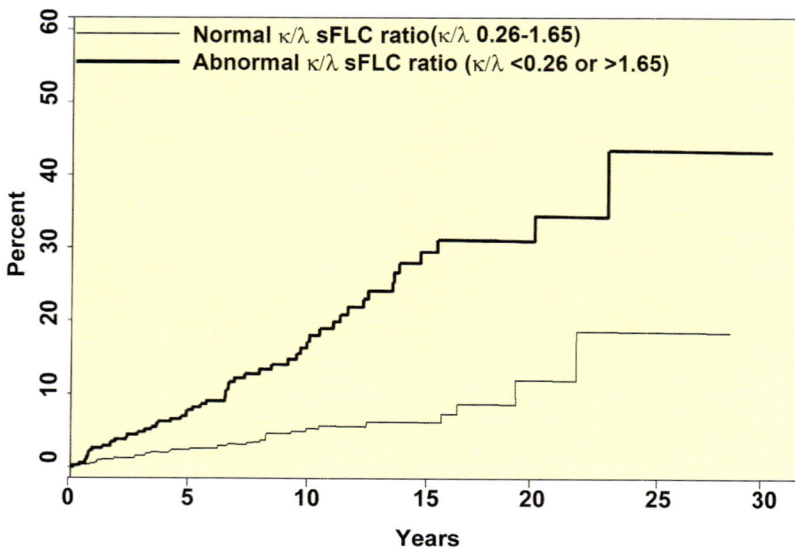

Figure 13.1. Risk of progression based upon the presence or absence of an abnormal κ/λ sFLC ratio. (This research was originally published in Blood[13] © the American Society of Hematology).

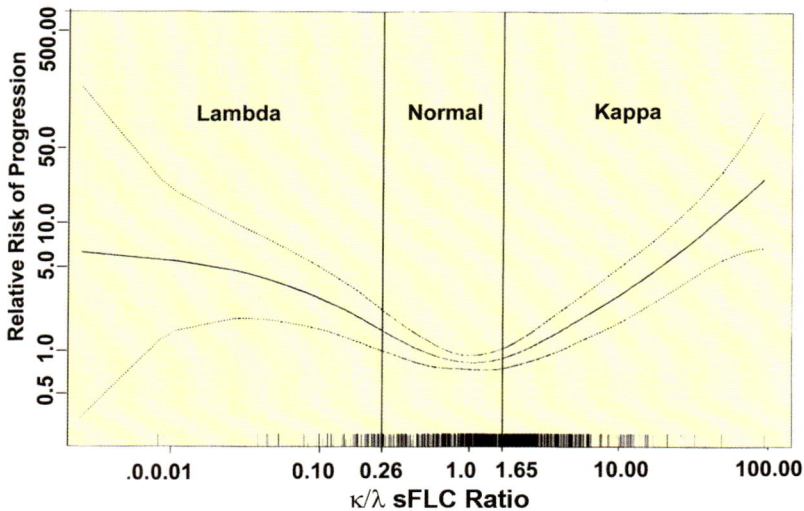

Figure 13.2. Effect of increasingly abnormal κ/λ sFLC ratios on the relative risk of progression of
MGUS. *(This research was originally published in Blood[13] © the American Society of Hematology).*

was significantly higher (hazard ratio 2.6) than in patients with normal ratios, and was independent of the size and type of the monoclonal protein *(Figure 13.1)*. Furthermore, the risk of progression increased as κ/λ ratios became more extreme *(Figure 13.2)*.

The prognostic value of baseline sFLC measurements has been validated in an independent study of 728 Swedish MGUS patients by Turesson et al.[18]. In this study, patients were monitored for up to 30 years (median 10 years), during which time 84 patients developed a lymphoid disorder, with MM accounting for the majority (53/84) of cases. The κ/λ sFLC ratio was abnormal in 47% of the study population at baseline. Three risk factors were significantly associated with progression: an abnormal κ/λ sFLC ratio, monoclonal protein concentration (>15 g/L) and a reduction of one or two uninvolved immunoglobulin isotypes (immunoparesis). No association was found between the monoclonal protein isotype and risk of progression, which is in contrast to some previous reports[1] [10,13], but in keeping with those of the Spanish PETHEMA group[16]. This Spanish group also previously identified immunoparesis as a significant risk factor for MGUS progression in univariate but not multivariate analysis[16].

Rajkumar et al.[13] constructed an MGUS risk stratification model based on the size and type of monoclonal protein, and the presence of an abnormal κ/λ sFLC ratio at diagnosis *(Table 13.2 and Figure 13.3)*. Using this model, low-risk patients were characterised as those with a small (<15 g/L) IgG monoclonal protein and a normal sFLC ratio. Such patients had a 2% absolute risk of disease progression at 20 years when competing causes of death were taken into account. Importantly, this low-risk group accounted for approximately 40% of the cohort. A smaller group of high-risk patients were identified as those with a large (>15 g/L) IgA or IgM monoclonal protein and an abnormal sFLC ratio. These patients had a 27% absolute risk of progression at 20 years.

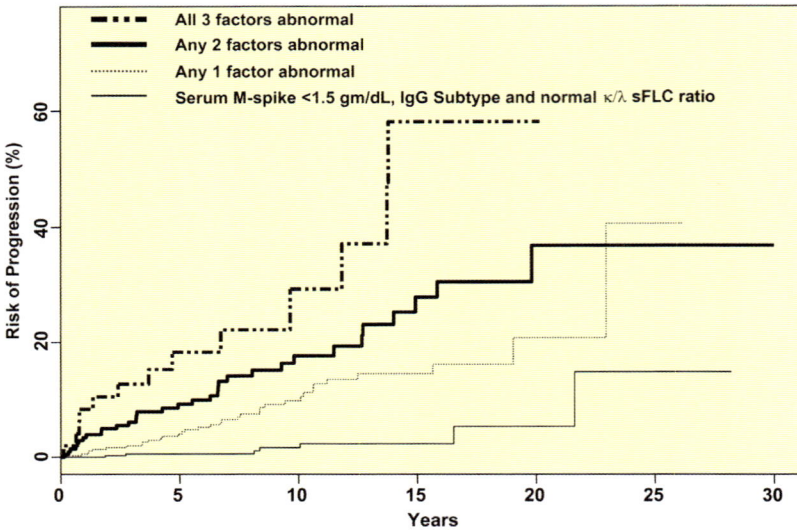

Figure 13.3. Risk of progression to myeloma or related condition in 1148 patients with MGUS. (This research was originally published in Blood[13] © the American Society of Hematology).

International Myeloma Working Group (IMWG) guidelines[9] recommend that patients with MGUS should be risk stratified at diagnosis to optimise counselling and follow-up, using the risk-stratification model outlined in Table 13.2 (see *Chapter 25, Table 25.3)*. For patients with low-risk MGUS, follow-up is recommended at 6 months initially and, if stable, every 2 - 3 years or when symptoms suggest evidence of a plasma cell malignancy. For these patients, a baseline bone marrow examination or skeletal radiography is not routinely indicated. For patients with intermediate- and high-risk MGUS, follow-up is recommended at 6 months initially, then annually and/or upon any change in the patient's clinical condition. A bone marrow aspirate and biopsy should also be carried out at baseline to rule out any underlying plasma cell malignancy[9].

Risk of progression	No. of abnormal risk factors	No. of patients	Absolute risk of progression at 20 years*
Low	0	449	2%
Low-intermediate	1	420	10%
High-intermediate	2	226	18%
High	3	53	27%
* Accounting for death as a competing risk. The three risk factors are defined as an abnormal κ/λ sFLC ratio (<0.26 or >1.65), a high serum monoclonal protein concentration (>15 g/L), and a non–IgG subtype (IgA or IgM).			

Table 13.2. Risk stratification model to predict progression of MGUS[13].

In future, additional markers may be added to risk stratification models to better define high-risk patients. Rawstron et al.[19] have recently showed that plasma cell phenotype (CD138/38/45 expression) and sFLCs provide independent and complementary prognostic information on the risk of progression. The use of additional genetic risk factors (including light chain gene rearrangements[20] and gene expression profiles[21]) are currently being investigated.

13.2.2. Prognostic value of Hevylite in MGUS

Suppression of uninvolved, polyclonal immunoglobulins (classical immunoparesis) has been identified as a risk factor of MGUS progression in some[11,12,18], but not in all studies[1]. With the availability of HLC immmunoassays, it is now possible to measure the isotype-specific suppression of the uninvolved HLC-pair (e.g. suppression of IgAλ in an IgAκ patient) (Section 11.2). Emerging evidence suggests that this 'HLC-pair suppression' may have prognostic importance in MGUS patients.

In a preliminary study, Katzmann et al.[22] analysed HLC results from 105 IgG and 28 IgA MGUS patients. For the purposes of analysis the samples were separated into 3 different groups: initial samples from patients with stable MGUS, initial samples from patients with MGUS which progressed, and samples collected shortly before progression was diagnosed (Table 13.3). For the IgG MGUS patients, HLC ratio abnormalities and HLC-pair suppression were increased in patients at greater risk of progression and the pair suppression was greater than the general immunoparesis. For the IgA MGUS patients the results were clearly different; ratio abnormalities were close to 100% in all groups and while HLC-pair suppression was higher in subjects at greater risk of progression, the frequency of general immunoparesis was almost identical (Table 13.3).

IgG MGUS	n	Abnormal IgGκ/IgGλ HLC ratio (%)	IgA or IgM suppression (%)	HLC-pair suppression (%)
MGUS stable Initial sample*	36	64	6	22
MGUS-progressed Initial sample*	30	83	7	53
MGUS-progressed Pre-progression sample**	39	87	46	90
IgA MGUS	n	Abnormal IgAκ/IgAλ HLC ratio (%)	IgG or IgM suppression (%)	HLC-pair suppression (%)
MGUS stable Initial sample*	4	100	25	25
MGUS-progressed Initial sample*	10	100	50	40
MGUS-progressed Pre-progression sample**	14	93	71	71

*Table 13.3. HLC-pair suppression compared to classical immunoparesis in IgG and IgA MGUS [22]. Suppression is defined as below the lower limit of the normal reference range. * Initial diagnostic sera from Olmsted County study of MGUS; ** pre-MM sample from NIH PLCO cohort.*

In a second and much larger study, Katzmann et al.[14] investigated the prognostic significance of HLC analysis utilising 999 MGUS patient samples taken at diagnosis. These were cryopreserved sera collected from the 1384 MGUS patients who had participated in the earlier, Kyle et al. MGUS study[1]. An abnormal HLC ratio was identified in two-thirds of patients. The frequency depended on the monoclonal protein isotype (Table 13.4): an abnormal HLC ratio was present in at least 90% of IgA and IgM MGUS patients, but in only 56% of IgG MGUS patients. The insensitivity of IgG HLC for IgG MGUS is thought to be due to the higher concentration of background polyclonal IgG compared with IgA and IgM (Section 11.5.3). HLC-pair suppression was present in 27% of patients overall, this represented a higher frequency than classical immunoparesis, which was present in only 11% of cases.

MGUS isotype	Monoclonal protein concentration (g/L)	n	Abnormal HLC ratio (%)	HLC-pair suppression (%)	Classical immunoparesis (%)
	Any	726	56	29	5
	≤5	83	7	53	53
IgG	6-10	150	57	35	7
	11-20	365	65	29	5
	21-30	50	90	50	10
	Any	117	97	36	33
	≤5	39	95	23	41
IgA	6-10	19	100	47	37
	11-20	55	96	44	27
	21-30	4	100	0	25
	Any	156	90	10	21
	≤5	49	84	2	18
IgM	6-10	28	93	14	21
	11-20	70	93	13	20
	21-30	9	100	22	33
All cases	Any	999	66	27	11

Table 13.4. Frequency of abnormal HLC ratios and HLC-pair suppression in IgG, IgA and IgM MGUS[14].

In univariate analysis, Katzmann et al.[14] showed that HLC-pair suppression and abnormal HLC ratios were both significantly associated with an increased risk of progression to MM (both p <0.001). On multivariate analysis, HLC-pair suppression remained significantly associated with progression to MM or a related condition, along with monoclonal protein size, type and an abnormal κ/λ sFLC ratio (Table 13.5). A risk-stratification model was developed to include these variables in which patients are categorised into five groups, according to the number of risk factors (0, 1, 2, 3 or 4) they possess. The probability of progression to MM increased with the number of risk factors (Figure 13.4).

Prognostic factor	Hazard ratio (95% CI)	P-value
HLC-pair suppression	1.8 (1.1-3.0)	0.018
Serum monoclonal protein size ≥15 g/L	2.3 (1.5-3.8)	<0.001
Abnormal κ/λ sFLC ratio	2.0 (1.2-3.4)	0.007
IgA or IgM heavy chain isotype	2.7 (1.6-4.6)	<0.001

Table 13.5. Prognostic factors for progression of MGUS to MM identified by multivariate analysis[14].

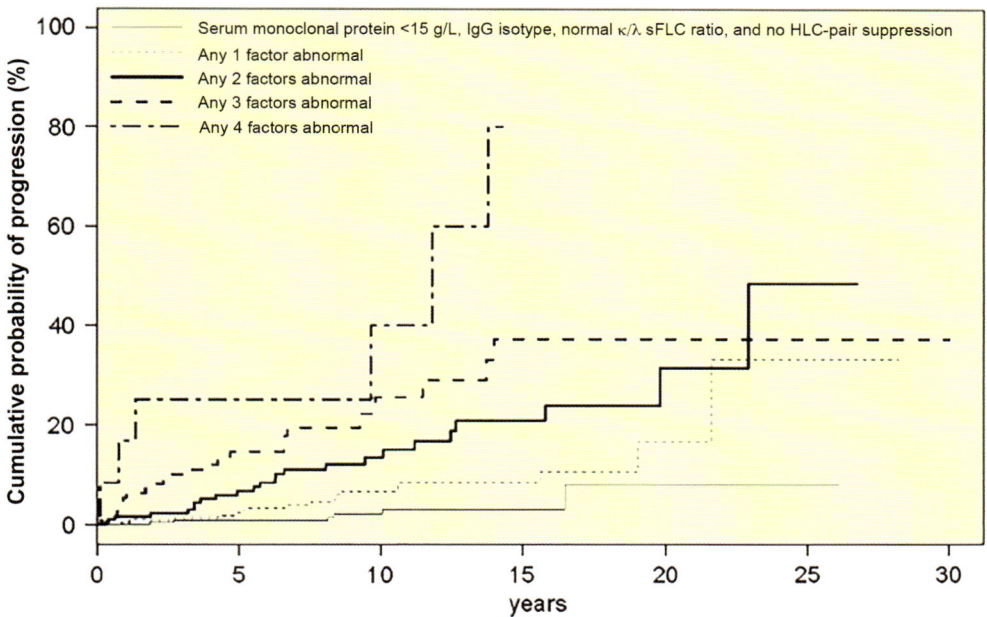

Figure 13.4. Risk of progression of MGUS to MM using a risk stratification model that incorporates HLC-pair suppression.
Prognostic factors defined in Table 13.5. (This research was originally published in Leukemia[14]. Reproduced with permission from nature.com).

Supportive data was reported by Jiménez et al.[23]. In this study, 248 MGUS patients were initially grouped as low- to high-risk based on the Rajkumar et al. MGUS risk stratification model[13]. The incidence of HLC-pair suppression increased with MGUS risk group *(Figure 13.5)*. Moreover, in IgG MGUS patients, both the HLC ratio and the degree of HLC-pair suppression became more extreme in higher risk groups *(Figure 13.6)*.

Espiño et al.[24] found that in IgG MGUS patients, the frequency of involved/uninvolved HLC ratios above 9.5 correlated with the classification of evolving/non-evolving MGUS proposed by Rosinal et al.[15] ($p<0.001$) *(Figure 13.7)*. Moreover, all patients that actually progressed to MM during the study had an involved/uninvolved HLC ratio above 9.5 at MGUS diagnosis. The authors speculated that suppression of normal plasma cells, indicated by HLC pair-suppression, may be a prerequisite for malignant transformation of MGUS. This may be particularly important for IgG MGUS, due to the high levels of normal IgG-secreting plasma cells that would otherwise prevent invasion of bone marrow niches by tumour cells[24]. In the future, HLC assays may be used routinely alongside sFLC analysis and other prognostic markers, to guide the optimal follow-up of MGUS patients.

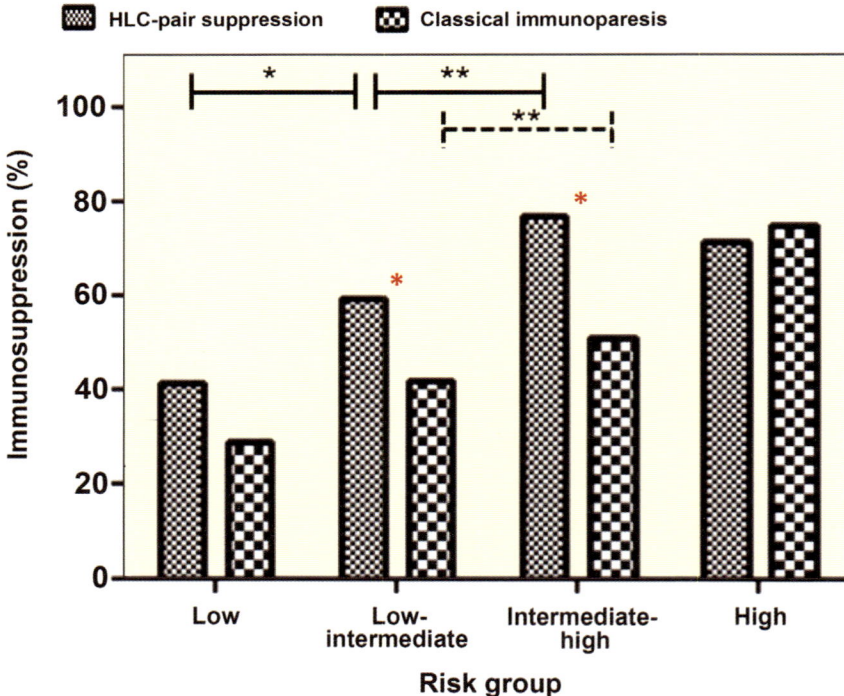

Figure 13.5. Incidence of HLC-pair suppression versus classical immunoparesis in MGUS patients, grouped according to Rajkumar et al.[13] MGUS risk stratification model. $*p<0.05$; $**p<0.005$. *There is a tendency for HLC-pair suppression to be more frequent than classical immunoparesis, reaching significance for two of the four risk groups,* $*p<0.05$[23]. *(Courtesy of J. Jimenez).*

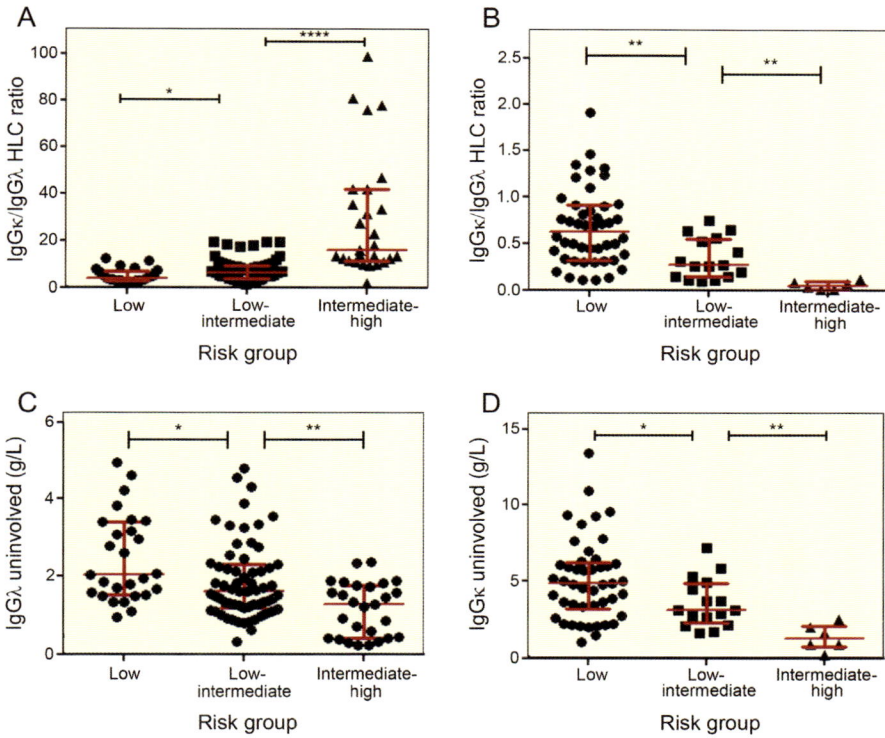

Figure 13.6. IgG HLC results in IgG MGUS patients, grouped according to Rajkumar et al.[13] MGUS risk stratification model. IgGκ/IgGλ HLC ratio in (A) IgGκ MGUS and (B) IgGλ MGUS. Uninvolved HLC concentration in (C) IgGκ MGUS and (D) IgGλ MGUS. *p<0.05; **p<0.005; ****p<0.0001[23]. (Courtesy of J. Jimenez).

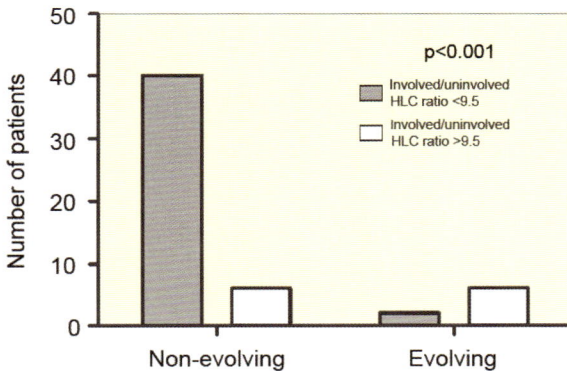

Figure 13.7. Patients with involved/uninvolved HLC ratios above 9.5 showed a higher risk of an evolving course in IgG MGUS patients than those with involved/uninvolved HLC ratios below 9.5. (Reproduced with permission from the British Journal of Haematology[24] and John Wiley & Sons Ltd).

13.3. MGUS as the precursor condition for MM and related disorders

Identification of factors that predict progression in MGUS, such as those described above, is important for individual patient management because the risk of transformation is life-long and the evolution of disease between individuals is variable. MGUS may evolve to other asymptomatic pre-malignant states with a significantly higher risk of progression (i.e. smouldering MM, smouldering WM, smouldering LCMM: *Section 12.3*). Disease evolution has been shown to be characterised by the acquisition of genetic mutations by tumour cell clones and associated changes in the bone marrow microenvironment *(Chapter 19)*[25,26].

13.3.1. MGUS consistently precedes MM

Two independent studies, by Landgren et al.[28] and Weiss et al.[29], addressed whether MGUS is consistently present prior to a diagnosis of MM. Landgren et al.[28] tested pre-diagnostic serum samples from 71 subjects who developed MM. Samples were available up to 10 years prior to the diagnosis of malignant disease. Using serum protein electrophoresis (SPE), serum immunofixation (sIFE) and sFLC analysis, it was shown that >80% of patients had detectable monoclonal protein ≥8 years before diagnosis, increasing to 100% 2 years before diagnosis. In approximately half of the patients who went on to develop MM, the involved/uninvolved sFLC ratio (defined as κ/λ in κ patients and λ/κ in λ patients) showed a year-by-year increase, whilst ratios in the other half remained largely stable. This is an important observation since an evolving MGUS phenotype (in which the monoclonal protein shows a steady increase, *Figure 13.8*) has been shown to identify patients with a high risk of malignant transformation[15,17], with transformation rates of 55% and 10% at 10 years of follow-up for evolving and stable phenotypes respectively[15].

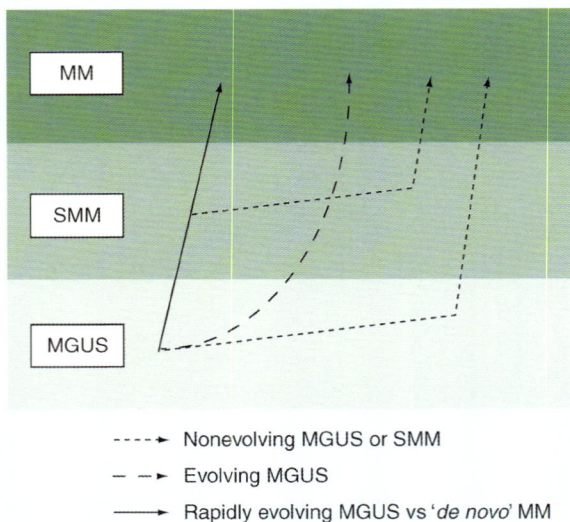

Figure 13.8. Proposed models for the patterns of progression from MGUS to MM[27]. (© 2010, Informa Healthcare. Reproduced with permission of Informa Healthcare).

In a separate group of patients, Weiss et al.[29] demonstrated that 27 of 30 MM diagnoses were preceded by MGUS. Monoclonal proteins were identified by SPE and/or IFE in 78% of patients and by an abnormal κ/λ sFLC ratio alone in 22% of patients. Of the 3 patients who had no MGUS detected, one patient with IgG myeloma had only one pre-diagnostic serum sample available at 9.5 years before diagnosis. The remaining 2 negative cases were IgD myeloma with sera available only 3 and 5 years before the diagnosis. Similarly to Landgren et al., the authors found that substantial increases in the involved sFLC ratio may precede the diagnosis of MM, with or without a corresponding change in the monoclonal intact immunoglobulin. It was notable that, in all four patients diagnosed with LCMM or NSMM, the disease evolved from light chain MGUS.

In a third study, also by Weiss et al.[30] and comprising 20 patients who went on to develop AL amyloidosis, MGUS was detected prior to diagnosis in all cases. A median of 3 pre-diagnostic samples were obtained up to 10 years prior to diagnosis. The monoclonal protein type was FLC in 55% of cases, and intact immunoglobulin in 45% of cases. The prevalence of MGUS was 100%, 80% and 42% at <4, 4 to 11, and >11 years prior to diagnosis.

Taken together, these findings confirm that a pre-malignant MGUS phase exists prior to disease emergence in most MM and AL amyloidosis patients. In a review of MGUS as a precursor condition, Weiss and Kuehl[27] included a model illustrating different patterns of MGUS progression comprising: non-evolving, evolving and rapidly evolving *(Figure 13.8)*. Measuring sFLC levels in routine MGUS follow-up may help to identify patients, with an evolving phenotype, who are at a higher risk of progression to malignant disease compared to patients with stable MGUS.

13.3.2. Light chain MGUS

Light chain MGUS was proposed by Dispenzieri et al.[8] as a separate clinical entity and the pre-malignant precursor of LCMM. The authors defined light chain MGUS as an abnormal κ/λ sFLC ratio with an increased concentration of the involved sFLC, no expression of monoclonal intact immunoglobulin, and an absence of end-organ damage that can be attributed to the plasma cell proliferative disorder. An example is shown in Figure 13.9. No abnormality was detected by SPE or urine protein electrophoresis (UPE), but an abnormal κ/λ sFLC ratio indicated the presence of monoclonal FLCs. This finding was confirmed by the detection of λ uBJP by urine IFE (uIFE).

In the study by Dispenzieri et al.[8] the prevalence and risk of progression of light chain MGUS amongst 18,357 residents of Olmstead County, Minnesota aged 50 years or older was assessed. 610 (3.3%) individuals had an abnormal κ/λ sFLC ratio, of whom 213 had an intact immunoglobulin MGUS. This included 57/213 additional patients whose monoclonal intact immunoglobulin had not previously been detected by screening with SPE, and so the prevalence of conventional MGUS in this population was revised from 3.2% to 3.4% (95% CI 3.2 - 3.7). Of the 397 individuals with an abnormal sFLC ratio but no abnormality detected by SPE, a total of 146 met the definition of light chain MGUS, equivalent to a prevalence of 0.8% (95% CI 0.7 - 0.9). This represented 19% of the total MGUS population; a proportion that matches the relative incidence of LCMM compared to all MM. The light chain type was identified as κ or λ in 108 and 38 individuals, respectively. Overall, involved sFLC concentrations tended to be low; only around 10% of patients had concentrations greater than 200 mg/L. It was noted that 23% of light chain MGUS patients either had or subsequently acquired, renal disease; an observation of relevance to the later proposal for monoclonal gammopathy of renal significance to be considerd as a separate entity *(Section 26.4.1)*. A similar incidence of light chain MGUS (0.7%) was confirmed by a European study of 4702 individuals aged 45 - 75 years[31].

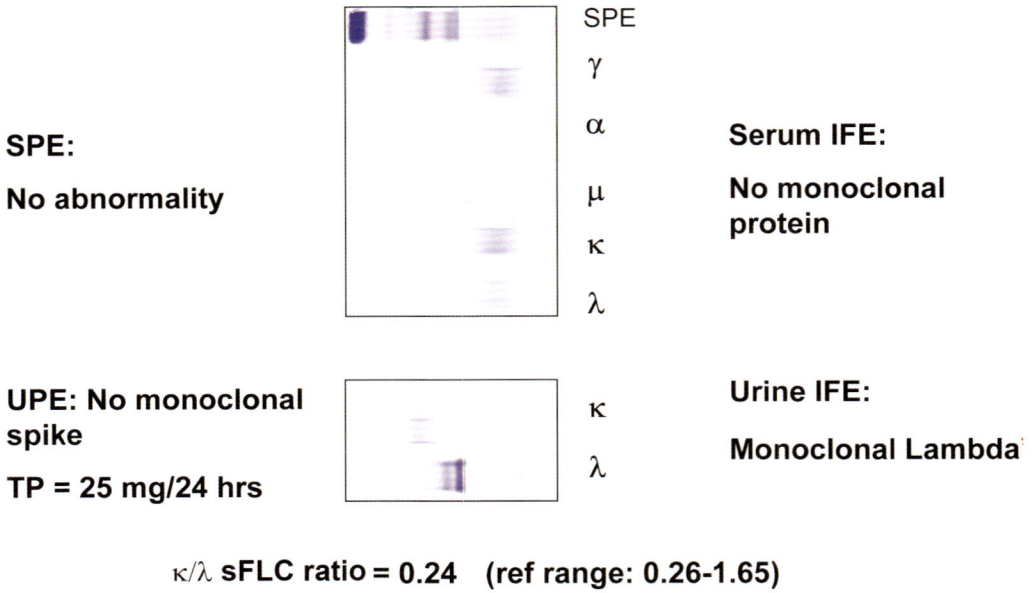

SPE

γ

α

μ

κ

λ

SPE:

No abnormality

Serum IFE:

No monoclonal protein

UPE: No monoclonal spike

TP = 25 mg/24 hrs

κ

λ

Urine IFE:

Monoclonal Lambda

κ/λ **sFLC ratio = 0.24** (ref range: 0.26-1.65)

Figure 13.9. Serum and urine IFE on a patient with isolated urine FLC excretion. Serum analysis for FLCs showed an abnormal κ/λ ratio. TP: urine protein excretion. (Courtesy of J.A. Katzmann).

Although a coexisting abnormal κ/λ sFLC ratio increased the risk of progression to MM and related disorders for patients with conventional MGUS, risk of progression of light chain MGUS did not differ from that for patients with low-risk conventional MGUS (i.e. those with no abnormal κ/λ sFLC ratio) (p=0.1822)[8]. Dispenzieri et al.[8] speculated that the transformation events resulting in either light chain MGUS or conventional MGUS may be the same, and that the presence of an abnormal sFLC ratio in patients with conventional MGUS indicate that two transformation events had occured and their disease was one step closer to malignant transformation.

Test Questions

1. Which MGUS risk factors are included in international guidelines?
2. What are the clinical benefits of MGUS risk stratification?
3. Why is light chain MGUS rarely seen with SPE and IFE testing of serum and urine?

Answers

1. International guidelines recommend risk stratification based on three risk factors: an abnormal k/λ sFLC ratio (<0.26 or >1.65), a high serum monoclonal protein concentration (>15 g/L), and a non-IgG subtype (IgA or IgM) (Section 13.2.1 and Chapter 25).

2. Patients at high risk of progression can be more closely monitored, while low-risk patients whose results are stable can be discharged from follow-up clinics (Section 13.2.1).

3. Because the amounts of FLCs produced are below the sensitivity of serum electrophoretic tests and are insufficient to exceed the proximal tubular reabsorption mechanisms and overflow into urine (Chapter 3).

References

1. Kyle RA, Therneau TM, Rajkumar SV, Offord JR, Larson DR, Plevak MF, Melton LJ, III. A long-term study of prognosis in monoclonal gammopathy of undetermined significance. N Engl J Med 2002;346:564-9

2. Leung N, Bridoux F, Hutchison CA, Nasr SH, Cockwell P, Fermand JP et al. Monoclonal gammopathy of renal significance (MGRS): when MGUS is no longer undetermined or insignificant. Blood 2012;120:4292-5

3. Kyle RA, Therneau TM, Rajkumar SV, Larson DR, Plevak MF, Offord JR et al. Prevalence of monoclonal gammopathy of undetermined significance. N Engl J Med 2006;354:1362-9

4. Landgren O, Gridley G, Turesson I, Caporaso NE, Goldin LR, Baris D et al. Risk of monoclonal gammopathy of undetermined significance (MGUS) and subsequent multiple myeloma among African American and white veterans in the United States. Blood 2006;107:904-6

5. Brown LM, Gridley G, Check D, Landgren O. Risk of multiple myeloma and monoclonal gammopathy of undetermined significance among white and black male United States veterans with prior autoimmune, infectious, inflammatory, and allergic disorders. Blood 2008;111:3388-94

6. Watters E, Calder M. MGUS. Myeloma UK Infosheet 2013

7. Kyle R, Larson D, Therneau T, Dispenzieri A, Benson J, Melton J et al. Idiopathic Bence Jones proteinuria (Smoldering monoclonal light-chain proteinuria): clinical course and prognosis. Clinical Lymphoma, Myeloma & Leukaemia 2013;13:O-18a

8. Dispenzieri A, Katzmann JA, Kyle RA, Larson DR, Melton LJ, III, Colby CL et al. Prevalence and risk of progression of light-chain monoclonal gammopathy of undetermined significance: a retrospective population-based cohort study. Lancet 2010;375:1721-8

9. Kyle RA, Durie BG, Rajkumar SV, Landgren O, Blade J, Merlini G et al. Monoclonal gammopathy of undetermined significance (MGUS) and smoldering (asymptomatic) multiple myeloma: IMWG consensus perspectives risk factors for progression and guidelines for monitoring and management. Leukemia 2010;24:1121-7

10. Blade J, Lopez-Guillermo A, Rozman C, Cervantes F, Salgado C, Aguilar JL et al. Malignant transformation and life expectancy in monoclonal gammopathy of undetermined significance. Br J Haematol 1992;81:391-4

11. Baldini L, Guffanti A, Cesana BM, Colombi M, Chiorboli O, Damilano I, Maiolo AT. Role of different hematologic variables in defining the risk of malignant transformation in monoclonal gammopathy. Blood 1996;87:912-8

12. Cesana C, Klersy C, Barbarano L, Nosari AM, Crugnola M, Pungolino E et al. Prognostic factors for malignant transformation in monoclonal gammopathy of undetermined significance and smoldering multiple myeloma. J Clin Oncol 2002;20:1625-34

13. Rajkumar SV, Kyle RA, Therneau TM, Melton LJ, 3rd, Bradwell AR, Clark RJ, et al. Serum free light chain ratio is an independent risk factor for progression in monoclonal gammopathy of undetermined significance. Blood 2005;106:812-7

14. Katzmann JA, Clark R, Kyle RA, Larson DR, Therneau TM, Melton LJ, III et al. Suppression of uninvolved immunoglobulins defined by heavy/light-chain pair suppression is a risk factor for progression of MGUS. Leukemia 2013;27:208-12

15. Rosinol L, Cibeira MT, Montoto S, Rozman M, Esteve J, Filella X, Blade J. Monoclonal gammopathy of undetermined significance: predictors of malignant transformation and recognition of an evolving type characterized by a progressive increase in M protein size. Mayo Clin Proc 2007;82:428-34

16. Perez-Persona E, Vidriales MB, Mateo G, Garcia-Sanz R, Mateos MV, de Coca AG et al. New criteria to identify risk of progression in monoclonal gammopathy of uncertain significance and smoldering multiple myeloma based on multiparameter flow cytometry analysis of bone marrow plasma cells. Blood 2007;110:2586-92

17. Perez-Persona E, Mateo G, Garcia-Sanz R, Mateos MV, de Las Heras N, de Coca AG et al. Risk of progression in smouldering myeloma and monoclonal gammopathies of unknown significance: comparative analysis of the evolution of monoclonal component and multiparameter flow cytometry of bone marrow plasma cells. Br J Haematol 2010;148:110-4

18. Turesson I, Kovalchik SA, Pfeiffer RM, Kristinsson SY, Goldin LR, Drayson MT, Landgren O. Monoclonal gammopathy of undetermined significance and risk of lymphoid and myeloid malignancies: 728 cases followed up to 30 years in Sweden. Blood 2014;123:338-45

19. Rawstron AC, Davis B, Denman S, de Tute RM, Kerr MA, Owen RG, Ashcroft AJ. Plasma cell phenotype and sFLC provide independent prognostic information in MGUS. Haematologica 2007;92:PO907a

20. Turkmen S, Binder A, Gerlach A, Niehage S, Theodora MM, Inandiklioglu N et al. High prevalence of immunoglobulin light chain gene aberrations as revealed by FISH in multiple myeloma and MGUS. Genes Chromosomes Cancer 2014;53:650-6

21. Dhodapkar MV, Sexton R, Waheed S, Usmani S, Papanikolaou X, Nair B et al. Clinical, genomic and imaging predictors of myeloma progression from asymptomatic monoclonal gammopathies (SWOG S0120). Blood 2014;123:78-85

22. Katzmann J, Clark R, Dispenzieri A, Kyle R, Landgren O, Bradwell AR, Rajkumar SV. Isotype-specific heavy/light chain (HLC) suppression as a predictor of myeloma development in monoclonal gammopathy of undetermined significance (MGUS). Blood 2009;114:1788a

23. Jimenez J, Campos L, Pais T, Barbosa N, Iarramendi C. Risk Stratification and Progression follow-up of MGUS Patients: value of the sFLC and Heavy Chain/Light Chain Pairs markers. Clinical Chemistry 2014;60:321a

24. Espino M, Medina S, Blanchard MJ, Villar LM. Involved/uninvolved immunoglobulin ratio identifies monoclonal gammopathy of undetermined significance patients at high risk of progression to multiple myeloma. Br J Haematol 2014;164:752-5

25. Korde N, Kristinsson SY, Landgren O. Monoclonal gammopathy of undetermined significance (MGUS) and smoldering multiple myeloma (SMM): novel biological insights and development of early treatment strategies. Blood 2011;117:5573-81

26. Morgan GJ, Walker BA, Davies FE. The genetic architecture of multiple myeloma. Nat Rev Cancer 2012;12:335-48

27. Weiss BM, Kuehl WM. Advances in understanding monoclonal gammopathy of undetermined significance as a precursor of multiple myeloma. Expert Rev Hematol 2010;3:165-74

28. Landgren O, Kyle RA, Pfeiffer RM, Katzmann JA, Caporaso NE, Hayes RB et al. Monoclonal gammopathy of undetermined significance (MGUS) consistently precedes multiple myeloma: a prospective study. Blood 2009;113:5412-7

29. Weiss BM, Abadie J, Verma P, Howard RS, Kuehl WM. A monoclonal gammopathy precedes multiple myeloma in most patients. Blood 2009;113:5418-22

30. Weiss BM, Hebreo J, Cordaro D, Roschewski MJ, Abbott KC, Olson SW. Monoclonal gammopathy of undetermined significance (MGUS) precedes the diagnosis of AL amyloidosis by up to 14 years. Blood 2011;118:1827a

31. Eisele L, Durig J, Huttmann A, Duhrsen U, Assert R, Bokhof B et al. Prevalence and progression of monoclonal gammopathy of undetermined significance and light-chain MGUS in Germany. Ann Hematol 2012;91:243-8

Smouldering multiple myeloma

In smouldering multiple myeloma:

- sFLCs are abnormal in approximately 80% of patients.
- Abnormal κ/λ sFLC ratios are associated with an increased risk of progression.
- In association with bone marrow plasma cell number and monoclonal immunoglobulin concentration, sFLCs can be used to produce a risk model for progression.
- Patients with very high risk factors (including extreme sFLC ratios) have been reclassified as active myeloma patients requiring treatment.

14.1. Introduction

Smouldering multiple myeloma (SMM) is an asymptomatic plasma cell disorder. A definitive diagnosis of SMM requires two criteria to be met: 1) the presence of a serum monoclonal protein (IgG or IgA) at a concentration of ≥30 g/L and/or 10 - 60% clonal bone marrow plasma cells (BMPC), and 2) the absence of diagnostic criteria for MM (myeloma-related end-organ damage and/or biomarkers of malignancy)[1] (*Section 14.3 and Section 25.2*). It carries a high risk of progression to symptomatic disease (10% per year for the first 5 years[2]), which is far higher than the risk of progression of monoclonal gammopathy of undetermined significance (MGUS, 1% per year, *Chapter 13*). As such, SMM represents the quintessential model for studying multiple myeloma precursor disease, and for developing early intervention strategies[3]. The time to disease progression (TTP) in SMM patients is typically between 2 and 4 years, so it is routine practice to monitor patients on a regular basis[2,4].

The progression rate amongst SMM patients is heterogeneous, and risk stratification is valuable for patient management, particularly since treatment intervention is now being considered for those at highest risk[5,6]. Early studies identified a variety of risk factors for progression, including a high percentage of BMPCs, a monoclonal protein concentration ≥30 g/L, an IgA isotype and Bence Jones proteinuria[2,7,8,9]. Subsequently, monoclonal serum free light chains (sFLCs) were identified as a significant, independent risk factor, as discussed below. Preliminary evidence suggests that immunoglobulin heavy/light chain (Hevylite®, HLC) assays may also have a role in SMM prognosis.

14.2. Monoclonal sFLCs and SMM progression

In an analysis of 43 SMM patients recruited to the UK MRC multiple myeloma (MM) trials between 1980 and 2000, Augustson et al.[10] observed that 84% of the patients had an abnormal κ/λ sFLC ratio at diagnosis, and that patients with normal sFLC ratios tended to progress more slowly than those with abnormal ratios. The difference was not significant, however, probably due to the small number of patients in the study.

Dispenzieri et al.[11] subsequently confirmed this finding in a larger study of sera obtained within 30 days of diagnosis from 273 SMM patients attending the Mayo clinic, Rochester, USA. At a median follow-up time of 12.4 years, transformation to active disease had occurred in 59% of patients. Abnormal κ/λ sFLC ratios were present in 90% of patients at baseline and were associated with adverse outcomes. The degree of ratio abnormality was independent of other SMM risk factors, including the number of BMPCs and the concentration of monoclonal immunoglobulin. The study concluded that an abnormal κ/λ sFLC ratio was an important additional determinant of clinical outcome; furthermore an increasingly abnormal ratio was associated with a higher risk of progression to active MM. Patients with a normal (0.26 - 1.65) or near normal (0.25 - 4) ratio had a rate of progression of 5% per year, while patients with markedly abnormal ratios (either ≤0.0312 [1/32] or >32) had a rate of progression of 8.1% per year *(Figure 14.1)*. This increased progression persisted after adjusting for competing causes of death. The best cut-off point for predicting risk of progression was a κ/λ sFLC ratio of <0.125 or >8, giving a hazard ratio for progression to active MM of 2.3 times that of patients with sFLC ratios between 0.125 and 8 *(Figure 14.2)*.

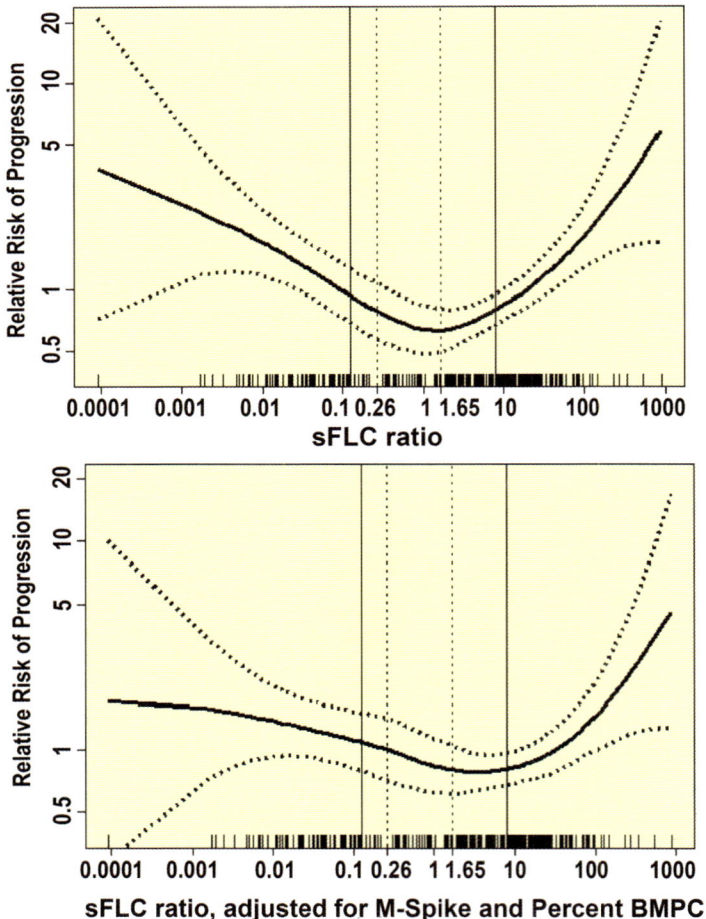

Figure 14.1. Effect of increasing abnormal sFLC ratios on the relative risk of progression of SMM to MM or related disorders.
BMPC: bone marrow plasma cells. *(This research was originally published in Blood[11] © the American Society of Hematology).*

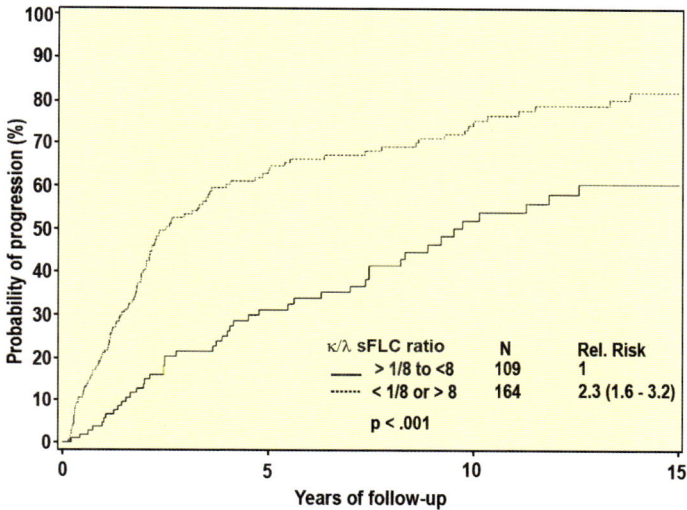

Figure 14.2. Risk of SMM progressing to MM using 2 different levels of sFLC κ/λ ratios. *(This research was originally published in Blood[11] © the American Society of Hematology).*

Combining κ/λ sFLC ratios with the percentage of BMPCs and monoclonal protein concentration produced a highly significant risk model *(Table 14.1)*[11]. The three risk factors were defined as: 1) an abnormal κ/λ sFLC ratio (<0.125 or >8); 2) BMPC ≥10%; and 3) serum monoclonal protein ≥30 g/L. The cumulative probability of progression at 10 years was 50% in patients with one risk factor; 65% for those with two risk factors; and 84% for those with three risk factors *(Figure 14.3)*. Correcting for death as a competing risk, the 10-year rates of progression were 35%, 54%, and 75%, respectively (p<0.001). Detection of a urinary monoclonal protein (>50 mg/24 hours) could not substitute for the κ/λ sFLC ratio in this model, indicating the value of using serum rather than urine for FLC analysis *(Chapter 24)*.

Number of risk factors*	Proportion of patients (%)	5-year progression (%)
1	28	25
2	42	51
3	30	76
* Risk factors: bone marrow plasma cells ≥10%; monoclonal protein ≥30 g/L; κ/λ sFLC ratio <0.125 or >8.		

Table 14.1.Mayo Clinic risk stratification model to predict progression of SMM[11].

The authors noted that unlike MGUS, in which the rate of progression remains constant over time *(Chapter 13)*, the overall risk of progression in SMM was greatly influenced by the length of time from diagnosis, with the highest rates of progression occurring in the first few years. The risk of SMM progression to MM or a related condition was 10% per year for the first 5 years, 3% per year for the next 5 years and 1 - 2% per year for the next 10 years. This was most notable in the high-risk group, in whom the probability of progression was about 26% per year for the first 2 years but reduced to 8% per year for the next 3 years *(Figure 14.3)*. In contrast, the rate of progression in the low-risk group was 6% per year for the first 2 years, and approximately 4% per year subsequently. It is possible that some patients classified as SMM are biologically identical to those with MGUS, and with increasing follow-up the cohort becomes enriched with such patients, resulting in progressively decreasing rates of progression. Why abnormal κ/λ sFLC ratios should predict a worse outcome in SMM is unclear, but the authors speculated that these patients might have immunoglobulin heavy chain translocations or other genetic disruptions associated with disease progression[12].

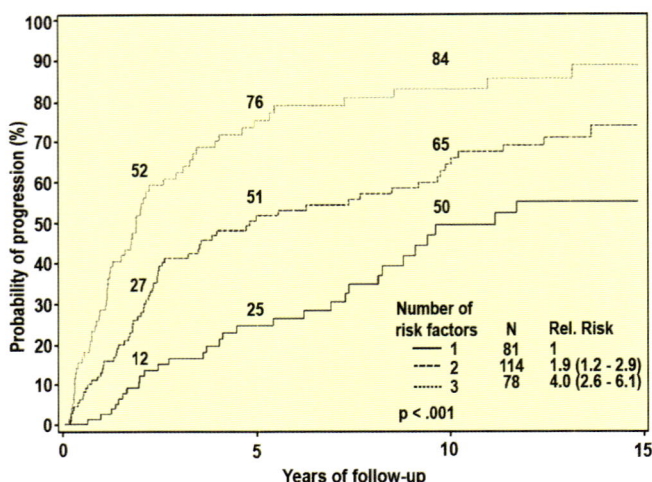

Figure 14.3. Risk of SMM progressing to MM with 1, 2 or 3 risk factors comprising: abnormal sFLC κ/λ ratios (<0.125 or >8); BMPC ≥10%; and serum monoclonal protein ≥30 g/L. (This research was originally published in Blood[11] © the American Society of Hematology).

In a very large follow-on study from the Mayo clinic (Larsen et al.[13]), baseline sFLC results were analysed retrospectively in 586 patients with newly diagnosed SMM. The κ/λ sFLC ratio was abnormal in 74% of patients. Receiver Operating Characteristic (ROC) analysis identified the optimal diagnostic cut-off for the sFLC ratio to identify patients at highest risk of progression to symptomatic disease within 2 years of diagnosis. A serum involved/uninvolved sFLC ratio ≥100 was used to define high-risk SMM (now considered one of the diagnostic criteria for MM; Section 14.3), and included 15% of the total cohort. This resulted in a specificity of 97% and a sensitivity of 16%. The risk of progression to MM within 2 years of diagnosis was 72% for SMM patients with an involved/uninvolved sFLC ratio ≥100 (Figure 14.4). This risk increased to 79% when progression to AL amyloidosis was included as an endpoint in addition to MM. In univariate analysis, BMPC content, serum monoclonal protein concentration and involved/uninvolved sFLC ratio ≥100 were all significant prognostic factors, and all remained significant on multivariate analysis. The authors concluded that patients with a markedly abnormal sFLC ratio should be monitored closely and may be considered candidates for early treatment intervention, especially as disease progression is associated with renal insufficiency in more than a quarter of cases. The prognostic value of extreme sFLC ratios (≥100) for progression from SMM was recently confirmed by Kastritis et al. in a study of 96 patients[14]. This study also identified extensive bone marrow infiltration (BMPCs ≥60%) as an additional risk factor. Rajkumar et al.[15] also identified that patients with BMPCs ≥60% progressed very rapidly and suggested that their disease should be treated as MM.

An alternative SMM risk stratification model developed by the Spanish PETHEMA study group incorporates the proportion of aberrant plasma cells (determined by multiparametric flow cytometry) and immunoparesis (suppression of uninvolved polyclonal immunoglobulins, i.e. suppression of IgA and/or IgM in an IgG patient) as risk factors for progression[16]. However, these criteria are limited by the requirement for fresh bone marrow aspirates from all patients and flow cytometry reagents that may not be available in all laboratories[17]. It is important to note that significant differences exist between the SMM risk stratification models of the Mayo Clinic and the Spanish PETHEMA group; a prospective study by Cherry et al.[18] identified only 28.6% overall concordance between the two models in defining low-, medium- and high-risk patients.

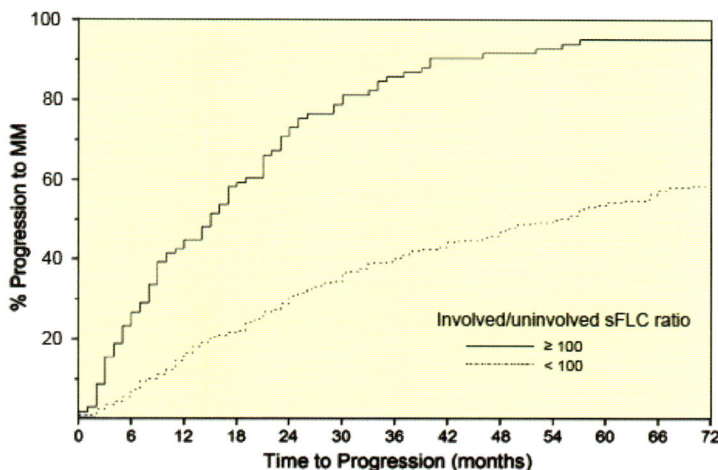

Figure 14.4. Extreme involved/uninvolved sFLC ratios identify SMM patients at risk of imminent progression to MM. (Reprinted by permission from Macmillan Publishers Ltd: Leukemia[13], copyright 2013).

14.3. sFLCs in the management of SMM

International guidelines recommend that sFLCs should be assessed at baseline in SMM, that patients should be risk stratified to optimise counselling and follow up, and that participation in clinical trials should be considered for patients at high risk of disease progression *(Chapter 25)*[19,20]. An initial report by Mateos et al.[21], of high-risk SMM patients treated with lenalidomide and dexamethasone provided the first evidence for a survival benefit resulting from early intervention in SMM patients. The authors described fewer myeloma-related events and significantly improved overall survival in treated patients (n=57) compared with patients who were assigned to the observation arm (n=62) (3-year survival rate of 94% versus 80%, p=0.03).

In a recent review article, Rajkumar and Kyle[6] discussed management options for SMM patients according to their risk factors. In patients with very high-risk factors (BMPCs ≥60%, involved/uninvolved sFLC ratio ≥100 or more than one focal lesion by magnetic resonance imaging [MRI]) the risk of progression within 2 years was at least 70%. The authors proposed that such patients should be treated regardless of the presence or absence of clinical symptoms, in order to prevent serious end-organ damage. Similarly, Dispenzieri et al.[5] recommended reclassifying patients with very high-risk SMM as having active MM, so that they receive therapy appropriate for a newly diagnosed MM patient *(Figure 14.5)*. The latest International Myeloma Working Group consensus for the diagnosis of MM[1] has revised the definition of MM to include the following as biomarkers of malignancy: 1) BMPCs ≥60%; 2) involved/uninvolved Freelite® sFLC ratio ≥100 (with involved sFLCs ≥100 mg/L); and 3) >1 focal lesion by MRI. A patient with one or more of these (and ≥10% BMPCs) is considered to have MM, requiring treatment, even in the absence of myeloma-related end organ damage *(Section 25.2)*.

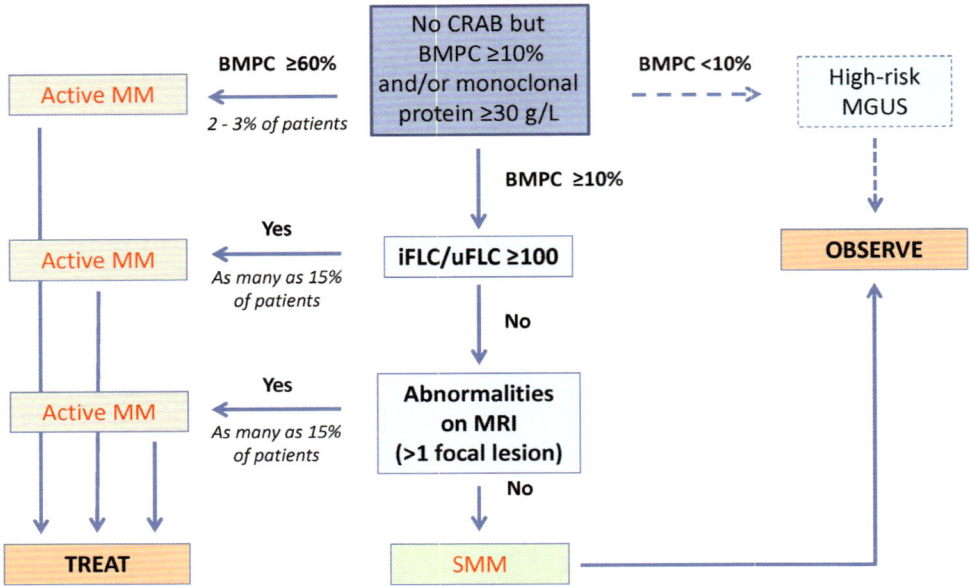

Figure 14.5. Algorithm for reclassifying SMM and active MM. (Figure based on[6]).

14.4. The prognostic value of HLC analysis

Hevylite assays allow the measurement of isotype-specific suppression of the uninvolved HLC-pair (i.e. suppression of IgGλ in an IgGκ patient) *(Section 11.2)*. As HLC-pair suppression has been identified as an adverse prognostic marker in MM and MGUS patients *(Chapters 13 and 20)*, it may also have prognostic significance in SMM. In the largest prospective study of HLC and SMM published to date, HLC-pair suppression was observed in 39/50 (78%) patients at diagnosis, compared with 32/50 (64%) patients who had conventional immunoparesis, i.e. suppression of uninvolved polyclonal immunoglobulins[22]. Of the 18 patients without immunoparesis, HLC-pair suppression was present in 8/18 cases and was associated with adverse biological features such as more skewed κ/λ sFLC ratios and a more pronounced distribution of abnormal/normal plasma cells. Further follow up is underway to determine the prognostic significance of HLC-pair suppression in SMM.

Test Questions

1. How frequently are sFLC ratios abnormal in SMM?
2. What is the recommended management for a patient with 20% BMPCs, Freelite κ sFLCs 250 mg/L, λ sFLCs 2 mg/L (κ/λ sFLC ratio 125) and no evidence of myeloma-related end organ damage?

Answers

1. An abnormal sFLC ratio is found in 74 - 90% of SMM patients at diagnosis *(Section 14.2)*.
2. An involved/uninvolved Freelite sFLC ratio of ≥100 (with involved sFLCs ≥100 mg/L) is considered a biomarker of malignancy. This patient would be classified as having active MM requiring treatment, even in the absence of myeloma-related symptoms *(Section 14.3)*.

References

1. Rajkumar SV, Dimopolous MA, Palumbo A, Blade J, Merlini G, Mateos MV et al. International Myeloma Working Group updated criteria for the diagnosis of multiple myeloma. Lancet Oncology 2014;15:e538-e548

2. Kyle RA, Remstein ED, Therneau TM, Dispenzieri A, Kurtin PJ, Hodnefield JM et al. Clinical course and prognosis of smoldering (asymptomatic) multiple myeloma. N Engl J Med 2007;356:2582-90

3. Korde N, Kristinsson SY, Landgren O. Monoclonal gammopathy of undetermined significance (MGUS) and smoldering multiple myeloma (SMM): novel biological insights and development of early treatment strategies. Blood 2011;117:5573-81

4. Rosinol L, Blade J, Esteve J, Aymerich M, Rozman M, Montoto S et al. Smoldering multiple myeloma: natural history and recognition of an evolving type. Br J Haematol 2003;123:631-6

5. Dispenzieri A, Stewart AK, Chanan-Khan A, Rajkumar SV, Kyle RA, Fonseca R et al. Smoldering multiple myeloma requiring treatment: time for a new definition? Blood 2013;122:4172-81

6. Rajkumar SV, Kyle RA. Haematological cancer: Treatment of smoldering multiple myeloma. Nat Rev Clin Oncol 2013;10:554-5

7. Dimopoulos MA, Moulopoulos A, Smith T, Delasalle KB, Alexanian R. Risk of disease progression in asymptomatic multiple myeloma. Am J Med 1993;94:57-61

8. Weber DM, Dimopoulos MA, Moulopoulos LA, Delasalle KB, Smith T, Alexanian R. Prognostic features of asymptomatic multiple myeloma. Br J Haematol 1997;97:810-4

9. Facon T, Menard JF, Michaux JL, Euller-Ziegler L, Bernard JF, Grosbois B et al. Prognostic factors in low tumour mass asymptomatic multiple myeloma: a report on 91 patients. The Groupe d'Etudes et de Recherche sur le Myelome (GERM). Am J Hematol 1995;48:71-5

10. Augustson BM, Reid SD, Mead GP, Drayson MT, Child JA, Bradwell AR. Serum free light chain levels in asymptomatic myeloma. Blood 2004;104:4880a

11. Dispenzieri A, Kyle RA, Katzmann JA, Therneau TM, Larson D, Benson J, et al. Immunoglobulin free light chain ratio is an independent risk factor for progression of smoldering (asymptomatic) multiple myeloma. Blood 2008;111:785–9

12. Kumar S, Fonseca R, Dispenzieri A, Katzmann JA, Kyle RA, Clark R, Rajkumar SV. High incidence of IgH translocations in monoclonal gammopathies with abnormal free light chain levels. Blood 2006;108:3514a

13. Larsen JT, Kumar SK, Dispenzieri A, Kyle RA, Katzmann JA, Rajkumar SV. Serum free light chain ratio as a biomarker for high-risk smoldering multiple myeloma. Leukemia 2013;27:941-6

14. Kastritis E, Terpos E, Moulopoulos L, Spyropoulou-Vlachou M, Kanellias N, Eleftherakis-Papaiakovou E et al. Extensive bone marrow infiltration and abnormal free light chain ratio identifies patients with asymptomatic myeloma at high risk for progression to symptomatic disease. Leukemia 2013;27:947-53

15. Rajkumar SV, Larson D, Kyle RA. Diagnosis of smoldering multiple myeloma. N Engl J Med 2011;365:474-5

16. Perez-Persona E, Vidriales MB, Mateo G, Garcia-Sanz R, Mateos MV, de Coca AG et al. New criteria to identify risk of progression in monoclonal gammopathy of uncertain significance and smoldering multiple myeloma based on multiparameter flow cytometry analysis of bone marrow plasma cells. Blood 2007;110:2586-92

17. Landgren O, Waxman AJ. Multiple myeloma precursor disease. JAMA 2010;304:2397-404

18. Cherry BM, Korde N, Kwok M, Manasanch EE, Bhutani M, Mulquin M et al. Modeling progression risk for smoldering multiple myeloma: results from a prospective clinical study. Leuk Lymphoma 2013;54:2215-8

19. Kyle RA, Durie BG, Rajkumar SV, Landgren O, Blade J, Merlini G et al. Monoclonal gammopathy of undetermined significance (MGUS) and smoldering (asymptomatic) multiple myeloma: IMWG consensus perspectives risk factors for progression and guidelines for monitoring and management. Leukemia 2010;24:1121-7

20. Dispenzieri A, Kyle R, Merlini G, Miguel JS, Ludwig H, Hajek R et al. International Myeloma Working Group guidelines for serum-free light chain analysis in multiple myeloma and related disorders. Leukemia 2009;23:215-24

21. Mateos MV, Hernandez MT, Giraldo P, de la Rubia J, de AF, Lopez CL et al. Lenalidomide plus dexamethasone for high-risk smoldering multiple myeloma. N Engl J Med 2013;369:438-47

22. Costello R, Espana K, Korde N, Kwok M, Zingone A, Yancey MA et al. Hevylite assays detect a hidden immunoparesis associated with adverse biology in myeloma precursor disease: A prospective clinical study. Blood 2011;118:5065a

Light chain multiple myeloma

In light chain multiple myeloma, sFLC concentrations are:

- Always elevated when urine FLCs are elevated.
- Diagnostically more sensitive than serum immunofixation electrophoresis.
- A better indicator of residual disease than urine measurements.
- Able to indicate disease changes more accurately than urine measurements.

15.1. Diagnosis of light chain multiple myeloma

Typical clinical features including bone pain, fractures, renal failure and anaemia may alert the physician to a possible diagnosis. Bence Jones protein in the urine, in the absence of intact monoclonal immunoglobulins in the serum, alongside a positive bone marrow biopsy, confirms the diagnosis of light chain multiple myeloma (LCMM). On occasions, symptoms and signs can be so obscure that urine tests for LCMM are not considered for some time. This leads to delays in diagnosis, as indicated by occasional published case reports[1,2,3], and illustrates the difficulties facing clinicians (Clinical case history 1).

Historically, the initial screening test for LCMM was commonly serum protein electrophoresis (SPE). This reveals a monoclonal free light chain (FLC) band in around 60% of patients[4,5] and may also show hypogammaglobulinaemia[4]. Serum immunofixation electrophoresis (sIFE) demonstrates monoclonal bands in most patients but ultimately a more sensitive test is required to identify and quantitate the monoclonal FLCs. Additionally, urine protein electrophoresis (UPE) and urine immunofixation (uIFE) has also been necessary, however monoclonal FLCs can also be measured in the serum using serum FLC (sFLC) immunoassays. Figure 15.1 shows some typical electrophoretic test results alongside the associated sFLC (Freelite®) results.

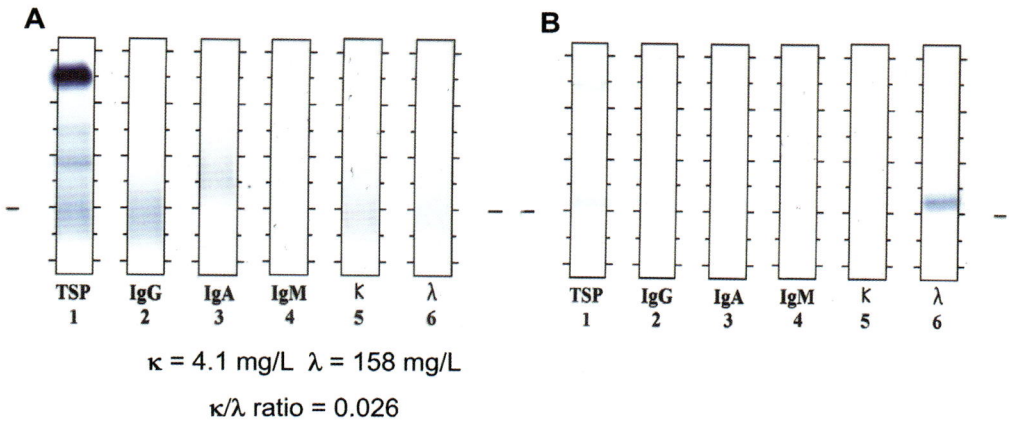

Figure 15.1. Serum and urine IFE from a patient with λ LCMM compared with sFLC immunoassay results. *SPE and IFE of (A) serum with no abnormality visible and (B) urine showing a λ FLC band.*

Since sFLC assays are more sensitive than electrophoretic tests *(Chapter 4)*, and considering the difficulties associated with urinalysis *(Chapter 24)*, could urine tests be avoided when a diagnosis of LCMM is being considered? The answer to this question was published in The Lancet in 2003 as a clear "Yes"[6]. This study was based on archived sera from 224 patients with LCMM entered into the UK MRC Myeloma trials between 1983 and 1999. The clinical diagnosis of LCMM had been established using bone marrow plasma cell content, the presence of monoclonal FLCs in the serum or urine (in the absence of intact monoclonal immunoglobulins), and the presence of lytic bone lesions. At the time of diagnosis, all patients had an abnormal concentration of the appropriate sFLC and an abnormal κ/λ sFLC ratio *(Figure 15.2)*. The non-tumour FLC concentrations produced by normal plasma cells were also abnormal in a high proportion of patients. Some were elevated as a result of renal impairment while others were low because of bone marrow suppression.

In 16 independent studies, which have included 692 LCMM patients, an abnormal κ/λ sFLC ratio was recorded in 100% of diagnostic samples *(Table 15.1)*. Only one study has reported a patient with a normal sFLC ratio at diagnosis[5]. In this case, although the involved λ sFLC concentration was highly abnormal (715 mg/L), an elevation of the uninvolved κ sFLC to 231 mg/L resulted in a normal ratio (0.32). At the next measurement (one month after diagnosis) the patients uninvolved κ sFLC concentration, although still abnormal, had dropped considerably to 99 mg/L. The λ sFLCs were still very high (686 mg/L) and the patient had an abnormal sFLC ratio (0.15), confirming the presence of monoclonal λ sFLCs. The reason for such a significant polyclonal elevation of the patient's FLCs at diagnosis was unknown to the authors (T. Jeong, personal communication).

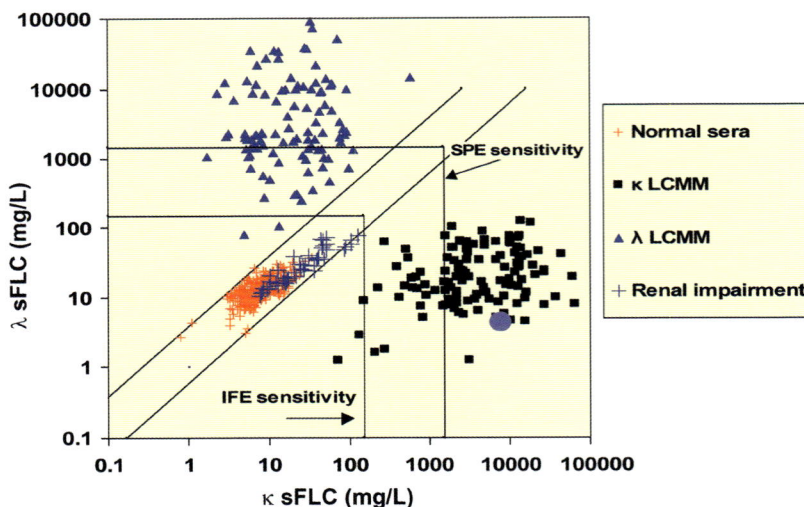

Figure 15.2. sFLC concentrations in normal individuals, patients with LCMM and patients with renal impairment but no plasma cell dyscrasia (Section 6.3). *Diagonal lines represent the limits of the reference interval for the κ/λ sFLC ratio (0.26-1.65, Chapter 6).*
● *Clinical case history 1.*

Study (year)	No. of patients	κ	λ	κ/λ ratio abnormal
Abraham (2002)[4]	28	9	19	100%
Bradwell (2003)[6]	224	123	101	100%
Kang (2005)[7]	23	14	9	100%
Nowrousian (2005)[8]	17	unknown	unknown	100%
Wolff (2006)[9]	5	unknown	unknown	100%
Giarin (2006)[10]	6	unknown	unknown	100%
Mösbauer (2007)[11]	9	5	4	100%
van Rhee (2007)[12]	49	unknown	unknown	100%
Hutchison (2008)[13]	13	5	8	100%
Piehler (2008)[14]	7	4	3	100%
Harding (2009)[15]	7	4	3	100%
Drayson (2009)[16]	223	unknown	unknown	100%
Kraj (2011)[17]	37	21	16	100%
Avet-Loiseau (2011)[18,19]	25	14	11	100%
Dogaru (2011)[20]	2	0	2	100%
Schneider (2013)[21]	17	unknown	unknown	100%

Table 15.1. sFLC measurements in studies of LCMM.

Jeong et al.[5] also assessed the diagnostic sensitivity of serum- and urine-based methods in screening panels for detecting monoclonal proteins. In their cohort of 231 MM patients, 49 (21%) had LCMM. The sFLC ratio alongside either SPE or sIFE were the only combinations that gave a diagnostic sensitivity of 100% for LCMM. By contrast, SPE in combination with UPE or uIFE gave a diagnostic sensitivity of 85.7% and 91.8%, respectively for LCMM. These results, and those of Katzmann et al.[22], highlight the benefits of a serum based screening algorithm for the detection of monoclonal FLCs *(Chapter 23)*. The sensitivity of sFLC analysis in LCMM patients is now reflected in international guidelines[23], which recommend the use of sFLC assays in combination with serum electrophoresis to screen for pathological monoclonal plasma cell proliferative disorders, including LCMM *(Chapter 25)*.

In The Lancet study mentioned above[6], all patients had elevated concentrations of both serum and urine involved FLCs, so it might be expected that the two variables would be highly correlated. In fact, there was only a modest association *(Figure 15.3)*. This may seem surprising, but can be explained by differences in renal tubular metabolism of FLCs. The amounts of FLCs observed in urine are highly dependent upon renal function *(Chapter 3)*. Hence, serum and urine FLC concentrations are frequently discordant, with serum being more representative of tumour mass than urine concentrations. The amount of sFLCs required to produce an abnormal urine test is discussed in Chapter 24.

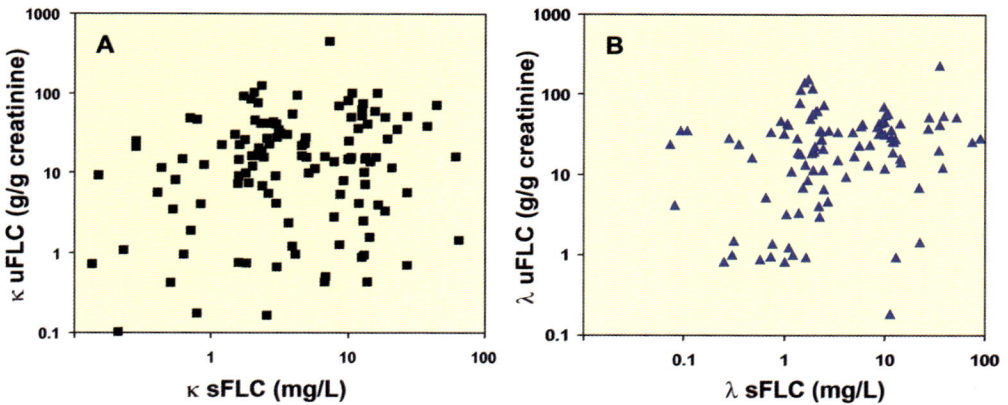

Figure 15.3. Relationship between serum and urine FLCs in 224 patients with LCMM at the time of diagnosis. (A) κ: r=0.29; p=0.0012. *(B)* λ: r=0.13; p=0.183. *Urine FLCs were measured by immunoassay and corrected for urine dilution using creatinine concentrations.*

Clinical case history 1

Unusual clinical features in a patient with LCMM.

A 63-year-old woman attended hospital with severe pain in her right shoulder. An X-ray showed minor erosive changes in the shoulder joint while blood tests were normal apart from a marginally elevated serum calcium of 2.69 mmol/L (normal range [NR]: 2.08 - 2.67). An orthopaedic surgeon recommended a hemiarthroplasty. At operation, the head of the humerus was eroded and the glenoid was almost entirely replaced by 'extremely soft bone' suggestive of malignancy or a metabolic cause. The operation was aborted and the tissue was sent for histological examination.

Re-examination of the patient failed to identify any additional clinical features. Investigations showed a normal chest X-ray while the serum calcium had increased further to 3.41 mmol/L and she was hypophosphataemic at 0.55 mmol/L (NR: 0.67 - 1.54). Other results included a raised alkaline phosphatase at 234 IU/L (NR: 30 - 115) and an increased parathyroid hormone-related peptide at 9.5 pmol/L (NR: 0.7 - 1.8) while parathyroid hormone levels were low at 9 ng/L (NR: 10 - 60). A metastatic tumour deposit was considered the most likely cause of her shoulder disease. The search for a primary tumour, however, was unsuccessful: CT scans of the abdomen and thorax were normal, as were the serum cancer markers, CA-199, CA-125 and CEA.

The possibility of multiple myeloma (MM) was considered. Bone histology from the surgically resected specimen showed osteoarthritis and osteopenia and there was no excess of plasma cells. A skeletal survey showed only osteoporotic bone with no discrete lytic lesions and no features of MM. Serum and urine electrophoretic tests showed no monoclonal gammopathy but assessment of immunoglobulins by nephelometry revealed hypogammaglobulinaemia: IgG 3.20 g/L (NR: 5.3 - 16.5), IgA 0.15 g/L (NR: 0.8 - 4.0) and IgM 0.26 g/L (NR: 0.5 - 2.0).

In view of the diagnostic difficulties, sFLC measurements were requested, with the following results: κ 7,840 mg/L (NR: 3.3 - 19.4); λ 4.4 mg/L (NR: 5.7 - 26.3); κ/λ ratio 1,782 (NR: 0.26 - 1.65) (Figure 15.4). Urinary FLC concentrations by immunoassay were as follows: κ 371 mg/L; λ 4.7 mg/L; κ/λ ratio 79. Subsequent bone marrow aspiration of the iliac crest indicated a high concentration of abnormal plasma cells. This established the diagnosis as κ LCMM with production of excess parathyroid hormone-related peptide leading to hypercalcaemia.

Several months after her initial clinical presentation, the patient was finally treated with chemotherapy. This resulted in a satisfactory reduction of the serum κ FLC concentrations and normalisation of serum calcium. Since then, her shoulder has remained unstable although pain free.

Comment. The diagnosis of LCMM can be difficult. In this case the clinical features were atypical and did not provide a clear suggestion as to the diagnosis, so tests for MM were not considered for some time. When electrophoretic analysis of serum and urine were eventually performed, the results showed no monoclonal proteins. Re-assessment of the original urine sample, showed a low concentration of monoclonal κ FLC by IFE, which had been overlooked on the earlier analysis. The final diagnosis was LCMM with limited plasma cell infiltration of the bone marrow. The response of the tumour to chemotherapy was good; serum κ FLC concentrations decreased for 45 weeks with a half-life of approximately 4 weeks (Figure 15.4). The patient is likely to have a good clinical course in the medium term.

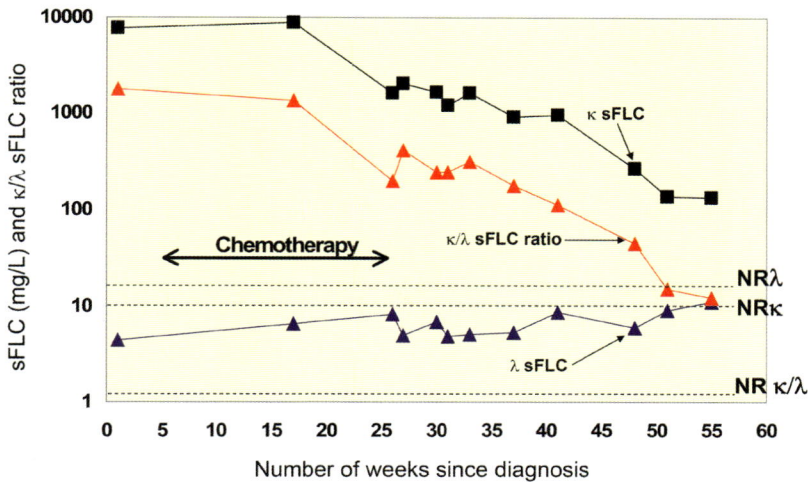

Figure 15.4. Clinical case history 1. sFLC concentrations in a patient with κ LCMM and unusual clinical features. NR: normal range.

15.2. Monitoring light chain multiple myeloma

Assays that are useful at disease diagnosis are typically useful for disease monitoring. This is particularly true for sFLC immunoassays. Not only are they quantitative but their analytical sensitivity is considerably better than measurements of monoclonal bands on electrophoretic gels (Chapter 4).

During the follow-up of LCMM patients who have detectable urinary monoclonal FLCs, changes in serum and urine FLC concentrations may show a good correlation. This is illustrated by two LCMM patients from the Mayo Clinic[4] (Figure 15.5). In both patients the concentrations of FLCs in serum and urine fell following chemotherapy (although in the first patient this was not in parallel, possibly due to inadequate 24-hour urine collections). In a further 71 LCMM patients, a good correlation was found between changes in serum and urine FLC concentrations[4] (Figure 15.6). The authors concluded that sFLC measurements provided a satisfactory alternative to 24-hour urine collections for monitoring patients with LCMM.

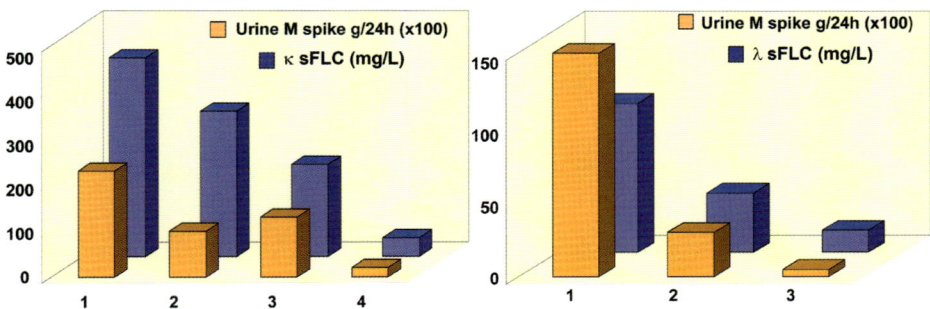

Figure 15.5. Comparison of 24-hour urinary monoclonal protein concentrations and sFLCs in 2 patients with LCMM, measured at different times after chemotherapy. (Courtesy of R.A. Kyle and J.A. Katzmann).

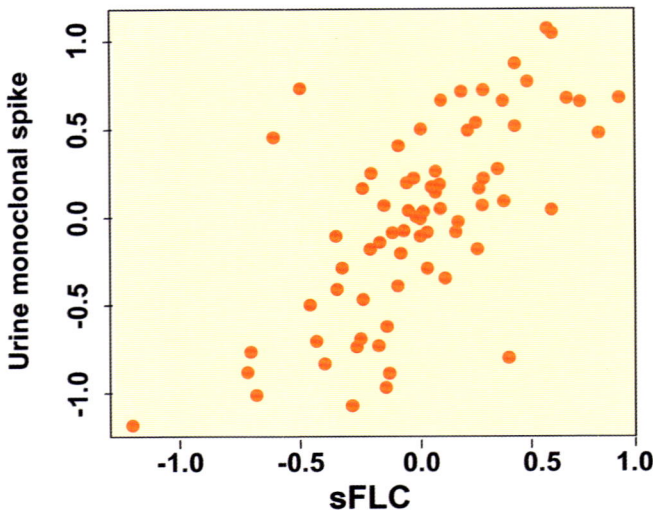

Figure 15.6. Correlation between changes in serum and urine FLCs during disease evolution in 71 patients with LCMM. Initial measurement values were changed to zero and transformed logarithmically for comparison purposes (p=0.0001). (Courtesy of R.A. Kyle and J.A. Katzmann).

However, there are considerable differences between serum and urine FLC measurements when assessing rates of remission. In The Lancet study[6], 32% (26/82) of patients were considered to be in complete remission when assessed by urine FLC concentrations compared with only 11% (9/82) upon sFLC assessment. In the same clinical trials, 10% (117/1189) of patients with intact immunoglobulin multiple myeloma (IIMM) had complete serological remission. Since the serum responses to chemotherapy were similar in IIMM and LCMM, the results indicated that urine FLC measurements were relatively insensitive for assessing residual disease. This has been substantiated in many other studies *(Chapter 24)* and is illustrated in Figure 15.7.

In many LCMM patients, urinary monoclonal protein becomes undetectable while serum tests remain abnormal. Reid et al.[24,25] assessed serological response in 35 LCMM patients judged to have achieved a complete response (CR) by negative serum and urine IFE. In 11 patients, the κ/λ sFLC ratio was normal, consistent with the definition of a stringent CR. In 24 patients however, an abnormal sFLC ratio suggested the presence of residual disease *(Figure 15.8)*. Other studies have similarly demonstrated that abnormal sFLC κ/λ ratios indicate residual disease in patients with negative serum and urine IFE[19,26].

The discrepancy between serum and urine results is mainly due to renal metabolism of FLCs *(Chapter 3)*. Other factors include increased sensitivity of the serum immunoassays and errors in the collection and measurement of urine samples *(Chapter 24)*. While urine testing can be uninformative in some patients, sFLC measurements may be a more reliable marker of treatment response, as demonstrated in Clinical case history 2[27].

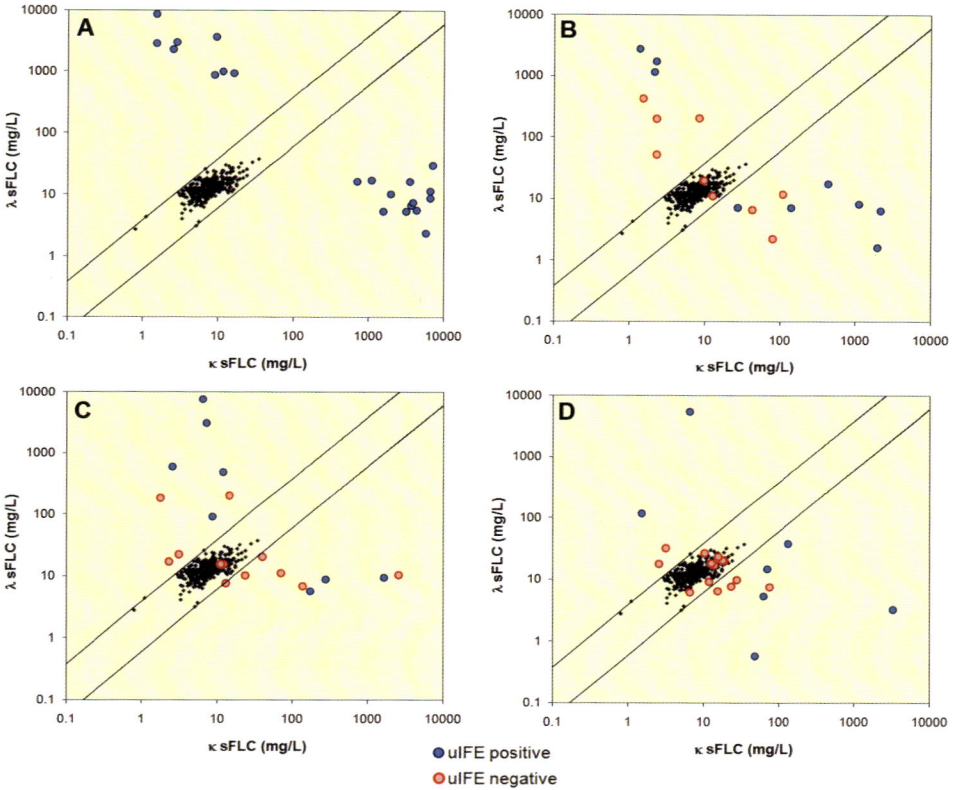

Figure 15.7. Comparison of sFLCs and urine electrophoresis for monitoring response to therapy for 25 patients with LCMM. At (A) presentation; (B) treatment cycle 2; (C) treatment cycle 4; and (D) post autologous stem cell transplant. After cycle 4 of therapy 9/21 patients with negative uIFE had an abnormal sFLC ratio, indicating residual disease. Black diamonds: 282 normal sera; parallel lines indicate the limits of the normal reference interval for the κ/λ sFLC ratio. (Courtesy of H. Avet Loiseau).

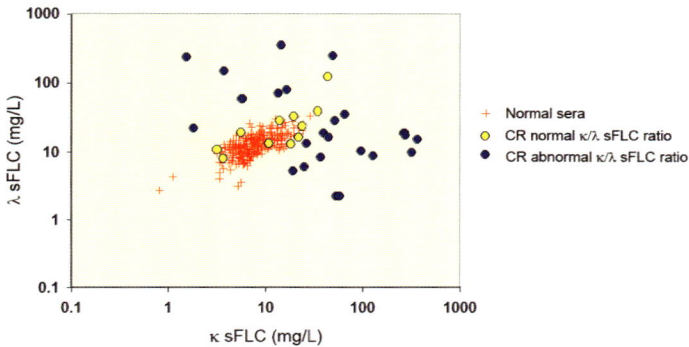

Figure 15.8. sFLC concentrations in 35 patients with LCMM at the time of complete response (CR; normal immunofixation tests). Normal sera are shown for comparison[24,25].

Clinical case history 2

Sensitivity of sFLCs for identifying poor response to treatment.[27]

A 59-year-old female, previously diagnosed with asymptomatic κ LCMM, was admitted to hospital because of increasing proteinuria. Haematological work-up reported a κ sFLC concentration of 200 mg/L and a λ sFLC concentration of 6.73 mg/L with a corresponding κ/λ sFLC ratio of 29.72. Urinary protein was reported as 6.5 g/24 hours and immunotyped as κ BJP. A bone marrow biopsy was hypocellular with 48.0% plasma cells. The patient was diagnosed with symptomatic κ LCMM (stage IIA [Durie and Salmon]; stage 2 [International Staging System]). The patient received induction therapy with high-dose dexamethasone (HDD), followed by four cycles of bortezomib/dexamethasone (BD). Over the course of treatment, urinary protein decreased from 6.5 to 0.1 g/24 hours (Figure 15.9).

Retrospective measurement of sFLCs twice weekly revealed additional information on FLC kinetics: sFLC levels initially fell during induction then markedly increased prior to starting BD therapy. Smaller changes in sFLC concentrations were also observed during each BD cycle, and the κ/λ sFLC ratio never entered the normal range. This case study and others[27] highlight that measurement of sFLCs allows early identification of patients responding poorly to treatment, whereas urine testing was uninformative. In future, such information could be adopted to allow early cessation of ineffective therapy and a switch to a more appropriate chemotherapeutic strategy.

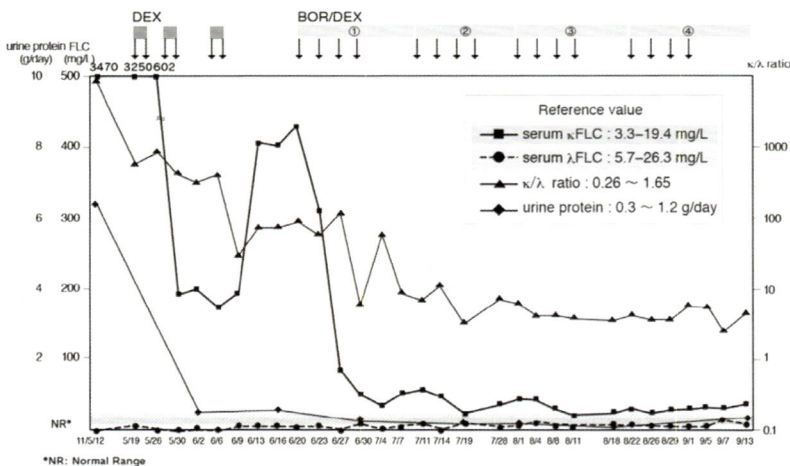

Figure 15.9. Serial sFLC and urine protein measurements in a patient with LCMM during treatment. DEX: dexamethasone; BOR/DEX: bortezomib and dexamethasone. (This research was originally published in International Journal of Hematology[27] © 2012 by The Japanese Society of Hematology).

15.3. Prognostic value of the sFLC response in light chain multiple myeloma

Reid et al. [24,25] determined the impact of abnormal sFLC ratios on survival. In a preliminary analysis including 35 LCMM patients, they showed that an abnormal κ/λ sFLC ratio in IFE-negative patients had a negative impact on overall survival. In a separate study, Boyle et al.[28] assessed the prognostic significance of the sFLC response in 122 LCMM patients. Following treatment, patients who achieved both a normal κ/λ sFLC ratio and a normal involved FLC concentration (32/122; 26%) had a significantly longer progression free survival and overall survival compared to those with a normalisation of their ratio only (50/122; 41%) ($p<0.001$ and $p=0.012$, respectively). Both these groups had a better survival than the remaining 40 patients judged to have had a suboptimal response ($p=0.012$). These studies highlight the prognostic relevance of sFLC measurements in LCMM, sFLC responses are similarly prognostic in patients with intact immunoglobulin MM and this is discussed in more detail in Chapter 20.

Test Questions

1. Describe the correlation between serum and urine concentrations of FLCs at diagnosis in patients with LCMM.

2. Do serum and urine FLC measurements always correlate during monitoring of LCMM?

3. What may account for the discrepancy between serum and urine FLC results?

Answers

1. A modest correlation (Section 15.1).

2. No. Although changes in serum and urine FLC concentrations often correlate when uBJP is present, sFLC measurements can indicate residual disease and/or provide an early indication of relapse in patients with undetectable uBJP (Section 15.2).

3. Renal metabolism of FLCs, increased sensitivity of sFLC assays and errors in the collection and measurement of urine samples (Section 15.2 and Chapter 24).

References

1. Bridgen ML, Webber D. Clinical Pathology Rounds: The case of the anaplastic carcinoma that was not - potential problems in the interpretation of monoclonal proteins. Lab Med 2000;31:661–5

2. Van Zaanen HC, Diderich PP, Pegels JG, Ruizeveld de Winter JA. [Renal insufficiency due to light chain multiple myeloma]. Ned Tijdschr Geneeskd 2000;144:2133–7

3. Chaves Lameiro P, Lazaro de la Osa J, Gonzalez J. Difficulties identifying a monoclonal component in a Bence-Jones multiple myeloma, a clinical case. Biochmica Clinica 2013;37:W249a

4. Abraham RS, Clark RJ, Bryant SC, Lymp JF, Larson T, Kyle RA, Katzmann JA. Correlation of serum immunoglobulin free light chain quantification with urinary Bence Jones protein in light chain myeloma. Clin Chem 2002;48:655-7

5. Jeong TD, Kim SY, Jang S et al. Diagnostic sensitivity of a panel of tests to detect monoclonal protein in Korean multiple myeloma patients. Clin Chem Lab Med 2013;51:e187-9

6. Bradwell AR, Carr-Smith HD, Mead GP, Harvey TC, Drayson MT. Serum test for assessment of patients with Bence Jones myeloma. Lancet 2003;361:489–91

7. Kang SY, Suh JT, Lee HJ, Yoon HJ, Lee WI. Clinical usefulness of free light chain concentration as a tumor marker in multiple myeloma. Ann Hematol 2005;84:588-93

8. Nowrousian MR, Brandhorst D, Sammet C, Kellert M, Daniels R, Schuett P, et al. Serum free light chain analysis and urine immunofixation electrophoresis in patients with multiple myeloma. Clin Cancer Res 2005;11:8706–14

9. Wolff F, Thiry C, Willems D. Assessment of the analytical performance and the sensitivity of serum free light chains immunoassay in patients with monoclonal gammopathy. Clin Biochem 2007;40:351-4

10. Giarin MM, Giaccone L, Caracciolo D, Bruno B, Falco P, Omedè P et al. Serum free light chains (SFLC) assay: a suggestive new criteria for evaluating disease response, progression and relapse in plasma-cell disorders (PD) and a prognostic factor in monoclonal gammopathy of undetermined significance (MGUS). Haematologica 2006;91:PO151a

11. Mösbauer U, Ayuk F, Schieder H, Lioznov M, Zander AR, Kroger N. Monitoring serum free light chains in patients with multiple myeloma who achieved negative immunofixation after allogeneic stem cell transplantation. Haematologica 2007;92:275–6

12. Van Rhee F, Bolejack V, Hollmig K, Pineda-Roman M, Anaissie E, Epstein J, et al. High serum-free light chain levels and their rapid reduction in response to therapy define an aggressive multiple myeloma subtype with poor prognosis. Blood 2007;110:827–32

13. Hutchison CA, Plant T, Drayson M, Cockwell P, Kountouri M, Basnayake K, et al. Serum free light chain measurement aids the diagnosis of myeloma in patients with severe renal failure. BMC Nephrol 2008;9:11

14. Piehler AP, Gulbrandsen N, Kierulf P, Urdal P. Quantitation of serum free light chains in combination with protein electrophoresis and clinical information for diagnosing multiple myeloma in a general hospital population. Clin Chem 2008;54:1823-30

15. Harding SJ, Mead GP, Bradwell AR, Berard AM. Serum free light chain immunoassay as an adjunct to serum protein electrophoresis and immunofixation electrophoresis in the detection of multiple myeloma and other B-cell malignancies. Clin Chem Lab Med 2009;47:302-4

16. Drayson MT, Morgan GJ, Jackson GH, Davies FE, Owen RG, Ross FM, et al. Prospective study of serum FLC and other M-protein assays: when and how to measure response? Clin Lymphoma Myeloma 2009;9:A346a

17. Kraj M, Kruk B, Poglod R, Szczepinski A. Correlation of serum free light chain quantification with serum and urine immunofixation in monoclonal gammopathies. Haematologica 2011;96:0861a

18. Avet Loiseau H, Mirbahai L, Young P, Mathiot C, Attal M, Moreau P et al. Nephelometric measurements of κFLC and λFLC for monitoring light chain multiple myeloma patients. Presented at Lymphoma and Myeloma 2011

19. Avet-Loiseau H, Young P, Mathiot C, Attal M, Harousseau J, Bradwell AR, Mirbahai L. Nephelometric measurements of ⬚FLC and λFLC for monitoring light chain myeloma patients. Haematologica 2011;96:0853a

20. Dogaru M, Lazar V, Coriu D. Assessing the efficiency of free light chain assay in monitoring patients with multiple myeloma before and after autologous stem cell transplantation along with serum protein electrophoresis and serum protein immunofixation. Roum Arch Microbiol Immunol 2011;70:15-22

21. Schneider N, Wynckel A, Kolb B, Sablon E, Gillery P, Maquart FX. [Comparative analysis of immunoglobulin free light chains quantification by Freelite (The Binding Site) and N Latex FLC (Siemens) methods]. Ann Biol Clin (Paris) 2013;71:13-19

22. Katzmann JA, Kyle RA, Benson J, Larson DR, Snyder MR, Lust JA et al. Screening panels for detection of monoclonal gammopathies. Clin Chem 2009;55:1517-22

23. Dispenzieri A, Kyle R, Merlini G, Miguel JS, Ludwig H, Hajek R, et al. International Myeloma Working Group guidelines for serum-free light chain analysis in multiple myeloma and related disorders. Leukemia 2009;23:215-24

24. Reid SD, Mead GP, Drayson MT, Bradwell AR. Comparison of immunofixation electrophoresis with serum free light chain measurement for determining complete remission in light chain multiple myeloma. Bone Marrow Transplant 2004;33:632a

25. Reid SD, Drayson MT, Mead GP, Augustson B, Bradwell AR. Serum free light chains are a more sensitive marker of serological remission in multiple myeloma patients. Clin Chem 2004;50:C34a

26. Lebovic D, Kendall T, Brozo C, McAllister A, Hari M, Alvi S et al. Serum free light chain analysis improves monitoring of multiple myeloma patients receiving first-line therapy with the combination of Velcade, Doxil, and Dexamethasone (VDD). Blood 2007;110:2736a

27. Fuchida SI, Okano A, Hatsuse M, Murakami S, Haruyama H, Itoh S, Shimazaki C. Serial measurement of free light chain detects poor response to therapy early in three patients with multiple myeloma who have measurable M-proteins. Int J Hematol 2012;96:664-8

28. Boyle E, Brioli A, Leleu X, Morgan G, Pawlyn C, Davies F et al. The value of serum free light chain monitoring compared to urinary Bence-Jones measurement in light chain only myeloma. Blood 2013;122:1895a

Nonsecretory multiple myeloma

In nonsecretory multiple myeloma, sFLC measurements:

- Are abnormal in the majority of patients and are important for diagnosis.
- Can be used for monitoring, without the need for frequent bone marrow biopsies or radiological scans.
- Are recommended by international guidelines for diagnosis and monitoring.
- Allow patients to be included in clinical trials from which they were previously excluded.

16.1. Introduction

Nonsecretory multiple myeloma (NSMM) accounts for 1 - 5% of all multiple myeloma (MM) cases [1,2]. The disease is characterised by the absence of detectable monoclonal proteins in serum and urine using immunofixation electrophoresis (IFE)[1,3,4]. However, monoclonal proteins can usually be detected immunohistochemically in bone marrow plasma cells (BMPCs) indicating that the patients have tumour cells that produce but may not secrete monoclonal immunoglobulins into the blood. Also, using highly sensitive tests such as isoelectric focusing, monoclonal proteins have been detected in the sera of some patients[5]. Ultimately, only 10 - 15% of NSMM patients are true "non-producers" in whom tumour plasma cells contain no detectable immunoglobulins[6].

As electrophoresis procedures for detecting monoclonal proteins have become more sensitive and reliable, fewer patients are now diagnosed with NSMM. Yet, even in expert hands, 2 - 3% of patients with MM have undetectable serum or urine monoclonal proteins by IFE and are classified as NSMM [3,7,8,9]. From a logical standpoint, such patients cannot be producing significant amounts of intact monoclonal immunoglobulins; IgG molecules accumulate in serum with a half-life of 3 - 4 weeks, so their production from even small clones of plasma cells can be visualised as monoclonal bands on serum protein electrophoresis (SPE) gels. By contrast, free light chains (FLCs) have a serum half-life of only 2 - 6 hours, 100- to 200-fold less *(Section 3.5)*. Clonal production of monoclonal FLCs, therefore, needs to be correspondingly much greater to produce similar serum concentrations of monoclonal protein to those found in IgG-producing MM. NSMM patients are therefore more likely to be producing low amounts of monoclonal FLC. Urinalysis may also be unhelpful because patients with NSMM usually have normal renal function. The modest monoclonal FLC production, typically seen, may not be sufficient to damage or overwhelm the reabsorption capacity of the kidneys and enter the urine *(Section 3.5.2)*. Hence, more sensitive methodologies are required when the production of FLCs is too low for detection by electrophoresis techniques.

16.2. Diagnosis of nonsecretory multiple myeloma

The above arguments suggest that sensitive assays for sFLCs might detect monoclonal proteins in a proportion of patients with NSMM. The results from a large study are shown in Table 16.1[1]. Archived sera were obtained from patients studied in MRC MM trials undertaken in the UK between 1983 and 1999. Of 2323 patients, 64 (2.8%) were diagnosed with NSMM and, of these, 28 were selected for study based on the availability of complete clinical records and the appropriate stored serum samples. In all patients, concentrations of κ and λ sFLCs were compared with results from SPE and IFE tests. The results showed that 19 of the 28 sera had abnormal κ/λ sFLC ratios and elevated κ or λ sFLC concentrations. A further four samples showed abnormally low levels of one or both sFLCs. sFLC concentrations in the remaining five samples were substantially normal *(Figure 16.1* and *Table 16.2).*

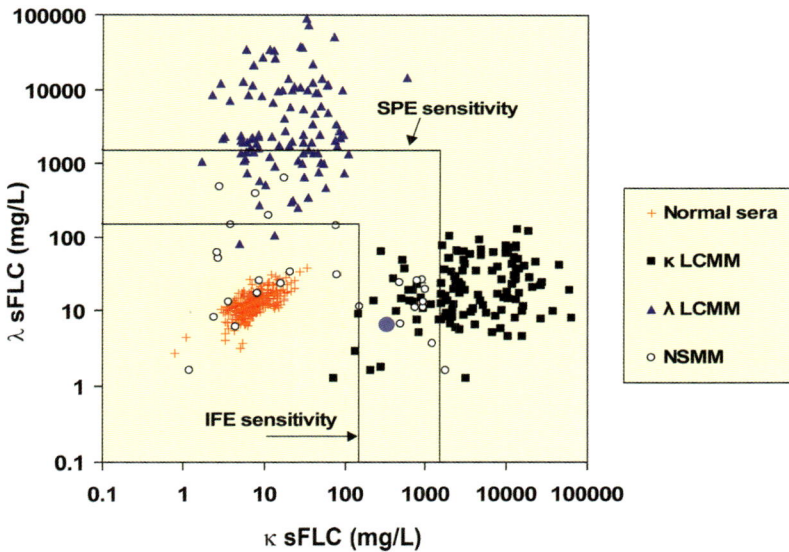

Figure 16.1. sFLC concentrations in patients with NSMM compared with normal individuals and patients with LCMM.
● *Clinical case history 1.*

Classification based on sFLCs		κ sFLC (mg/L)	λ sFLC (mg/L)	κ/λ sFLC ratio	BMPC %	Other Results
Serum reference interval		3.6 - 16	8.1 - 33	0.36 - 1.0		
12 patients: elevated free κ and increased κ/λ ratio	1	1754	1.6	1096	85	IFE κ +/-
	2	1201	3.6	333	82	BJP κ +/-
	3	935	11	85	70	ND
	4	487	6.6	74	20	ND
	5	931	13.2	71	>90	IFE κ +/-
	6	730	11.1	65	35	ND
	7	978	19.4	50	65	ND
	8	920	26.3	35	14*	ND
	9	789	25.6	31	>50	BJP κ +/-
	10	480	23.8	20	30	ND
	11	151	11.5	13	66	Hist κ +
	12	79.8	30.8	2.6	50	ND
7 patients: elevated free λ with reduced κ/λ ratio	13	11.2	196	0.057	20	IFE λ +
	14	2.7	50.9	0.053	74	ND
	15	2.6	61	0.043	6*	ND
	16	17.8	624	0.029	8	IFE λ, BJP +/-
	17	3.8	144	0.026	70	ND
	18	7.7	389	0.019	60	ND
	19	2.8	481	0.005	29	IFE λ +
4 patients: suppression of either κ, λ or both FLCs	20	4.5	6	0.75	21	ND
	21	1.2	1.6	0.75	55	ND
	22	2.4	8.1	0.296	34	ND
	23	3.6	13.1	0.274	70	ND
5 patients: κ or λ normal or elevated and κ/λ ratios normal or borderline	24	16.2	23.4	0.692	67	ND
	25	20.7	33	0.627	73	ND
	26	77	142	0.543	18	IFE λ +
	27	8.3	17.4	0.477	9*	ND
	28	8.6	25.2	0.341	80	ND

BMPC: bone marrow plasma cell; Hist: immunohistochemical confirmation of MM; IFE +/-: weak diffuse bands; IFE +: weak narrow band; BJP +/-: low concentrations of urine FLCs; ND not detected; *trephine biopsy +ve for MM.

Table 16.1. sFLC concentrations in 28 patients with NSMM[1]. Serum reference intervals were the 95% ranges in use at the time of publication.

Careful repeat testing of the 28 sera by IFE, using optimal sensitivity *(Table 16.1)*, showed monoclonal sFLCs in six, but the monoclonal bands were mostly weak and diffuse. Rather surprisingly, in nine of the 28 patients no monoclonal bands were seen using IFE even though the immunoassays indicated sFLC concentrations of >200 mg/L. In many of these samples, the elevated FLC concentrations should have been easily detectable by IFE. IFE gels from five of the serum samples containing high concentrations of κ sFLCs are shown in Figure 16.2. These are compared with three samples from patients with typical κ light chain multiple myeloma (LCMM). The sFLCs in the NSMM samples failed to focus into the same narrow monoclonal bands seen in the LCMM sera.

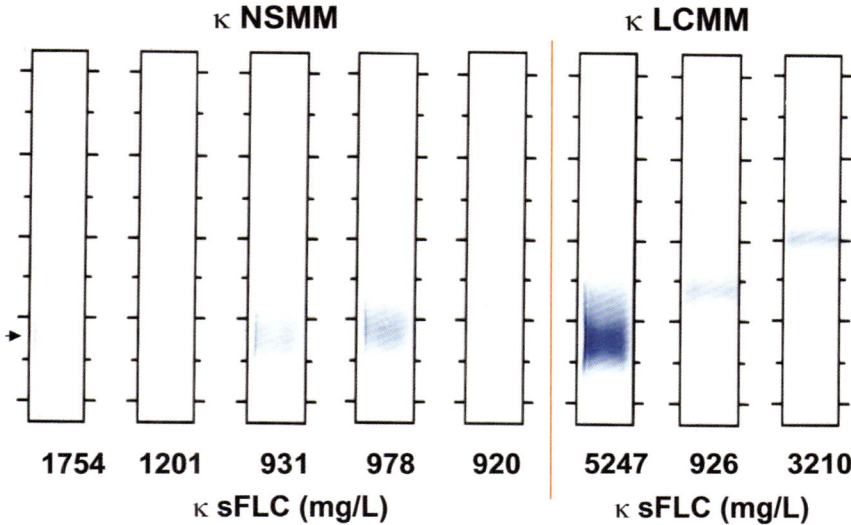

κ NSMM   κ LCMM

| 1754 | 1201 | 931 | 978 | 920 | | 5247 | 926 | 3210 |

κ sFLC (mg/L)   κ sFLC (mg/L)

Figure 16.2. Serum IFE from five patients with κ NSMM and three patients with κ LCMM. Samples were applied at similar FLC concentrations.

Two sera from NSMM patients with substantial concentrations of sFLCs measured by nephelometry (980 mg/L and 1700 mg/L), were subjected to size-separation gel chromatography and found to contain highly polymerised FLCs (40 - 200 kDa) *(Figure 16.3)*. This suggested that variable polymerisation caused the monoclonal bands to smear on the SPE gels and this could account for their absence or diffuse appearance. Such large polymers would have minimal renal clearance compared with monomeric FLCs. Good renal function would be maintained (typical of these patients) and little FLC would enter the urine. These observations concur with other reports that describe polymerised or structurally abnormal FLCs in some patients with MM *(Section 7.5)*[10,11,12].

Of additional interest, it was found that diffuse bands were more common in κ FLC-producing patients *(Table 16.1)*. Hence, λ patients with low FLC production are more likely to produce discrete monoclonal bands and be classified as "secretory" LCMM. At one time, the lack of λ NSMM led to the suggestion that such patients may not exist. Moreover, the observed higher frequency of κ FLC polymerisation probably explains the 4:1 ratio of κ to λ NSMM patients reported in the literature[3].

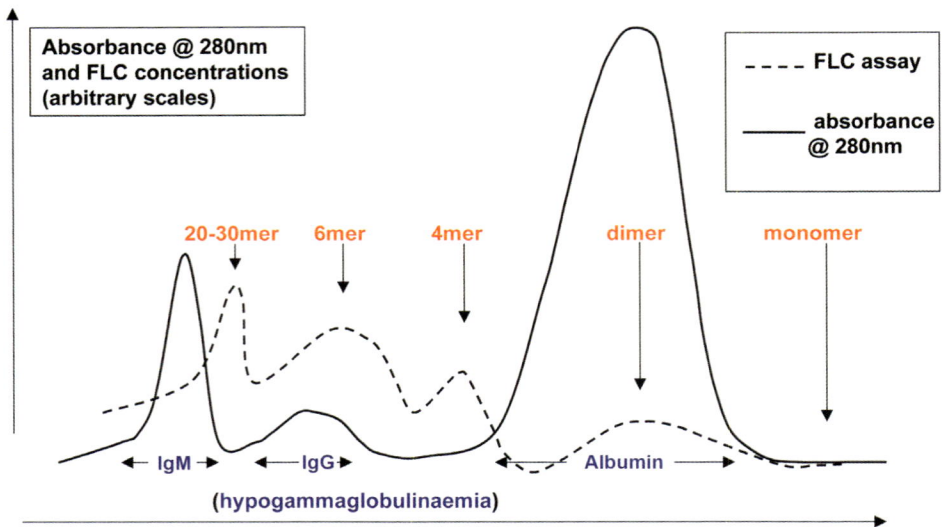

Figure 16.3. Size-separation gel chromatography showing the FLC size variation in a serum sample from a patient with NSMM. The sample contained 1754 mg/L of κ FLCs by Freelite® immunoassay but was negative by SPE and IFE (Figure 16.2).

There has only been one other large study of sFLC measurements in NSMM: Chawla et al.[13] found an abnormal κ/λ sFLC ratio in 19/29 (65%) NSMM patients at diagnosis. In addition, the authors reported that overall survival was worse in patients with an abnormal sFLC ratio at baseline compared to patients with a normal ratio, similar to findings for MM patients in general (Section 20.2).

Other reports have confirmed the diagnostic sensitivity of the sFLC ratio in smaller groups of NSMM patients. Cavallo et al.[14] reported that four of five NSMM patients had abnormal FLC concentrations. Most recently, Jeong et al.[15] found abnormal κ/λ sFLC ratios in two NSMM patients with normal serum and urine electrophoresis and immunofixation results. They commented that a combination of SPE and sFLC analysis was effective in screening for monoclonal gammopathies, including NSMM (Chapter 23).

Whilst elevated sFLC concentrations are found in a high proportion of patients conventionally thought of as non-secretory, normal sFLC results can be indicative of true non-secretory patients or non-producing patients. Papanikolaou et al.[16] reviewed flow cytometry data for 210 NSMM patients and identified 19 that had no cytoplasmic immunoglobulin detected. sFLC analysis of these patients revealed normal sFLC ratios for 18/19, demonstrating concordance with the flow cytometry results. In the one patient with an abnormal sFLC ratio, elevated sFLCs were attributable to grade 3 renal failure. Application of the renal reference interval for the κ/λ sFLC ratio may aid interpretation of results in such cases (Section 6.3). Ma et al.[17] also reported a true 'non-producing' NSMM patient in whom normal sFLC results were in agreement with electrophoretic and immunohistochemical analysis.

The widespread routine use of sFLC immunoassays has made the identification of true NSMM even rarer than previously observed, with a frequency in the order of only one in 200 myeloma cases[18].

16.3. Monitoring nonsecretory multiple myeloma

The assessment of disease burden using routine marrow histology and flow cytometry is notoriously inaccurate, due in large part to the patchy nature of marrow involvement and issues with sampling[2]. The sFLC assays facilitate disease response assessment in most NSMM patients, and can be done with routine blood testing rather than requiring imaging or bone marrow assessment[2]. As sFLC concentrations assess FLC production from all of the bone marrow and extramedullary sites, they are likely to provide a better indication of overall tumour activity than bone marrow aspirations or skeletal surveys. The use of sFLC analysis for monitoring oligosecretory patients including those previously classified as NSMM, is now recommended in international guidelines *(Chapter 25)*.

In the first study of sFLCs in NSMM patients, limited monitoring samples were available from six patients, and revealed elevated sFLC levels at clinical presentation, reduced concentrations during plateau phase, and increased levels at relapse *(Figure 16.4)*[1]. One patient (no. 2) showed some discordance between the clinical assessment and sFLC concentrations; whilst still being classified as being in remission, rising concentrations of sFLCs indicated imminent disease relapse.

Historically, randomised trials have generally tended to exclude patients with NSMM because they do not have easily measurable disease[19]. However, since the incorporation of sFLC analysis into the International Uniform Response Criteria (IURC) *(Chapter 25)*, the majority of NSMM patients can now be enrolled into clinical trials. For example, in the study of 28 NSMM patients described above, 17/28 (61%) patients had measurable monoclonal sFLC concentrations (defined as involved sFLCs >100 mg/L)[1]. Many patients with NSMM have been studied prospectively since sFLC analysis has been routinely available. Two examples are described in the clinical case histories below.

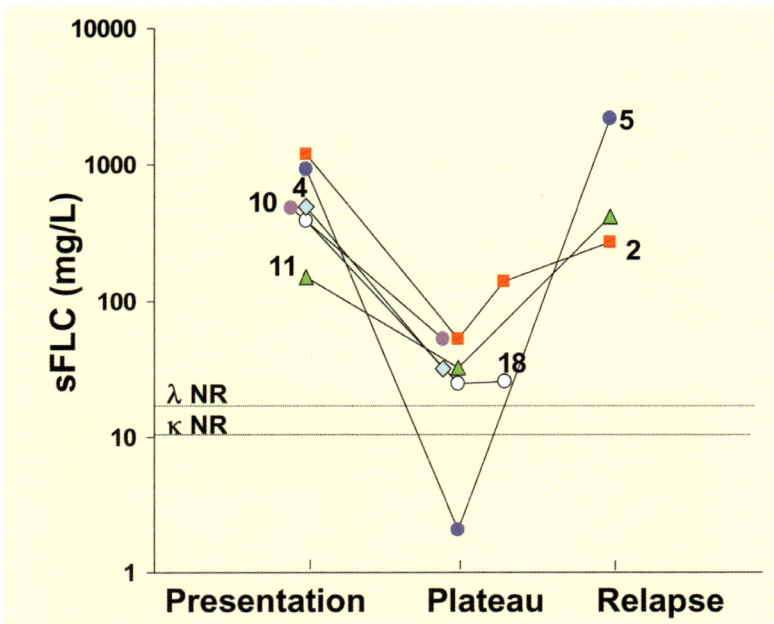

Figure 16.4. Changes in sFLCs and clinical status in 6 patients with NSMM. Numbers refer to patients in Table 16.1. NR: upper limit of normal range. (This research was originally published in Blood[1] © the American Society of Hematology).

Clinical case history 1

NSMM with "difficult to assess" symptoms during clinical relapse.

A 38-year-old woman presented with a fractured rib following mild trauma. Over the following months, the pain subsided but non-specific symptoms including breathlessness, vague chest pains and tiredness persisted. During this time, full blood counts, erythrocyte sedimentation rate (ESR) and biochemistry were all normal, as were chest X-rays and lung function tests. In the absence of a diagnosis, the general practitioner considered a psychiatric assessment.

Seven months after the initial presentation, she remained symptomatic and was re-investigated, whereupon bone scans and X-rays showed extensive osseous lesions. Immunoglobulin measurements showed immunoparesis, but no serum monoclonal protein was detected. She was noted to have hypercalcaemia (2.85 mmol/L - NR: 2.08 - 2.67) but had normal renal function. In view of the absence of monoclonal immunoglobulins, MM was still considered unlikely. However, a skull X-ray and CT scan showed osteolytic lesions *(Figure 16.5)* so a skull biopsy was performed which was reported as 'plasmacytoma/NSMM'. She was given chemotherapy for the following 8 months that resulted in clinical remission.

Seven months later, and over 2 years after the initial presentation, she re-attended hospital because of chest pains and breathlessness. Again, clinical examination was normal, as were routine biochemistry and haematology tests. Immunology tests showed reduced immunoglobulins but no detectable monoclonal protein by serum electrophoresis. A bone marrow biopsy showed 5% plasma cells that were morphologically normal. Chest X-ray, a ventilation perfusion scan and lung function tests revealed no evidence of pulmonary disease. Blood tests were requested for sFLCs, the results of which were: κ 330 mg/L, λ 6.5 mg/L and an abnormal κ/λ ratio of 51 *(Figures 16.1 and 16.6* [week 67]). Doubt was expressed regarding the validity of the results so sFLC measurements were repeated 2 and 3 weeks later and showed κ increases to 470 mg/L and then 525 mg/L with a rising κ/λ ratio, confirming disease recurrence.

sFLC concentrations were assessed retrospectively from archived samples and then the patient was monitored prospectively. Figure 16.6 shows that the κ sFLC concentrations had increased rapidly during the tumour recurrence, with an apparent doubling time of 30 days as indicated by the κ/λ ratio. κ sFLC concentrations subsequently reduced during treatment. During the period of relapse, the λ sFLC concentration increased suggesting reduced renal clearance of FLCs from impaired glomerular filtration *(Section 6.3)*. After a peripheral blood stem cell transplant (PBSCT) κ and λ sFLC concentrations and the κ/λ sFLC ratio returned towards normal as the patient went into clinical remission.

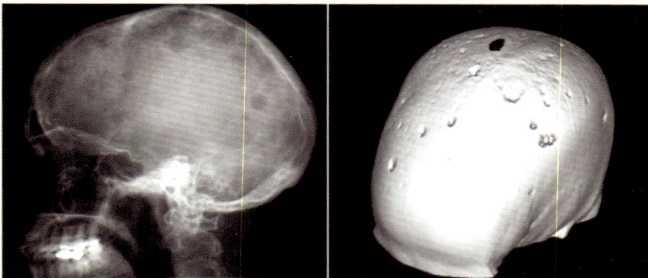

Figure 16.5. X-ray and computerised tomography (CT) scans of the skull in NSMM.

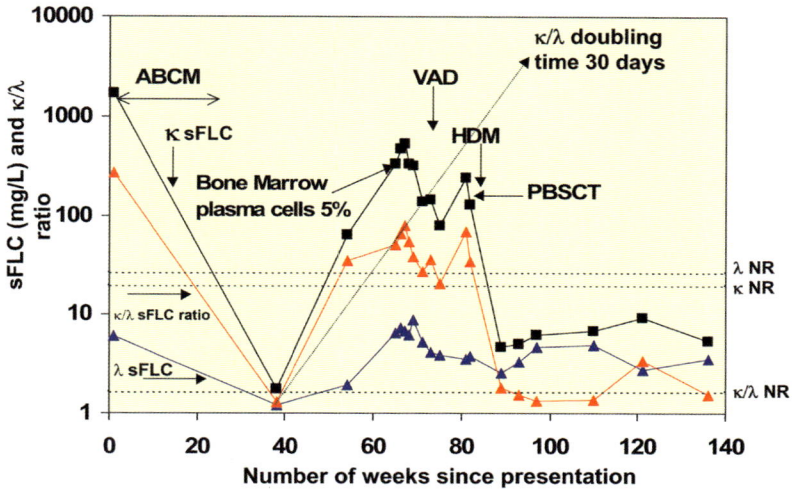

Figure 16.6. sFLC concentrations during the course of the disease in a patient with NSMM.
The changing κ/λ sFLC ratio is related to the tumour growth. ABCM: adriamycin (doxorubicin),
busulphan, cyclophosphamide, melphalan; VAD: vincristine, adriamycin (doxorubicin),
dexamethasone; HDM: high dose melphalan; PBSCT: peripheral blood stem cell transplant.

Clinical case history 2

A patient with NSMM/plasmacytoma who was excluded from clinical trials.

A 37-year-old man with pelvic pain was found to have a solitary plasmacytoma located in the right iliac crest. Bone marrow biopsy of the opposite iliac crest was normal and no monoclonal protein was identified in serum or urine. Treatment comprised surgical resection followed by irradiation (5,000 Gy). Subsequently, he remained asymptomatic, but 5 years later a routine skeletal survey showed a thoracic spine lesion at T2, which was irradiated. Over the following 7 years further painful lesions developed. These were identified using different scanning techniques (particularly positron emission tomography) and were treated with irradiation or melphalan and prednisolone.

Throughout this period, and in spite of repeated testing, no monoclonal protein was identified by SPE and UPE. Finally, 12 years after the initial presentation, sFLC immunoassays became available and showed κ 7.5 mg/L, λ 632 mg/L and a κ/λ ratio of 0.01. These results identified a λ-producing tumour with no associated suppression of the κ sFLCs *(Figure 16.7)*. One month later, λ sFLC concentrations had increased to 700 mg/L, prompting treatment with thalidomide (50 mg/day) and dexamethasone (40 mg/week). Over the subsequent 7 months, the λ sFLC concentration gradually fell to 33 mg/L and the κ/λ sFLC ratio began to normalise. Based on the sFLC results, dexamethasone was reduced to 12 mg/week and he remained well and in complete remission.

Figure 16.7 shows the changes in sFLC concentrations over a 12-month period. The effectiveness of the drugs and the doses required can all be monitored during this period of therapy. This has produced clear benefits for the patient and avoided costly scans and painful bone marrow biopsies. Furthermore, since the patient has measureable monoclonal sFLCs (>100 mg/L[19,20]) he can be entered into clinical trials of new treatments. The patient has been monitored successfully using sFLC assays for many years since the original tests were performed.

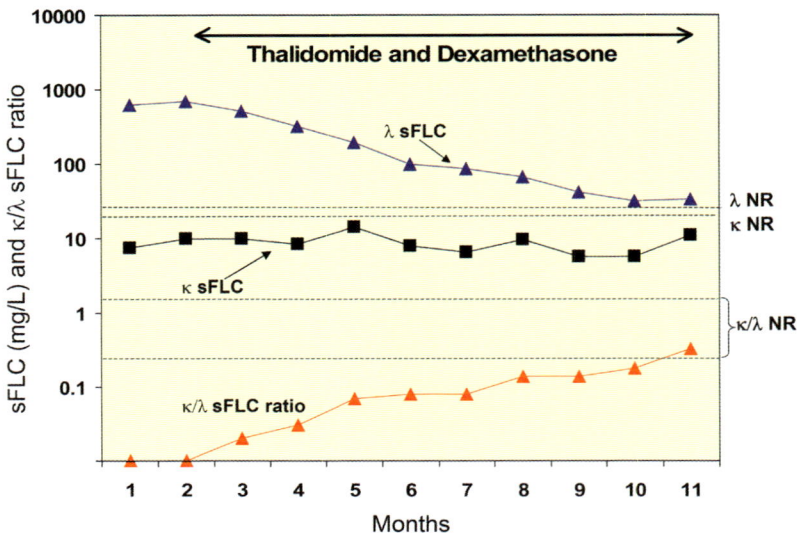

Figure 16.7. sFLC concentrations during treatment for NSMM. NR: normal range.

Test Questions

1. What proportion of patients classified as non-secretory, have abnormal sFLC ratios?

2. Do international guidelines recommend sFLC analysis for NSMM patients?

Answers

1. In the largest study to date, 68% had abnormal κ/λ sFLC ratios. Other smaller studies suggest that it could be higher.

2. Yes, sFLC analysis is recommended by international guidelines for the diagnosis and monitoring of NSMM (*Chapter 25*).

References

1. Drayson M, Tang LX, Drew R, Mead GP, Carr-Smith H, Bradwell AR. Serum free light-chain measurements for identifying and monitoring patients with nonsecretory multiple myeloma. Blood 2001;97:2900–2

2. Lonial S, Kaufman JL. Non-secretory myeloma: a clinician's guide. Oncology (Williston Park) 2013;27:924-8, 930

3. Blade J, Kyle RA. Nonsecretory myeloma, immunoglobulin D myeloma and plasma cell leukemia. Hematol/Oncology Clinics of North America 1999;13:1259–72

4. Dreicer R, Alexanian R. Nonsecretory multiple myeloma. Am J Hematol 1982;13:313–8

5. Sheehan T, Sinclair D, Tansey P, O'Donnell JR. Demonstration of serum monoclonal immunoglobulin in a case of non-secretory myeloma by immunoisoelectric focusing. J Clin Pathol 1985;38:806–9

6. Raubenheimer EJ, Dauth J, Senekal JC. Non-secretory IgA kappa myeloma with distended endoplasmic reticulum: a case report. Histopathology 1991;19:380–2

7. Reilly BM, Clarke P, Nikolinakos P. Clinical problem-solving. Easy to see but hard to find. N Engl J Med 2003;348:59–64

8. Katzmann JA, Abraham RS, Dispenzieri A, Lust JA, Kyle RA. Diagnostic performance of quantitative kappa and lambda free light chain assays in clinical practice. Clin Chem 2005;51:878–81

9. van Rhee F, Bolejack V, Hollmig K, Pineda-Roman M, Anaissie E, Epstein J, et al. High serum-free light chain levels and their rapid reduction in response to therapy define an aggressive multiple myeloma subtype with poor prognosis. Blood 2007;110:827–32

10. Abdalla IA, Tabbara IA. Nonsecretory multiple myeloma. South Med J 2002;95:761–4

11. Coriu D, Weaver K, Schell M, Eulitz M, Murphy CL, Weiss DT, Solomon A. A molecular basis for nonsecretory myeloma. Blood 2004;104:829–31

12. Émond JP, Harding S, Lemieux B. Aggregation of serum free light chains (FLC) causes overestimation of FLC nephelometric results as compared to serum protein electrophoresis (SPE) while preserving clinical usefulness. Blood 2007;110:4767a

13. Chawla SS, Kumar SK, Dispenzieri A, Greenberg AJ, Larson DR, Kyle RA et al. Clinical course and prognosis of non-secretory multiple myeloma. Eur J Haematol 2014 In press

14. Cavallo F, Rasmussen E, Zangari M, Tricot G, Fender B, Fox M et al. Serum free-lite chain (sFLC) assay in multiple myeloma (MM): Clinical correlates and prognostic implications in newly diagnosed MM patients treated with Total Therapy 2 or 3 (TT2/3). Blood 2005;106:3490a

15. Jeong TD, Kim SY, Jang S, Park CJ, Chi HS, Lee W et al. Diagnostic sensitivity of a panel of tests to detect monoclonal protein in Korean multiple myeloma patients. Clin Chem Lab Med 2013;e187-9

16. Papanikolaou X, Zhang Q, Heuck C, Waheed S, Atrash S, Singh Z et al. Non-producing multiple myeloma (MM) is a distinct subset of non-secretory MM characterized by high Cyclin D1 experession and decreased progression free survival. Blood 2013;122:1911a

17. Ma ES, Shek TW, Ma SY. Non-secretory plasma cell myeloma of the true non-producer type. Br J Haematol 2007;138:561

18. Shaw GR. Nonsecretory plasma cell myeloma-becoming even more rare with serum free light-chain assay: a brief review. Arch Pathol Lab Med 2006;130:1212-5

19. Durie BG, Harousseau JL, Miguel JS, Blade J, Barlogie B, Anderson K et al. International uniform response criteria for multiple myeloma. Leukemia 2006;20:1467-73

20. Rajkumar SV, Harousseau JL, Durie B, Anderson KC, Dimopoulos M, Kyle R et al. Consensus recommendations for the uniform reporting of clinical trials: report of the International Myeloma Workshop Consensus Panel 1. Blood 2011;117:4691-5

Intact immunoglobulin multiple myeloma - monoclonal immunoglobulins at presentation

In intact immunoglobulin multiple myeloma:

- IgG is the most common disease isotype, followed by IgA, IgD, IgM and IgE.
- An abnormal κ/λ sFLC ratio is detected in around 95% of patients.
- Monitoring concentration changes in the intact immunoglobulin is essential for assessing patient response.
- An abnormal IgG or IgA Hevylite® ratio (corresponding to the monoclonal immunoglobulin type) is found in 97 - 100% of both IgG and IgA multiple myeloma patients at diagnosis.
- Hevylite assays offer an alternative method to densitometric quantification in cases where small monoclonal proteins are obscured by other serum proteins.

17.1. Introduction

Approximately 80% of all multiple myeloma (MM) patients produce monoclonal intact immunoglobulins, with 95% of these also producing monoclonal serum free light chains (sFLCs). IgG intact immunoglobulin multiple myeloma (IIMM) accounts for more than half of all MM patients, and IgA IIMM accounts for a further 20% of cases *(Table 17.1)*[1,9]. Only around 1 - 2% of patients have IgD IIMM[1,2] and monoclonal IgM is present in less than 1% of MM patients[1] (more commonly found in Waldenström's macroglobulinaemia, *Chapter 32*). IgE MM is extremely rare, with fewer than 50 cases reported in the literature[2].

Measurement of the monoclonal intact immunoglobulin and sFLC are essential for diagnosis and follow-up of IIMM, and form the basis of response criteria[3,4,5,6,7,8]. This chapter reviews intact immunoglobulin and sFLC measurements at diagnosis. The limitations of serum electrophoretic techniques used to quantify monoclonal intact immunoglobulins are discussed, along with immunoglobulin heavy/light chain assays (Hevylite, HLC).

Type	% of MM patients*
IgGκ	34
IgGλ	18
IgAκ	13
IgAλ	8
IgMκ	0.3
IgGλ	0.2
IgDκ	1
IgDλ	1
κ FLC only	9
λ FLC only	7
Biclonal	2
Negative	7

*Table 17.1. Types of serum monoclonal proteins in 1027 patients with multiple myeloma[9]. *Total does not equal 100% due to rounding.*

17.2. FLCs at diagnosis

Although IIMM is characterised by the secretion of monoclonal intact immunoglobulins, around 95% of patients have abnormal sFLC concentrations *(Table 17.2)*[10,11,12,13,14,15,16]. Mead et al.[14] assessed the frequency of sFLC abnormalities at presentation of IIMM according to immunoglobulin isotype. The study comprised 314 patients with IgG MM, 142 with IgA MM, 36 with IgD MM and 5 with IgE MM. Generally, sFLC concentrations were higher in IgA than in IgG patients, but highest in IgD patients *(Figures 17.1A and B)*. Overall, 89% had abnormally high sFLCs, with the following breakdown: IgG 84%, IgA 92%, IgD 94%, and all five of the IgE MM patients[17]. Some patients had normal or reduced concentrations of FLCs, but abnormal κ/λ ratios, indicating monoclonality in association with bone marrow suppression.

Publication	Number of patients	% of patients with an abnormal κ/λ sFLC ratio
Mead et al. (2004)[14,17]	497	89
Orlowski et al. (2007)[11]	487	94
Owen et al. (2007)[15]	207	95
Snozek et al. (2008)[16]	576	95
Dispenzieri et al. (2008)[10]	399	96
Katzmann et al. (2009)[13]	467	97
Jeong et al. (2013)[12]	159	87

Table 17.2. Summary of studies showing the percentage of IIMM patients with abnormal κ/λ sFLC ratios.

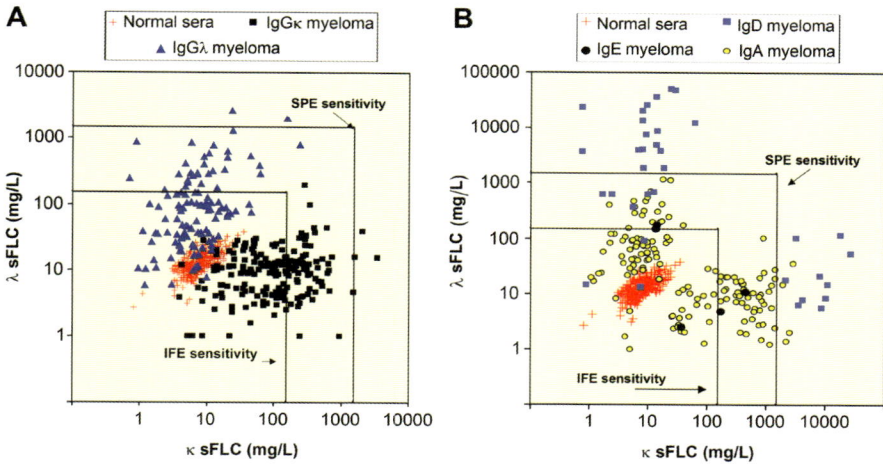

Figure 17.1. sFLC concentrations in IIMM. *(A)* *314 patients with IgG MM compared with 282 normal sera.* *(B)* *142 IgA, 36 IgD and 5 IgE MM patients compared with 282 normal sera.*

It is noteworthy that the concentration of monoclonal immunoglobulins and monoclonal FLCs are not correlated in IIMM patients *(Figure 17.2)*. However, in the majority of cases, changes in the intact immunoglobulin and the FLC are concordant *(Chapter 18)*. Importantly, discordant responses may indicate the presence of multiple clones, which have been identified by Ayliffe et al.[18,19] in a proportion of MM patients, using dual staining immunocytochemistry. In 82% of MM patients, single populations of cells were present that expressed either intact monoclonal immunoglobulin (with or without monoclonal FLC co-expression [74%]) or monoclonal FLC alone (8%). However, 18% of the samples contained a mixture of both cell populations[18]. Therefore, measurement of both monoclonal intact immunoglobulins and sFLCs in IIMM patients provides information on the underlying tumour cell clones, which may evolve differentially over the course of the disease *(Chapter 19)*.

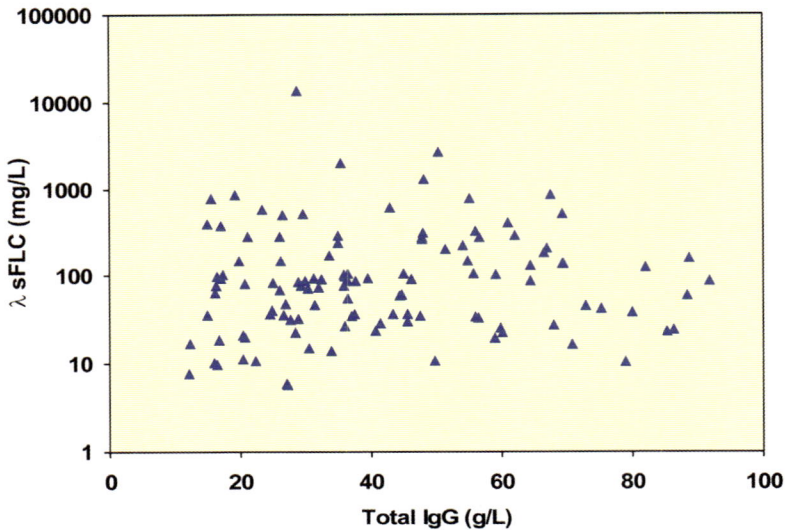

Figure 17.2. Serum IgG and λ sFLC concentrations in 116 IgGλ MM patients. (Pearson rank correlation r = -0.0037).

17.3. International guidelines for the quantification of monoclonal immunoglobulins in IIMM

Once a monoclonal intact immunoglobulin is identified in a patient's serum, guidelines recommend that it is quantified using scanning densitometry of serum protein electrophoresis (SPE) gels (or capillary zone electrophoresis [CZE]), alongside nephelometric/turbidimetric quantitation of total immunoglobulins *(Chapter 25)*[20]. The serum concentration of the monoclonal intact immunoglobulin is an important determinant in choosing the correct method to monitor disease course. Whilst it is preferred that monoclonal proteins are monitored by densitometric quantification, in cases where small monoclonal proteins are obscured by other serum proteins (e.g. transferrin), nephelometric measurements may be more accurate[20,21].

Additionally, international guidelines recommend performing sFLC analysis at presentation as it provides important prognostic information *(Chapter 20)*. This also gives a baseline measurement for monitoring oligosecretory patients (serum monoclonal protein <10 g/L and urine monoclonal protein <200 mg/24 hours[3]) and all patients to allow early detection of relapse by FLC escape *(Chapter 18)*[22].

17.4. Limitations of electrophoresis

Whilst serum electrophoresis and total immunoglobulin assays are both well-established techniques for the diagnosis and monitoring of IIMM, users should be aware of their limitations.

Firstly, monoclonal immunoglobulins can co-migrate with other major serum protein bands in gel electrophoresis, making identification and quantification inaccurate. This is often the case for monoclonal IgA, since its anodal electrophoretic migration positions it over other bands such as transferrin and complement component 3 (C3) in the β-region of gels in approximately 40% of cases [26,27,28]. Co-migration with other serum proteins may also affect monoclonal IgM[29] and to a lesser extent monoclonal IgG[28].

Secondly, quantification of monoclonal proteins at low concentrations (1 - 10 g/L) can be inaccurate[23]. In the case of monoclonal proteins that migrate in the γ-region, it is usually impossible to avoid including a proportion of polyclonal IgG in the densitometric measurement. Whilst the coefficient of variation (CV) of SPE quantitation for intact immunoglobulin >10 g/L is acceptable (at less than 10%), for monoclonal proteins of <10 g/L that are detectable by SPE, the CV rises sharply and can be as high as 35% *(Figure 17.3)*[21,23]. At presentation, approximately 10% of MM patients are classified as having oligosecretory disease[30]. Below these thresholds, monoclonal proteins are deemed unmeasurable because quantification by electrophoretic techniques is unreliable. In addition, small monoclonal bands may be completely undetectable by SPE/CZE[20]; this is a particular problem for monoclonal immunoglobulin concentrations of <3 g/L[31,32].

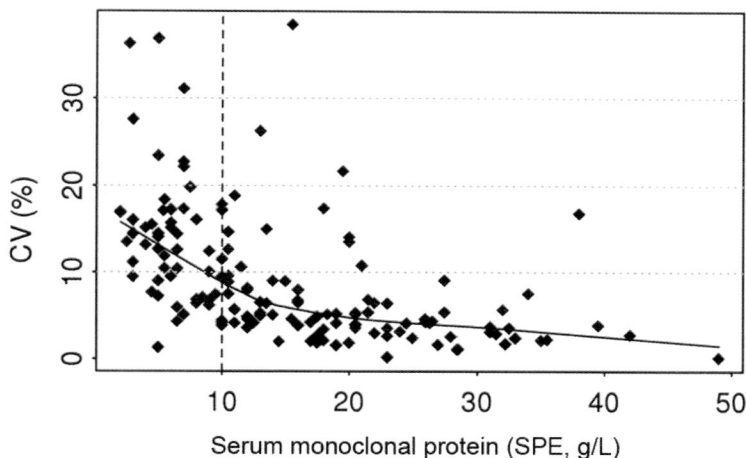

Figure 17.3. Median serum monoclonal protein concentration by SPE plotted against the coefficient of variation (CV) for individual patient's serial samples. Dashed lines indicate current recommendations for minimal values for monitoring. *(Republished with permission of Clinical Chemistry[23]; permission conveyed through Copyright Clearance Center, Inc.).*

Thirdly, changes in plasma cell populations in IgG IIMM patients may not be accurately reflected by changes in monoclonal IgG concentrations quantified by SPE. The correlation between monoclonal IgG measurements by SPE and nephelometry is non-linear above 20 g/L *(Figure 17.4)*[24]. This is attributed to dye saturation of dense, narrow monoclonal IgG bands in the SPE gel[33] and leads to an underestimation of tumour burden by SPE at high monoclonal protein concentrations *(Figure 17.5)*. Furthermore, assessments of monoclonal IgG are affected by concentration dependent catabolism via FcRn recycling receptors *(Sections 3.5.3 and 18.4.5)*.

Finally, IgM monoclonal proteins may self-aggregate and precipitate at the point of application, making quantification by SPE inaccurate *(Chapter 32)*. In some instances, IgM and IgA monoclonal proteins migrate as broadly restricted bands in the γ-region after electrophoresis, making them difficult to distinguish from polyclonal background immunoglobulins[34]. In particular, IgA monoclonal proteins may be relatively broad because they are heavily glycosylated and can exist as monomers, dimers or multimers[1]. In such cases, HLC assays offer an alternative means of monitoring response *(Chapter 18,* Clinical case history 2).

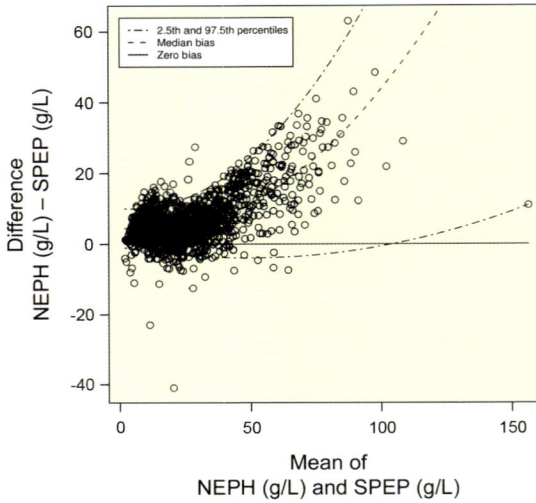

Figure 17.4. Bland-Altman plot comparing SPE monoclonal protein values and quantitative immunoglobulins assessed by nephelometry for IgG monoclonal proteins. (Republished with permission of Clinical Chemistry[24]; permission conveyed through Copyright Clearance Center, Inc.).

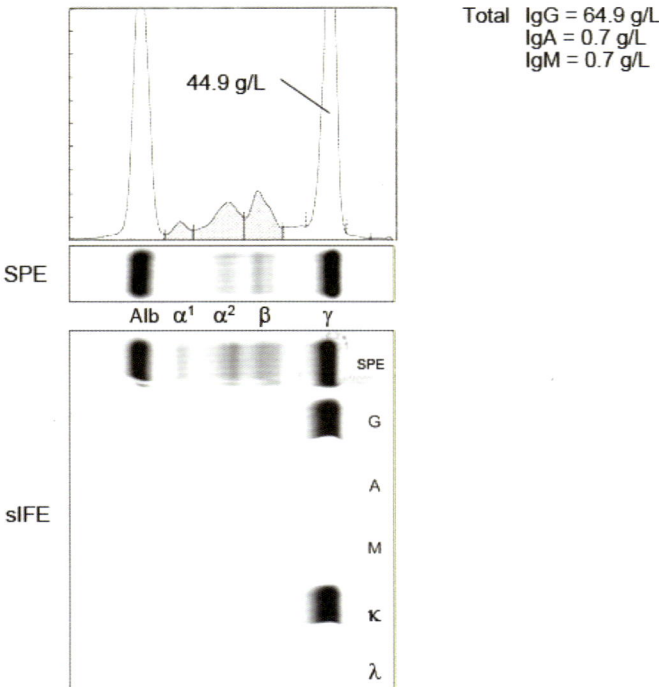

Figure 17.5. IgG monoclonal protein concentration by SPE compared with total IgG by nephelometry. (Republished with permission from ASM press, Washington, DC[25]).

17.5. Limitations of total immunoglobulin measurements

Total immunoglobulin measurements are unable to distinguish monoclonal from polyclonal immunoglobulin concentrations of the same isotype. Therefore, when IIMM patient samples contain significant concentrations of non-tumour polyclonal immunoglobulins, nephelometric results are inaccurate.

Nephelometry is also known to grossly overestimate monoclonal IgM concentrations. In one study, IgM values obtained by SPE and nephelometry were linearly correlated with a slope of 1.8 (CI 1.68 – 1.92), showing a systematic bias for higher values by nephelometry[24].

17.6. Immunoglobulin HLC immunoassays (Hevylite) at diagnosis

HLC immunoassays provide an additional tool for the management of patients with IIMM. The assays separately quantify the different light chain types of each immunoglobulin isotype (i.e. IgGκ, IgGλ, IgAκ, IgAλ, IgMκ and IgMλ, *Chapter 9*). The molecules are assessed in pairs to produce HLC ratios (e.g. IgGκ/IgGλ) in the same manner as κ/λ sFLC ratios. The HLC ratio provides information on both the involved (monoclonal) immunoglobulin (e.g. IgGκ in an IgGκ patient) and the uninvolved (polyclonal) HLC-pair (e.g. IgGλ in an IgGκ patient). When the concentration of the HLC-pair is below the normal reference interval, alongside an abnormal HLC ratio, this is termed "HLC-pair suppression".

HLC assays are less labour-intensive and less subjective than serum electrophoretic techniques[35,36], and may overcome many of the known limitations of serum electrophoresis discussed above (including co-migration, dye saturation and broadly migrating monoclonal proteins) *(Section 17.4)*. For example, in Figure 17.6 the monoclonal protein co-migrated with other β-region serum proteins, whereas HLC assays provided a quantitative result.

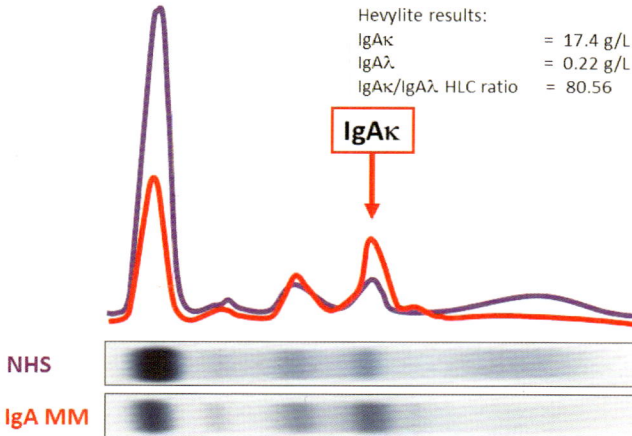

Figure 17.6. Monoclonal proteins may co-migrate with other serum proteins in an SPE gel. A normal human serum (NHS) SPE gel is shown above the SPE for a patient with IgA MM. The corresponding densitometric traces for NHS (purple) and IgA MM (red) are also shown. The IgAκ monoclonal protein co-migrates with serum proteins in the β-region, making densitometric quantification inaccurate. Hevylite provides quantitative results for the same patient.

HLC assays were assessed in a large cohort of IIMM patients recruited to the IFM 2005-01 MM trial[26]. A total of 339 patients, comprising 245 with IgG (166 IgGκ, 79 IgGλ) and 94 with IgA (60 IgAκ, 34 IgAλ) isotypes were evaluated at presentation. The HLC data are summarised in Figures 17.7 A and B, using Ig'κ/Ig'λ dot plots. The involved HLC concentration was greater than the upper limit of the normal range in the majority of patients (Tables 17.3 and 17.4), and all IIMM patients had the corresponding abnormal HLC ratio. Thirty-three percent (31/94) of the IgA patients could not be accurately quantified by SPE, due to co-migration with other serum proteins.

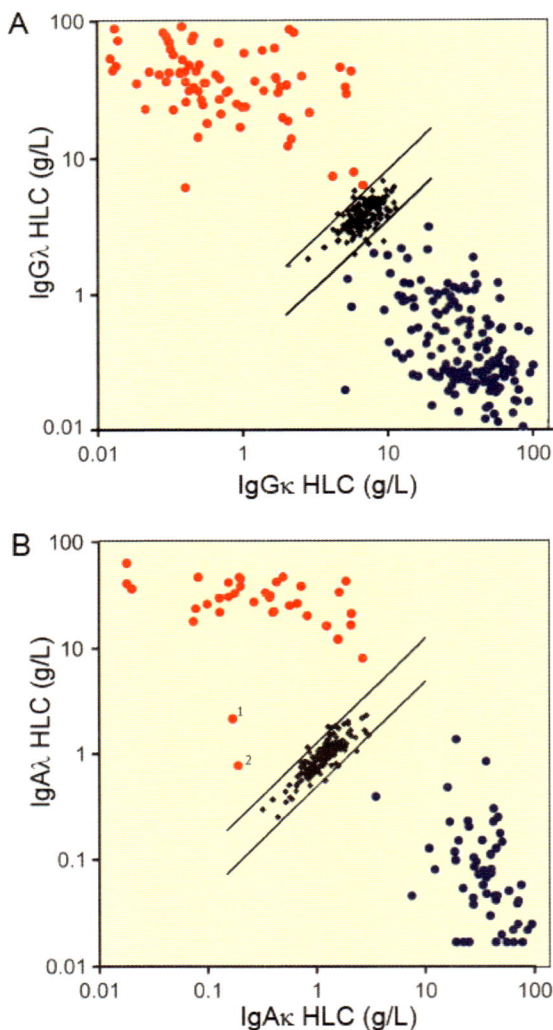

Figure 17.7. Serum HLC concentrations in MM patients at presentation. (A) 166 IgGκ patients (blue circles) and 79 IgGλ patients (red circles). (B) 60 IgAκ patients (blue circles) and 34 IgAλ patients (red circles). Concentrations of λ sFLCs in samples 1 and 2 were 103,000 mg/L and 8,500 mg/L, respectively. Healthy blood donors (black diamonds) and 95% confidence limits (diagonal lines) are shown. (Reprinted by permission from Macmillan Publishers Ltd: Leukemia[26], copyright 2013).

		IgGκ MM	IgGλ MM
Monoclonal Ig by SPE (g/L)	Median 95% range Total range	40.5 8.02 - 90 (4.9 - 109)	46.0 10.86 - 85.02 (5.7 - 86.0)
IgGκ HLC (g/L)	Median 95% range Total range	33.0 5.60 - 91.81 (4.07 - 107)	0.41 0.12 - 5.84 (0.09 - 6.76)
IgGλ HLC (g/L)	Median 95% range Total range	0.33 0.072 - 2.03 (0.04 - 3.19)	35.5 4.77 - 91.12 (4.58 - 97.3)
IgGκ/IgGλ HLC ratio	Median 95% range Total range	93.52 5.13 - 864 (3.94 - 1334)	0.018 0.001 - 0.878 (0.001 - 1.05)

Table 17.3. Concentrations of IgG monoclonal proteins and IgG HLC in 245 patients with IgG MM[26].

		IgAκ MM	IgAλ MM
Monoclonal Ig by SPE (g/L)	Median 95% range Total range	34.0 11.35 - 88.55 (10.0 - 98.0)	28.0 3.46 - 62.1 (2.2 - 67.0)
IgAκ HLC (g/L)	Median 95% range Total range	36.7 5.36 - 110.2 (3.49 - 125)	0.3 0.018 - 2.17 (0.018 - 2.65)
IgAλ HLC (g/L)	Median 95% range Total range	0.072 0.017 - 1.13 (0.017 - 1.38)	30.1 1.95 - 49.9 (0.78 - 64.1)
IgAκ/IgAλ HLC ratio	Median 95% range Total range	462 11.2 - 6020 (8.8 - 7352)	0.01 0.018 - 0.255 (0.001 - 0.32)

Table 17.4. Concentrations of IgA monoclonal proteins and IgA HLC in 94 patients with IgA MM[26].

Ludwig et al.[28] evaluated the HLC assays in 100 IgG and 56 IgA MM patients, all of whom had corresponding abnormal HLC ratios at diagnosis. Of note, accurate quantitation of the monoclonal immunoglobulin by SPE densitometry was not possible in 46% (26/56) of IgA patients and 4% (4/100) of IgG patients due to co-migration with other serum proteins. Similarly, in a study by Mirbahai et al. comparing HLC data with SPE results at diagnosis of IgA MM[37], all 210 patients had abnormal HLC ratios as determined by HLC assays (Figure 17.8A). However, accurate quantitation of the monoclonal protein was not possible in 40% (83/210) of patients by SPE; three of these are shown in Figure 17.8B.

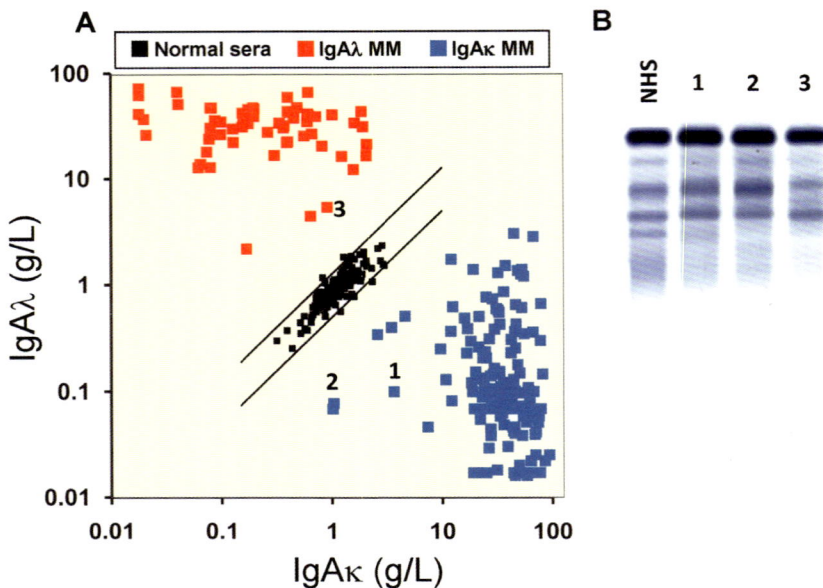

Figure 17.8. HLC results for IgA MM at disease presentation. (A) Serum IgA HLC concentrations in 210 IgA MM patients (145 IgAκ [blue squares] and 65 IgAλ [red squares]). Healthy blood donors (black squares) and 95% confidence limits (diagonal lines) are shown. All patients had abnormal HLC ratios, including three samples with unquantifiable monoclonal protein by SPE (numbered). (B) SPE gel of normal human sera (NHS) and the 3 IgA MM samples highlighted in (A) where the monoclonal protein was not quantifiable by SPE densitometry[37].

Katzmann et al.[38] assessed the diagnostic sensitivity of HLC ratios in 365 IgG and 153 IgA MM patients at presentation. An abnormal HLC ratio was present in 97% of both IgG (354/365) and IgA (148/153) diagnostic samples. In IgA MM, the HLC ratio was more sensitive for detecting a monoclonal intact immunoglobulin than SPE (Section 4.2.5), and the authors recognised the utility of HLC assays in patients whose monoclonal protein migrates in the β-region.

In the IFM 2005-01 MM trial[26], the majority of IIMM patients had HLC-pair suppression (i.e. reduced concentrations of IgGκ in a patient with IgGλ IIMM). For IgGκ, IgGλ, IgAκ and IgAλ MM patients HLC-pair suppression was present in 99%, 92%, 93% and 69% of cases, respectively. In one IgAλ patient, whose IgAλ HLC concentration was within the normal range (labelled 2 in Figure 17.7B), IgAκ HLC-pair suppression was present and the IgAκ/IgAλ ratio was abnormal. Interestingly, this patient and one additional patient (labeled 1 in Figure 17.7B) had highly elevated λ sFLC concentrations (8,500 mg/L and 103,000 mg/L, respectively). This was consistent with monoclonal λ sFLCs being the dominant monoclonal protein produced by the tumour. In such cases, sFLC analysis may be more informative for monitoring disease status (Chapter 18).

The degree of HLC-pair suppression varied greatly between patients, although suppression was generally greater in patients with IgA-producing tumours than in IgG-producing tumours (Tables 17.3 and 17.4). In addition, patients with higher concentrations of involved HLCs tended to have lower concentrations of uninvolved HLCs. This negative correlation between suppression and production was more significant in IgG patients (IgGκ: $r = -0.456$; $p=8.7 \times 10^{-10}$, IgGλ: $r = -0.310$; $p=0.005$) than in IgA patients (IgAκ: $r = -0.28$; $p=0.031$, IgAλ: $r = -0.33$; $p=0.05$). Emerging evidence suggests that HLC-pair suppression may have important prognostic significance in a number of monoclonal gammopathies including MM. This is described in more detail in Chapter 20.

Test Questions

1. How often are sFLC ratios abnormal in IIMM?

2. How frequently is quantitation of IgA monoclonal proteins not possible by SPE densitometry?

3. How often are IgAκ/IgAλ HLC ratios abnormal in IgA MM patients at disease presentation?

Answers

1. In approximately 95% of patients at clinical presentation (Section 17.2).

2. Accurate quantitation by SPE is not possible in around 40% of IgA MM patients (Section 17.6).

3. In 4 studies comprising 508 patients, IgAκ/IgAλ HLC ratios were abnormal in 99% of cases at clinical presentation (Section 17.6).

References

1. Keren DF. Serum protein electrophoresis evaluation of monoclonal gammopathies (M-proteins). J Ligand Chem 2005;27:218-26

2. Pandey S, Kyle RA. Unusual myelomas: a review of IgD and IgE variants. Oncology (Williston Park) 2013;27:798-803

3. Durie BG, Harousseau JL, Miguel JS, Blade J, Barlogie B, Anderson K et al. International uniform response criteria for multiple myeloma. Leukemia 2006;20:1467-739

4. Gertz MA, Merlini G. Definition of organ involvement and response to treatment in AL amyloidosis: an updated consensus opinion. Amyloid 2010;17:CP-Ba

5. Kyle RA, Rajkumar SV. Criteria for diagnosis, staging, risk stratification and response assessment of multiple myeloma. Leukemia 2009;23:3-9

6. Palladini G, Dispenzieri A, Gertz MA, Wechalekar A, Hawkins P, Schonland SO et al. Validation of the criteria of response to treatment in AL amyloidosis. Blood 2010;116:1364a

7. Palladini G, Dispenzieri A, Gertz MA, Kumar S, Wechalekar A, Hawkins PN et al. New criteria for response to treatment in immunoglobulin light chain amyloidosis based on free light chain measurement and cardiac biomarkers: impact on survival outcomes. J Clin Oncol 2012;30:4541-9

8. Rajkumar SV, Harousseau JL, Durie B, Anderson KC, Dimopoulos M, Kyle R et al. Consensus recommendations for the uniform reporting of clinical trials: report of the International Myeloma Workshop Consensus Panel 1. Blood 2011;117:4691-5

9. Kyle RA, Gertz MA, Witzig TE, Lust JA, Lacy MQ, Dispenzieri A et al. Review of 1027 patients with newly diagnosed multiple myeloma. Mayo Clin Proc 2003;78:21-33

10. Dispenzieri A, Zhang L, Katzmann JA, Snyder M, Blood E, DeGoey R et al. Appraisal of immunoglobulin free light chain as a marker of response. Blood 2008;111:4908-15

11. Orlowski R, Sutherland H, Blade J, Miguel JS, Hajek R, Nagler A et al. Early normalization of serum free light chains is associated with prolonged time to progression following bortezomib {+/-} pegylated liposomal doxorubicin treatment of relapsed/ refractory multiple myeloma. Blood 2007;110:2735a

12. Jeong TD, Kim SY, Jang S, Park CJ, Chi HS, Lee W et al. Diagnostic sensitivity of a panel of tests to detect monoclonal protein in Korean multiple myeloma patients. Clin Chem Lab Med 2013;e187-e189

13. Katzmann JA, Kyle RA, Benson J, Larson DR, Snyder MR, Lust JA et al. Screening panels for detection of monoclonal gammopathies. Clin Chem 2009;55:1517-22

14. Mead GP, Carr-Smith HD, Drayson MT, Morgan GJ, Child JA, Bradwell AR. Serum free light chains for monitoring multiple myeloma. Br J Haematol 2004;126:348-54

15. Owen RG, Child JA, Rawstron AC, Bell S, Cocks K, Davies FE et al. Defining complete response in multiple myeloma: Role of the serum free light chain assay and multiparameter flow cytometry. Blood 2007;110:1479a

16. Snozek CL, Katzmann JA, Kyle RA, Dispenzieri A, Larson DR, Therneau TM et al. Prognostic value of the serum free light chain ratio in newly diagnosed myeloma: proposed incorporation into the international staging system. Leukemia 2008;22:1933-7

17. Pratt G. The evolving use of serum free light chain assays in haematology. Br J Haematol 2008;141:413-22

18. Ayliffe MJ, Davies FE, de Castro D, Morgan GJ. Demonstration of changes in plasma cell subsets in multiple myeloma. Haematologica 2007;92:1135-8

19. Ayliffe MJ, Behrens J, Stern S, Sumar N. Association of plasma cell subsets in the bone marrow and free light chain concentrations in the serum of monoclonal gammopathy patients. J Clin Pathol 2012;65:758-61

20. Dimopoulos M, Kyle R, Fermand JP, Rajkumar SV, San MJ, Chanan-Khan A et al. Consensus recommendations for standard investigative workup: report of the International Myeloma Workshop Consensus Panel 3. Blood 2011;117:4701-5

21. Tate J, Caldwell G, Daly J, Gillis D, Jenkins M, Jovanovich S et al. Recommendations for standardized reporting of protein electrophoresis in Australia and New Zealand. Ann Clin Biochem 2012;49:242-56

22. Dispenzieri A, Kyle R, Merlini G, Miguel JS, Ludwig H, Hajek R et al. International Myeloma Working Group guidelines for serum-free light chain analysis in multiple myeloma and related disorders. Leukemia 2009;23:215-24

23. Katzmann JA, Snyder MR, Rajkumar SV, Kyle RA, Therneau TM, Benson JT, Dispenzieri A. Long-term biologic variation of serum protein electrophoresis M-spike, urine M-spike, and monoclonal serum free light chain quantification: implications for monitoring monoclonal gammopathies. Clin Chem 2011;57:1687-92

24. Murray DL, Ryu E, Snyder MR, Katzmann JA. Quantitation of serum monoclonal proteins: relationship between agarose gel electrophoresis and immunonephelometry. Clin Chem 2009;55:1523-9

25. Katzmann JA, Kyle RA. Immunochemical characterization of immunoglobulins in serum, urine, and cerebrospinal fluid. Manual of Molecular and Clinical Laboratory Immunology. ASM Press, 2006

26. Bradwell A, Harding S, Fourrier N, Mathiot C, Attal M, Moreau P et al. Prognostic utility of intact immunoglobulin Ig'kappa/Ig'lambda ratios in multiple myeloma patients. Leukemia 2013;27:202-7

27. Wang H, Gao CF, Xu LL, Yang ZX, Zhao WJ, Kong XT. Laboratory characterizations on 2007 cases of monoclonal gammapathies in East china. Cell Mol Immunol 2008;5:293-8

28. Ludwig H, Milosavljevic D, Zojer N, Faint JM, Bradwell AR, Hubl W, Harding SJ. Immunoglobulin heavy/light chain ratios improve paraprotein detection and monitoring, identify residual disease and correlate with survival in multiple myeloma patients. Leukemia 2013;27:213-9

29. Tseng CH, Chang CY, Liu KS, Liu FJ. Accuracy of serum IgM and IgA monoclonal protein measurements by densitometry. Ann Clin Lab Sci 2003;33:160-6

30. Larson D, Kyle RA, Rajkumar SV. Prevalence and monitoring of oligosecretory myeloma. N Engl J Med 2012;367:580-1

31. Lippi G, Battistelli L, Vernocchi A, Mussap M. Analytical evaluation of the novel Helena V8 capillary electrophoresis system. J Med Biochem 2013;32:245-9

32. Poisson J, Fedoriw Y, Henderson MP, Hainsworth S, Tucker K, Uddin Z, McCudden CR. Performance evaluation of the Helena V8 capillary electrophoresis system. Clin Biochem 2012;45:697-9

33. Katzmann JA, Clark R, Wiegert E, Sanders E, Oda RP, Kyle RA et al. Identification of monoclonal proteins in serum: a quantitative comparison of acetate, agarose gel, and capillary electrophoresis. Electrophoresis 1997;18:1775-80

34. Donato LJ, Zeldenrust SR, Murray DL, Katzmann JA. A 71-year-old woman with multiple myeloma status after stem cell transplantation. Clin Chem 2011;57:1645-8

35. Bradwell AR, Harding SJ, Fourrier NJ, Wallis GL, Drayson MT, Carr-Smith HD, Mead GP. Assessment of monoclonal gammapathies by nephelometric measurement of individual immunoglobulin kappa/lambda ratios. Clin Chem 2009;55:1646-55

36. Keren DF. Heavy/light-chain analysis of monoclonal gammapathies. Clin Chem 2009;55:1606-8

37. Mirbahai L, Fourrier NJ, Harper J, Harris J, Bradwell AR, Harding SJ. Monoclonal IgA proteins migrating into the b region of serum protein electrophoresis gels can be easily identified and quantified using IgAk and IgAl measurements. Clin Chem 2011;57:C-64a

38. Katzmann JA, Willrich MA, Kohlhagen MC, Kyle RA, Murray DL, Snyder MR et al. Monitoring IgA Multiple Myeloma: Immunoglobulin Heavy/Light Chain Assays. Clin Chem 2014 *In press*

Intact immunoglobulin multiple myeloma - monitoring monoclonal immunoglobulins

In intact immunoglobulin multiple myeloma:

- Routine measurement of monoclonal immunoglobulins and monoclonal FLCs is necessary for effective disease monitoring.

- Oligosecretory patients may be monitored with sFLC or Hevylite® assays.

- sFLC analysis is required for early detection of relapse with light chain escape and to define a stringent complete response.

- sFLC measurements allow rapid assessment of response, prediction of overall response and early detection of ineffective therapy.

- Hevylite assays offer an alternative method to densitometric quantification in cases where small monoclonal proteins are obscured by other serum proteins.

- Quantitative Hevylite assays can provide clarity when monitoring patients with ambiguous electrophoresis results.

- Hevylite ratios are more sensitive than SPE and IFE in some patients.

18.1. Introduction

Serum protein electrophoresis (SPE), serum immunofixation (sIFE) and serum free light chain (sFLC) analysis are all required to monitor intact immunoglobulin multiple myeloma (IIMM) patients. These tests form the basis of response criteria that are discussed below[1,2,3,4,5,6]. Immunoglobulin heavy/light chain analysis (Hevylite, HLC) may overcome many of the limitations of SPE (including co-migration and dye saturation issues, *Section 17.4)*, and can provide clarity for patients with ambiguous electrophoresis results. HLC ratios are more sensitive than SPE and sIFE in some patients, and may improve the detection of residual disease and/or disease relapse. In this chapter the roles for sFLC and HLC assays in the routine monitoring of IIMM patients are discussed.

18.2. Current guidelines for monitoring IIMM

International Myeloma Working Group (IMWG) guidelines state that serum monoclonal proteins (including intact immunoglobulins) should be quantified using scanning densitometry on SPE (or capillary zone electrophoresis [CZE]) *(Section 17.4)*[1,6]. If monoclonal protein quantitation by SPE is not available or considered to be unreliable during follow-up (e.g. in patients with monoclonal IgA migrating in the β-region), then quantitative immunoglobulin assays performed by nephelometry or turbidimetry are recommended[1].

Monitoring patients with oligosecretory disease (defined as a serum monoclonal protein <10 g/L and a urine monoclonal protein <200 mg/24 hours[1,6]) presents a significant challenge to laboratory staff and physicians. However, sFLC measurement provides a quantitative assessment of response in more than 70% of patients[7] and its use is recommended in international guidelines[8]. Clinical trial protocols often allow inclusion of oligosecretory patients with measurable sFLCs (e.g. IFM 2009-02[9] and IFM/DFCI 2009 NCT01208662). In addition, sFLC analysis is required in all patients with IIMM in order to detect relapse with free light chain escape (FLC escape) and define a stringent complete response (sCR)[1]. These uses are described in more detail below.

18.2.1. Detection of free light chain escape

The frequency at which IIMM patients relapse with FLC escape may be as high as 20%[10], when FLC escape is defined as an increase in monoclonal FLCs without a corresponding increase in monoclonal intact immunoglobulins. A typical example is shown in Figure 18.1. Guidelines state that periodic assessment of sFLCs should be made to avoid missing such events[8].

The first published observation of FLC escape was made in 1969 by J.R. Hobbs while monitoring patients in the first UK myeloma trial[11]. He noted that 5% of patients producing intact monoclonal immunoglobulins relapsed with only Bence Jones proteinuria. In addition, the relative proportion of monoclonal urine FLCs increased in a further 35% of patients at relapse.

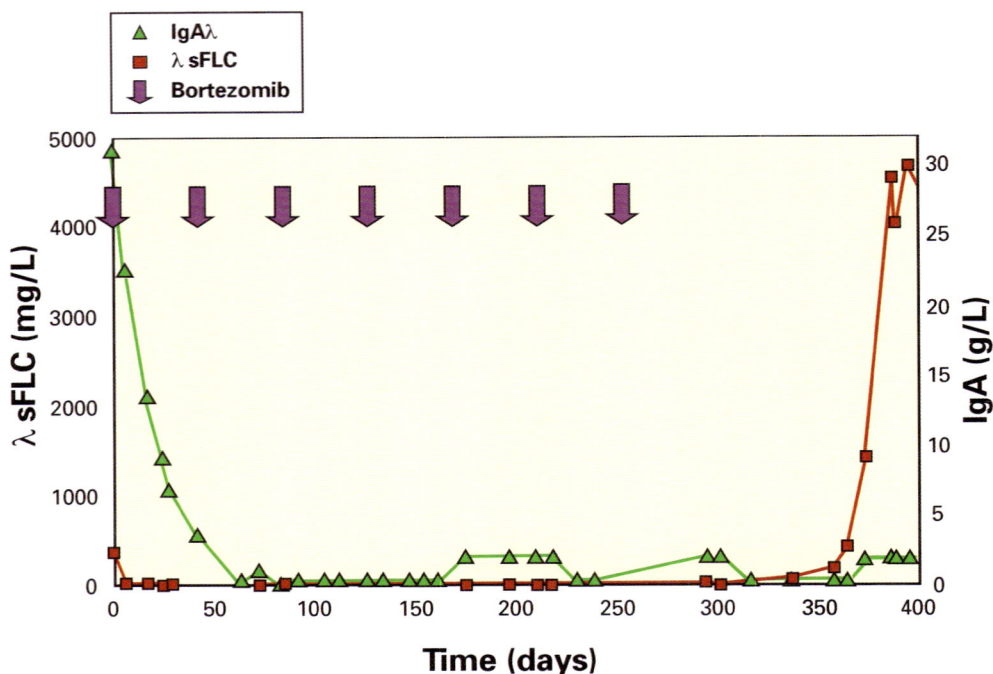

Figure 18.1. Serum λ FLCs and IgAλ in a patient showing FLC escape. FLC escape was apparent as a conversion from IgA production to FLC only. (Courtesy of Christie Hospital).

The true incidence of FLC escape is higher than is indicated by evidence from urine analysis [12,13]. The increased use of sensitive sFLC immunoassays has resulted in an increase in the observed incidence of FLC escape[10,13,14,15,16,17,18,19,20]. For example, in a large study comprising 520 multiple myeloma (MM) patients, FLC escape was reported in 10% of patients at disease relapse[10]. The authors classified FLC escape as a failure to meet the IMWG criteria for relapse by a change in intact immunoglobulin levels, but satisfied IMWG criteria for changes in sFLC levels *(Chapter 25)*[6]. These patients represented 6.5% (24/369) of IgG patients and 19.9% (30/151) of IgA patients. In 85% of FLC escape patients, the increase in the involved sFLC was >200 mg/L, which is the minimum level recommended for defining a relapse that requires treatment in the absence of clinical symptoms[6]. Interestingly, any patients relapsing with sFLC involvement (either FLC escape alone or with intact immunoglobulin) experienced significantly shorter survival times than those relapsing with intact immunoglobulin only[10]; this is discussed further in Section 20.3.3.

Kuhnemund et al.[18] reported renal impairment in 50% of patients with FLC escape. As renal impairment is associated with significant morbidity and mortality *(Chapter 26)*, it is important to identify FLC escape early, and thus avoid serious complications. A typical example that demonstrates the use of sFLC measurements to provide early detection of FLC escape is described in the clinical case below.

Insight into the mechanism of FLC escape has been proposed by Ayliffe et al.[21,22], who identified dual plasma cell clones in a proportion of patients with IIMM, with some cells expressing intact immunoglobulin (with or without FLC co-expression) and others expressing FLC alone. Disease relapse may be associated with the selective outgrowth of one of the clones, influenced by a combination of factors, including the tumour microenvironment and the patient's treatment regimen *(Chapter 19)*. In line with this, a number of researchers have proposed that FLC escape has become a more frequent occurrence with modern and more aggressive chemotherapy[15,18].

Another form of disease relapse, termed clonal change, was proposed by Hobbs et al.[14] and describes an alteration in the relative proportions of intact immunoglobulins and FLCs produced. Such changes are consistent with evolving tumour cell clones during the course of disease, and are demonstrated for an IgAκ MM patient in Figure 18.2. Zamarin et al.[20] studied the incidence of changes in monoclonal protein type at relapse or disease progression in MM patients who had achieved a complete response (CR) after an autologous stem cell transplant (ASCT). A total of 54% (29/54) of IIMM patients had a change in their monoclonal protein type at relapse or progression of disease *(Chapter 19)*. These observations highlight the importance of using both FLC and intact immunoglobulin measurements to monitor disease progression.

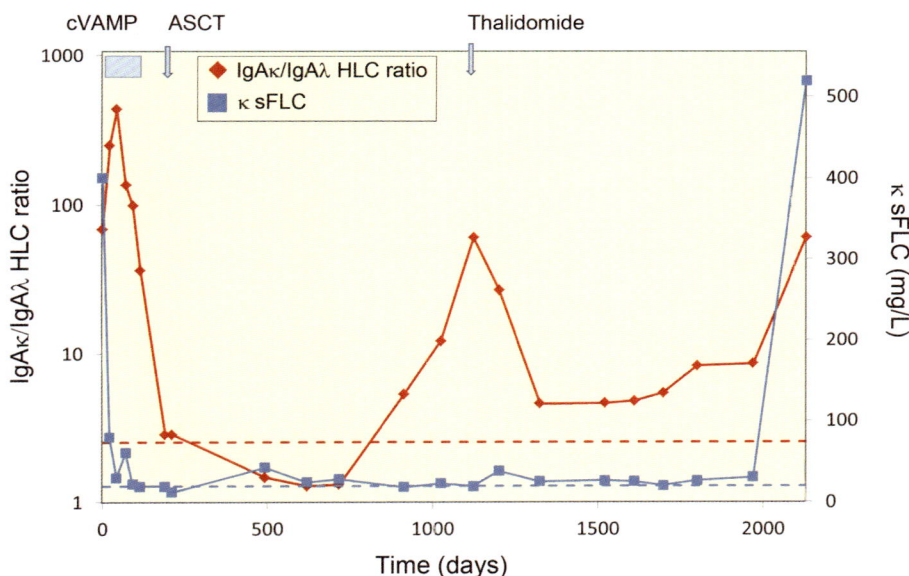

Figure 18.2. Clonal changes during the course of disease assessed using a combination of HLC and FLC analysis. The κ sFLC concentration (blue) and IgAκ/IgAλ HLC ratio (red) are shown. Dashed lines indicate the upper limits of the respective reference ranges. The patient presents with clones expressing IgAκ and κ sFLC and achieves a CR around 500 days after treatment, at which time both IgAκ/IgAλ and κ/λ sFLC ratios normalise. After around 750 days, a clone emerges that expresses IgAκ but not κ sFLC. The IgAκ clone is reduced but not eradicated after a second round of treatment. After approximately 2000 days, the patient relapses with clones expressing both IgAκ and κ sFLC.

Clinical case history 1

An IgAλ multiple myeloma patient exhibiting FLC escape[23].

A 48-year-old man with IgAλ MM and monoclonal λ sFLCs was monitored for 3 years following treatment with vincristine, doxorubicin and dexamethasone (VAD) plus high dose melphalan followed by autologous stem cell transplant (ASCT). Laboratory tests included serum and urine electrophoresis, sFLC (Freelite®) and HLC (Hevylite) immunoassays. The patient's clinical course is shown in Figure 18.3.

After ASCT, the patient achieved a CR and was stable for 330 days. Subsequently, relapse was characterised by a substantial increase in sFLCs only; the κ/λ sFLC ratio became abnormal, the dFLC (λ [involved] FLC minus κ [uninvolved] FLC) concentration began to increase and a trace of λ Bence Jones protein (BJP) was detected by urine immunofixation (IFE). However, both SPE and serum IFE (sIFE) were normal and the HLC ratio (IgAκ/IgAλ) was within the normal range. The dFLC continued to increase over the following months.

At 27 months post ASCT, the patient sustained a pathological fracture of the tibia and 4 months later the dFLC peaked at 3168 mg/L. λ BJP was detectable by both serum and urine IFE. However, there was still no detectable monoclonal intact immunoglobulin by serum IFE or HLC analysis. A bone marrow biopsy revealed 15% involvement of λ-restricted plasma cells and a bone survey identified osteolysis. The patient was diagnosed with progression of MM and received further treatment that included a second ASCT.

In this case study an increase in dFLC levels was an early indication of disease progression and emphasises the importance of monitoring IIMM patients with sFLC assays for detection of FLC escape.

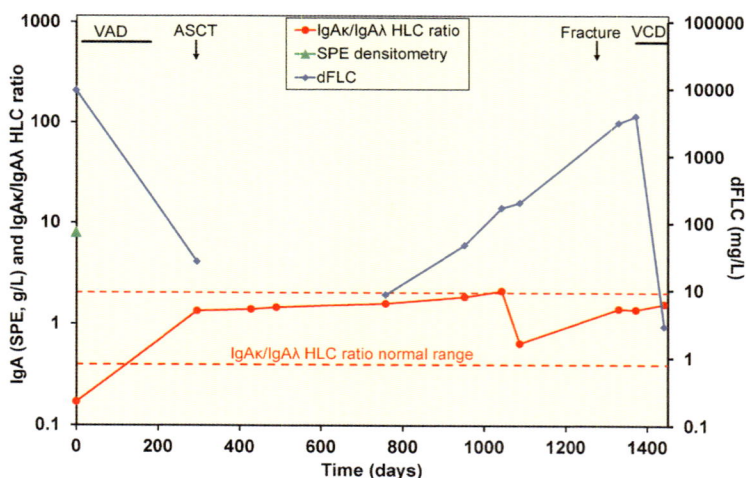

Figure 18.3. Relapse in a patient with IgAλ MM was characterised by an increase in monoclonal sFLCs only. The patient achieved a complete response (CR) following treatment, which was stable for 330 days. Relapse by FLC escape was characterised by a substantial increase in dFLC from 8.61 mg/L to 3168 mg/L, with no change in the intact immunoglobulins (by either HLC assays or SPE)[23]. VAD: vincristine, doxorubicin and dexamethasone; ASCT: autologous stem cell transplant; VCD: bortezomib, cyclophosphamide, dexamethasone. (Courtesy of M. Kraj).

18.2.2. Definition of a stringent complete response

An abnormal κ/λ sFLC ratio indicates residual disease in a proportion of IIMM patients classified as having achieved a complete response (CR) *(Figure 18.4)*[24]. This has led to the incorporation of the κ/λ sFLC ratio in the definition of a stringent complete response (sCR) in the International Uniform Response Criteria (IURC) for MM[1]. In addition to the criteria for a CR (absence of monoclonal protein by IFE and <5% clonal bone marrow plasma cells (BMPCs) by immunohistochemistry/immunofluorescence), a sCR requires the absence of BMPCs and normalisation of the κ/λ sFLC ratio[1].

IMWG guidelines recommend that sFLCs are measured in all patients who have achieved a CR, in order to detect residual disease and therefore determine whether they have attained a sCR *(Section 25.3.5)*[8]. Attainment of a sCR has prognostic significance, as it identifies patients with improved long-term outcome *(Section 20.3.1)*[25].

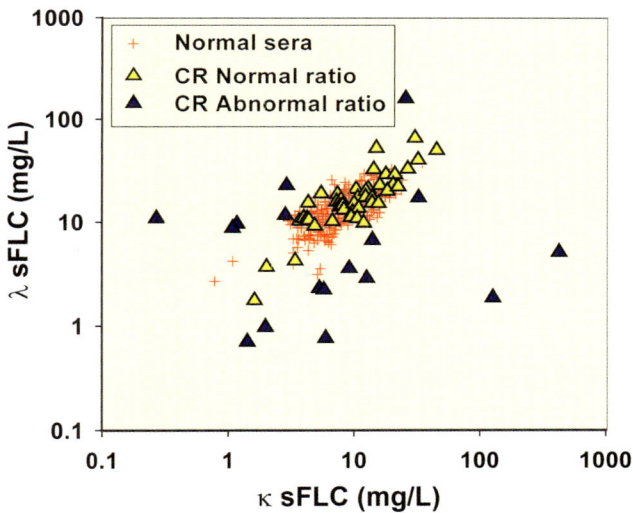

Figure 18.4. sFLC concentrations in 54 patients with IIMM whilst in complete remission, both clinically and by serum and urine IFE. CR: complete response.

18.3. Other uses of sFLC analysis in IIMM response assessment

18.3.1. Rapid assessment of response

The short serum half-life of sFLCs (2 – 6 hours) compared with that of intact immunoglobulins (5 – 7 days for IgA/IgM, or several weeks for IgG; *Chapter 3*) means that they often provide an earlier indication of response to treatment. In addition, at low serum IgG concentrations, the half-life of IgG is prolonged by FcRn receptor recycling *(Chapter 3)*. In such cases, serum IgG levels are particularly slow to indicate responses to treatment, and sIFE may remain positive long after a tumour has been eradicated (as demonstrated by bone marrow immunophenotyping)[27,28].

Early sFLC responses to chemotherapy have been reported by many researchers[28,29,30,31,32,33,34,35]. Such responses are most apparent in IIMM patients treated with drugs that produce a rapid tumour response, such as bortezomib (Velcade). As an example, IgGλ and λ FLC levels for a patient with IgGλ MM are shown in Figure 18.5[26]. During initial therapy with bortezomib, doxorubicin and dexamethasone (VDD), the serum λ FLC concentration fell rapidly, and had normalised by 21 days following treatment. In contrast, IgGλ only gradually decreased (with a serum half-life of around 30 days), and treatment was continued.

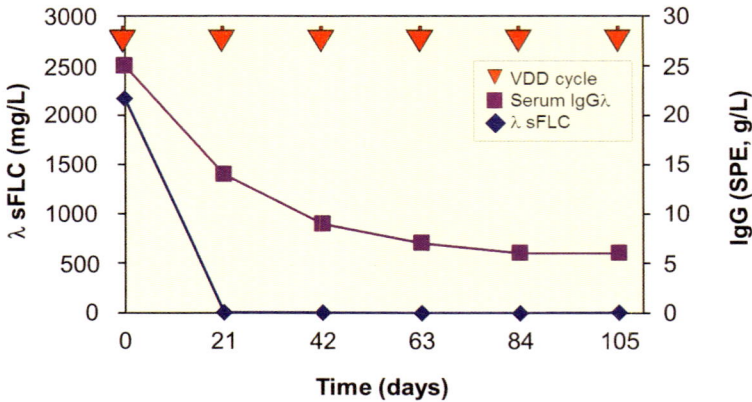

Figure 18.5. *A rapid decrease in λ sFLCs gives an earlier indication of response than intact immunoglobulin measurements in a patient with IgGλ IIMM*[26]. *VDD: Velcade, doxorubicin and dexamethasone.*

Measurement of sFLCs at short time intervals can provide additional information on the kinetics of response to treatment. For example, Das et al.[29] reported rapid responses to bortezomib in 6 of 8 patients, 3 of whom exhibited repeated falls and rises of sFLCs co-incident with treatment cycles *(Figure 18.6)*. The sFLC relapse was very rapid, with doubling times of less than 10 days. By comparison, the intact monoclonal immunoglobulin did not show the same peaks and troughs. Similar observations have been made in other studies using bortezomib[30,36,37,38]. These rapid patterns of response can only be observed with the use of tumour markers - such as sFLCs - that are quickly cleared from the serum, together with short sampling intervals. Early indication of tumour responses by sFLCs could facilitate changes of treatment strategy, which may have a major bearing on cost of treatment and utilisation of resources[29].

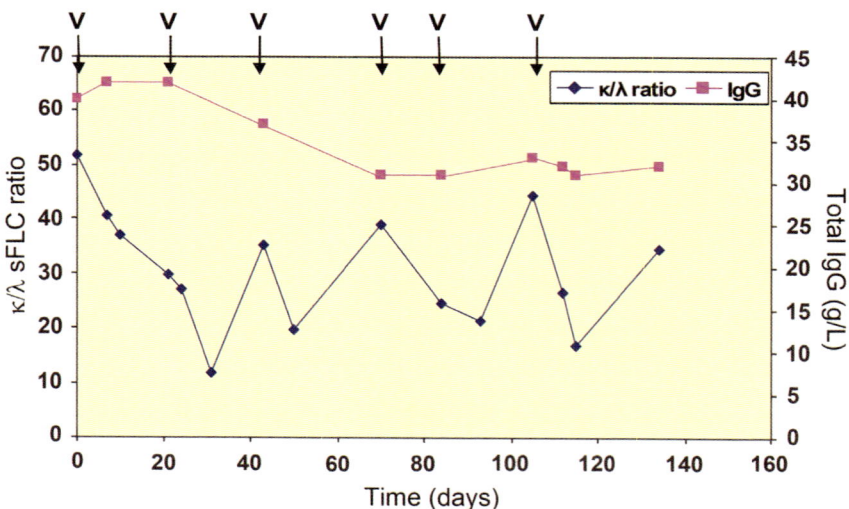

Figure 18.6. *Changes in κ/λ sFLC ratio during 6 cycles of bortezomib (V) showing rapid responses to treatment and subsequent relapses.*

The validity of sFLC measurements as a marker of tumour response has been illustrated by comparison with bone marrow plasma cell counts. In a study comprising 45 IgG MM patients, Mead et al.[27] showed that, during treatment, monoclonal plasma cell counts correlated better with changes in sFLCs (and serum β_2-microglobulin) than they did with intact monoclonal IgG *(Figure 18.7)*. κ/λ sFLC ratios had the highest concordance with bone marrow plasma cell counts, and were more accurate than both urine FLCs and SPE/sIFE for assessing disease status *(Table 18.1)*.

Patient	A	B	C	D	E
Monoclonal IgG by densitometry (g/L)	6.1	9.4	1.7	3.0	7.8
SPE	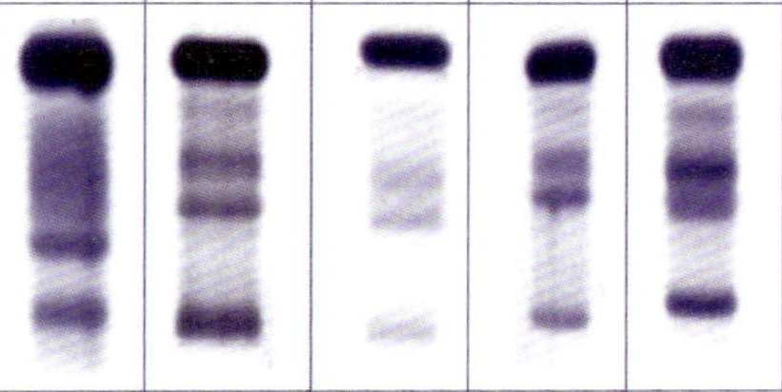				
sFLC (mg/L) (95% Normal range < 26mg/L)	11.9	7.4	15.3	12.9	34.5
% plasma cells in bone marrow	0%	0.1%	<5%	7%	<5%
$\beta2$ microglobulin (mg/L)	3.0	3.5	4.0	3.0	3.0

Figure 18.7. Accuracy of different blood tests for assessing bone marrow plasma cell volume in MM. Because of slow catabolism, IgG concentrations lag behind reductions in bone marrow plasma cell content during treatment.

		Bone Marrow		Concordance (%)
		Normal	Abnormal	
Serum FLCs	Normal	19	4	88
	Abnormal	5	47	
Urine FLCs	Normal	21	21	68
	Abnormal	3	30	
Serum IFE	Normal	10	5	75
	Abnormal	14	46	

sFLCs were classified as abnormal if the κ/λ sFLC ratio was outside the normal range; urine FLCs >40 mg/L were classified as abnormal; and bone marrow assessment was classified as abnormal if there were $\geq$5% plasma cells.

Table 18.1. Comparison of bone marrow plasma cell counts in MM using different tests for monoclonal proteins [27].

18.3.2. Prediction of overall response

Many studies have indicated that the reduction in sFLCs after one or two cycles of treatment is highly predictive of overall response. For example, Dispenzieri et al.[39] reported that a 90% reduction in sFLCs (90% reduction in the difference between the involved and uninvolved FLC [dFLC]) within 7 days post-ASCT predicted for haematologic complete response (p<0.001). Other studies have similarly highlighted the value of early sFLC reductions in predicting overall response[31,32,33,40,41]. Looking at a different measure of outcome, Orlowski et al.[42] reported that rapid normalisation of the FLC κ/λ ratio - after the first or second cycle of therapy - was highly predictive of prolonged time to progression. The prognostic value of the sFLC response is discussed further in Chapter 20.

18.3.3. Early detection of ineffective therapy

Monitoring with sFLCs allows early detection of ineffective treatment, and the identification of patients who may benefit from alternative chemotherapy regimens. One such example is shown in Figure 18.8. In this patient with IgGλ MM, the sFLC concentration initially decreased in response to treatment, with a negligible corresponding change in IgG concentration. Subsequently, λ sFLC levels stabilised, indicating that the patient was no longer responding to treatment. This was in contrast to the IgG levels, which were continuing to fall, suggesting a continuing response. Only after several months did IgG levels start to increase, signifying a tumour regrowth.

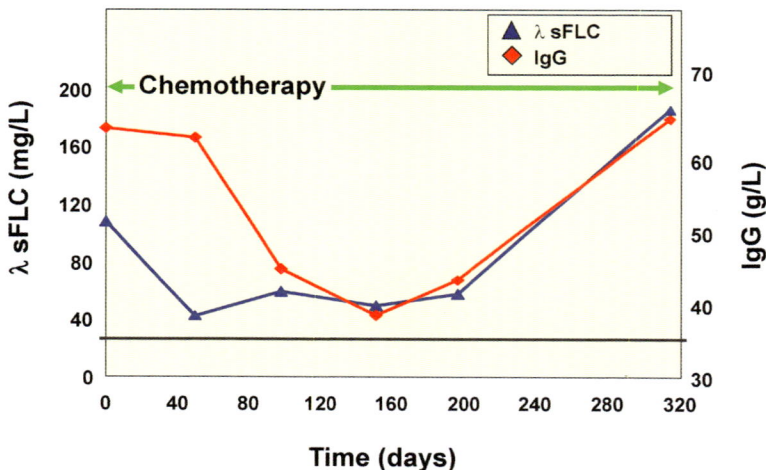

Figure 18.8. A rapid drop in λ sFLCs provides an early indication of response to treatment. By contrast, IgG levels remained high for almost 2 months. Subsequently, a lack of treatment effect was indicated by stable λ sFLC levels despite decreasing IgG levels. Several months later, relapse was confirmed by an increase in both λ sFLC and IgG concentrations.

18.3.4. Early detection of disease relapse

Since sFLC assays are intrinsically more sensitive than sIFE for detection of monoclonal FLC production (Chapter 4), earlier detection of tumour relapse should be possible in IIMM patients who relapse with FLCs alone or potentially, a proportion of those who relapse with intact immunoglobulins and FLCs. In a study of 187 MM patients, Willenbacher et al.[44] found that relapse was detected a median of 3 months earlier by sFLC levels than by conventional monoclonal protein measurements. In a smaller study by Mösbauer et al.[43], relapse was identified earlier in eight of nine IIMM patients when sFLC ratios were used rather than IFE (median, 98 days; range 35 - 238 days) (Figure 18.9).

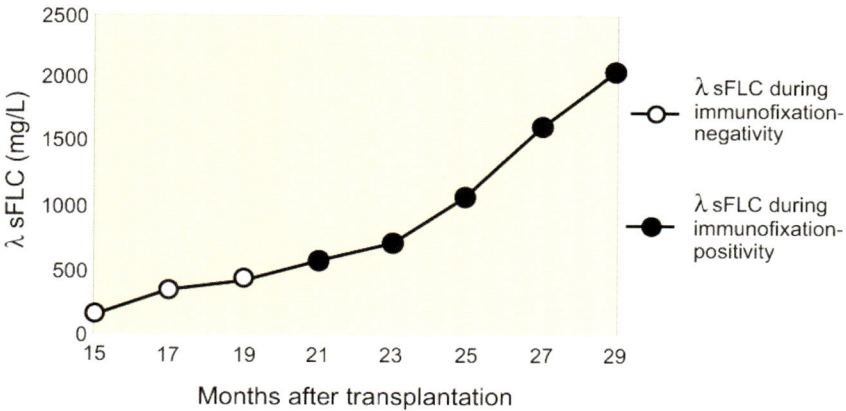

Figure 18.9. sFLCs and IFE during relapse of patient with MM[43]. *(Obtained from Haematologica Journal website: haematologica.org).*

In situations where relapse occurs relatively rapidly after successful treatment (i.e. within a few months), due to their relatively long half-life, monoclonal IgG levels may not normalise before relapse. Therefore, falling concentrations of IgG hide the early increases caused by tumour relapse. In contrast, because of their short half-life, an increase in sFLCs at relapse occurs from lower baseline levels and can be more readily detected. This is illustrated in a case study by Fuchida et al.[36] *(Figure 18.10).*

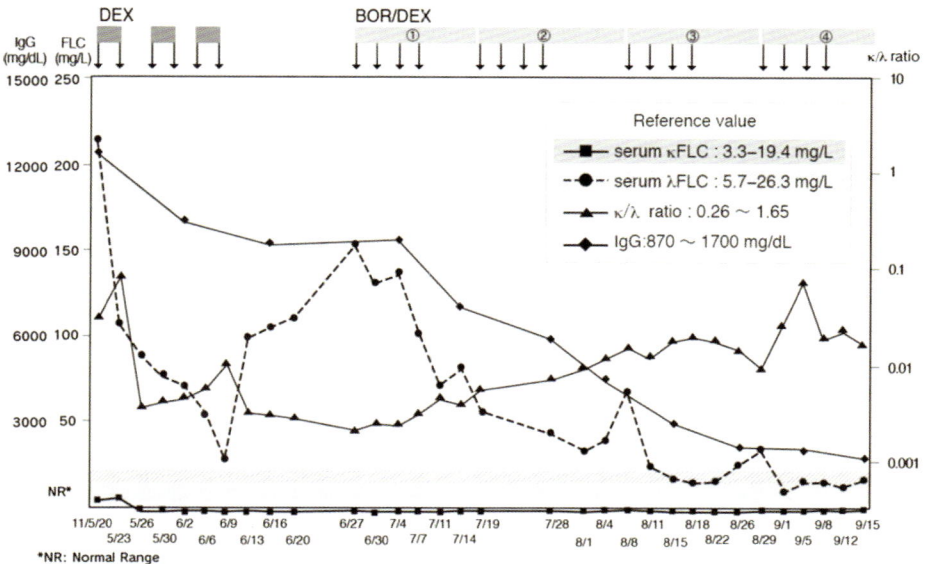

Figure 18.10. λ sFLC levels decrease more rapidly than IgG levels in a patient with IgGλ IIMM treated with dexamethasone (Dex). *Relapse from initial treatment was masked by slowly decreasing IgG levels but detected by an increase in λ sFLC. The patient was subsequently treated with bortezomib/dexamethasone (Bor/Dex) and short term falls and rises in sFLC levels correlated with treatment cycles. Such changes were not evident from IgG levels. (This research was originally published in International Journal of Hematology[36] © 2012 by The Japanese Society of Hematology).*

18.4. Monitoring IIMM patients using HLC assays

Immunoglobulin heavy/light chain (Hevylite, HLC) assays separately quantify the different light chain types of each immunoglobulin isotype (i.e. IgGκ, IgGλ, IgAκ, IgAλ, IgMκ and IgMλ, *Chapter 9*), and are assessed in pairs to produce HLC ratios (e.g. IgGκ/IgGλ) in the same manner as κ/λ sFLC ratios. The assays offer several advantages over SPE/CZE and sIFE for monitoring patients with IIMM, as discussed below.

18.4.1. HLC assays are quantitative and non-subjective

HLC assays provide numerical results, are less labour-intensive and interpretation is less subjective compared with electrophoretic techniques. For patients with a measurable monoclonal protein by SPE (M-spike), the relative change in the involved HLC concentration has been shown to be equivalent to the relative change in the M-spike *(Section 11.5.2)*[45]. However, for many patients, accurate quantitation of monoclonal proteins by SPE is not possible for a variety of reasons (such as co-migration or dye saturation issues, *Section 17.4*). In such cases, HLC assays can provide clarity for monitoring patients. One such patient is described in the clinical case history below.

Clinical case history 2

Confirmation of disease progression in a patient with a broadly migrating IgA monoclonal protein.

A 71-year-old female with a 9-year history of MGUS presented with anaemia and hypercalcaemia in January 2006[46]. SPE showed a 48 g/L broadly migrating monoclonal protein in the γ-region. The monoclonal protein was identified as an IgAκ intact immunoglobulin by sIFE *(Figure 18.11)*. Total IgA levels were 47.2 g/L and there was an abnormal sFLC κ/λ ratio (7.0). A bone marrow biopsy indicated 40% monoclonal κ-restricted plasma cells. A bone survey revealed diffuse osteopenia, multiple small lytic lesions and a lesion consistent with plasmacytoma in one of the thoracic vertebrae. The patient was diagnosed with MM (Durie Salmon stage IIIA).

The patient was successfully treated and achieved a serum and urine IFE CR, which was sustained for 18 months. Subsequently, the patient relapsed with monoclonal IgAκ (39.2 g/L), as detected by electrophoresis. She was successfully treated with Revlimid and dexamethasone, achieving a second CR *(Figure 18.11, August 2010)*. Between August and October 2010, although electrophoresis remained negative, total IgA levels increased steadily and became abnormal. Concurrently, the patient developed a lung infection *(Figure 18.11, October 2010)*. The elevation of serum IgA may have been attributable to the infection or, given the patient's history, due to disease relapse. However, IFE did not identify a monoclonal protein until January 2011.

Retrospective HLC analysis was performed on the equivocal samples taken between January 2008 and January 2011 *(Figure 18.12)*. The IgAκ/IgAλ HLC ratio decreased in response to treatment after the first relapse (January 2008) but did not normalise, possibly indicating residual disease. In the following months, HLC ratios increased steadily, supporting the existence of an abnormal clone despite the apparently normal IFE results.

The authors concluded that IgA HLC assays were particularly beneficial for monitoring this broadly migrating monoclonal protein, which was difficult to identify and quantify by serum electrophoretic techniques. In addition, IgA HLC was more sensitive than electrophoresis measurements for detecting disease relapse.

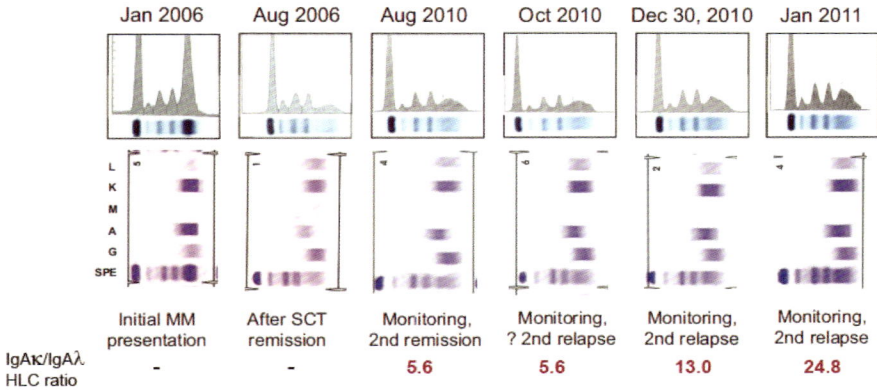

Figure 18.11. SPE, IFE and HLC analysis during the disease course. (Republished with permission of Clinical Chemistry, from[46]; permission conveyed through Copyright Clearance Center, Inc.).

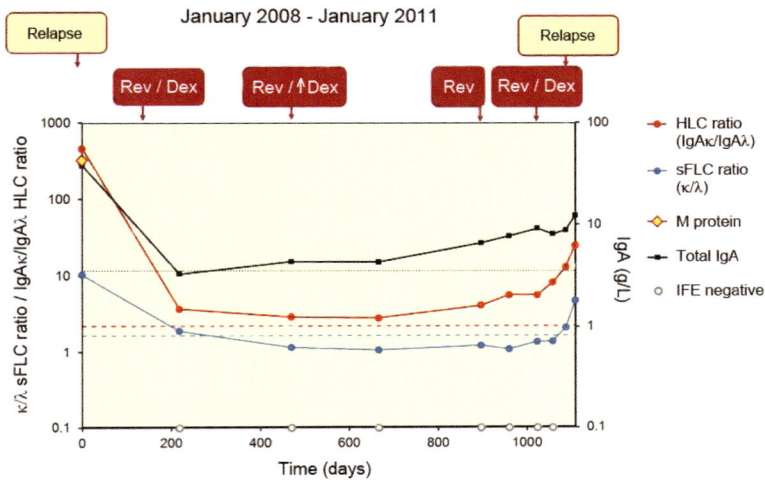

Figure 18.12. HLC and FLC results following the first relapse of disease. Dashed lines indicate the upper limits of the reference ranges for total IgA (black), IgAκ/IgAλ HLC ratio (red) and κ/λ sFLC ratio (blue). (Graph generated using published data[46]).

197

18.4.2. HLC assays to monitor oligosecretory patients

New evidence, reported by Ludwig et al.[48] shows that HLC assays can offer an additional means of monitoring oligosecretory patients. In a study of 156 MM patients, an abnormal HLC ratio was identified at presentation in all 18 oligosecretory patients (7 IgG and 11 IgA). Similar findings were reported by Boyle et al.[49]. In a study by Young and colleagues[47] IgG and IgA HLC analysis was performed on serial samples from 8 oligosecretory patients (5 IgA, 3 IgG) with sFLC <100 mg/L. In all 8 patients, the HLC ratio was abnormal at presentation and changes in the HLC ratio were in concordance with clinical assessment during follow-up. An example of an IgAκ oligosecretory MM patient is shown in Figure 18.13. Although the patient initially responded to therapy (indicated by a fall in the IgAκ/IgAλ HLC ratio), the HLC ratio remained abnormal. A subsequent increase in the HLC ratio suggested disease progression 445 days before a clinical relapse was confirmed.

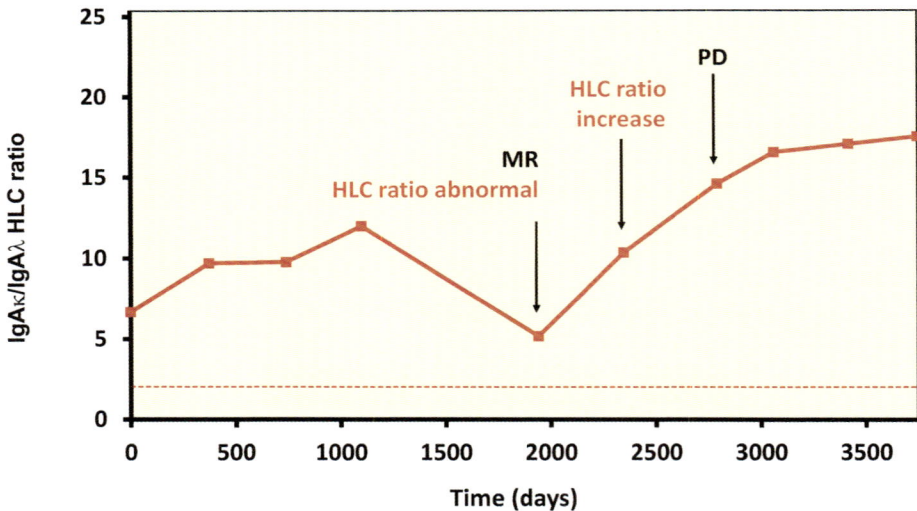

Figure 18.13. An increase in the HLC ratio indicates disease progression 445 days before relapse is clinically confirmed in a patient with oligosecretory IgAκ MM[47]. The upper limit for the IgA HLC ratio reference range is indicated by the dashed line. MR: maximum response, PD: progressive disease.

18.4.3. HLC assays improve detection of residual disease

According to IMWG response criteria[1], the current definition of CR requires the absence of the monoclonal protein by IFE and <5% bone marrow plasma cells[6]. However, this definition is not satisfactory for several reasons. Firstly, monoclonal protein quantification by electrophoresis measures only the product of the secreting clone, and not all MM plasma cells are secretory[50]. Secondly, recycling of IgG by the FcRn receptor may prolong the persistence of IgG monoclonal proteins in the serum, causing IFE to remain positive long after the tumour has been eradicated *(Section 3.5.3)*[51]. Finally, IFE is a subjective technique, and interpretation can be difficult, leading to discordance in the response category assigned by different operators[52].

With the introduction of highly effective, novel therapies to treat MM, assays with increased sensitivity are required to improve the definition of CR. This will allow more precise comparisons of treatment responses and the detection of clinically relevant minimal residual disease[25,53]. A more rigorous sCR has been defined, which incorporates sFLC analysis *(Section 18.2.2)*[1], and in future, inclusion of Hevylite analysis may further improve the definition of CR. A number of studies show that abnormal HLC ratios may indicate residual disease in IIMM patients whose electrophoresis results have normalised following therapy[48,54,55,56,57].

Ludwig et al.[48] used Hevylite to assess response in IgG and IgA MM patients. A total of 100 IgG and 56 IgA patients were followed for a median of 46.1 months. Hevylite results were compared with data from SPE, IFE, nephelometry and sFLC assays. Following induction therapy, a CR or sCR was observed in 31 patients. Residual disease was indicated by an abnormal HLC ratio in 8/31 patients – in four of these HLC was the only abnormality, and in the remaining four, abnormal HLC and sFLC ratios were observed. Figure 18.14A shows an example of an IgAκ MM patient who achieved a CR during follow-up[48]. The monoclonal IgAκ became undetectable by IFE, but the IgAκ/IgAλ HLC ratio remained abnormal. After further follow-up, the HLC ratio normalised. In this case, the κ/λ sFLC ratio showed a similar trend to the HLC ratio throughout the study.

It has been reported that patients with an abnormal HLC ratio at maximum response have a significantly worse outcome than patients in whom the HLC ratio normalises (Chapter 20)[48,58]. An abnormal HLC ratio may be the result of HLC-pair suppression (as illustrated in the case by Ludwig et al. discussed above). HLC-pair suppression is an important prognostic marker, and has been shown to identify patients with inferior progression-free survival[58] and overall survival (Chapter 20)[59].

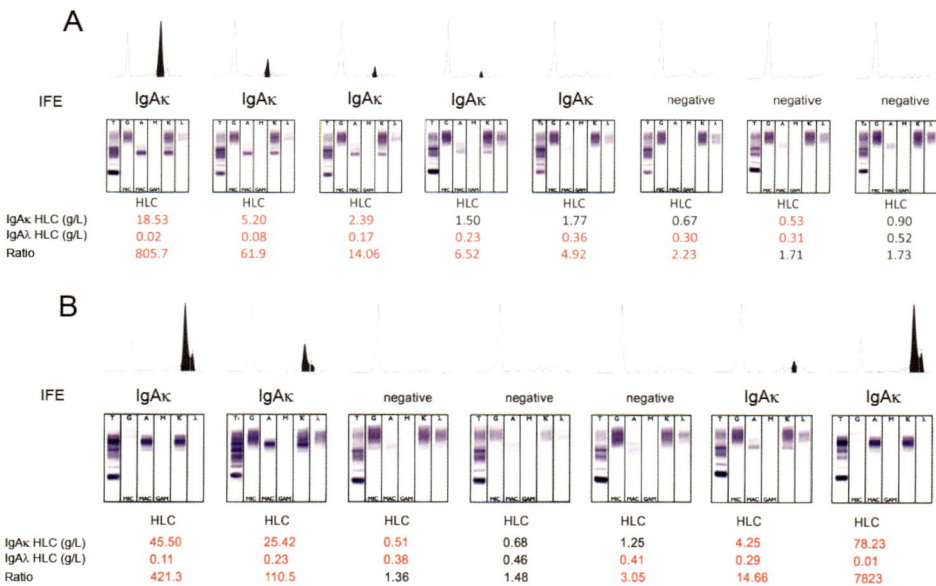

Figure 18.14. Utility of IgA HLC for monitoring IgA MM. (A) IFE became negative when an abnormal IgAκ/IgAλ HLC ratio indicated residual disease. The HLC ratio became normal with further follow up. **(B)** IFE and the IgAκ/IgAλ HLC ratio became normal at the same time, but on subsequent follow up, IgA HLC ratio became abnormal, indicating relapse when IFE was still normal. (Reprinted by permission from Macmillan Publishers Ltd: Leukemia[48], copyright 2013).

18.4.4. HLC assays improve detection of relapse

Ludwig et al.[48] reported three MM patients in whom a HLC abnormality pointed to imminent relapse while IFE was still negative. Data from one of the three patients is shown in Figure 18.14B. Following induction therapy, the patient with IgAκ MM initially achieved a CR and the IgAκ/IgAλ HLC ratio was normal[48]. Seven months later, the HLC ratio became abnormal due to pair-suppression of IgAλ (IgAκ was still within the normal range). Subsequently, IgAκ became elevated, with further reductions in the uninvolved HLC-pair, confirming disease evolution. IFE became positive 5.5 months after the HLC ratio became abnormal. It is noteworthy that, although the κ/λ sFLC ratio was abnormal in this patient at diagnosis, it normalised following treatment and remained normal at relapse. This highlights the importance of measuring both FLCs and intact immunoglobulins during follow-up.

Other examples where HLC ratios have provided an early indication of relapse have been published elsewhere[56,60,61,62,63,64]. Bradwell et al.[56] reported on 5 IgG MM patients who achieved a CR by IFE with normalisation of the IgGκ/IgGλ HLC ratio. In 3 of 5 patients, subsequent relapse was indicated earlier by abnormal HLC ratios. In an IgA patient, abnormal HLC ratios indicated a slow relapse more than a year before IFE became positive.

18.4.5. Discrepancies between HLC and IFE during follow-up

Ludwig et al.[48] observed a normal HLC ratio in 12 of 35 MM patients who achieved a near complete response (nCR: 100% monoclonal protein reduction by electrophoresis, but IFE-positive), or a very good partial response (VGPR: at least 90% serum and urine monoclonal protein reduction) following treatment. This discrepancy between HLC analysis and IFE may be due to the recovery of polyclonal immunoglobulins producing a normal HLC ratio, despite the persistence of small amounts of monoclonal immunoglobulin. While continuing low levels of a monoclonal protein may reflect residual disease, it has been shown that a normal HLC ratio predicts a good patient outcome, irrespective of IFE positivity *(Chapter 20)*.

In IgG patients specifically, persistence of small amounts of monoclonal IgG is partly the result of a prolonged half-life due to recycling by FcRn receptors, causing IFE to remain positive after the tumour has been eradicated. This is an issue previously reported by Waldmann et al.[66] *(Chapter 3)* and demonstrated in Figure 18.15. Consistent with this, discrepancies between IFE and bone marrow immunophenotypic responses can be observed during follow-up[50].

HLC ratios are not affected by the variable metabolism of IgG and for the detection of residual disease, they demonstrate a better agreement than sIFE with flow cytometry results *(Figure 18.16)*[65]. Others have similarly found a good correlation between HLC and flow cytometry[54].

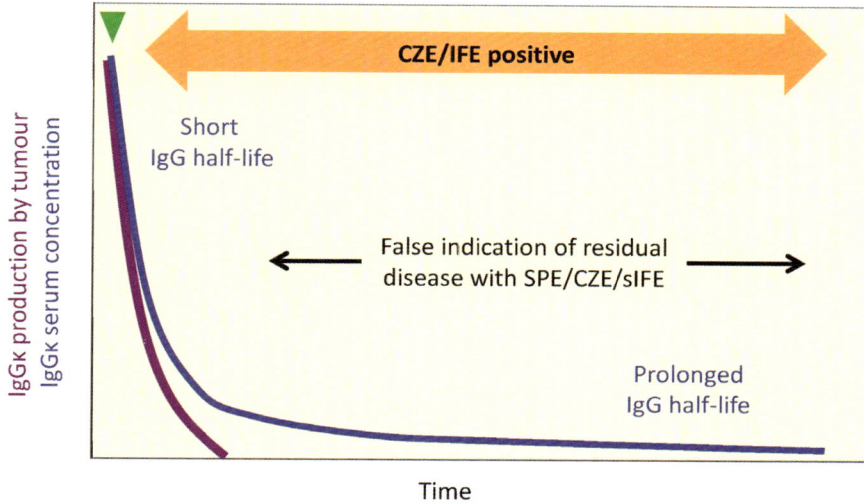

Figure 18.15. Theoretical patient with persistence of low-level monoclonal IgG due to FcRn receptor recycling. *Although monoclonal IgGκ production by the tumour ceases following treatment, low levels of IgGκ are still detected by CZE/IFE due to prolonged IgG half-life.*

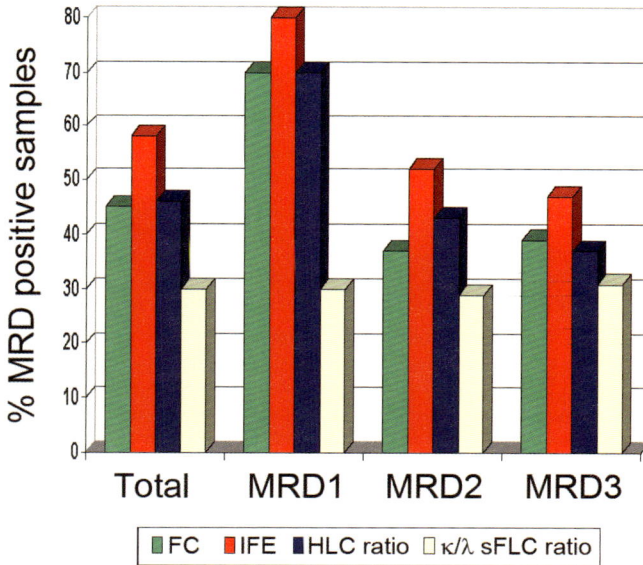

Figure 18.16. Comparison between flow cytometry (FC), serum immunofixation (IFE), HLC ratios (Hevylite) and κ/λ sFLC ratios (Freelite) for assessment of minimal residual disease (MRD) in IIMM patients [65]. *Results analysed at 3 time-points (pre-ASCT, MRD1; post-ASCT, MRD2; and post-consolidation, MRD3) showed a good correlation between HLC ratios and FC. At each time-point, sIFE assigned a greater percentage of MRD-positive patients than HLC or FC. (Obtained from Haematologica Journal website: haematologica.org).*

Test Questions

1. Why can sFLC measurements be used as an early marker of relapse in IIMM?

2. Can sFLC measurements help when assessing residual disease in MM?

3. Following treatment, why do HLC ratios occasionally normalise when IFE remains positive in patients with intact immunoglobulin MM?

Answers

1. sFLCs may increase before intact immunoglobulins because sFLC assays are more sensitive; or the relative proportion of monoclonal FLC production to intact immunoglobulin changes (FLC escape); or FLCs may relapse from the normal range while immunoglobulins have not normalised (Sections 18.2.1 and 18.3.4).

2. Some patients are normal by serum and urine electrophoretic tests but have abnormal sFLC concentrations. Statistically, these patients are more likely to have residual disease and shorter survival (Section 18.2.2 and Chapter 20).

3. This may be due to recovery of polyclonal immunoglobulins producing a normal HLC ratio despite the persistence of low levels of monoclonal immunoglobulin. The persistence of low concentrations of a monoclonal protein may reflect residual disease that has not been cleared by treatment, or in IgG patients this may also be due to the persistence of small amounts of monoclonal IgG with a prolonged half-life due to recycling by FcRn receptors (Section 18.4.5).

References

1. Durie BG, Harousseau JL, Miguel JS, Blade J, Barlogie B, Anderson K et al. International uniform response criteria for multiple myeloma. Leukemia 2006;20:1467-73

2. Gertz MA, Merlini G. Definition of organ involvement and response to treatment in AL amyloidosis: an updated consensus opinion. Amyloid 2010;17:CP-Ba

3. Kyle RA, Rajkumar SV. Criteria for diagnosis, staging, risk stratification and response assessment of multiple myeloma. Leukemia 2009;23:3-9

4. Palladini G, Dispenzieri A, Gertz MA, Wechalekar A, Hawkins P, Schonland SO et al. Validation of the criteria of response to treatment in AL amyloidosis. Blood 2010;116:1364a

5. Palladini G, Dispenzieri A, Gertz MA, Kumar S, Wechalekar A, Hawkins PN et al. New criteria for response to treatment in immunoglobulin light chain amyloidosis based on free light chain measurement and cardiac biomarkers: impact on survival outcomes. J Clin Oncol 2012;30:4541-9

6. Rajkumar SV, Harousseau JL, Durie B, Anderson KC, Dimopoulos M, Kyle R et al. Consensus recommendations for the uniform reporting of clinical trials: report of the International Myeloma Workshop Consensus Panel 1. Blood 2011;117:4691-5

7. Larson D, Kyle RA, Rajkumar SV. Prevalence and monitoring of oligosecretory myeloma. N Engl J Med 2012;367:580-1

8. Dispenzieri A, Kyle R, Merlini G, Miguel JS, Ludwig H, Hajek R et al. International Myeloma Working Group guidelines for serum-free light chain analysis in multiple myeloma and related disorders. Leukemia 2009;23:215-24

9. Leleu X, Attal M, Arnulf B, Moreau P, Traulle C, Marit G et al. Pomalidomide plus low-dose dexamethasone is active and well tolerated in bortezomib and lenalidomide-refractory multiple myeloma: Intergroupe Francophone du Myelome 2009-02. Blood 2013;121:1968-75

10. Brioli A, Giles H, Pawlyn C, Campbell J, Kaiser M, Melchor L et al. Serum free light chain evaluation as a marker for the impact of intra-clonal heterogeneity on the progression and treatment resistance in multiple myeloma. Blood 2014;123:3414-9

11. Hobbs JR. Growth rates and responses to treatment in human myelomatosis. Br J Haematol 1969;16:607-17

12. Hobbs JA, Kilvington F, Sharp K, Harding S, Drayson M, Bradwell AR, Mead GP. Incidence of light chain escape in UK MRC Myeloma VII Trial. Clin Chem 2008;54:C109a

13. Qu X, Zhang L, Fu W, Zhang H, Xiang X, Qiu L, Hou J. An infrequent relapse of multiple myeloma predominantly manifesting as light chain escape: clinical experience from two Chinese centers. Leuk Lymphoma 2010;51:1844-9

14. Hobbs JA, Drayson MT, Sharp K, Harding S, Bradwell AR, Mead GP. Frequency of altered monoclonal protein production at relapse of multiple myeloma. Br J Haematol 2009;148:659-61

15. Dawson MA, Patil S, Spencer A. Extramedullary relapse of multiple myeloma associated with a shift in secretion from intact immunoglobulin to light chains. Haematologica 2007;92:143-4

16. Dierge L, Lutteri L, Chauvet D, Hastir D, Chapelle J, Cavalier E. Heavy/Light chain (HLC) and free light chain (FLC) analysis allow sensitive monitoring of multiple myeloma patients and aid detection of clonal changes. Biochmica Clinica 2013;37:W251a

17. Graubaum K, Heymann GA, Hunger T, Ostapowicz B. Case report: Shift in secretion from intact immunoglobulin to free light chains in multiple myeloma at relapse: early detection by free light chain assay. Hematology meeting reports 2008;2:D26a

18. Kuhnemund A, Liebisch P, Bauchmuller K, Zur Hausen A, Veelken H, Wasch R, Engelhardt M. 'Light-chain escape-multiple myeloma'-an escape phenomenon from plateau phase: report of the largest patient series using LC-monitoring. J Cancer Res Clin Oncol 2009;135:477-84

19. Teleanu V, Kull M, Kuchenbauer F, Leibisch P, Graf M, Steinbach G et al. Heavy/light chain (HLC) and free light chain (FLC) analysis allow sensitive monitoring of multiple myeloma patients and aid detection of potential clonal changes. Onkologie 2013;36:P530a

20. Zamarin D, Giralt S, Landau H, Lendvai N, Lesokhin A, Chung D et al. Patterns of relapse and progression in multiple myeloma patients after auto-SCT: implications for patients' monitoring after transplantation. Bone Marrow Transplant 2013;48:419-24

21. Ayliffe MJ, Davies FE, de Castro D, Morgan GJ. Demonstration of changes in plasma cell subsets in multiple myeloma. Haematologica 2007;92:1135-8

22. Ayliffe MJ, Behrens J, Stern S, Sumar N. Association of plasma cell subsets in the bone marrow and free light chain concentrations in the serum of monoclonal gammopathy patients. J Clin Pathol 2012;65:758-61

23. Kraj M, Kruk B, Warzocha K, Szczepinski A, Endean K, Harding S. An intact immunoglobulin IgA lambda multiple myeloma patient exhibiting light chain escape. Blood 2012;120:5008a

24. Reid SD, Drayson MT, Mead GP, Augustson B, Bradwell AR. Serum free light chains are a more sensitive marker of serological remission in multiple myeloma patients. Clin Chem 2004;50:C34a

25. Kapoor P, Kumar SK, Dispenzieri A, Lacy MQ, Buadi F, Dingli D et al. Importance of achieving stringent complete response after autologous stem-cell transplantation in multiple myeloma. J Clin Oncol 2013;31:4529-35

26. Lebovic D, Kendall T, Brozo C, McAllister A, Hari M, Alvi S et al. Serum free light chain analysis improves monitoring of multiple myeloma patients receiving first-line therapy with the combination of Velcade, Doxil, and Dexamethasone (VDD). Blood 2007;110:2736a

27. Mead GP, Reid SD, Augustson BM, Drayson MT, Bradwell AR, Child JA. Correlation of serum free light chains and bone marrow plasma cell infiltration in multiple myeloma. Blood 2004;104:4865a

28. Tang G, Snyder M, Rao LV. Assessment of serum free light chain (FLC) assays with immunofixation electrophoresis (IFE) and bone marrow (BM) immunophenotyping in the diagnosis of plasma cell disorders. Clin Chem 2008;54:A96a

29. Das M, Mead GP, Sreekanth V, Anderson J, Blair S, Howe T et al. Serum free light chain (sFLC) concentration kinetics in patients receiving bortezomib: temporary inhibition of protein synthesis and early biomarker for disease response. Blood 2005;106:5094a

30. Giarin MM, Giaccone L, Bruno B, Omedè P, Battaglio S, Falco P et al. Serum free light chains: a potential useful marker for diagnosis and early assessment of response to treatment and relapse in plasma cell disorders. Haematologica Reports 2006;2:4a

31. Hassoun H, Reich L, Klimek VM, Dhodapkar M, Cohen A, Kewalramani T et al. The serum free light chain ratio after one or two cycles of treatment is highly predictive of the magnitude of final response in patients undergoing initial treatment for multiple myeloma. Blood 2005;106:972a

32. Hassoun H, Reich L, Klimek VM, Dhodapkar M, Cohen A, Kewalramani T et al. Doxorubicin and dexamethasone followed by thalidomide and dexamethasone is an effective well tolerated initial therapy for multiple myeloma. Br J Haematol 2006;132:155-61

33. Patten PE, Ahsan G, Kazmi M, Fields PA, Chick GW, Jones RR et al. The early use of the serum free light chain assay in patients with relapsed refractory myeloma receiving treatment with thalidomide analogue (CC-4047). Blood 2003;102:1640a

34. Pratt G, Mead GP, Godfrey KR, Hu Y, Evans ND, Chappell MJ et al. The tumor kinetics of multiple myeloma following autologous stem cell transplantation as assessed by measuring serum-free light chains. Leuk Lymphoma 2006;47:21-8

35. Pratt G. Using serum free light chain concentrations as rapid response markers in multiple myeloma. Hematology meeting reports 2008;2:p2

36. Fuchida SI, Okano A, Hatsuse M, Murakami S, Haruyama H, Itoh S, Shimazaki C. Serial measurement of free light chain detects poor response to therapy early in three patients with multiple myeloma who have measurable M-proteins. Int J Hematol 2012;96:664-8

37. Kyrtsonis MC, Sachanas S, Vassilakopoulos TP, Kafassi N, Tzenou T, Papadogiannis A et al. Bortezomib in patients with relapsed-refractory multiple myeloma (MM). Clinical observations. Blood 2005;106:5193a

38. Robson E, Mead G, Das M, Cavet J, Liakpoulou E. Free light chain analysis in patients receiving Bortezomib. Haematologica 2007;92:PO1019a

39. Dispenzieri A, Rajkumar SV, Plevak MF, Katzmann JA, Kyle RA, Larson D et al. Early immunoglobulin free light chain (FLC) response post autologous peripheral blood stem cell transplant predicts for hematologic complete response in patients with multiple myeloma. Blood 2006;108:3097a

40. Cavallo F, Rasmussen E, Zangari M, Tricot G, Fender B, Fox M et al. Serum free-lite chain (sFLC) assay in Multiple Myeloma (MM): Clinical correlates and prognostic implications in newly diagnosed MM patients treated with Total Therapy 2 or 3 (TT2/3). Blood 2005;106:3490a

41. Nakorn TN, Watanaboonyongcharoen P, Suwannabutra S, Theerasaksilp S, Paritpokee N. Early reduction of serum free light chain can predict therapeutic responses in multiple myeloma. Blood 2007;110:4742a

42. Orlowski R, Sutherland H, Blade J, Miguel JS, Hajek R, Nagler A et al. Early normalization of serum free light chains is associated with prolonged time to progression following bortezomib {+/-} pegylated liposomal doxorubicin treatment of relapsed/ refractory multiple myeloma. Blood 2007;110:2735a

43. Mösbauer U, Ayuk F, Schieder H, Lioznov M, Zander AR, Kroger N. Monitoring serum free light chains in patients with multiple myeloma who achieved negative immunofixation after allogeneic stem cell transplantation. Haematologica 2007;92:275–6

44. Willenbacher E, Gasser S, Gastl G, Willenbacher W. Serum & urine free light chain analysis compared to conventional paraprotein measurements: usefulness for clinical decision making in real life haematology. Blood 2009;114:2889a

45. Katzmann JA, Willrich MA, Kohlhagen MC, Kyle RA, Murray DL, Snyder MR et al. Monitoring IgA Multiple Myeloma: Immunoglobulin Heavy/Light Chain Assays. Clin Chem 2014 In press

46. Donato LJ, Zeldenrust SR, Murray DL, Katzmann JA. A 71-year-old woman with multiple myeloma status after stem cell transplantation. Clin Chem 2011;57:1645-8

47. Young P, Ludwig H, Zojer N, Milosavljevic D, Harding S. Use of heavy/light chain (HLC) and free light chain (FLC) ratios for monitoring oligosecretory multiple myeloma patients. Clinical Lymphoma, Myeloma & Leukaemia 2013;13:P-236a

48. Ludwig H, Milosavljevic D, Zojer N, Faint JM, Bradwell AR, Hubl W, Harding SJ. Immunoglobulin heavy/light chain ratios improve paraprotein detection and monitoring, identify residual disease and correlate with survival in multiple myeloma patients. Leukemia 2013;27:213-9

49. Boyle EM, Fouquet G, Guidez S, Bonnet S, Demarquette H, Dulery R et al. IgA kappa/IgA lambda heavy/light chain assessment in the management of patients with IgA myeloma. Cancer 2014;120:3952-7

50. Paiva B, Martinez-Lopez J, Vidriales MB, Mateos MV, Montalban MA, Fernandez-Redondo E et al. Comparison of immunofixation, serum free light chain, and immunophenotyping for response evaluation and prognostication in multiple myeloma. J Clin Oncol 2011;29:1627-33

51. Roopenian DC, Akilesh S. FcRn: the neonatal Fc receptor comes of age. Nat Rev Immunol 2007;7:715-25

52. Caillon H, Dejoie T, Le Loupp AG, Azoulay-Fauconnier C, Masson D, Moreau P et al. Difficulties in immunofixation analysis: a concordance study on the IFM 2007-02 trial. Blood Cancer J 2013;3:e154

53. Munshi NC, Anderson KC. Minimal residual disease in multiple myeloma. J Clin Oncol 2013;31:2523-6

54. Matsue K, Sugihara H, Nishida Y, Yamakura M, Takeuchi M. Heterogeneity of IMWG defined response assessed by FLC assay, multicolor flow cytometry, and heavy/light chain analysis. Clinical Lymphoma, Myeloma & Leukaemia 2013;13:P-203a

55. Lakomy D, Lemaire-Ewing S, Lafon I, Bastie JN, Borgeot J, Guy J et al. IgA heavy/light chain analysis - a new marker for the diagnosis and monitoring of myeloma patients. Haematologica 2012;97:590

56. Bradwell AR, Harding SJ, Fourrier NJ, Wallis GL, Drayson MT, Carr-Smith HD, Mead GP. Assessment of monoclonal gammopathies by nephelometric measurement of individual immunoglobulin kappa/lambda ratios. Clin Chem 2009;55:1646-55

57. Lakomy D, Dejoie T, Lafon I, Bastie JN, Lemaire-Ewing S, Caillot D. Hevylite™ IgA assay - a promising tool for the diagnosis and monitoring of myeloma patients. Haematologica 2011;96:P-043a

58. Drayson MT, Berlanga O, Plant T, Newnham NJ, Young P, Harding S. Immunoglobulin heavy/light chain measurements during monitoring provide prognostic information of relapse after therapy in myeloma patients. Blood 2012;120:3964a

59. Ludwig H, Slavka G, Hubl W, Carr-Smith H, Milosavljevic D, Hughes R et al. Usage of HLC-ratio, FLC-ratio, IFE, PBMC infiltration and isotype suppression at best response reveals isotype suppression as most powerful parameter for identification of multiple myeloma patients with long survival. Blood 2012;120:1817a

60. Amolak B, Dale P, Simon S, Judith B, Pinika P, Lauren H. Assessment of IgA Heavy/Light chain immunoassays utility in multiple myeloma patients. Biochmica Clinica 2013;37:W233a

61. Bengoufa D, Arnulf B, Bugnot L, Charron D, Fermand JP. Usefulness of a Hevylite immunoassay in serum for the diagnosis and the follow up of IgA monoclonal gammopathy. Hematology Reports 2010;2:G68a

62. Decaux O, Besnard S, Beaumont MP, Collet N, Sebillot M, Grosbois B, Guenet L. Serial sample analysis of 15 multiple myeloma patients using heavy/light chain specific immunoglobulin ratios (HevyliteTM). Contribution to the evaluation of response to treatment. Haematologica 2011;96:P-039a

63. Harding S, Koulieres E, Kyrtsonis MC, Levoguer A, Mirbahai L, Drayson M et al. Hevylite Ig'k/Ig'l lambda ratios in multiple myeloma correlate with clinical status. Hematology Reports 2010;2:G65a

64. Margetts C, Drayson M, Sharp K, Harper J, Fourrier N, Harding S. Serial sample analysis of 3 IgA multiple myeloma patients using a novel immunoassay measuring IgA kappa and IgA lambda. Hematology meeting reports 2008;2:F46a

65. Olivero B, Robillard N, Wuilleme S, Avet-Loiseau H, Attal M, Roussel M, Dejoie T. Heavy/light chain assay, potential new tool in minimal residual disease assessment. A biological study from IFM 2008 trial. Haematologica 2011;96:P-079a

66. Waldmann TA, Strober W. Metabolism of immunoglobulins. Prog Allergy 1969;13:1-110

Clonal evolution in multiple myeloma

Summary:

- Multiple myeloma is a clonally diverse disease, with multiple clones present at diagnosis.
- Clones may express intact immunoglobulin, FLCs, both, or rarely, neither.
- Changes in clonal dominance may be reflected by changes in monoclonal immunoglobulin production.
- FLC escape is an example of clonal evolution, first characterised over 40 years ago.

19.1. Introduction

Monoclonal gammopathy of undetermined significance (MGUS; *Chapter 13*) and smouldering multiple myeloma (SMM; *Chapter 14*) are asymptomatic plasma cell dyscrasias, with a propensity to progress to symptomatic multiple myeloma (MM). Genetic analysis has demonstrated that the pre-malignant conditions share some of the mutations associated with MM, and that multiple genetic "hits" are required for the progression to symptomatic disease[1]. Such mutations are not acquired in a linear fashion *(Figure 19.1A)*, but instead through branching, non-linear pathways *(Figure 19.1B)*[2].

During the evolution of MM, tumour clones may acquire further genetic abnormalities, e.g. to allow them to further expand or compete for stromal niches within the bone marrow, such that within an individual patient, multiple genetically distinct clones may be present. Furthermore, the clonal composition changes during the course of the disease, giving rise to "tides" of myelomic clones which compete for dominance in a landscape that is continually changed by therapy[2]. In this chapter we review the current understanding of myeloma clonal evolution and discuss the importance of monoclonal protein measurements in surveying these changes.

19.2 Clonal populations in multiple myeloma

MM patients can be classified according to their monoclonal protein type, i.e. intact immunoglobulin MM (IIMM; *Chapter 17*), light chain MM (LCMM; *Chapter 15*) and nonsecretory MM (NSMM; *Chapter 16*)[4]. At presentation, 95% of IIMM patients also have an abnormal κ/λ serum free light chain (sFLC) ratio *(Section 17.2)*. The simplest interpretation is that most IIMM patients have a single MM clone producing monoclonal intact immunoglobulin plus free light chains (FLCs). However, specific methods of plasma cell staining have challenged this idea. Ayliffe et al.[3,5] performed double immunofluorescence staining to study immunoglobulin heavy chain and light chain expression by plasma cells in bone marrow biopsies. The majority of patients had a single tumour cell population that expressed either monoclonal intact immunoglobulins and FLCs (42%), intact immunoglobulins alone

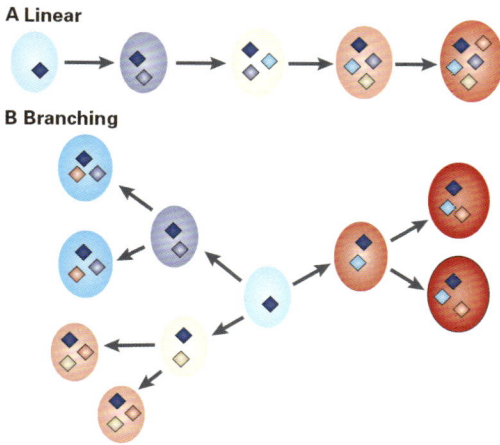

A Linear

B Branching

Figure 19.1. (A) Linear and (B) branching transformation of MGUS to MM. Genetic events conferring a selective advantage are shown as diamonds. (Reprinted by permission from Macmillan Publishers Ltd: Nature Reviews Cancer[1], copyright 2012).

(32%), or FLCs alone (8%). However, in the remaining 18% of patients, separate clones expressing either intact immunoglobulin or FLC only were identified *(Figure 19.2)*. These dual clonal populations were the first indicators that, within a single patient, multiple clones expressing different monoclonal proteins could be found. Subsequently, using array comparative genomic hybridisation (aCGH) and fluorescence in situ hybridisation (FISH), Keats et al.[6] elegantly demonstrated the presence of multiple clones in a patient with IgA MM. The impact of these multiple clones is illustrated in the clinical case history below.

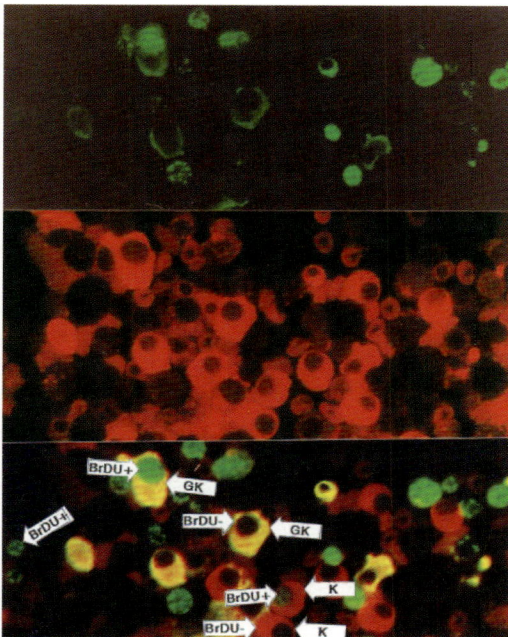

Figure 19.2. The same microscope field of an IgGκ MM bone marrow sample showing dual populations stained with anti-IgG fluorescein isothiocyanate (FITC, green) and anti-κ tetramethylrhodamine isothiocyanate (TRITC, red). In addition, anti-bromo deoxyuridine (BrdU) FITC (green) staining of nuclei has been performed to show cells in S-phase of the cell cycle. Upper panel shows anti-IgG FITC cytoplasmic and anti-BrdU FITC nuclear staining, middle shows the same field with anti-κ TRITC staining and lower shows a double exposure of the 2 upper plates superimposed to demonstrate double stained IgGκ cells (yellow), κ only cells (red) and S-phase cells with green nuclei. Arrows indicate BrdU+ and BrdU- intact immunoglobulin + cells, BrdU+ and BrdU- κ only cells together with non-plasma cells in S-phase[3]. (Obtained from Haematologica Journal website: haematologica.org).*

207

19.3. Clonal changes and clonal escape in multiple myeloma

The earliest observation of changes in monoclonal protein production during MM disease evolution was published by J. R. Hobbs in 1969 from his analysis of the first MRC MM trial[8]. He described the phenomenon of Bence Jones escape (FLC escape) in 15 patients at disease relapse, in which the serum intact immunoglobulin concentration reduced, but Bence Jones proteinuria dramatically increased. This phenomenon is further discussed in Section 18.2.1.

In accord with Ayliffe's phenotyping of clones based on their protein expression[3], both Hobbs[7] and Brioli[10] used serum protein measurements as indicators of clonal change during the course of a patient's disease. In an analysis of the MRC VII trial, Hobbs[7] suggested three classifications of clonal evolution: 1) light chain escape - an increase in sFLC concentrations without a corresponding increase in intact immunoglobulins; 2) intact immunoglobulin escape - an increase in monoclonal intact immunoglobulin without an associated increase in sFLC; and 3) clonal change - a change in the relative proportion of monoclonal intact immunoglobulin and sFLCs *(Figure 19.3)*.

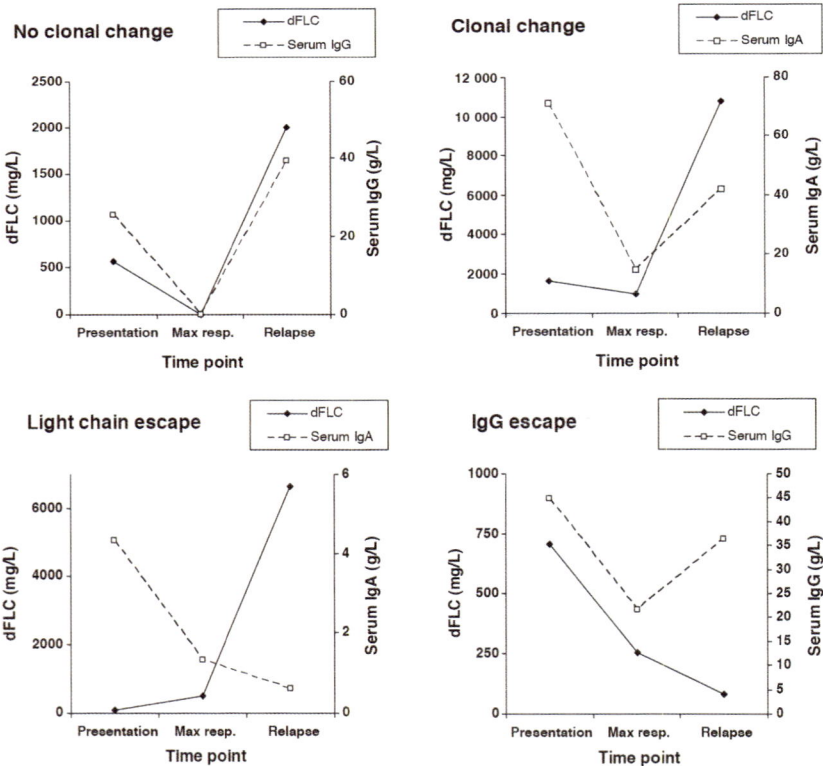

Figure 19.3. Changes in monoclonal protein expression at MM relapse. dFLC: difference between involved and uninvolved FLC levels. (Reproduced with permission from the British Journal of Haematology[7] and John Wiley & Sons Ltd).

In a larger study of 520 IIMM patients at relapse, Brioli et al.[10] reported that 183 (35%) had a significant increase in intact immunoglobulin and sFLC levels, 258 (50%) had an increase in intact immunoglobulin only and 54 (10%) had light chain escape. Similar patterns of serum protein changes were reported by Zamarin et al.[9] in a study of 66 patients (Figure 19.4). Importantly, this study included patients with LCMM. There was no evidence of clonal change in the LCMM patients, suggesting that loss of heavy chain production represented a terminal genetic event.

Genotypic analysis can identify changes in the clonal architecture of the disease and identify if disease progression is due to acquired genetic mutations or due to the presence of multiple clones. However, this technique is not readily available outside of clinical studies and academic centres of excellence. The case report by Keats et al.[6] and Egan et al.[11] described below provides evidence of the relationship between the genotype and phenotype of the disease. The assessment of monoclonal protein production using sFLC analysis and intact immunoglobulin measurements are simple, widely available techniques that allow patients to be monitored for evidence of clonal evolution.

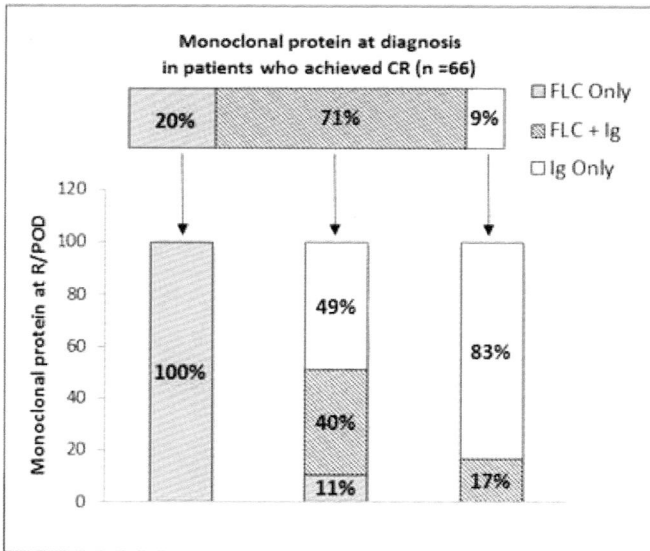

Figure 19.4. Changes in monoclonal protein type at relapse or progression of disease (R/POD). (Reprinted by permission from Macmillan Publishers Ltd: Bone Marrow Transplantation[9], copyright 2013).

Clinical case history

Alternating dominance of competing myeloma clones[6,11].

Both Keats et al.[6] and Egan et al.[11] described the case of a 67-year-old woman with MM who was monitored closely during the course of her disease using sFLC analysis and total IgA assays. In addition, at 7 time points, genetic analysis of tumour plasma cells was performed using array comparative genomic hybridisation (aCGH) and fluorescence in situ hybridisation (FISH). This enabled the comparison of genetic changes in the competing tumour clones with the serological monoclonal protein changes (Figure 19.5).

At diagnosis, a bone marrow biopsy revealed a plasma cell content of 25%. Tumour cells were comprised primarily of one clone (termed '1.1') but minor sub-clones (1.2 and 2.1) were also detected, both with a frequency of approximately 10% of the myeloma cells. At this point, both total IgA and the κ/λ sFLC ratio were abnormal.

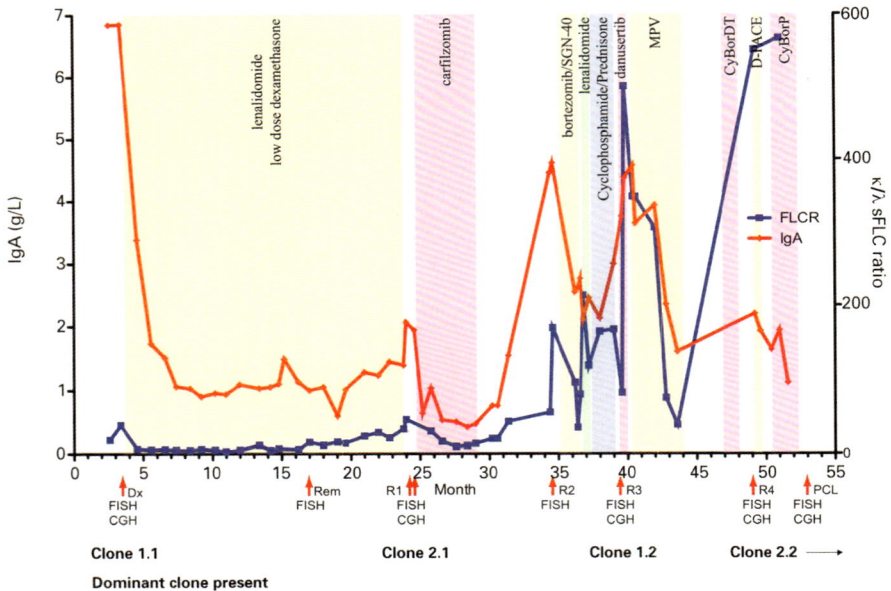

Figure 19.5. sFLC analysis and total IgA concentrations over the course of treatment and disease relapse. The dominant clone present at each disease stage is shown. Red arrows indicate relapse (R1-R4) and remission (Rem). SGN-40: dacetuzemab; MPV: melphalan, prednisone, bortezomib; CyBorDT: cyclophosphamide, bortezomib, dexamethasone; D-PACE: dexamethasone, thalidomide, cisplatin, doxorubicin, cyclophosphamide, etoposide; CyBorP: cyclophosphamide, bortezomib, prednisone. (This research was originally published in Blood[6] © the American Society of Hematology).

The patient responded to treatment with lenalidomide and low-dose dexamethasone, achieving a partial response. Relapse (R1; *Figure 19.5*) occurred after 22 months, with a change in clonal dominance (clone 2.1; 64%) and a subtle increase in both monoclonal IgA and FLC. During 2 subsequent relapses (R2 and R3; *Figure 19.5*), changes in the clonal composition of the patient's disease were characterised by an increase in monoclonal IgA, and a gross increase in the sFLC ratio. Interestingly, the dominant clone at R3 was 1.2, which shared a common progenitor with the original tumour clone. A final relapse occurred at 49 months (R4), characterised by the emergence of clone 2.2 and a dramatic increase in the κ/λ sFLC ratio. At 53 months, the patient progressed to secondary plasma cell leukemia (PCL; *Chapter 22*) with a further increase in the κ/λ sFLC ratio but no further change in the dominant clone present.

The detailed study of this patient revealed that, at each relapse, a clone emerged which was distinct from the previously dominant clone. In some instances the new clone was related to a preceding one, with which it shared a common progenitor. Clones related to sub-clone progenitor 1 were present at diagnosis and relapse R3. Clones related to sub-clone progenitor 2 represented the majority of the tumour population at R1 and R4/PCL progression. The authors termed this pattern of progression as the "alternating dominance of two major clones".

In conclusion, for this patient, it can be seen that sub-clones present at diagnosis were responsible for the relapsing pattern of disease and the relative abundance of each clone appeared to be modulated by the therapy received.

Test Questions

1. What is the incidence of FLC escape?

References

1. Morgan GJ, Walker BA, Davies FE. The genetic architecture of multiple myeloma. Nat Rev Cancer 2012;12:335-48

2. Bahlis NJ. Darwinian evolution and tiding clones in multiple myeloma. Blood 2012;120:927-8

3. Ayliffe MJ, Davies FE, de Castro D, Morgan GJ. Demonstration of changes in plasma cell subsets in multiple myeloma. Haematologica 2007;92:1135–8

4. Rajkumar SV, Kyle RA, Buadi FK. Advances in the diagnosis, classification, risk stratification, and management of monoclonal gammopathy of undetermined significance: implications for recategorizing disease entities in the presence of evolving scientific evidence. Mayo Clin Proc 2010;85:945-8

5. Ayliffe MJ, Behrens J, Stern S, Sumar N. Association of plasma cell subsets in the bone marrow and free light chain concentrations in the serum of monoclonal gammopathy patients. J Clin Pathol 2012;65:758-61

6. Keats JJ, Chesi M, Egan JB, Garbitt VM, Palmer SE, Braggio E et al. Clonal competition with alternating dominance in multiple myeloma. Blood 2012;120:1067-76

7. Hobbs JA, Drayson MT, Sharp K, Harding S, Bradwell AR, Mead GP. Frequency of altered monoclonal protein production at relapse of multiple myeloma. Br J Haematol 2009;148:659-61

8. Hobbs JR. Growth rates and responses to treatment in human myelomatosis. Br J Haematol 1969;16:607-17

9. Zamarin D, Giralt S, Landau H, Lendvai N, Lesokhin A, Chung D et al. Patterns of relapse and progression in multiple myeloma patients after auto-SCT: implications for patients' monitoring after transplantation. Bone Marrow Transplant 2013;48:419-24

10. Brioli A, Giles H, Pawlyn C, Campbell J, Kaiser M, Melchor L et al. Serum free light chain evaluation as a marker for the impact of intra-clonal heterogeneity on the progression and treatment resistance in multiple myeloma. Blood 2014;123:3414-9

11. Egan JB, Shi CX, Tembe W, Christoforides A, Kurdoglu A, Sinari S et al. Whole-genome sequencing of multiple myeloma from diagnosis to plasma cell leukemia reveals genomic initiating events, evolution, and clonal tides. Blood 2012;120:1060-6

Multiple myeloma prognosis

Summary:

- sFLC and Hevylite® ratios plus sFLC and Hevylite absolute values can provide prognostic information for multiple myeloma patients, independently of other prognostic markers.

- Prognostic value has been reported at all stages of the disease process and in association with various treatment regimens.

- sFLC and Hevylite analysis can improve prognostic power when used alongside other markers, e.g. in association with the International Staging System.

20.1. Introduction

The outcome for patients with multiple myeloma (MM) is highly variable, and understanding the prognosis for a particular patient can help when selecting the intensity of treatment to be used and the frequency of review, as well as being necessary for stratifying patients before entry into trials. This is true during and after treatment as well as at the initial diagnosis. The International Myeloma Working Group (IMWG) guidelines for risk stratification published in 2011[1] state that the International Staging System (ISS)[2] is applicable as a prognostic system in the majority of settings *(Table 20.1 and Section 25.3.4)*.

Stage	Criteria	Median Survival
I	Serum β_2M <3.5 mg/L and serum albumin ≥35 g/L	62 months
II	Serum β_2M <3.5 mg/L but serum albumin <35 g/L; or serum β_2M between 3.5 and <5.5 mg/L, irrespective of the serum albumin level	44 months
III	Serum β_2M ≥5.5 mg/L	29 months

Table 20.1. International Staging System[2]. *β_2M: β_2-microglobulin.*

The authors of the ISS[2], published in 2005, proposed the use of just serum albumin and β_2-microglobulin (β_2M) measurements, with the intention of making the system inexpensive and available to the maximum number of institutes. The authors' analysis did show, however, that many other serum markers (e.g. creatinine, calcium, platelet count, lactate dehydrogenase, type and size of monoclonal protein) and physical factors (age, extent of lytic lesions, bone marrow plasma cell [BMPC] infiltration) were also prognostic to varying degrees. However, serum free light chain (sFLC; *Chapter 5*) and immunoglobulin heavy/light chain (Hevylite, HLC; *Chapter 9*) assays were not available when the study was initiated and cytogenetic data was only available for a small subset of the study population. The prognostic value of genetic abnormalities has now been studied widely, and their assessment by techniques such as fluorescence in situ hybridization (FISH) has shown that they can have greater prognostic power than more traditional markers[3,4,5]. IMWG guidelines recognise that cytogenetics and FISH analysis play an important and independent role in risk stratification[1]. Nevertheless, such analyses are still relatively expensive and available only at specialist centres.

The monoclonal protein size and type has frequently been investigated as a potential predictor of patient outcome in MM. Before the development of the ISS, the most widely used staging system was that devised by Durie and Salmon[6] and this incorporated the size of the monoclonal protein as one of the prognostic variables. In an analysis of data from 2592 patients who had participated in UK myeloma trials[7], Drayson and colleagues corroborated results from earlier studies[2,8,9,10] by demonstrating that patients with light chain MM (LCMM) had shorter survival than those with intact immunoglobulin MM (IIMM). The authors' conclusion was that this could be attributed to delays in diagnosis and increased mortality due to renal failure *(Chapter 26)*. Increased renal failure and shortened survival times were also seen in IIMM patients who had elevated urine FLC concentrations similar to those in LCMM.

Therefore, since previous studies have found that levels of both serum monoclonal immunoglobulin and urine FLCs are related to MM patient survival, serum HLC and sFLC analysis may provide better predictions. The purpose of this chapter is to present the studies that have investigated sFLC and HLC analysis as prognostic markers at each stage of MM development.

20.2. sFLCs at diagnosis

There are now a number of published studies which have assessed the relationship between sFLCs at disease presentation and subsequent outcome. Kyrtsonis et al.[12] investigated the prognostic value of baseline sFLC ratios in 94 MM patients. The median baseline κ/λ ratio for κ MM was 3.57 and λ/κ ratio for λ MM was 45.1. Importantly, the 5-year disease specific survival for patients with involved/uninvolved (iFLC/uFLC) sFLC ratios < or ≥ median values was 82% or 30%, respectively (p<0.001; *Figure 20.1*).

In a similar study of 790 patients at the Mayo Clinic, Snozek et al.[13] found that abnormal sFLC ratios at presentation were again important, independent markers of outcome. The authors calculated κ/λ ratios for all patients and showed that those with ratios <0.03 or >32 had a median survival of 30 months compared with 48 months for those with ratios within the normal range (0.26 - 1.65; p<0.001).

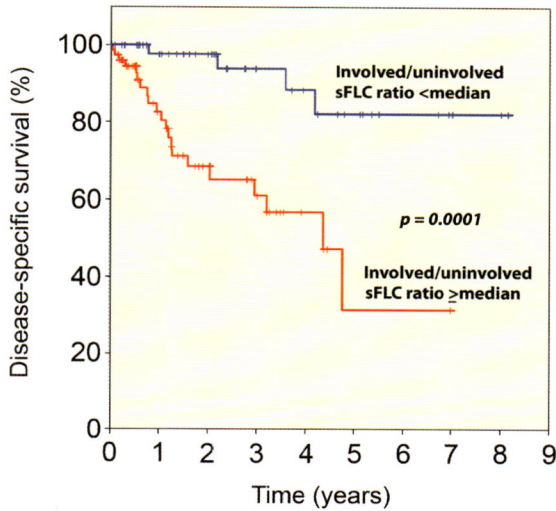

Figure 20.1.Disease-specific survival of MM patients according to baseline κ/λ sFLC ratios. *(Courtesy of M.C. Kyrtsonis).*

Dispenzieri et al.[14] divided their study population (n=399) into tertiles based upon the patients' sFLC concentration (iFLC or dFLC [difference between the iFLC and uFLC concentrations]) or sFLC ratio. In all analyses, the lowest tertile had the best event free and overall survival although outcomes for the upper two tertiles were very similar. van Rhee et al.[11] also divided their study population (n=301; all intensively treated) into tertiles but solely based upon the concentration of sFLCs. They observed good separation of the survival curves for all three tertiles, with the highest concentrations predicting the worst outcomes *(Figure 20.2)*.

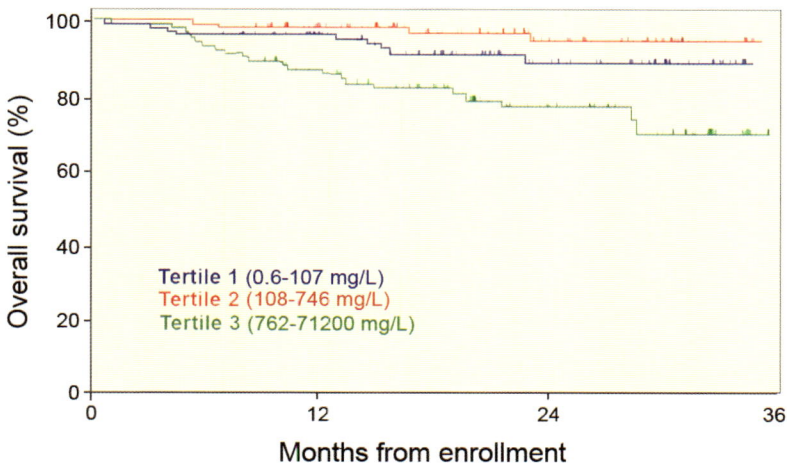

Figure 20.2. Kaplan-Meier overall survival plot according to terciles of baseline concentrations of sFLCs. *Outcome was inferior among patients with top-tercile sFLC baseline levels. (This research was originally published in Blood[11] © the American Society of Hematology).*

Preliminary analyses of more recent studies have further supported the prognostic value of sFLC measurements. More extreme ratios at diagnosis independently predicted worse overall and progression-free survival in 118 consecutive patients treated between 2002 and 2008[15]. Taccheti and colleagues[16] analysed the outcomes for 110 patients treated with first-line therapy including bortezomib. They concluded that a baseline sFLC concentration >100 mg/L was associated with more aggressive disease, characterized by a lower probability of achieving a complete response (CR) and shorter progression-free survival.

20.2.1. sFLCs combined with the ISS

In current myeloma practice, patients are categorized at presentation using the ISS, based upon serum albumin and β_2M measurements alone[1,2]. Kyrtsonis et al.[12] found that within each ISS stage, patients with an elevated involved/uninvolved sFLC ratio (>median) had reduced survival compared with those with less elevated values (<median). Furthermore, by combination of the ISS with sFLC ratios it was possible to divide the patient population into three groups with clearly divergent disease-specific survival (Table 20.2 and Figure 20.3).

Patient subgroup	No. (%) of patients	3 year DSS (%)	5 year DSS (%)
sFLC ratio <median and ISS I or II	61 (29)	95	90
Either sFLC ratio >median or ISS III	96 (46)	82	56
sFLC ratio >median and ISS III	50 (24)	37	24

Table 20.2. Disease specific survival (DSS) in 207 newly diagnosed patients with MM according to the combined sFLC κ/λ ratios and the ISS comprising serum albumin and β_2-microglobulin[12]. (Courtesy of M.C. Kyrtsonis).

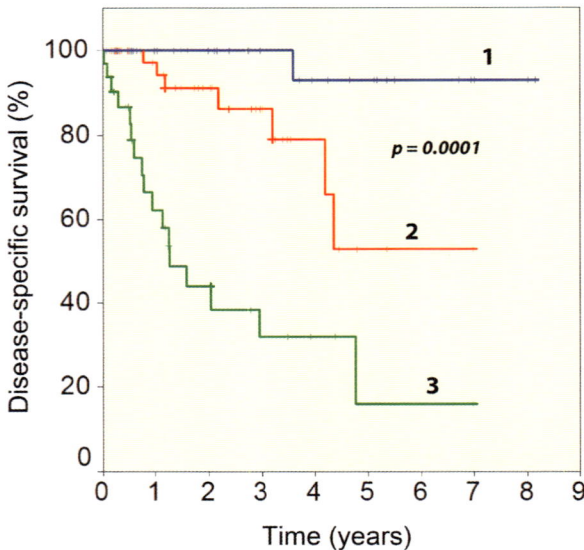

Figure 20.3. Disease-specific survival of MM patients according to abnormalities of baseline sFLC κ/λ ratios, serum albumin or β_2-microglobulin as used in the ISS. Group 1 (blue): lower than median involved/uninvolved sFLC ratio and ISS stage I or II; group 2 (red): either higher than median involved/uninvolved sFLC ratio or ISS stage III; group 3 (green): higher than median involved/uninvolved sFLC ratio and ISS stage III. (Courtesy of M.C. Kyrtsonis).

Snozek et al.[13] used extreme κ/λ sFLC ratios (<0.03 or >32) as an additional risk factor to those of the ISS (serum β_2M >3.5 g/L, serum albumin <35 g/L) to separate patients (n=790) into four groups with 0, 1, 2, or 3 risk factors. These groups had median overall survival of 51, 39, 30 and 22 months, respectively (p<0.001). Because these data provided additional outcome information, it was suggested that sFLC ratios should be incorporated into the ISS to provide a new risk stratification model. In a study including 122 Chinese MM patients, Xu et al.[17] used similar κ/λ sFLC ratio boundaries (<0.04 or >25) to add a third risk factor to the ISS. This produced four patient groups with clearly separate survival curves *(Figure 20.4)* and the authors again concluded that the prognostic potential of the ISS could be improved by incorporating sFLC ratios.

Further evidence of the independence of sFLC ratios as a risk factor was provided by Esteves and colleagues[18], who used abnormal κ/λ ratios (<0.03 or >32) to separate patients within the ISS stage II into groups with different overall survival. In this study, however, the ratio did not provide further discrimination for patients in ISS stages I or III.

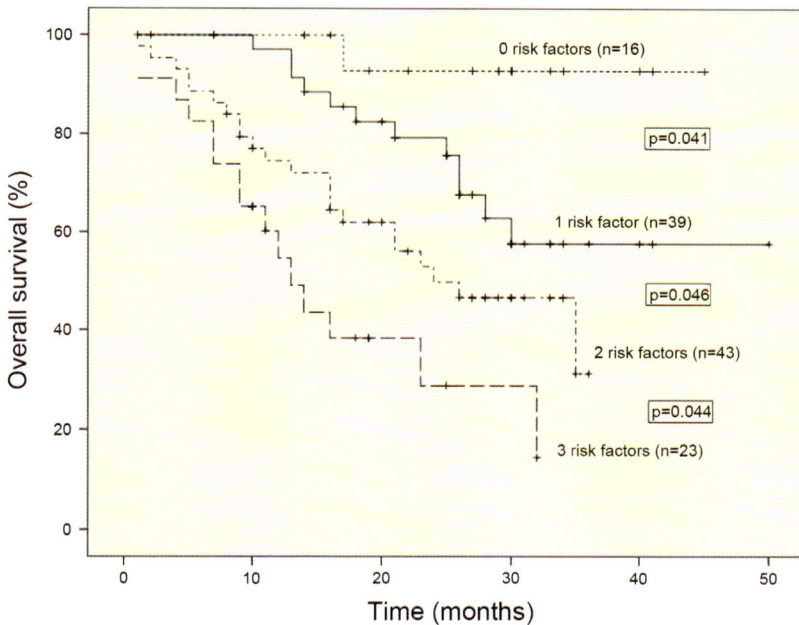

Figure 20.4. Risk stratification model using the ISS combined with κ/λ sFLC ratios[17]. *Three risk factors were: abnormal sFLC ratio (<0.04 or >25), high serum β_2-microglobulin (>3.5 mg/L) and low serum albumin (<35 g/L).*

20.2.2. Association between sFLCs and other prognostic markers

Most of the studies discussed in this chapter have sought to establish whether FLC analysis is prognostic independently of other markers. However, it would also be of value if a simple serum test could replace a more expensive and/or invasive investigation such as multi-parameter flow cytometry or cytogenetic analysis.

Kumar et al.[19] studied the relationship between sFLC results and the presence of IgH translocations in 314 MM patients at diagnosis. The median κ/λ sFLC ratio and dFLC were higher in patients with IgH translocations, particularly t(14;16), but multivariate analysis indicated that sFLC abnormalities were independent risk factors and better prognosis was obtained using a combination of both the genetic and sFLC risk factors.

20.3. sFLCs during response assessment

Various studies have highlighted the prognostic significance of both the depth and rate of sFLC response following treatment of MM. In addition, patients relapsing with FLC production appear to have an adverse prognosis. These aspects are now considered separately.

20.3.1. Normalisation of the sFLC ratio and importance of a sCR

International Uniform Response Criteria published in 2006[21] introduced the designation of "stringent complete response" (sCR) requiring a normal sFLC ratio in addition to other criteria (*Section 18.2.2 and Chapter 25*).

Kapoor et al.[20] analysed outcomes for 445 patients who underwent an autologous stem cell transplant (ASCT) within 12 months of MM diagnosis. Five-year overall survival for patients with a sCR (n=109), conventional CR (n=37) and "near CR" (nCR; n=91) were 80%, 53% and 47% respectively. Progression-free and overall survival curves are shown in Figures 20.5A and B. It was also observed that overall survival was superior in patients who maintained their sCR status for at least 6 months compared to those who had a sCR which was maintained for less than 6 months (*Figure 20.5C*). The authors concluded that myeloma trials reporting response rates should identify those achieving sCR and conventional CR separately owing to their markedly disparate outcomes.

A further indication of the independent prognostic value of achieving a normal κ/λ sFLC ratio was provided by Iwama et al.[22], who reported that ratio normalisation identified patients with improved overall and progression-free survival whether they had achieved a conventional CR, a very good partial response (VGPR) or a partial response (PR) (n=126; p<0.001). Several other publications have also reported a survival advantage after achieving normal κ/λ sFLC ratios[16,23,24].

In a study of LCMM patients only[25] (n=122), those who normalised both their κ/λ sFLC ratio and iFLC values had significantly longer progression-free survival (PFS) and overall survival (OS) compared to patients that normalised their ratio only. Both these groups had better survival than those failing to normalise either parameters (median PFS 43.3, 33.0 vs. 18.8 months, respectively [p<0.001]; median OS 85.3, 69.9 vs. 45.5 months, respectively [p=0.012]).

An alternative prognostic use of sFLC analysis was made by Singh and colleagues[26] who monitored the uFLC concentration in patients after reduced–intensity allogeneic transplant. Both uFLC and iFLC concentrations were suppressed immediately after transplant, and the patients (n=47) were divided into 3 groups according to whether their uFLC concentrations failed to recover, recovered early or recovered late. Progression-free survival was significantly longer in the late uFLC recovery group (median PFS not reached at 5 years vs. 11.8 months for early recovery and 4.6 months for no recovery; p=0.0001). The authors concluded that late uFLC recovery might indicate better graft versus MM effect and that monitoring uFLC may help in managing immune suppression strategies.

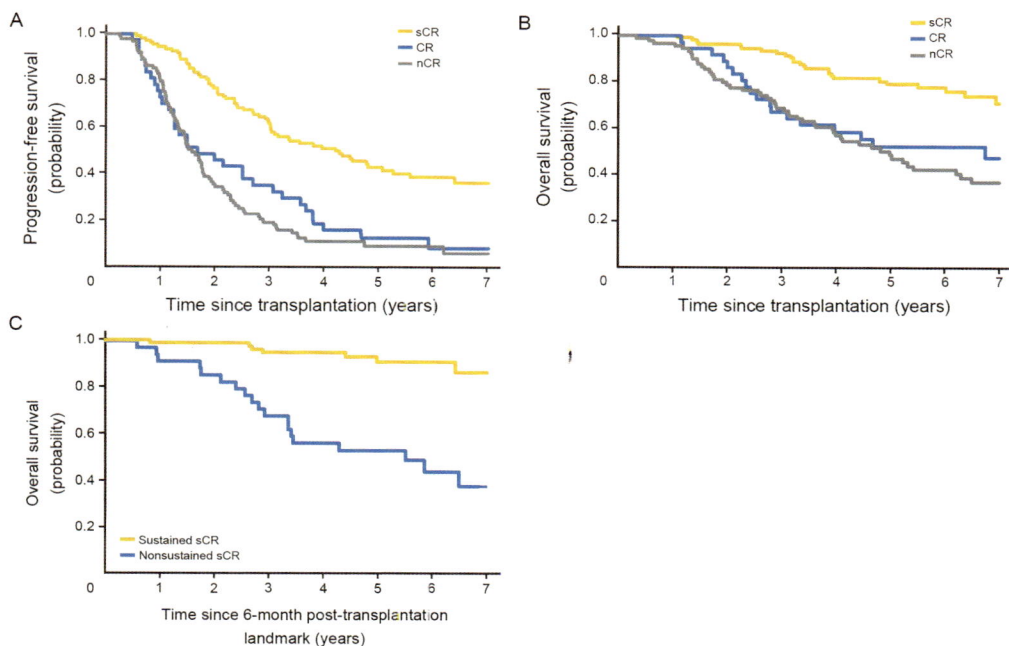

Figure 20.5. Progression-free and overall survival of patients achieving varying degrees of CR. (A) *Median time to progression of patients achieving sCR (n=109) is 50 months compared with 20 months and 19 months for groups attaining a CR (n=37) and near CR (nCR; n=91), respectively (p<0.001).* **(B)** *Those with sCR had a marked improvement in overall survival (median not-reached) compared with patients achieving CR (median 81 months) or nCR (median 60 months).* **(C)** *Median overall survival of patients with sustained sCR at 6 months from ASCT (n=75) was significantly longer than for those with a non-sustained sCR (n=34) (not reached vs. 5.5 years, respectively; p<0.001). (Originally published by the American Society of Clinical Oncology [20]).*

20.3.2. Early sFLC response predicts outcome

The short serum half-life of FLCs means that concentrations can fall rapidly if therapeutic treatment has been successful *(Section 18.3.1)*. A number of studies have investigated the prognostic implications of an early sFLC response.

Hassoun et al.[27] monitored response in 42 MM patients and found that normalisation of the sFLC ratio after just one or two cycles of therapy was highly predictive for achieving CR or nCR (p=0.003). Dytfeld et al.[28] reported that a scoring system including ≥90% reduction in monoclonal immunoglobulin, ≥90% reduction in iFLC, or κ/λ sFLC ratio normalisation had >90% sensitivity and specificity for predicting patients going on to achieve a VGPR (n=40). Similarly, Hansen et al.[29] found an 80% reduction in iFLC at day 21 (after 1 cycle of treatment) gave a sensitivity of 87.5% and specificity of 100% for predicting VGPR (n=36) but noted that changes in the monoclonal immunoglobulin over the same period were not significantly different for those achieving VGPR or PR. Supportive data has also been published in various studies encompassing a number of different treatment modalities, with measurements taken during induction therapy[30,31,32], post ASCT[33,34] and in relapsed/refractory patients[33,34,35,36].

20.3.3. Prognostic implications of relapse with FLC escape

"Light chain escape" or "FLC escape" is the term used to describe the phenomenon when a patient, who presented with MM producing monoclonal intact immunoglobulin, relapses with just monoclonal FLC production. This is examined in more detail in Section 18.2.1 but here, the prognostic implications of FLC escape are considered.

A study of 104 patients who relapsed after bortezomib-based salvage therapy[37] found that 15 (14%) relapsed with an altered disease phenotype, of whom 9 (9%) had plasmacytoma/plasma cell leukaemia and 6 (6%) showed FLC escape. The transformed group had significantly worse median overall survival (10.7 vs. 32.7 months; p<0.001) *(Figure 20.6)*. A separate investigation of relapse in 232 patients[39] reported changes of immunoglobulin production in 39 (17%) patients, of whom 15 (6%) had FLC escape and 7 (3%) had monoclonal immunoglobulin escape. Both of these groups had similarly short survival after the change in production (approximately 3 months).

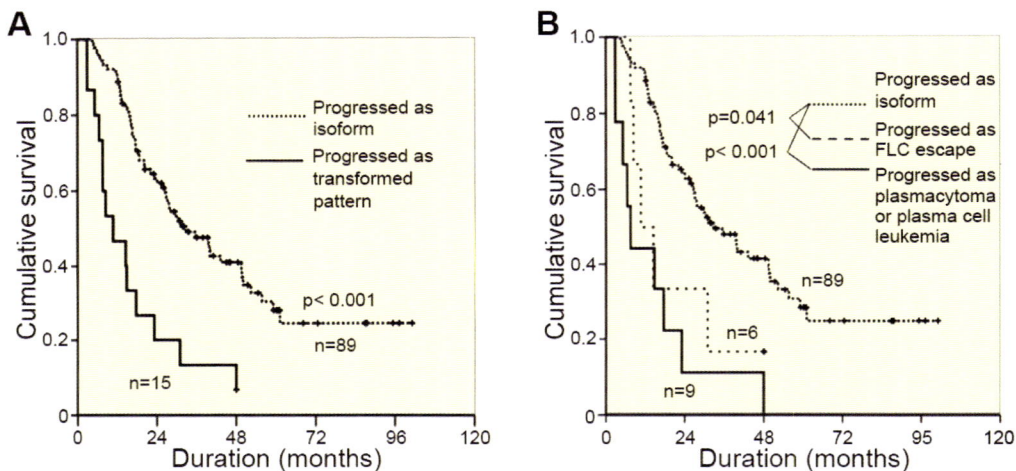

Figure 20.6. Overall survival according to patterns of relapse or progression. (A) Patients with a transformed pattern at relapse or progression had a significantly inferior overall survival to those who progressed with their original isoform (p<0.001). (B) In a subanalysis, patients with FLC escape and other transformed progression exhibited significantly inferior overall survival (p<0.05). (Reproduced from[37] Copyright 2014, with permission from Elsevier).

Brioli and colleagues[38] have, to date, published the largest analysis of clonal change at relapse and reported that 10.4% (54/520) patients relapsed with FLC escape, 35.2% (183/520) relapsed with rising intact immunoglobulin plus FLC, while 49.6% (258/520) relapsed with significant rises in their intact immunoglobulin alone. Interestingly, they found that patients who relapsed with FLC alone or FLC plus immunoglobulin had similarly reduced survival after relapse compared to those without rising FLC (p=0.002; *Figure 20.7*). Tacchetti et al.[16] reported FLC escape in a similar proportion of patients (11/110; 10%) but did not observe reduced time to treatment or overall survival unless the sFLC concentration was >100 mg/L.

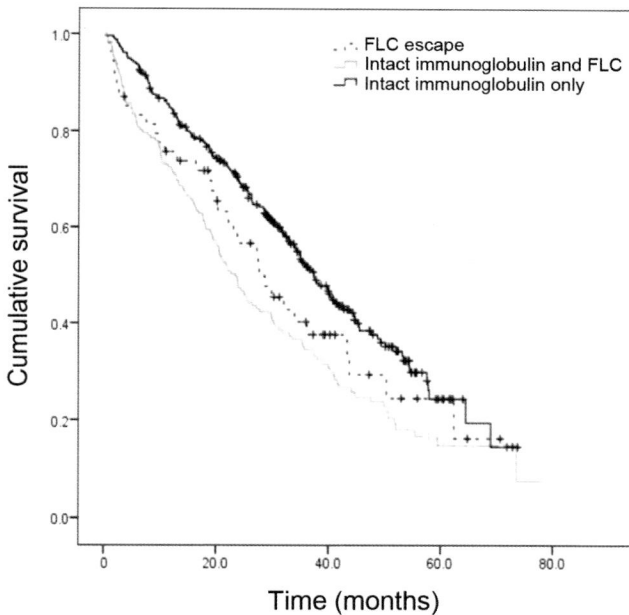

Figure 20.7. Kaplan-Meier curves of survival from first relapse according to patterns of relapse. Median overall survival from relapse was 37.4 months, 23.5 months and 27.7 months for patients relapsing with intact immunoglobulin only, both intact immunoglobulin and FLCs, and FLC only (FLC escape), respectively (p=0.002). (This research was originally published in Blood[38] © the American Society of Hematology).

20.4. HLC analysis at diagnosis

Recent studies have assessed the relationship between HLC ratios and outcome in MM, both at presentation and at maximum response. Ludwig et al.[40] investigated the prognostic value of baseline HLC ratios in 156 patients with IgG or IgA MM. The median survival of the entire cohort was 53.5 months. Extreme HLC ratios (<0.022 or >45) at presentation were significantly associated with shorter overall survival (OS) times; hazard ratio [HR] 2.07, 95% confidence interval [CI] 1.15-3.75; p=0.016) (Figure 20.8).

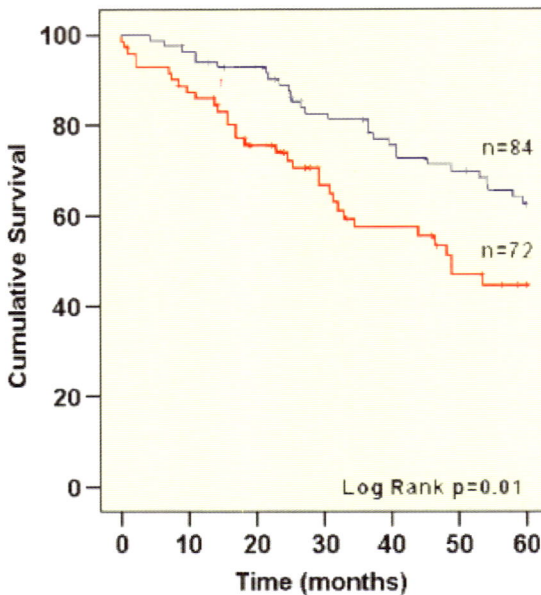

Figure 20.8. Overall survival of MM patients stratified by HLC ratio at baseline. *Median survival was 40.5 months in patients with a highly abnormal HLC ratio at baseline (<0.022 or >45; red line) and was not reached in patients with a less abnormal ratio (blue line; p=0.016). (Reprinted by permission from Macmillan Publishers Ltd: Leukemia[40], copyright 2013).*

Bradwell et al.[41] studied the prognostic value of baseline HLC ratios in 339 MM patients comprising 245 with IgG (166 IgGκ, 79 IgGλ) and 94 with IgA (60 IgAκ, 34 IgAλ). During the study period, 125 patients (37%) had disease progression and 46 patients (14%) died. When patients were grouped according to baseline monoclonal protein concentrations determined by SPE (grouped according to either above/below median values or by tertiles of concentration), no significant differences in progression-free survival (PFS) or OS were observed. By contrast, there was a significant correlation between HLC ratios and outcome. When patients were categorised with HLC ratios above/below median (using Ig'κ/Ig'λ ratios for Ig'κ patients and Ig'λ/Ig'κ ratios for Ig'λ patients), a significant difference in PFS was observed (p=0.022; Figure 20.9A). This significance increased when patients were grouped according to extreme HLC ratios (<0.01 or >200 compared to 0.01 - 200). Approximately one-third of the patients had extreme HLC ratios, which were associated with significantly shorter PFS (HR 1.9, p=0.0002; Figure 20.9B). Whilst there was a tendency for patients with extreme ratios at baseline to have shorter overall survival, this did not reach significance.

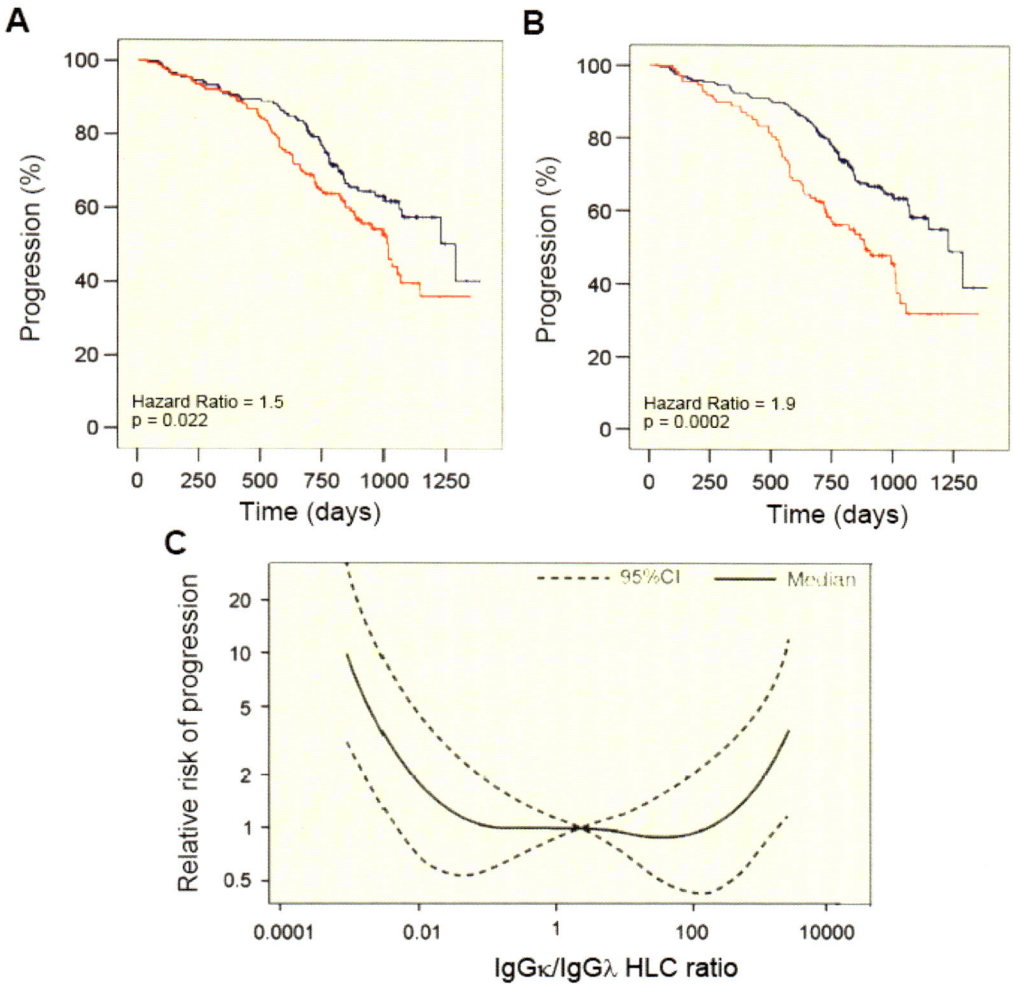

Figure 20.9. Progression-free survival of MM patients stratified by HLC ratio at baseline. (A) *HLC ratios above (red, n=163) or below (blue, n=162) median values.* **(B)** *Extreme HLC ratios (<0.01 or >200, red, n=116) or less extreme values (>0.01 to <200, blue, n=209).* **(C)** *Relationship between baseline IgG HLC ratios and progression in IgG MM patients. (Reprinted by permission from Macmillan Publishers Ltd: Leukemia[41], copyright 2013).*

Bradwell et al.[41] also analysed IgG and IgA HLC ratios individually to predict the relative risk of progression. Increasingly abnormal IgG HLC ratios were associated with an increased risk of progression (p<0.001; *Figure 20.9C*), but this did not apply to IgA HLC ratios (p=0.32). It is likely that the IgA HLC ratios would have been associated with poorer survival if more patients had been included.

The contribution of baseline values of involved HLC (iHLC) and uninvolved HLC (uHLC) to the risk of progression was also studied[41]. When IgG and IgA patients were grouped together and categorised by tertiles of iHLC or uHLC concentrations, patients who had iHLC concentrations in the top tertile had significantly shorter PFS (HR 1.4, p=0.039; *Figure 20.10A*). However, suppressed concentrations of uHLC concentrations were even more significantly associated with shorter PFS (HR 1.8, p=0.002; *Figure 20.10B*). No significant association was observed between PFS and concentrations of the non-tumour immunoglobulin isotypes (i.e. classical immunoparesis).

The current ISS for MM relies upon serum $\beta_2 M$ and albumin measurements *(Section 20.1)*[2]. The correlation between these measurements and PFS is shown in Figure 20.10C (p=0.017)[41]. In univariate analysis, extreme HLC ratios had a greater prognostic significance (p=0.017) than albumin (p=0.153) on PFS. Concordant with this, in multivariate analysis, elevated $\beta_2 M$ (>3.5 mg/L) and extreme HLC ratios (<0.01 or >200) were the only independent variables to identify patients with reduced PFS, whereas other variables (albumin <35 g/L; κ/λ sFLC ratios, and cytogenetic abnormalities [Del:13, t4:14, Del:17p]) did not reach significance. A risk-stratification model was developed in which patients were grouped into three categories: low risk ($\beta_2 M$ <3.5 mg/L and HLC ratio 0.01 - 200), intermediate risk (either $\beta_2 M$ >3.5 mg/L or HLC ratio <0.01 or >200), or high risk (both $\beta_2 M$ >3.5 mg/L and HLC ratio <0.01 or >200) *(Figure 20.10D)*. In this model, the high risk group was more significantly associated with shorter PFS than ISS stage III disease (p=0.000002).

20.5. HLC analysis during response assessment

Research has indicated that HLC analysis can provide prognostic information when performed early in a treatment regimen or at the time of maximum response. From a study of 44 MM patients treated with carfilzomib, lenalidomide and dexamethasone, Bhutani et al.[43] reported that normalisation of the HLC ratio after 2 cycles of therapy was significantly associated with achieving a sCR (p=0.001). In a multivariate model that initially included monoclonal immunoglobulin, dFLC, normalised sFLC ratio, difference between involved and uninvolved HLC concentration (dHLC) and normalised HLC ratio; only dHLC (<2.6 g/L vs. ≥2.6 g/L) remained as an independent factor after 2 treatment cycles. A preliminary analysis of 70 patients treated with bortezomib[44] suggested that the HLC ratio was a more sensitive monitoring tool than the monoclonal immunoglobulin and suppression of the uninvolved HLC isotype (HLC-pair suppression) was associated with poor PFS and OS.

A greater number of studies have investigated the prognostic value of HLC analysis at the time of maximal response. Ludwig et al.[40] analysed outcomes in 156 patients with IgG or IgA MM. Patients with HLC ratios that remained abnormal at maximal response (PR or better) had a significantly shorter survival than those achieving a normal HLC ratio (HR 2.8, CI 0.99 - 8.3; p<0.03) *(Figure 20.11A)*. In a separate study of 65 patients at maximal response, Ludwig and colleagues[42] compared immunofixation electrophoresis (IFE), BMPC infiltration, sFLC ratio, HLC concentrations and HLC ratio, and concluded that HLC-pair suppression was the most powerful predictor for OS *(Figure 20.11B)*. Drayson et al.[45] studied the prognostic value of IgA HLC analysis at maximal response in 195 IgA MM patients treated in the UK, MRC IX myeloma trial. At maximal response, an abnormal HLC ratio was associated with shorter PFS in both the intensive (p=0.002) and non-intensive (p=0.032) treatment arms. HLC-pair suppression was also associated with shorter PFS in all patients achieving a CR (p=0.061). By contrast, classical immunoparesis of either IgG or IgM was not associated with PFS (p=0.525 and p=0.964, respectively). Koulieris et al.[46] found that HLC ratio normalisation was predictive of improved PFS (p=0.046) irrespective of the treatment used.

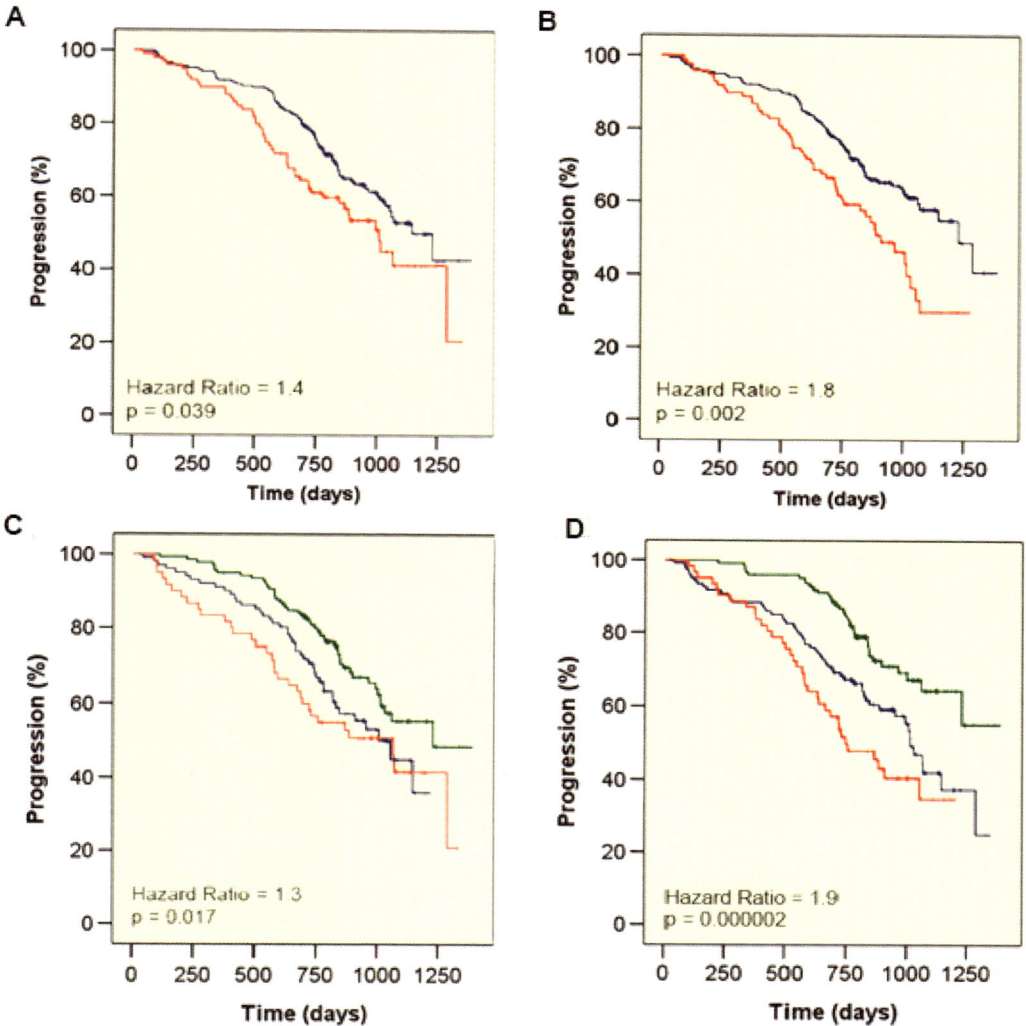

Figure 20.10. *Progression-free survival of MM patients stratified by (A) involved HLC concentrations at baseline, (B) uninvolved HLC concentrations at baseline, (C) the ISS, and (D) β₂-microglobulin (β₂M) and HLC ratios.* Patients in (A) and (B) grouped as upper 1/3rd (red, n=116) or lower 2/3rds (blue, n=209). (C) ISS Stage I (green, n=140), Stage II (blue, n=102), Stage III (red, n=60). (D) Low risk: β₂M <3.5 mg/L and HLC ratio 0.01 - 200 (green, n=124), intermediate risk: either β₂M >3.5 mg/L or HLC ratio <0.01 or >200 (blue, n=122), high risk: β₂M >3.5 mg/L and HLC ratio <0.01 or >100 (red, n=62). (Reprinted by permission from Macmillan Publishers Ltd: Leukemia[41], copyright 2013).

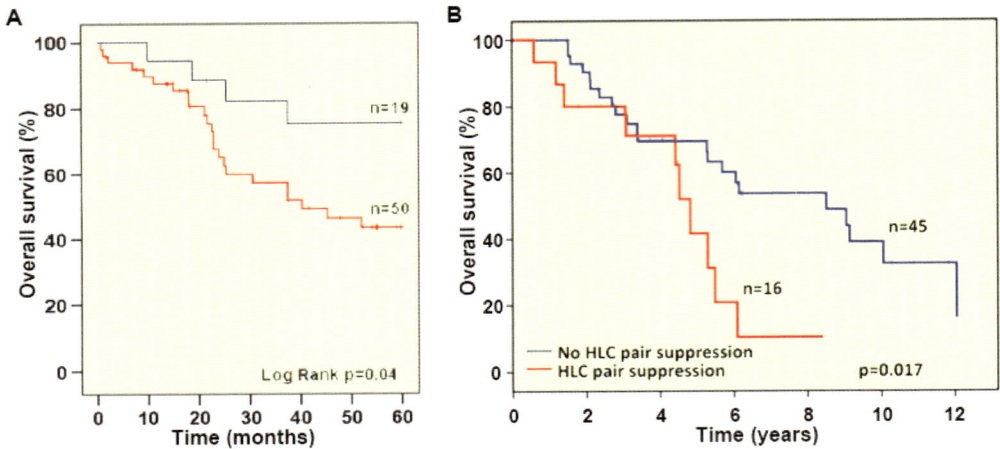

Figure 20.11. The prognostic value of HLC analysis at maximum response. (A) Overall survival of MM patients achieving a partial response or better, stratified at best response according to HLC ratios. Blue line: patients with normal HLC ratio; red line: patients with abnormal HLC ratio. (Reprinted by permission from Macmillan Publishers Ltd: Leukemia[40], copyright 2013). (B) Overall survival was significantly shorter in patients with HLC pair suppression than patients with no HLC-pair suppression (median 4.8 years vs. 8.5 years, respectively; p<0.02). (This research was originally published in Blood[42] © the American Society of Hematology).

20.6. Prognostic value of combining sFLC and HLC measurements

In their retrospective analysis of 195 IgA patients, Drayson et al.[45] also demonstrated that patients achieving a CR but still having both HLC and FLC ratios abnormal (n=7) had a worse outcome than those having just one of those ratios abnormal (n=62) (median PFS 18 months vs. not reached after 25 months; p=0.006) *(Figure 20.12)*. The authors suggested that a response category based upon normalisation of FLC and HLC ratios may be more valuable than the current sCR category of response criteria[21].

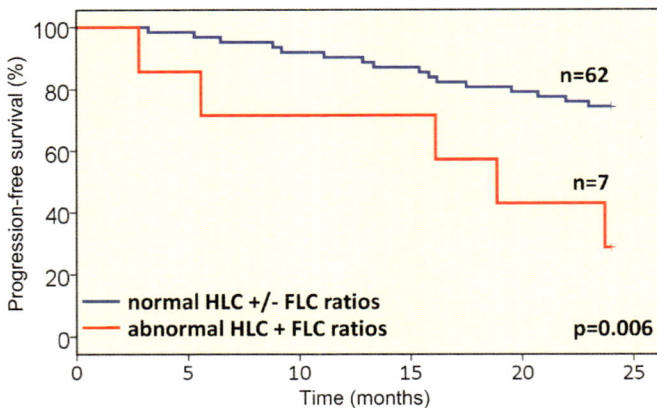

Figure 20.12. Prognostic role of HLC and sFLC ratios in patients achieving at least a complete response. Patients with abnormal HLC and sFLC ratios had significantly shorter 2-year progression-free survival (PFS) than patients with either HLC or sFLC ratios normal. (Courtesy of M.T. Drayson).

Test Questions

1. What prognostic markers are used in the ISS?
2. What is the benefit of achieving a sCR?
3. At what MM stage can HLC analysis provide prognostic information?

References

1. Munshi NC, Anderson KC, Bergsagel PL, Shaughnessy J, Palumbo A, Durie B et al. Consensus recommendations for risk stratification in multiple myeloma: report of the International Myeloma Workshop Consensus Panel 2. Blood 2011;117:4696-700

2. Greipp PR, San Miguel J, Durie BG, Crowley JJ, Barlogie B, Blade J et al. International staging system for multiple myeloma. J Clin Oncol 2005;23:3412-20

3. Avet-Loiseau H. Role of genetics in prognostication in myeloma. Best Pract Res Clin Haematol 2007;20:625-35

4. Avet-Loiseau H, Li C, Magrangeas F, Gouraud W, Charbonnel C, Harousseau JL et al. Prognostic significance of copy-number alterations in multiple myeloma. J Clin Oncol 2009;27:4585-90

5. Fonseca R, Bergsagel PL, Drach J, Shaughnessy J, Gutierrez N, Stewart AK et al. International Myeloma Working Group molecular classification of multiple myeloma: spotlight review. Leukemia 2009;23:2210-21

6. Durie BG, Salmon SE. A clinical staging system for multiple myeloma. Correlation of measured myeloma cell mass with presenting clinical features, response to treatment, and survival. Cancer 1975;36:842-54

7. Drayson M, Begum G, Basu S, Makkuni S, Dunn J, Barth N, Child JA. Effects of paraprotein heavy and light chain types and free light chain load on survival in myeloma: an analysis of patients receiving conventional-dose chemotherapy in Medical Research Council UK multiple myeloma trials. Blood 2006;108:2013-9

8. Shustik C, Bergsagel DE, Pruzanski W. Kappa and lambda light chain disease: survival rates and clinical manifestations. Blood 1976;48:41-51

9. Irish AB, Winearls CG, Littlewood T. Presentation and survival of patients with severe renal failure and myeloma. QJM 1997;90:773-80

10. Goranova V, Spassov E. Prognostic significance of the immunological variant in patients with multiple myeloma. Folia Med (Plovdiv) 1999;41:164-7

11. van Rhee F, Bolejack V, Hollmig K, Pineda-Roman M, Anaissie E, Epstein J et al. High serum-free light chain levels and their rapid reduction in response to therapy define an aggressive multiple myeloma subtype with poor prognosis. Blood 2007;110:827-32

12. Kyrtsonis MC, Vassilakopoulos TP, Kafasi N, Sachanas S, Tzenou T, Papadogiannis A et al. Prognostic value of serum free light chain ratio at diagnosis in multiple myeloma. Br J Haematol 2007;137:240-3

13. Snozek CL, Katzmann JA, Kyle RA, Dispenzieri A, Larson DR, Therneau TM et al. Prognostic value of the serum free light chain ratio in newly diagnosed myeloma: proposed incorporation into the international staging system. Leukemia 2008;22:1933-7

14. Dispenzieri A, Zhang L, Katzmann JA, Snyder M, Blood E, DeGoey R et al. Appraisal of immunoglobulin free light chain as a marker of response. Blood 2008;111:4908-15

15. Sobh M, Morisset S, Ducastelle S, Barraco F, Chelghoum Y, Thomas X et al. Serum free light chain ratio (sFLCr): an independent prognostic factor for overall survival and progression free survival in multiple myeloma. Haematologica 2011;96:P-027a

16. Tacchetti P, Rocchi S, Pezzi A, Zamagni E, Pantani L, Zannetti B et al. Prognostic imapct of serum free light chain (sFLC) assay in newly diagnosed multiple myeloma (MM) treated with bortezomib. Blood 2013;122:1859a

17. Xu Y, Sui W, Deng S, An G, Wang Y, Xie Z et al. Further stratification of multiple myeloma patients by the International Staging System in combination with the ratio of serum free kappa to lambda light chains (rFLC). Leuk Lymphoma 2012;54:123-32

18. Esteves C, Neves M, Martins H, Costa M, Valle S, Raposo J et al. Serum free light chain ratio (FLCr) is a powerful prognostic factor for survival in newly diagnosed multiple myeloma (MM) in the era of new agents namely on ISS Stage II patients. Blood 2013;122:1873a

19. Kumar S, Zhang L, Dispenzieri A, Van WS, Katzmann JA, Snyder M et al. Relationship between elevated immunoglobulin free light chain and the presence of IgH translocations in multiple myeloma. Leukemia 2010;24:1498-505

20. Kapoor P, Kumar SK, Dispenzieri A, Lacy MQ, Buadi F, Dingli D et al. Importance of achieving stringent complete response after autologous stem-cell transplantation in multiple myeloma. J Clin Oncol 2013;31:4529-35

21. Durie BG, Harousseau JL, Miguel JS, Blade J, Barlogie B, Anderson K et al. International uniform response criteria for multiple myeloma. Leukemia 2006;20:1467-73

22. Iwama KI, Chihara D, Tsuda K, Ugai T, Sugihara H, Nishida Y et al. Normalization of free light chain kappa/lambda ratio is a robust prognostic indicator of favorable outcome in patients with multiple myeloma. Eur J Haematol 2012;90:134-41

23. Reid SD, Drayson MT, Mead GP, Augustson B, Bradwell AR. Serum free light chains are a more sensitive marker of serological remission in multiple myeloma patients. Clin Chem 2004;50:C34a

24. Matsue K, Sugihara H, Nishida Y, Yamakura M, Takeuchi M. Heterogeneity of IMWG defined response assessed by FLC assay, multicolor flow cytometry, and heavy/light chain analysis. Clinical Lymphoma, Myeloma & Leukaemia 2013;13:P-203a

25. Boyle E, Brioli A, Leleu X, Morgan G, Pawlyn C, Davies F et al. The value of serum free light chain monitoring compared to urinary Bence-Jones measurement in light chain only myeloma. Blood 2013;122:1895a

26. Singh V, Cornell FF, Paruchuri S, Sala M, Saad A, Bredeson C et al. Patterns of serum free light chain (FLC) recovery after reduced intensity conditioning (RIC) allogeneic transplant for multiple myeloma (MM) predict long term outcomes. Blood 2010;116:1301a

27. Hassoun H, Reich L, Klimek VM, Dhodapkar M, Cohen A, Kewalramani T et al. The serum free light chain ratio after one or two cycles of treatment is highly predictive of the magnitude of final response in patients undergoing initial treatment for multiple myeloma. Blood 2005;106:972a

28. Dytfeld D, Griffith KA, Friedman J, Lebovic D, Harvey C, Kaminski MS, Jakubowiak AJ. Superior overall survival of patients with myeloma achieving very good partial response or better to initial treatment with bortezomib, pegylated liposomal doxorubicin, and dexamethasone, predicted after two cycles by a free light chain- and M-protein-based model: extended follow-up of a phase II trial. Leuk Lymphoma 2011;52:1271-80

29. Hansen CT, Pedersen PT, Nielsen LC, Abildgaard N. Evaluation of the serum free light chain (sFLC) analysis in prediction of response in symptomatic multiple myeloma patients; rapid profound reduction in involved FLC predicts achievement of VGPR. Eur J Haematol 2014;93:407-13

30. Cavallo F, Rasmussen E, Zangari M, Tricot G, Fender B, Fox M et al. Serum free-lite chain (sFLC) assay in multiple myeloma (MM): Clinical correlates and prognostic implications in newly diagnosed MM patients treated with Total Therapy 2 or 3 (TT2/3). Blood 2005;106:3490a

31. Nakorn TN, Watanaboonyongcharoen P, Suwannabutra S, Theerasaksilp S, Paritpokee N. Early reduction of serum free light chain can predict therapeutic responses in multiple myeloma. Blood 2007;110:4742a

32. Watanaboonyongcharoen P, Suwannabutra S, Theerasaksilp S, Paripokee N, Na Nakorn T. The roles of serum free light chain assay on the prognosis of multiple myeloma. Clin Lymphoma Myeloma 2009;9:A420a

33. Barley K, Tindle S, Bagiella E, Jagannath S, Chari A. Lack of a response by serum free light chains performed early post stem cell transplantation in patients with multiple myeloma predicts inferior progression free and overall survival. Blood 2012;120:3127a

34. Dispenzieri A, Rajkumar SV, Plevak MF, Katzmann JA, Kyle RA, Larson D et al. Early immunoglobulin free light chain (FLC) response post autologous peripheral blood stem cell transplant predicts for hematologic complete response in patients with multiple myeloma. Blood 2006;108:3097a

35. Orlowski R, Sutherland H, Blade J, Miguel JS, Hajek R, Nagler A et al. Early normalization of serum free light chains is associated with prolonged time to progression following bortezomib {+/-} pegylated liposomal doxorubicin treatment of relapsed/ refractory multiple myeloma. Blood 2007;110:2735a

36. Popat R, Oakervee H, Williams C, Cook M, Craddock C, Basu S et al. Bortezomib, low dose intravenous melphalan and dexamethasone for patients with relapsed multiple myeloma. Haematologica 2008;93:918a

37. Ahn JS, Jung SH, Yang DH, Bae SY, Kim YK, Kim HJ, Lee JJ. Patterns of relapse or progression after bortezomib-based salvage therapy in patients with relapsed/refractory multiple myeloma. Clin Lymphoma Myeloma Leuk 2014;14:389-94

38. Brioli A, Giles H, Pawlyn C, Campbell J, Kaiser M, Melchor L et al. Serum free light chain evaluation as a marker for the impact of intra-clonal heterogeneity on the progression and treatment resistance in multiple myeloma. Blood 2014;123:3414-9

39. Nikolaou E, Panayiotidis P, Sarris K, Maltezas D, Koulieris E, Iliakis T et al. Evaluation of immunoglobulin variations (clonal changes) in symptomatic multiple myeloma (MM) patient's course. Blood 2013;122:3137a

40. Ludwig H, Milosavljevic D, Zojer N, Faint JM, Bradwell AR, Hubl W, Harding SJ. Immunoglobulin heavy/light chain ratios improve paraprotein detection and monitoring, identify residual disease and correlate with survival in multiple myeloma patients. Leukemia 2013;27:213-9

41. Bradwell A, Harding S, Fourrier N, Mathiot C, Attal M, Moreau P et al. Prognostic utility of intact immunoglobulin Ig'kappa/Ig'lambda ratios in multiple myeloma patients. Leukemia 2013;27:202-7

42. Ludwig H, Slavka G, Hubl W, Carr-Smith H, Milosavljevic D, Hughes R et al. Usage of HLC-ratio, FLC-ratio, IFE, PBMC infiltration and isotype suppression at best response reveals isotype suppression as most powerful parameter for identification of multiple myeloma patients with long survival. Blood 2012;120:1817a

43. Bhutani M, Costello R, Korde N, Manasanch E, Kwok M, Tageja N et al. Serum heavy-light chains (HLC) and free light chains (FLC) as predictors for early CR in newly diagnosed myeloma patients treated with carfilzomib, lenalidomide, and dexamethasone (CRd). Blood 2013;122:762a

44. Murillo-Florez I, Andrade-Campos M, Montes-Limon A, Quintero-Gutierrez J, Grasa J, Giraldo P, Rubio D. Predictive value of light and heavy chain analysis in multiple myeloma patients treated with bortezomib. Haematologica 2013;98:B1519a

45. Drayson MT, Berlanga O, Plant T, Newnham NJ, Young P, Harding S. Immunoglobulin heavy/light chain measurements during monitoring provide prognostic information of relapse after therapy in myeloma patients. Blood 2012;120:3964a

46. Koulieris E, Maltezas D, Eytychia N, Bartzis V, Tzenou T, Karali V et al. Impact of novel M-component based biomarkers on to progression free survival after treatment in intact immunoglobulin multiple myeloma. Blood 2012;120:2927a

Plasmacytoma

Summary:

- An abnormal κ/λ sFLC ratio at baseline is associated with increased risk of progression to multiple myeloma and reduced overall survival in patients with solitary plasmacytoma of bone.

- Risk stratification models incorporating sFLC analysis identify solitary plasmacytoma patients at greater risk of progression to multiple myeloma.

21.1. Introduction

Plasmacytomas are isolated clonal proliferations of plasma cells. They are localised to a specific site and do not elicit the typical clinical symptoms associated with multiple myeloma (MM). The estimated incidence rate of all plasmacytomas is 0.34 per 100,000 person years, meaning it is approximately 16-fold less common than MM[1].

In 2003, the International Myeloma Working Group (IMWG) published criteria for the classification of solitary plasmacytoma of bone (SPB), extramedullary plasmacytoma and multiple solitary plasmacytoma as distinct disease entities[2]. These were subsequently adopted by the British Committee for Standards in Haematology[3]. The incidence of SPB has been estimated to be 40% higher than that of extramedullary plasmacytoma[1] and there are distinct differences in the probable outcomes for patients with these diseases.

21.2. Solitary plasmacytoma of bone

SPB represents 3 - 5% of plasma cell neoplasms and is approximately twice as common in men as in women[1]. The majority (83%) of tumours occur in the axial skeleton, particularly the vertebrae[1]. An example of a tumour affecting the mandible is presented in Figure 21.1. The diagnostic criteria for SPB are listed below.

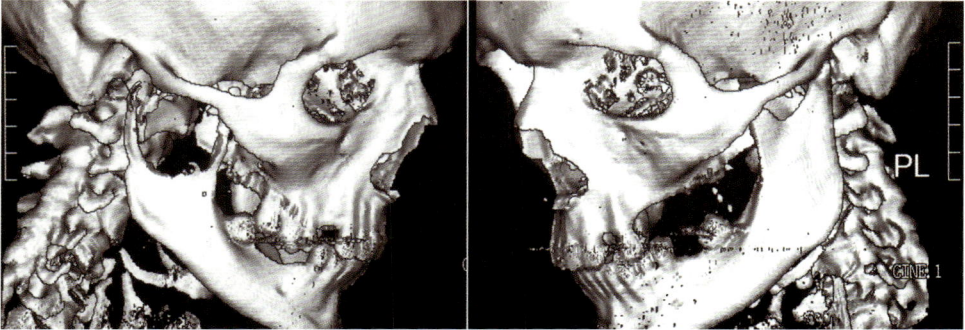

Figure 21.1. Solitary plasmacytoma of the right ramus of the mandible. (Courtesy of Ade Olujohungbe).

Criteria for the diagnosis of solitary plasmacytoma of bone[3]
• Low concentration or absence of monoclonal protein in serum and/or urine
• Single area of bone destruction due to clonal plasma cells
• Bone marrow not consistent with MM
• Normal skeletal survey (and magnetic resonance imaging [MRI] of spine and pelvis if performed)
• No related organ or tissue impairment (no end organ damage other than a solitary bone lesion)

The outcome for patients with SPB is varied. Progression to MM is most frequent and has been reported to occur in approximately 50% of patients, with a median time to progression of 21 months. In 13% of patients, recurrence of the disease is at the site of the original lesion[4] but some patients develop new bone lesions with normal intervening bone marrow, consistent with a 'macrofocal' pattern of growth[5]. Other patients may remain clinically stable for more than a decade[5]. The 10-year disease free survival for SPB is reported to be between 25 and 46% and the median overall survival between 7 and 12 years[6].

21.2.1. Monoclonal proteins in patients with solitary plasmacytoma of bone

From a review of seven different studies, it was reported that immunofixation electrophoresis (IFE) of serum and/or concentrated urine identified a small monoclonal protein in between 24 - 72% of patients with SPB[5]. When present, a monoclonal protein can be useful for guiding therapy. In most patients, the monoclonal protein is markedly reduced upon completion of local radiotherapy but it only disappears entirely in a minority of patients. Persistence of the monoclonal protein may indicate the presence of a tumour outside the field of radiotherapy[5]. The potential utility of sFLC analysis has been investigated in a growing number of studies, the most comprehensive of which was performed retrospectively by Dingli et al.[4] at the Mayo Clinic. Of 116 patients with a serum sample taken at diagnosis and prior to any therapy, the κ/λ sFLC ratio was abnormal in 54 (47%). Three smaller studies have reported abnormal κ/λ sFLC ratios in 30 - 68% of patients at diagnosis[7,8,9].

21.2.2. Prognostic factors in patients with solitary plasmacytoma of bone

Many attempts have been made to identify prognostic factors associated with disease-free survival and progression to MM. Tumour location, presence of a monoclonal protein at diagnosis[10], persistence of a serum monoclonal protein[11] and low levels of uninvolved immunoglobulins[12] have each been reported to be associated with progression. However, the relatively small number of patients studied has limited the ability to draw robust conclusions[13]; moreover, the prognostic utility of many factors has not been consistent between series. One of the more reliable predictors of progression is the persistence of a serum monoclonal protein[4,14]. However, as this can only be assessed at 1 or 2 years following therapy, there is a clear need for reliable prognostic markers that can be measured at diagnosis[4].

The prognostic utility of baseline sFLC measurements was evaluated by Dingli et al.[4]. A total of 43/116 patients progressed to MM with a median time to progression of 1.8 years. An abnormal κ/λ sFLC ratio was associated with a 44% risk of progression at 5 years compared with a 26% risk in patients with a normal κ/λ sFLC ratio (p=0.039) (Figure 21.2). Patients with an abnormal κ/λ sFLC ratio also had a shorter overall survival (Figure 21.3). At 1 - 2 years after therapy, a persistent serum monoclonal immunoglobulin concentration of $\geq$5 g/L was an additional risk factor for progression to MM. A risk stratification model was therefore constructed based on these two risk factors (an abnormal κ/λ sFLC ratio at baseline and a monoclonal protein concentration of >5 g/L at 1 - 2 years following diagnosis). Low-, intermediate- and high-risk groups of progression to MM corresponded to none, one or two risk factors, and these gave 5-year progression rates of 13%, 26% and 62% respectively (Figure 21.4). The authors commented that sFLC analysis provided an important prognostic indicator in these patients.

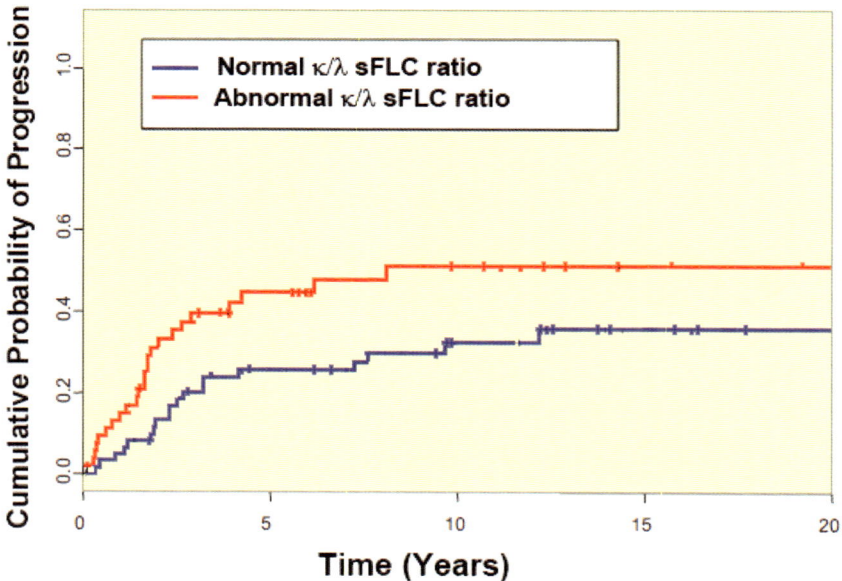

Figure 21.2. Kaplan-Meier plots for time to progression to multiple myeloma in 116 patients with solitary bone plasmacytoma and normal (n=62) or abnormal (n=54) κ/λ sFLC ratios. (This research was originally published in Blood[4] © the American Society of Hematology).

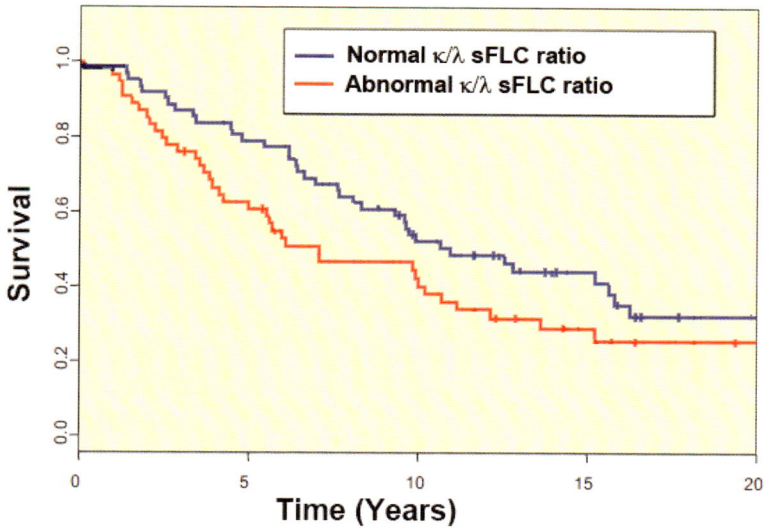

Figure 21.3. Kaplan-Meier plots for survival in 116 patients with solitary bone plasmacytoma and normal (n=62) or abnormal (n=54) κ/λ sFLC ratios. (This research was originally published in Blood[4] © the American Society of Hematology).

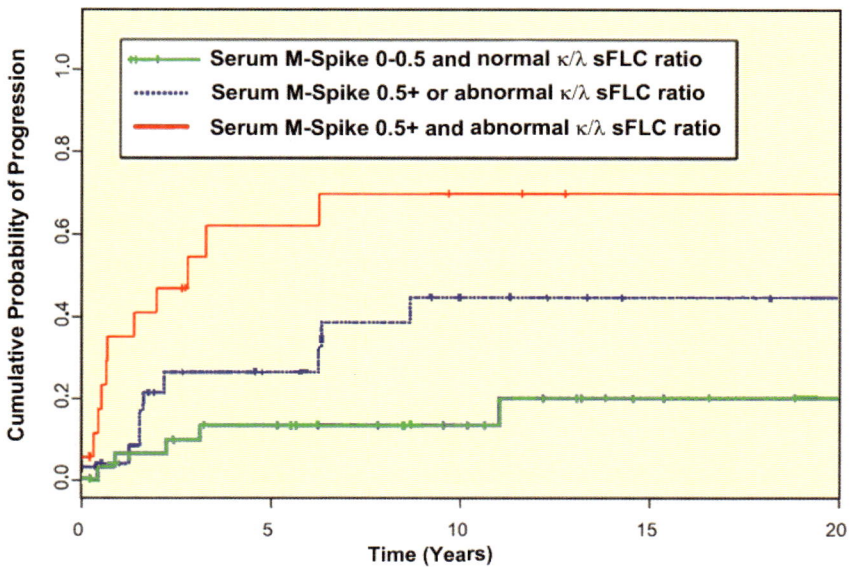

Figure 21.4. Risk of progression in solitary plasmacytoma of bone using sFLCs and serum monoclonal immunoglobulins. Low, intermediate and high risk groups correspond to 0, 1 or 2 positive risk factors, respectively. (This research was originally published in Blood[4] © the American Society of Hematology).

Subsequent studies have further highlighted the prognostic potential of sFLC analysis. Koch et al.[7] reported that 17/32 (53%) patients with an abnormal sFLC ratio at diagnosis progressed to MM compared with 2/17 (12%) patients with a normal κ/λ sFLC ratio at diagnosis. The authors concluded that an abnormal baseline κ/λ sFLC ratio was significantly associated with progression to MM (p=0.012). Most recently, Fouquet and colleagues[9] proposed a risk stratification model that incorporates an abnormal involved FLC (iFLC) concentration and whole body, fluorodeoxyglucose positron emission tomography – computed tomography (FDG-PET CT) at diagnosis. This model was constructed using patients with both bone and extramedullary plasmacytomas and is discussed in detail in Section 21.3.

In summary, these reports indicate that baseline sFLC abnormalities are consistently associated with increased risk of progression from SPB to MM, and sFLC analysis is recommended in IMWG guidelines for all patients with solitary plasmacytoma (Section 25.3.1).

21.2.3. Monitoring solitary plasmacytoma of bone using sFLCs

There is some data to support the use of sFLC analysis to monitor patients with SBP. Leleu et al.[15] monitored 10 patients and observed a trend to shorter time to progression (to MM) in patients with no change in sFLCs following radiotherapy. The same group[16] also described a patient with monoclonal κ FLCs in whom sFLCs were abnormal at disease relapse while electrophoresis and MRI were both 'unremarkable'. A subsequent MRI investigation and biopsy confirmed relapse 6 months later, whilst serum and urine electrophoresis results remained normal.

National Comprehensive Cancer Network® (NCCN®) guidelines recommened sFLC analysis alongside serum protein electrophoresis (SPE) and serum IFE in a panel of tests for surveillance/follow-up of solitary plasmacytoma after primary treatment (Section 25.7)[17].

21.3. Solitary extramedullary plasmacytoma

Solitary extramedullary plasmacytomas are plasma cell tumours that arise outside the bone marrow and are defined by the criteria listed below. They are predominantly found in the head and neck mucosa, especially within the upper respiratory tract, although they can occur in any organ. Local tumour irradiation is the treatment of choice, with nearly all patients successfully achieving local control.

Criteria for the diagnosis of extramedullary plasmacytoma[3]
• Low concentration or absence of monoclonal protein in serum and/or urine
• Extramedullary tumour of clonal plasma cells
• Normal bone marrow
• Normal skeletal survey
• No related organ or tissue impairment (no end organ damage including bone lesions)

The outcome of patients with a solitary extramedullary plasmacytoma is varied, with a 5-year survival rate of 78.9%[1]. As with SPB, the most common outcome is progression to MM, which is reported to occur in 30 - 50% of patients, with a median time to progression of 1.5 - 2.5 years. In fewer than 10% of patients, there is recurrence of disease at the site of the original lesion[6]. A monoclonal protein (typically IgA[2]) is detected in the serum or urine of approximately 25% of patients[12]. Although there is limited evidence, sFLC measurements should also prove useful in monitoring patients with abnormal iFLCs[18], particularly those previously classified as having nonsecretory disease[6].

Fouquet et al.[9] assessed the prognostic utility of sFLCs and whole body FDG-PET CT in 43 patients with solitary plasmacytoma. This comprised 33 patients with solitary plasmacytoma of bone and 10 patients with extramedullary plasmacytoma. At diagnosis, 21/43 (49%) patients had an abnormal iFLC concentration and 11/43 (26%) had an abnormal κ/λ sFLC ratio. By univariate analysis, an abnormal iFLC concentration, an abnormal κ/λ sFLC ratio or the presence of ≥ 2 hypermetabolic lesions on initial PET CT were associated with significantly shorter time to MM progression (Figure 21.5, p=0.002; and data not shown). On multivariate analysis, an abnormal initial iFLC concentration and the presence of ≥ 2 hypermetabolic lesions on PET-CT were the strongest independent prognostic factors to identify patients at greatest risk of progression to MM. A risk stratification model was constructed in which patients were grouped into 3 categories, based on the presence of 0, 1, or 2 of these risk factors, and median time to MM progression was "Not reached", 41 or 21 months, respectively (Figure 21.6).

IMWG guidelines recommend baseline measurements of sFLCs in all solitary plasmacytomas to identify patients at increased risk of progression to MM (Section 25.3.1)[19].

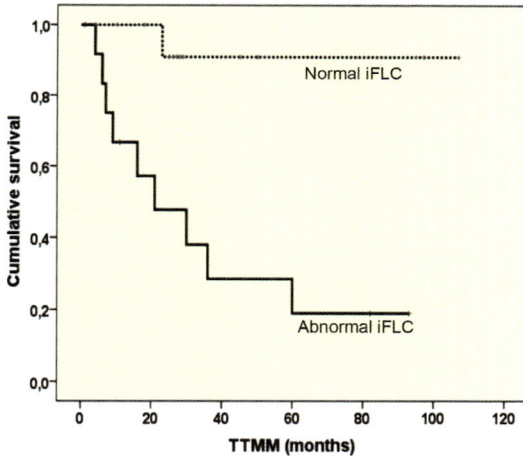

Figure 21.5. Time to progression towards MM (TTMM) in patients with solitary plasmacytoma and a normal or abnormal iFLC concentration at baseline. (Reprinted by permission from the American Association for Cancer Research[9]).

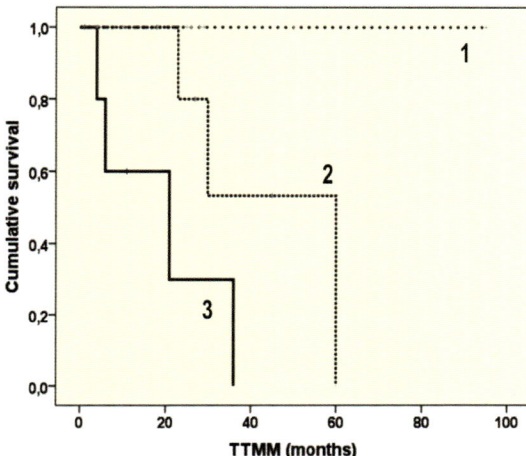

Figure 21.6. Solitary plasmacytoma risk stratification model. The three categories (1 - 3) are defined by the presence of 0, 1 or 2 risk factors (an abnormal iFLC concentration and ≥ 2 hypermetabolic lesions on initial PET CT). (Reprinted by permission from the American Association for Cancer Research[9]).

235

21.4. Multiple solitary plasmacytoma

Up to 5% of patients presenting with solitary plasmacytomas go on to develop multiple lesions in the bone or elsewhere, without evidence of MM[2]. The criteria for diagnosing patients with multiple solitary plasmacytomas are shown below. As with solitary plasmacytoma, sFLC measurements may be helpful in managing these patients.

Criteria for the diagnosis of multiple solitary plasmacytomas (± recurrent)[2]
• Low concentration or absence of monoclonal protein in serum and/or urine
• More than one localised area of bone destruction or extramedullary tumour of clonal plasma cells, which may be recurrent
• Normal bone marrow
• Normal skeletal survey and MRI of spine and pelvis if done
• No related organ or tissue impairment (no end organ damage other than the localised bone lesions)

Test Questions

1. What is the reported 5-year risk of progression to MM in SPB patients with an abnormal κ/λ sFLC ratio?

2. Based on the risk stratification model reported by Dingli et al.[4], which two factors can effectively discriminate SPB patients at low, medium and high risk of progression to MM?

3. Which two risk factors were defined by Fouquet et al.[9] to identify solitary plasmacytoma patients at risk of progression to MM?

Answers

1. 44% (Section 21.2.2).

2. The κ/λ sFLC ratio at baseline and the persistence of a monoclonal immunoglobulin after 1 - 2 years (Section 21.2.2).

3. An abnormal involved sFLC concentration and the presence of ≥2 lesions by PET CT at baseline (Section 21.3).

References

1. Dores GM, Landgren O, McGlynn KA, Curtis RE, Linet MS, Devesa SS. Plasmacytoma of bone, extramedullary plasmacytoma, and multiple myeloma: incidence and survival in the United States, 1992-2004. Br J Haematol 2009;144:86-94

2. Kyle R, Child JA, Anderson K, Barlogie B, Bataille R, Bensinger W et al. Criteria for the classification of monoclonal gammopathies, multiple myeloma and related disorders: a report of the International Myeloma Working Group. Br J Haematol 2003;121:749-57

3. Hughes M, Soutar R, Lucraft H, Owen R, Bird J. Guidelines on the diagnosis and management of solitary plasmacytoma of bone, extramedullary plasmacytoma and multiple solitary plasmacytomas: 2009 update. BCSH guidelines available online at www.bcshguidelines.com

4. Dingli D, Kyle RA, Rajkumar SV, Nowakowski GS, Larson DR, Bida JP et al. Immunoglobulin free light chains and solitary plasmacytoma of bone. Blood 2006;108:1979-83

5. Dimopoulos MA, Moulopoulos LA, Maniatis A, Alexanian R. Solitary plasmacytoma of bone and asymptomatic multiple myeloma. Blood 2000;96:2037-2044

6. Weber DM. Solitary bone and extramedullary plasmacytoma. Hematology Am Soc Hematol Educ Program 2005;373-376

7. Koch A, Shain K, Alsina M, Sullivan D, Nishihori T, Ochoa-Bayona J, Baz R. Outcome of patients with solitary plasmacytomas (SP) in the era of PET imaging and serum-free light chain (sFLC) testing: A single institution experience. J Clin Oncol 2013;31:8608a

8. Fouquet G, Guidez S, Herbaux C, Van de Wyngaert Z, Bonnet S, Beauvais D et al. Imapct of initial FGD-PET CT and serum free light chain on transformation of solitary plasmacytoma to MM. Blood 2013;122:1888a

9. Fouquet G, Guidez S, Herbaux C, Van de Wyngaert Z, Bonnet S, Beauvais D et al. Impact of initial FGD-PET CT and Serum Free Light Chain on transformation of conventionally defined Solitary Plasmacytoma to Multiple Myeloma. Clin Cancer Res 2014;20:3254-60

10. Reed V, Shah J, Medeiros LJ, Ha CS, Mazloom A, Weber DM et al. Solitary plasmacytomas: Outcome and prognostic factors after definitive radiation therapy. Cancer 2011;117:4468-74

11. Wilder RB, Ha CS, Cox JD, Weber D, Delasalle K, Alexanian R. Persistence of myeloma protein for more than one year after radiotherapy is an adverse prognostic factor in solitary plasmacytoma of bone. Cancer 2002;94:1532-1537

12. Soutar R, Lucraft H, Jackson G, Reece A, Bird J, Low E, Samson D. Guidelines on the diagnosis and management of solitary plasmacytoma of bone and solitary extramedullary plasmacytoma. Br J Haematol 2004;124:717-26

13. Guo SQ, Zhang L, Wang YF, Sun BC, Zhang LY, Zhang J et al. Prognostic factors associated with solitary plasmacytoma. Onco Targets Ther 2013;6:1659-66

14. Wilder RB, Ha CS, Cox JD, Weber D, Delasalle K, Alexanian R. Persistence of myeloma protein for more than one year after radiotherapy is an adverse prognostic factor in solitary plasmacytoma of bone. Cancer 2002;94:1532-1537

15. Leleu X, Moreau AS, Coiteux V, Guieze R, Hennache B, Facon T et al. Serum free light chain assays in solitary bone plasmacytoma. Clin Chim Acta 2005;355:TP4.02a

16. Leleu X, Moreau AS, Coiteux V, Guieze R, Hennache B, Facon T et al. Serum free light chain assays in solitary bone plasmacytoma. Br J Haematol 2005;129:186a

17. Anderson KC, Alsina M, Bensinger W, Biermann JS, Chanan-Khan A, Cohen AD et al. NCCN Clinical practice guidelines in oncology for multiple myeloma. J Natl Compr Canc Netw 2011;9:1146-83

18. Mayo MM, Johns GS. Serum free light chains in the diagnosis and monitoring of patients with plasma cell dyscrasias. Contrib Nephrol 2007;153:44-65

19. Dispenzieri A, Kyle R, Merlini G, Miguel JS, Ludwig H, Hajek R et al. International Myeloma Working Group guidelines for serum-free light chain analysis in multiple myeloma and related disorders. Leukemia 2009;23:215-24

Plasma cell leukaemia

Summary:

- Plasma cell leukaemia is a rare leukaemic variant of multiple myeloma with a more aggressive clinical course.

- sFLC analysis and serum protein electrophoresis is an effective screen for plasma cell leukaemia.

- International Myeloma Working Group guidelines recommend the use of general multiple myeloma response criteria for monitoring plasma cell leukaemia, which includes sFLC analysis.

22.1. Introduction

Plasma cell leukaemia (PCL) is a rare and aggressive variant of multiple myeloma (MM), accounting for 2 - 4% of cases. It is defined by the presence of >20% plasma cells in the peripheral blood and/or an absolute plasma cell count >2 x 10^9/L[1]. It can occur without evidence of MM (primary PCL; 60 - 70%), or may develop from leukaemic transformation of a pre-existing myeloma clone (secondary PCL; 30 - 40%) in 1 - 2% of advanced and refractory patients[2].

Both primary and secondary PCL have distinct clinical and biological features. The median age of primary PCL patients is approximately 10 years younger than both the general myeloma and secondary PCL populations[1]. Primary PCL also has a more aggressive clinical presentation, with a higher tumour burden and an increased incidence of extramedullary and light-chain only disease (26 - 44%)[1]. Both forms of PCL have very poor outcomes, with the worst prognosis associated with secondary PCL[3]. Overall survival for primary PCL patients is still inferior to that of patients with MM, but has significantly improved in recent years[4].

22.2. Diagnosis and monitoring of plasma cell leukaemia using sFLCs

Monoclonal proteins are present in the majority of PCL patients. In some cases, a monoclonal protein may be undetectable by serum protein electrophoresis, but clearly indicated by sFLC analysis[5]. A combination of serum protein electrophoresis (SPE) and sFLC analysis has been shown to be an effective screen for MM, including plasma cell leukaemia[6], and sFLC analysis should form part of the initial diagnostic work-up of these patients *(Chapter 23)*[7].

As there are no specific response criteria for assessing response to treatment in PCL, the International Myeloma Working Group recommend the application of the MM response criteria[1]. These criteria incorporate sFLC analysis in the definitions of stringent complete response for all patients, and very good partial response and partial response for patients whose monoclonal protein is not measurable by serum or urine electrophoresis *(Chapter 25.3.5.)*.

A number of case reports highlight the utility of sFLC analysis for the diagnosis and monitoring of PCL [8,9,10,11,12,13,14]. An example of primary PCL is described in the clinical case history below and a case of MM progressing to secondary PCL is presented in the clinical case history in Section 19.3.

Clinical case history

Successful treatment of primary plasma cell leukaemia expressing monoclonal light chains[11]

A 40-year-old female presented with conjunctival haemorrhage. She also reported giddiness, fatigue, and weight loss. On examination she was afebrile, and had no organomegaly. Peripheral blood counts revealed she was anaemic (haemoglobin 10.6 g/dL) with a markedly raised total leukocyte count (39.6 x 10^9/L) and severe thrombocytopaenia (platelet count 1.0 x 10^9/L). A peripheral blood smear showed a prominence of plasma cells with occasional binucleate cells (Figure 22.1).

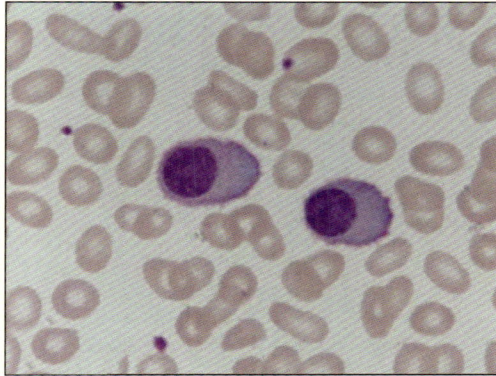

Figure 22.1. Peripheral blood smear showing marked prominence of plasma cells. These cells have abundant basophilic cytoplasm and an eccentrically placed nucleus with clumped chromatin (Leishman stain, × 1000 magnification). (Reproduced with permission from Indian J Med Paediatr Oncol [11]).

A bone marrow aspirate and biopsy revealed an almost complete replacement of normal marrow elements by sheets of plasma cells. By flow cytometry, these cells were CD38+, CD138+, CD117+ and expressed cytoplasmic λ light chain.

Serum total protein was low (46.0 g/L) and albumin, calcium and creatinine concentrations were normal. Serum β$_2$-microglobulin was elevated (12.95 mg/L). No monoclonal protein was detectable by serum protein electrophoresis and total immunoglobulins were all low (IgG 3.3 g/L; IgA 0.09 g/L and IgM 0.08 g/L). sFLC analysis showed markedly elevated λ sFLCs (3527 mg/L) with suppressed κ sFLCs (1.15 mg/L), resulting in a highly abnormal κ/λ sFLC ratio (0.00033).

Interphase fluorescence in situ hybridization analysis revealed IgH gene translocations and 13q deletions. Radiographs of the skull, dorsal spine, lumbar spine and femora did not reveal any lytic lesions.

After a diagnosis of primary PCL was made, treatment with RVd (lenalidomide, bortezomib and dexamethasone) was commenced. Following four cycles of therapy, the patient achieved a complete response with normalisation of κ sFLCs (8.1 mg/L), λ sFLCs (5.5 mg/L) and the κ/λ sFLC ratio (1.47).

She subsequently underwent high-dose chemotherapy with melphalan and autologous stem cell transplantation, and was reported to be in complete remission 9 months after her initial diagnosis.

Test Questions

1. Can sFLC analysis help in the diagnosis of PCL?

1. Yes, in some patients sFLC analysis can be abnormal when SPE is negative, and sFLC analysis should form part of the initial diagnostic work-up for PCL.

References

1. Fernandez de LC, Kyle RA, Durie BG, Ludwig H, Usmani S, Vesole DH et al. Plasma cell leukemia: consensus statement on diagnostic requirements, response criteria and treatment recommendations by the International Myeloma Working Group. Leukemia 2013;27:780-91

2. Usmani SZ, Heuck C, Mitchell A, Szymonifka J, Nair B, Hoering A et al. Extramedullary disease portends poor prognosis in multiple myeloma and is over-represented in high-risk disease even in the era of novel agents. Haematologica 2012;97:1761-7

3. Tiedemann RE, Gonzalez-Paz N, Kyle RA, Santana-Davila R, Price-Troska T, Van Wier SA et al. Genetic aberrations and survival in plasma cell leukemia. Leukemia 2008;22:1044-52

4. Gonsalves WI, Rajkumar SV, Go RS, Dispenzieri A, Gupta V, Singh PP et al. Trends in survival of patients with primary plasma cell leukemia: a population based analysis. Blood 2014;124:907-12

5. Kar R. Dutta S, Bhargava R, Kumar R, Pati HP. Immunoglobulin free light chains: do they have a role in plasma cell leukemia? Hematology 2008;13:344-7

6. Katzmann JA, Kyle RA, Benson J, Larson DR, Snyder MR, Lust JA et al. Screening panels for detection of monoclonal gammopathies. Clin Chem 2009;55:1517-22

7. van de Donk NW, Lokhorst HM, Anderson KC, Richardson PG. How I treat plasma cell leukemia. Blood 2012;120:2376-2389

8. Ueda S, Kubo M, Matsuura N, Matsunaga H, Kataoka S, Maeda T et al. Stringent complete remission of primary plasma cell leukemia with reduced-dose bortezomib, lenalidomide and dexamethasone: a case report and review of the literature. Intern Med 2013;52:1235-8

9. Gozzetti A, Musto P, Defina M, D'Auria F, Papini G, Statuto T et al. Efficacy of bortezomib, lenalidomide and dexamethasone (VRD) in secondary plasma cell leukaemia. Br J Haematol 2012;157:497-8

10. Kruger WH, Kiefer T, Schuler F, Lotze C, Busemann C, Dolken G. Complete remission and early relapse of refractory plasma cell leukemia after bortezomib induction and consolidation by HLA-mismatched unrelated allogeneic stem cell transplantation. Onkologie 2007;30:193–5

11. Goyal M, Mohammad N, Palanki SD, Vaniawala SN. Primary plasma cell leukemia with light chain secretion and multiple chromosomal abnormalities: How successfully treated? Indian J Med Paediatr Oncol 2010;31:96-100

12. Tamura S, Koyama A, Shiotani C, Kurihara T, Nishikawa A, Okamoto Y, Fujimoto T. Successful bortezomib/dexamethasone induction therapy with lenalidomide in an elderly patient with primary plasma cell leukemia complicated by renal failure and pulmonary hypertension. Intern Med 2014;53:1171-5

13. Egan JB, Shi CX, Tembe W, Christoforides A, Kurdoglu A, Sinari S et al. Whole-genome sequencing of multiple myeloma from diagnosis to plasma cell leukemia reveals genomic initiating events, evolution, and clonal tides. Blood 2012;120:1060-6

14. Keats JJ, Chesi M, Egan JB, Garbitt VM, Palmer SE, Braggio E et al. Clonal competition with alternating dominance in multiple myeloma. Blood 2012;120:1067-76

Screening studies using serum free light chain analysis

Summary:

- Screening symptomatic patients using serum protein electrophoresis and sFLCs is a clinically sensitive strategy for identifying patients with monoclonal gammopathies.
- The inclusion of sFLC analysis in routine screening can identify additional patients with plasma cell malignancies and B-cell leukaemia/lymphoma.
- Adding urine tests to the initial screen is only necessary if AL amyloidosis is suspected.

23.1. Introduction

Whether or not serum free light chains (sFLCs) should be measured as part of an initial diagnostic request for "possible myeloma - please investigate" is an important issue. Traditionally, serum protein electrophoresis (SPE) and/or serum immunofixation electrophoresis (sIFE) tests have been performed first, sometimes alongside total immunoglobulin (IgG, IgA and IgM) measurements. SPE can detect monoclonal proteins with sensitivities down to 500 - 2000 mg/L *(Chapter 4)*, which is adequate to identify most intact immunoglobulin multiple myeloma (IIMM) patients. However, many patients with light chain multiple myeloma (LCMM) will not be identified. Some centres screen using sIFE: although this technique is 10 times more sensitive than SPE, it is time-consuming, non-quantitative and occasionally monoclonal FLCs are not detected. Furthermore, additional low-level monoclonal gammopathy of undetermined significance (MGUS) patients are detected that are unlikely to progress to malignancy, provided sFLC levels are also normal *(Chapter 13)*[1]. A few laboratories measure total serum κ and λ in the initial screen, but this is clinically inadequate as the assay is insensitive for the detection of monoclonal FLCs *(Chapter 4)*[2].

As a consequence of the inadequacy of serum electrophoretic procedures for identifying monoclonal FLC production, urine protein electrophoresis (UPE) and urine IFE (uIFE) have, historically, been performed alongside serum tests, but many patients with nonsecretory multiple myeloma (NSMM), AL amyloidosis and other FLC-associated disorders are still missed. Furthermore, only a minority of patients have accompanying urine samples (14% in a recent UK pathology review) *(Table 23.5)*[3]. It is therefore logical to test for sFLCs on receipt of the first blood sample. The results will also provide baseline values for subsequent disease monitoring.

A strategy of using SPE/sIFE combined with sFLC analysis in an initial screen increases the identification of clinically significant monoclonal gammopathies, facilitates risk assessment for disease progression in MM *(Chapter 20)*, MGUS *(Chapter 13)*, smouldering multiple myeloma (SMM, *Chapter 14*) and plasmacytomas *(Chapter 21)*, as well as aiding appropriate clinical decisions for monitoring patients.

This chapter discusses the current and potential screening options for identifying monoclonal proteins. As a general rule, intact monoclonal immunoglobulins can be identified using serum electrophoretic tests while monoclonal light chain diseases should be identified using sFLC assays. The combination of the two procedures produces good diagnostic accuracy and this has been recognised in the current International Myeloma Working Group (IMWG) guidelines. These state that, with the exception of light chain amyloidosis (AL amyloidosis), serum electrophoretic and sFLC assays are sufficient to screen for all pathological plasmaproliferative disorders *(Chapters 25 and 28)*[4].

23.2. Screening panels for the detection of monoclonal gammopathies

The largest study that compared the relative diagnostic contributions of serum and urine assays in the detection of plasma cell proliferative disorders was reported by Katzmann and colleagues[5]. Samples from 1,877 untreated patients diagnosed with various plasmaproliferative diseases underwent a full panel of five screening tests (SPE, UPE, sIFE, uIFE and sFLCs; *Table 23.1)*. This allowed different screening protocols to be compared, and addressed the question of whether sFLC analyses could replace urine studies.

Diagnosis	n	Diagnostic performance (% sensitivity)						
		All 5 tests	SPE, sIFE & uIFE	SPE, sIFE & sFLC	SPE & sFLC	sIFE	SPE	sFLC
All	1877	98.6	97.0	97.4	94.3	87.0	79.0	74.3
MM	467	100.0	98.7	100.0	100.0	94.4	87.6	96.8
WM	26	100.0	100.0	100.0	100.0	100.0	100.0	73.1
SMM	191	100.0	100.0	100.0	99.5	98.4	94.2	81.2
MGUS	524	100.0	100.0	97.1	88.7	92.8	81.9	42.4
Plasmacytoma	29	89.7	89.7	89.7	86.2	72.4	72.4	55.2
POEMS syndrome	31	96.8	96.8	96.8	74.2	96.8	74.2	9.7
Extramedullary plasmacytoma	10	20.0	20.0	10.0	10.0	10.0	10.0	10.0
Primary AL amyloidosis	581	98.1	94.2	97.1	96.2	73.8	65.9	88.3
LCDD	18	83.3	77.8	77.8	77.8	55.6	55.6	77.8

Table 23.1. Sensitivity of monoclonal gammopathy screening panels[5]. MM: multiple myeloma; WM: Waldenström's macroglobulinaemia; SMM: smouldering multiple myeloma; MGUS: monoclonal gammopathy of undetermined significance; LCDD: light chain deposition disease.

The combined results from all five tests identified 1,851 (98.6%) samples as abnormal. Of those not detected, 11 were AL amyloidosis (1.9% of total), 8 extramedullary plasmacytoma (80%), 3 plasmacytoma (10.3%), 3 light chain deposition disease (LCDD, 16.7%) and 1 POEMS syndrome (3%).

The same data are used to produce a simpler comparison of different potential screening panels in Table 23.2. The table quantifies the nature and number of additional diagnoses that would have been missed if alternative screening panels had been used (compared with the use of all five tests). The major differences were that omission of sFLC analysis from the panel resulted in six additional MM and 23 additional primary amyloidosis patients being undetected, whereas the inclusion of sFLCs but omission of urine analysis resulted in 15 additional MGUS and six amyloidosis patients being undetected.

Diagnosis	n	Alternative test panels with associated missed diagnoses			
		SPE, sIFE, UPE, uIFE, sFLC	SPE, sIFE, UPE, uIFE	SPE, sIFE & sFLC	SPE (with reflex sIFE) & sFLC
MM	467	0	6	0	0
WM	26	0	0	0	0
SMM	191	0	0	0	1
MGUS	524	0	0	15	59
Plasmacytoma	29	0	0	0	1
POEMS syndrome	31	0	0	0	7
Extramedullary plasmacytoma	10	0	0	1	1
Primary AL amyloidosis	581	0	23	6	11
LCDD	18	0	1	1	2

Table 23.2. Diagnoses that would have been missed using alternative test panels compared with the use of all five diagnostic tests[5]. MM: multiple myeloma; WM: Waldenström's macroglobulinaemia; SMM: smouldering multiple myeloma; MGUS: monoclonal gammopathy of undetermined significance; LCDD: light chain deposition disease.

Palladini et al.[6] also found that uIFE, sIFE and sFLCs are necessary for the optimal detection of amyloidosis. Katzmann and colleagues commented that MGUS patients with negative SPE results and normal sFLC ratios (i.e. the 15 detected only by urinalysis) would all be defined as having a low risk of progression, and the consequences of failing to identify them were unlikely to be severe[1,5]. Furthermore, the authors concluded that because urine studies and sIFE gave only a small incremental increase in sensitivity, SPE plus sFLCs provide an efficient initial diagnostic screen for monoclonal gammopathies with a high tumour burden such as MM, SMM and Waldenström's macroglobulinaemia (with sIFE used only as a reflex test).

An earlier, smaller study was designed specifically to address whether sFLC analysis could eliminate the need for urine testing when screening for monoclonal gammopathies[7]. In this investigation, records from 428 patients with a monoclonal gammopathy and positive uIFE (at presentation) were examined to determine whether sIFE and sFLC analysis had also been positive. Only two (0.5%) patients were negative by both sIFE and sFLC, and further investigation indicated that the urine of one had almost certainly been contaminated with monoclonal immunoglobulin in the laboratory, while the other patient had a light chain MGUS and did not require medical intervention. This suggested that the addition of sFLC analysis to SPE and sIFE made the inclusion of urine tests unnecessary in a screening algorithm for monoclonal gammopathies.

The overall findings of both studies provide significant support for the IMWG recommendations, which state that initial screening should use a combination of serum electrophoresis and sFLC tests, with uIFE required only to maximise sensitivity when AL amyloidosis is suspected *(Chapter 25)*[4].

23.3. Incorporation of sFLC analysis into routine screening for monoclonal gammopathies

In addition to the two studies discussed above, there have been a considerable number of published reports examining the value of incorporating sFLC analysis in routine screening programmes *(Table 23.3)*. Inevitably, there is a degree of repetition between many studies and only selected results are discussed in detail, with the aim of illustrating different aspects of the overall data.

Publication	Number of patients	Screening tests utilised	Location of study (country)
Hofman et al. (2004)[8]	107	sIFE, sFLC. uIFE, total light chains	Germany
Bakshi et al. (2005)[9]	1003	CZE. sFLC	USA
Foray et al. (2005)[10]	273	CZE, sIFE, sFLC, UPE, uIEP	France
Abadie & Bankson (2006)[11]	312	SPE, sFLC	USA
Hill et al. (2006)[12]	923	SPE, sIFE, sFLC, UPE, uIFE	UK
Reid et al. (2006)[13]	971	SPE, sIFE, sFLC, UPE, uIFE	UK
Beetham at al. (2007)[14]	932	SPE, sIFE, sFLC, uIFE	UK
Piehler et al. (2008)[15]	1067	SPE, sFLC, Igs	Norway
Vermeersch et al. (2008)[16]	833	CZE, sIFE, sFLC, uIFE	Belgium
Fulton & Fernando (2009)[17]	890	SPE, sIFE, sFLC, UPE, uIFE	Australia
Katzmann et al. (2009)[5]	1020	SPE, sIFE, sFLC, UPE, uIFE	USA
Robson et al. (2009)[18]	653	SPE, sIFE, sFLC, UPE, uIFE	UK
Holding et al. (2011)[3]	753	SPE/CZE, sIFE, sFLC, UPE, uIFE	UK
Park et al. (2012)[19]	471	SPE, sFLC, Igs, UPE	Korea
Jeong et al. (2013)[20]	231	SPE, sIFE, sFLC, UPE, uIFE	Korea
McTaggart et al. (2013)[21]	2799	SPE, sIFE, sFLC, UPE, uIFE	UK

Table 23.3. Published screening studies investigating the contribution of sFLC analysis in routine screening for monoclonal gammopathies. CZE: capilliary zone electrophoresis; uIEP: urine immunoelectrophoresis: Igs: Immunoglobulins.

The number/proportion of additional symptomatic plasma cell malignancies detected by sFLC analysis in the screening studies was very variable. Numbers would have been influenced by diverse factors such as the referral population, whether sIFE was used on all sera or only as a reflex test when there was an abnormal SPE result, and the proportion of sera that had an accompanying urine sample. However, the nature of the additional malignancies detected was similar, with a majority producing modest amounts of monoclonal FLC only (i.e. LCMM, NSMM, AL amyloidosis and LCDD). This pattern is unsurprising because every study employed either SPE or capillary zone electrophoresis (CZE) on all sera, so patients with large amounts of monoclonal immunoglobulin production were less likely to have escaped detection. By way of example, Hill et al.[12] reported the detection of two additional LCMM patients, Piehler et al.[15] reported five LCMM, one NSMM and one AL amyloidosis patients, while McTaggart et al.[21] identified two additional patients, one with LCDD and one with multiple plasmacytomas.

While the diagnostic use of sFLC analysis is principally for the detection of plasma cell malignancies, B-cell leukaemias and lymphomas may also produce monoclonal FLCs. In many of the screening studies *(Table 23.3)*, further investigation of patients with abnormal sFLC ratios but normal electrophoresis identified the presence of a B-cell leukaemia or lymphoma *(Chapters 33 and 31)*. Of the nine additional gammopathy patients identified by Bakshi et al.[9], three had diagnoses of B-CLL/small cell lymphoma and one had an atypical B-cell lymphoma, while Holding et al.[3] reported two B-CLL patients in whom a serum abnormality was identified only by sFLC analysis.

In some instances, patients found to have abnormal sFLC ratios but apparently normal SPE results were ultimately diagnosed with IIMM. This was illustrated by Robson et al.[18] who published the SPE results for 2 patients which appeared unremarkable but sIFE was requested due to the presence of abnormal sFLC ratios *(Figure 23.1)*. sIFE revealed the presence of monoclonal IgD in one patient (MM) and a monoclonal IgA band in the other, that was hidden in the β-region of the gel (IgA MGUS). Similarly, Fulton and Fernando[17] reported 3 patients whose sera contained IgA paraproteins that were not visible by SPE but were identified by abnormal sFLC ratios. A common observation in screening populations is the number of patients with borderline elevations of the κ/λ ratio (i.e. ratios of ~ 1.66 – 3.0) but no evidence of a monoclonal process on further investigation. Such results are seen in Figure 23.2. Reduced FLC clearance when renal function is impaired can cause this elevation and a renal reference range has been derived for use with such patients (κ/λ sFLC ratio 0.37 – 3.1; *Section 6.3*) [22,23].

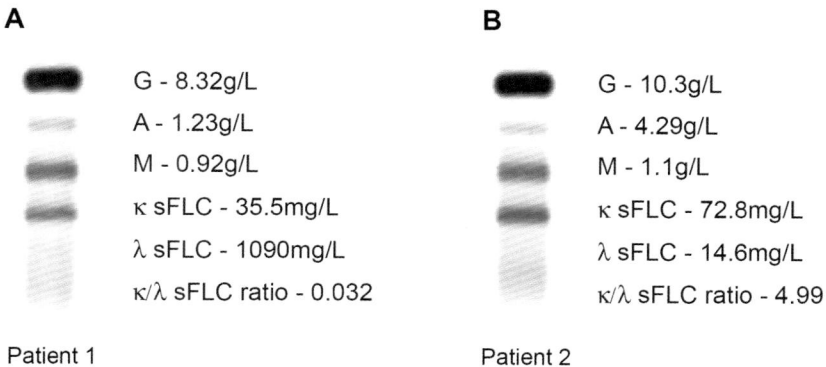

A

G - 8.32g/L
A - 1.23g/L
M - 0.92g/L
κ sFLC - 35.5mg/L
λ sFLC - 1090mg/L
κ/λ sFLC ratio - 0.032

Patient 1

B

G - 10.3g/L
A - 4.29g/L
M - 1.1g/L
κ sFLC - 72.8mg/L
λ sFLC - 14.6mg/L
κ/λ sFLC ratio - 4.99

Patient 2

Figure 23.1. Monoclonal intact immunoglobulins identified by sFLC analysis. (A) Patient 1 displayed no suppression of IgG, IgA, or IgM, and SPE was not sufficiently abnormal to initiate immunofixation. An abnormal serum κ/λ sFLC ratio of 0.032 triggered sIFE, leading to the patient subsequently being diagnosed with IgDλ MM. *(B)* Patient 2 had minimal elevation of IgA concentration with normal IgG and IgM concentrations, and an SPE gel that did not initiate sIFE. sFLC analysis indicated monoclonal κ FLC production (κ/λ sFLC ratio 4.99), and subsequent sIFE revealed an IgAκ band. *(Reproduced with permission from Lab Med[18]).*

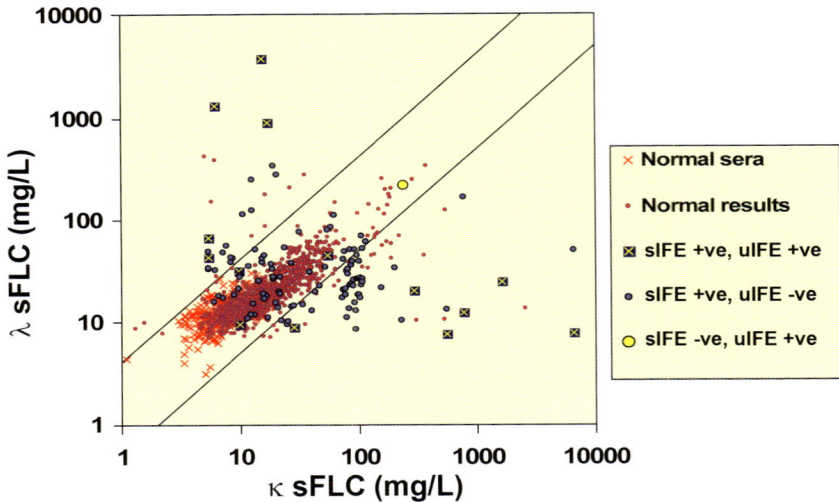

Figure 23.2. sFLCs in 925 sera screened at Derby, UK. *Normal results are the FLC levels in samples with normal SPE.* *(Courtesy of P Hill).*

23.3.1 Screening for monoclonal gammopathy in patients presenting with renal dysfunction

Screening for monoclonal gammopathy in patients with renal impairment is associated with distinct challenges: patients may become anuric, in which case urine measurements become irrelevant, and urine samples are often not provided. For example in one renal screening study, urine samples were only obtained from 24 of 41 myeloma patients[23].

The increased sensitivity of sFLC analysis over urine testing identifies additional monoclonal gammopathies associated with renal disease; Gerth et al.[24] performed a retrospective analysis of a cohort of patients with light-chain associated kidney disease comprising 143 patients with myeloma cast nephropathy, 12 patients with LCDD and 53 patients with AL amyloidosis. The authors reported that UPE alone detected 96.4% of cast nephropathy patients, 76.9% of AL amyloidosis patients and 55% LCDD patients. This compared with the sFLC ratio sensitivity of 96.8% for cast nephropathy, 100% for AL amyloidosis and 71.4% for LCDD patients.

Use of a renal reference interval for the κ/λ sFLC ratio in routine clinical practice may lead to increased diagnostic accuracy for the diagnosis of monoclonal gammopathy *(Section 6.3)*. The diagnostic utility of the renal reference interval was assessed in combination with SPE/UPE by Park et al.[19] in a retrospective analysis of 471 patients who visited a nephrologist due to unexplained renal impairment. A total of 110 patients (23.4%) were diagnosed with MM, 346 were classed as "non-MM" and the remaining 15 patients had other plasma cell dyscrasias or lymphoproliferative diseases and were excluded from further study. sFLC analysis was particularly effective for screening patients for LCMM (diagnostic sensitivity: 100%), compared with SPE or UPE (diagnostic sensitivity: 58.6% or 69.0% respectively) *(Table 23.4)*. The authors also commented on the difficulty in obtaining 24-hour urine collections *(Chapter 24)*, and the benefit of including sFLC analysis in the initial diagnostic screen: an additional 24/252 (9.5%) CKD patients were newly diagnosed with MM following the introduction of routine sFLC analysis. The authors concluded that a combination of SPE and sFLC analysis (using the renal reference range for the sFLC ratio) was the optimal screening algorithm for detection of MM in patients presenting with renal impairment.

		SPE	UPE	Conventional sFLC ratio (0.26 - 1.65)	Renal sFLC ratio (0.37 - 3.1)	Combined analysis: SPE + renal sFLC ratio (0.37 - 3.1)
All MM (n=110)	Sensitivity (%)	81.8	70.2	90.9	91.8	98.2
	Specificity (%)	97.5	98.6	89.9	95.1	95.1
IIMM (n=81)	Sensitivity (%)	90.1	70.7	87.7	88.9	97.5
	Specificity (%)	97.5	98.6	89.9	95.1	95.1
LCMM (n=29)	Sensitivity (%)	58.6	69.0	100	100	100
	Specificity (%)	97.5	98.6	89.9	95.1	95.1

*Table 23.4. Diagnostic sensitivity and specificity of routine laboratory screening tests for MM in patients with renal impairment[19].
IIMM: intact immunoglobulin MM; LCMM: light chain MM.*

23.3.2 Interpretation of borderline sFLC ratios

Modest sFLC ratio elevations (but no monoclonal FLC) are not exclusive to patients with renal impairment but are also observed in patients with polyclonal inflammatory and autoimmune conditions *(Section 6.2 and Chapter 35)*, suggesting a possible increased bias towards κ sFLC production in these instances[12,25,26]. Indeed, application of the renal range has been found to improve specificity when screening general populations[18,25]. Whilst borderline sFLC results can be problematic, it should be remembered that urine electrophoresis can produce greater numbers of equivocal results[27]. Analysis of a screening population by McTaggart and colleagues[28] led them to conclude that addition of UPE into their screening panel decreased the specificity through the identification of more "false-positive" results.

Apart from application of the renal reference range, other authors have similarly explored the influence on specificity/positive predictive value (PPV) of categorising patients into groups with different degrees of ratio abnormality. Hill et al.[12] found that κ/λ sFLC ratios of >3 or >5 were successively more predictive of finding a monoclonal gammopathy (by sIFE) or diagnosing a B-cell disorder. Vermeersch and colleagues[29] proposed the use of different sFLC ratio intervals to give likelihood ratios as an aid for interpreting screening results. In the screening population studied by Piehler et al.[15], sFLC ratios of <0.05 or >10 were found to be 100% specific for haematological disorders. However, as with any diagnostic test, sFLC results should always be interpreted in the context of the patient's symptoms and other test results *(Chapter 7)*.

23.4. The sensitivity of abnormal sFLC ratios for Bence Jones proteinuria

As indicated in the IMWG guidelines[4], the logical use of sFLC analysis in screening is as a replacement for urinalysis, and a number of studies have directly analysed the sensitivity of serum assays for identifying patients with urinary Bence Jones protein (uBJP). The largest study is discussed above *(Section 23.2)* and reported that serum tests (including sFLC) identified almost all patients requiring medical intervention, with the exception of some patients with AL amyloidosis[5].

Results from other studies have also reached this conclusion: Hill et al. reported 15 patients with uBJP, of whom 12 were detected by SPE plus sFLC[12]. The remaining three patients all had uBJP concentrations measured at ~50mg/L, and only 1 of these had persistent uBJP; however, as a skeletal survey and bone marrow biopsy were negative, this was consistent with a diagnosis of FLC-only MGUS. Beetham and colleagues[14] concluded that uIFE should still be included in a screening algorithm, but of the 34 patients found to have uBJP in their screening study, 26 had abnormal κ/λ ratios, and of the remaining eight, only one MGUS patient (with uBJP <50 mg/L) did not have a serum monoclonal protein identified.

Finally, Holding et al.[3] reviewed 126 patients who had a newly diagnosed monoclonal gammopathy with uBJP and found that 124 had abnormal sFLC results, while the remaining 2 also had IgGκ paraproteins detected by SPE, so serum analysis would have identified all 126 cases. Holding et al.[3] also presented a detailed review of similar studies, highlighting how the use of concentrated versus unconcentrated urine or uIFE versus UPE (as an initial test) would have influenced the results. In addition, it was also noted that when uBJP had been identified in patients with normal sFLC ratios, the concentration of urinary FLC determined by electrophoretic methods was always low, indicating that the discrepant results were unlikely to have been caused by the polyclonal antibodies (in the sFLC assays) failing to recognise the patients' FLCs (Section 24.9).

23.5. Issues with urine compliance

When screening for plasma cell disorders, the desirability of obtaining urine samples to test for uBJP has long been recognised, and included in diagnostic guidelines for more than a decade (e.g. IMWG guidelines, 2003[30]). In spite of this, published audits and studies have usually indicated that less than 50% of sera that were sent to laboratories to screen for monoclonal gammopathies had an accompanying urine sample. Table 23.5 records the urine compliance from recent screening studies. Irrespective of the relative sensitivities of urine electrophoresis and sFLC analysis for monoclonal FLC detection, urine can only be examined if it is provided. Table 23.5 demonstrates that one very clear, practical advantage of using sFLC analysis is the fact that it can be performed on the same sample that is provided for SPE/sIFE analysis.

Screening study	Number of sera	Urine compliance
Hill et al. (2006)[12]	923	40%
Beetham et al. (2007)[14]	932	52%
Abadie et al. (2009)[11]	-	35%
Robson et al. (2009)[18]	653	<5%
Holding et al. (2011)[3]	753	17%
McTaggart et al. (2011)[21]	2799	21%

Table 23.5. Published urine compliance rates.

23.6. Organisational and cost implications of screening algorithms

Hill et al.[12] compared the costs of urine electrophoretic tests with sFLC immunoassays in routine screening. On a per-patient basis, costs increased by £4.73 if sFLC tests were used. However, this figure compared sFLC analysis in 100% of the patients with urine analysis in only 40% (due to poor compliance). Furthermore, savings made due to the reduction of time spent interpreting urine electrophoresis gels were unquantified and the authors concluded in favour of sFLC analysis, as better clinical governance was achieved with more clinical diagnoses. Potential organisational benefits, through replacing urine electrophoresis with sFLC assays, were also identified at the Christie Hospital, Manchester, UK; this study considered monitoring as well as screening and the data is presented in Section 24.10. The combination of CZE plus sFLC (e.g. Bakshi et al.[9], Holding et al.[3], Vermeersch et al.[16]) gives the opportunity of a more automated screening procedure, and may further reduce operating costs.

McTaggart et al.[21] noted that testing all patients for FLC production by urine analysis would require more staff than currently employed, whereas 100% testing with sFLC analysis did not require extra staff as the technique was less labour-intensive. Fulton and Fernando[17] reached similar conclusions in their review of screening strategies, and suggested that incorporation of sFLC analysis in the screening algorithm could reduce the volume of "labour-intensive" sIFE and urine electrophoresis while still increasing the detection of monoclonal proteins.

Katzmann et al.[7] compared the costs of sFLC screening with urine testing in the USA. The 2006 Medicare reimbursement for sFLCs was $38 compared with $71 for urine assays (total protein, UPE and uIFE). As sFLC tests cost approximately half that of urine tests, considerable laboratory savings could be made. Zia & Singh[31] reviewed testing patterns from an inner-city hospital in Midwestern USA (2009-2012) and found that costs could be reduced in spite of increased sFLC testing by more selective use of sIFE and UPEP/uIFE analysis.

Direct assessments of clinical cost benefits are difficult to make. However, one relatively simple clinical situation that may benefit by measuring sFLCs is the determination of underlying pathology in patients presenting with acute kidney injury *(Chapter 27)*. If MM is suspected, the normal procedure has been to perform SPE/IFE and UPE. A simpler and better approach would be to perform SPE and sFLCs, which provides a rapid screen for monoclonal disease. Early diagnosis is essential in these patients and would allow the prompt initiation of disease-specific treatment and prevent irreversible renal damage and the need for long-term dialysis[23]. Data from a health economics study of this particular diagnostic issue has now been published by Cook et al.[32] who reported that there were economic gains (for the use of SPE + Freelite®) at both diagnostic and treatment stages. The use of sFLC analysis reduced the time to diagnosis and treatment and thereby improved the probability of both renal recovery and survival.

Test Questions

1. How do sFLC assays fit into routine testing for monoclonal proteins?
2. When should urine electrophoresis still be included in a monoclonal gammopathy screening algorithm?

2. If AL amyloidosis is suspected (Section 23.2)

1. sFLC tests should be added to SPE/IFE tests (Section 23.2).

Answers

References

1. Rajkumar SV, Kyle RA, Therneau TM, Melton LJ, III, Bradwell AR, Clark RJ et al. Serum free light chain ratio is an independent risk factor for progression in monoclonal gammopathy of undetermined significance. Blood 2005;106:812-7

2. Marien G, Oris E, Bradwell AR, Blanckaert N, Bossuyt X. Detection of monoclonal proteins in sera by capillary zone electrophoresis and free light chain measurements. Clin Chem 2002;48:1600-1

3. Holding S, Spradbery D, Hoole R, Wilmot R, Shields ML, Levoguer AM, Dore PC. Use of serum free light chain analysis and urine protein electrophoresis for detection of monoclonal gammopathies. Clin Chem Lab Med 2011;49:83-8

4. Dispenzieri A, Kyle R, Merlini G, Miguel JS, Ludwig H, Hajek R et al. International Myeloma Working Group guidelines for serum-free light chain analysis in multiple myeloma and related disorders. Leukemia 2009;23:215-24

5. Katzmann JA, Kyle RA, Benson J, Larson DR, Snyder MR, Lust JA et al. Screening panels for detection of monoclonal gammopathies. Clin Chem 2009;55:1517-22

6. Palladini G, Russo P, Bosoni T, Verga L, Sarais G, Lavatelli F et al. Identification of amyloidogenic light chains requires the combination of serum-free light chain assay with immunofixation of serum and urine. Clin Chem 2009;55:499-504

7. Katzmann JA, Dispenzieri A, Kyle RA, Snyder MR, Plevak MF, Larson DR et al. Elimination of the need for urine studies in the screening algorithm for monoclonal gammopathies by using serum immunofixation and free light chain assays. Mayo Clin Proc 2006;81:1575-8

8. Hofmann W, Garbrecht M, Bradwell AR, Guder WG. A new concept for detection of Bence Jones proteinuria in patients with monoclonal gammopathy. Clin Lab 2004;50:181-5

9. Bakshi NA, Gulbranson R, Garstka D, Bradwell AR, Keren DF. Serum free light chain (FLC) measurement can aid capillary zone electrophoresis in detecting subtle FLC-producing M proteins. Am J Clin Pathol 2005;124:214-8

10. Foray V, Chapuis-Cellier C. Contribution of serum free light chain immunoassays in diagnosis and monitoring of free light chain monoclonal gammopathies. Immuno-analyse et Biologie Specialisee 2005;20:385-93

11. Abadie JM, Bankson DD. Assessment of serum free light chain assays for plasma cell disorder screening in a Veterans Affairs population. Ann Clin Lab Sci 2006;36:157-62

12. Hill PG, Forsyth JM, Rai B, Mayne S. Serum free light chains: an alternative to the urine Bence Jones proteins screening test for monoclonal gammopathies. Clin Chem 2006;52:1743-8

13. Reid SD, Katsavara H, Augustson BM, Hutchison CA, Mead GP, Shirfield M et al. Screening for monoclonal gammopathy: inclusion of serum free light chain immunoassays produce an increased detection rate. Clin Chem 2006;52:E37a

14. Beetham R, Wassell J, Wallage MJ, Whiteway AJ, James JA. Can serum free light chains replace urine electrophoresis in the detection of monoclonal gammopathies? Ann Clin Biochem 2007;44:516-22

15. Piehler AP, Gulbrandsen N, Kierulf P, Urdal P. Quantitation of serum free light chains in combination with protein electrophoresis and clinical information for diagnosing multiple myeloma in a general hospital population. Clin Chem 2008;54:1823-30

16. Vermeersch P, Van Hoovels L, Delforge M, Marien G, Bossuyt X. Diagnostic performance of serum free light chain measurement in patients suspected of a monoclonal B-cell disorder. Br J Haematol 2008;143:496-502

17. Fulton RB, Fernando SL. Serum free light chain assay reduces the need for serum and urine immunofixation electrophoresis in the evaluation of monoclonal gammopathy. Ann Clin Biochem 2009;46:407-12

18. Robson EJD, Taylor J, Beardsmore C, Basu S, Mead G, Lovatt T. Utility of serum free light chain analysis when screening for lymphoproliferative disorders. Lab Med 2009;40:325-9

19. Park JW, Kim YK, Bae EH, Ma SK, Kim SW. Combined analysis using extended renal reference range of serum free light chain ratio and serum protein electrophoresis improves the diagnostic accuracy of multiple myeloma in renal insufficiency. Clin Biochem 2012;45:740-4

20. Jeong TD, Kim SY, Jang S, Park CJ, Chi HS, Lee W et al. Diagnostic sensitivity of a panel of tests to detect monoclonal protein in Korean multiple myeloma patients. Clin Chem Lab Med 2013;e187-e189

21. McTaggart MP, Kearney EM. Evidence-based use of serum protein electrophoresis in laboratory medicine. Clin Chem Lab Med 2013;51:e113-e115

22. Hutchison CA, Harding S, Hewins P, Mead GP, Townsend J, Bradwell AR, Cockwell P. Quantitative assessment of serum and urinary polyclonal free light chains in patients with chronic kidney disease. Clin J Am Soc Nephrol 2008;3:1684-90

23. Hutchison CA, Plant T, Drayson M, Cockwell P, Kountouri M, Basnayake K et al. Serum free light chain measurement aids the diagnosis of myeloma in patients with severe renal failure. BMC Nephrol 2008;9:11

24. Gerth J, Sachse A, Busch M, Illner N, Muegge LO, Grone HJ, Wolf G. Screening and differential diagnosis of renal light chain-associated diseases. Kidney Blood Press Res 2011;35:120-8

25. Abadie JM, van Hoeven KH, Wells JM. Are renal reference intervals required when screening for plasma cell disorders with serum free light chains and serum protein electrophoresis? Am J Clin Pathol 2009;131:166-71

26. Marshall G, Tate J, Mollee P. Borderline high serum free light chain k/l ratios are seen not only in dialysis patients but also in non-dialysis-dependent renal impairment and inflammatory states. Am J Clin Pathol 2009;132:309

27. Beetham R. Detection of Bence-Jones protein in practice. Ann Clin Biochem 2000;37:563-70

28. McTaggart MP, Lindsay J, Kearney EM. Replacing urine protein electrophoresis with serum free light chain analysis as a first-line test for detecting plasma cell disorders offers increased diagnostic accuracy and potential health benefit to patients. Am J Clin Pathol 2013;140:890-7

29. Vermeersch P, Vercammen M, Holvoet A, Broeck IV, Delforge M, Bossuyt X. Use of interval-specific likelihood ratios improves clinical interpretation of serum FLC results for the diagnosis of malignant plasma cell disorders. Clin Chim Acta 2009;410:54-8

30. Kyle R, Child JA, Anderson K, Barlogie B, Bataille R, Bensinger W et al. Criteria for the classification of monoclonal gammopathies, multiple myeloma and related disorders: a report of the International Myeloma Working Group. Br J Haematol 2003;121:749-57

31. Zia HM, Singh G. Optimization of utilization of serum protein analysis: role of the electronic medical record in promoting consultation by pathology. Am J Clin Pathol 2013;139:793-7

32. Cook M, Cockwell P, Almond C, Cranmer H, Harding S, Hughes R et al. Serum free light chain assays in the early detection of cast nephropathy in patients presenting with unexplained acute kidney injury (AKI): Results from a pharmacoeconomic evaluation. Blood 2014;124:2612a

Serum versus urine tests for free light chains

Summary:

- Normal renal tubular metabolism prevents urine excretion of significant amounts of monoclonal FLCs. This mechanism ensures that some patients have abnormal sFLCs but normal urine.

- Urine is not usually supplied at initial patient screening, whereas a serum sample is available.

- Methodology for urine electrophoresis varies considerably between laboratories, and interpretation can be challenging.

- Further benefits of sFLC analysis over urine tests include improved clinical sensitivity and a more rapid reporting turnaround time.

24.1. Introduction

Most of the issues relating to the use of serum versus urine for the measurement of free light chains (FLCs) have been detailed individually in preceding chapters. This chapter summarises these arguments and attempts to provide a coherent discussion of the relative merits of serum versus urine testing. Some laboratories continue to favour urine over serum measurements: this chapter aims to persuade them otherwise. An analogy with diabetes mellitus is helpful: 50 years ago, all patients were monitored using urine glucose tests, whereas now they are monitored using blood glucose due to its overwhelming clinical advantages. As glucose and FLCs are handled in a similar manner by the kidneys, similar benefits accrue from testing serum over urine for FLC analysis.

"If free light chains are in the urine they are always in the serum first".

24.2. Renal threshold for FLC excretion

As described in Chapter 3, serum FLCs (sFLCs) are cleared primarily through the renal glomeruli and then metabolised in the proximal tubules of the nephrons. Only when the tubular absorptive capacity is exceeded are significant amounts of FLCs observed in the urine as "overflow proteinuria". Since normal production is about 500 mg/day and the renal absorptive capacity is 10 - 30 g/day, production must increase many times before urine contains measurable quantities of FLCs[1].

The clinical effect of renal tubular absorption on urine FLC concentrations is shown in Figure 24.1. Serum and urine FLC concentrations were compared in four patients undergoing treatment[2]. Patients 1 and 2 had large amounts of serum and urine FLCs with good correlations between changes in concentrations. In patients 3 and 4, urine FLC excretion was minimal and unchanging over many months, while serum levels could be used to monitor the changing tumour burden. Despite similar sFLC concentrations, there were no urine FLCs in these latter patients because there was no renal impairment, and therefore, no overflow proteinuria.

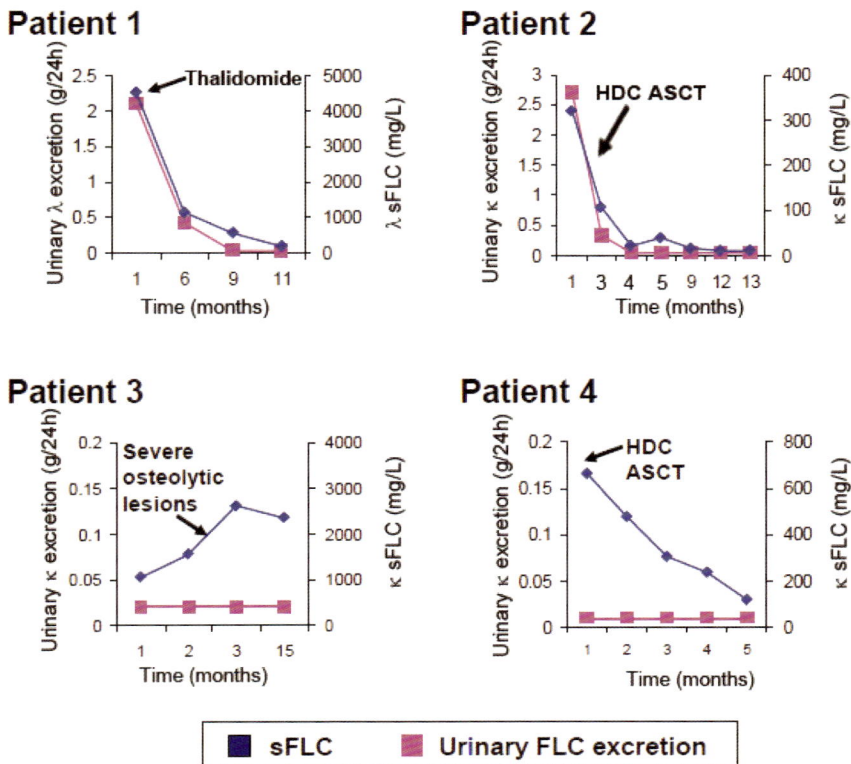

Figure 24.1. Serum and urine FLCs in four patients with light chain multiple myeloma (LCMM) or AL amyloidosis. Serum tests (blue) were useful even when urine FLC excretion (pink) was minimal in patients 3 and 4. HDC ASCT: high-dose chemotherapy autologous stem cell transplant. (Reproduced with permission from the American Journal of Hematology[2] and John Wiley and Sons).

Nowrousian et al.[3] studied the concentrations of sFLCs necessary to cause overflow proteinuria and a positive urinary immunofixation electrophoresis (uIFE) test result, in a group of patients attending a myeloma clinic. Of 98 serum samples with monoclonal κ sFLCs, the corresponding urine was positive for monoclonal FLCs (urinary Bence Jones protein; uBJP) by uIFE in 51% of cases. The median κ sFLC concentration associated with positive uBJP was 113 mg/L (range 7 - 39,500), and 40 mg/L (range 6 - 710) for negative urine *(Figure 24.2)*. Of the 107 serum samples with monoclonal λ sFLCs, the corresponding urine was positive for uBJP in 35% of cases. The median λ sFLC concentration associated with positive uBJP was 278 mg/L (range 5 - 7,060), and 44 mg/L (range 3 - 561) for negative urine. The large overlap of sFLC concentrations between patients with/without uBJP presumably reflects differences in renal reabsorptive capacity and the extent of renal damage between individuals.

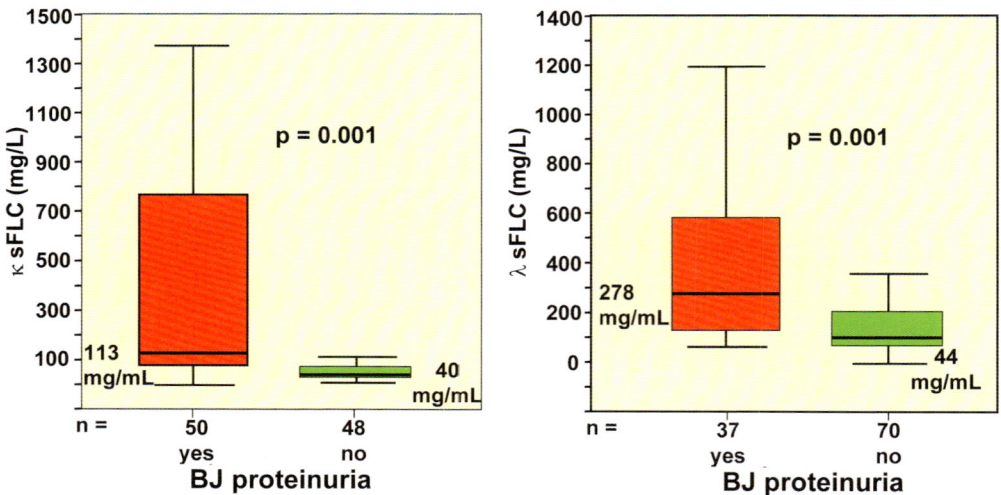

Figure 24.2. Amounts of sFLCs required to produce light chain proteinuria for κ and λ myelomas. The median (line), 95% ranges (boxes) and 100% ranges (whiskers) are shown. (Courtesy of MR Nowrousian).

Thus, median sFLC levels associated with uBJP were 5-fold above normal for κ-producing patients (upper limit of normal range: 19.4 mg/L) and 10-fold for λ patients (upper limit of normal range: 26.3 mg/L) when the urine contained uBJP. The higher serum levels necessary for λ overflow proteinuria can be explained by the dimerisation of λ molecules. This reduces glomerular filtration compared with monomeric κ molecules *(Chapter 3)*. Therefore, when FLC production is below the renal reabsorptive capacity, serum tests are more sensitive than urinalysis for detecting monoclonal FLC[2,4].

24.3. Problems measuring urine samples

Urinary FLC measurements are normally based upon electrophoretic tests: urine protein electrophoresis (UPE) and uIFE *(Chapter 4)*. The methodology employed for urine electrophoresis varies considerably between laboratories, and contributes to quantitative differences in the results reported. In addition, the visual interpretation of electrophoretic gels presents many challenges even to experienced users. These include "ladder banding" and high background staining in the presence of proteinuria.

Furthermore, difficulties of 24-hour urine collection include: 1) collections are cumbersome for patients with painful or fractured bones; 2) accurate timing of a 24-hour collection is important but may be difficult for ill patients; 3) large volumes of urine are produced in polyuric patients - perhaps larger than the bottle volume; 4) problems can occur handling and storing large volumes of urine at the laboratory; 5) collections may be embarrassing in front of friends or work colleagues.

Consistent with the various issues described above, Siegel et al.[5] reported that urine electrophoresis results can be highly susceptible to error. Analysis of laboratory results from 207 monoclonal gammopathy patients, monitored during treatment and follow-up, revealed fluctuating urine electrophoresis results and 19% of urine samples were reported to have unexpectedly high monoclonal protein levels. The samples with these elevated results had correspondingly high creatinine clearance data suggesting that errors in the measurement of 24-hour urine volumes had occurred. No such fluctuations were observed for sFLC values. An example is shown in Figure 24.3.

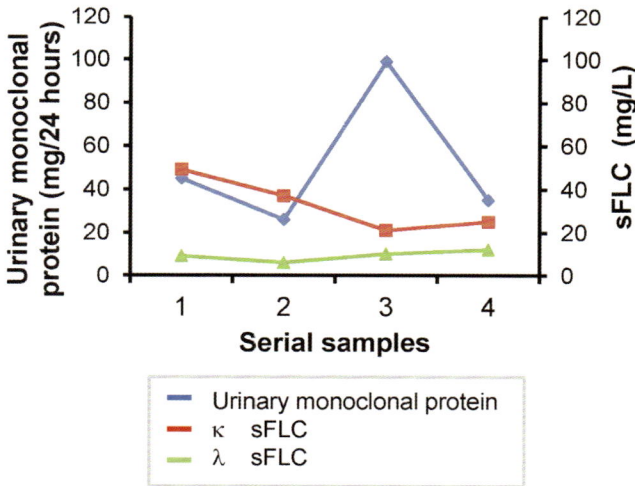

Figure 24.3. Example of a clinically unexpected increase in 24-hour urine protein.
Graph based on data supplied in[5].

Figure 24.4 compares serum and urine results in a patient with relapsing light chain multiple myeloma (LCMM). The FLC concentrations in both fluids are considerably elevated, indicating that the renal threshold is exceeded (compare with patients 3 and 4 in *Figure 24.1*). However, the urine measurements are variable and do not show a definitive rise until day 160. By contrast, the steady rise in sFLC concentrations from day 40 indicates relapse of the tumour 3 to 4 months earlier.

In addition to the analytical issues described above, biological variation of FLCs may contribute to variations in both serum and urine measurements *(Section 7.2.6)*.

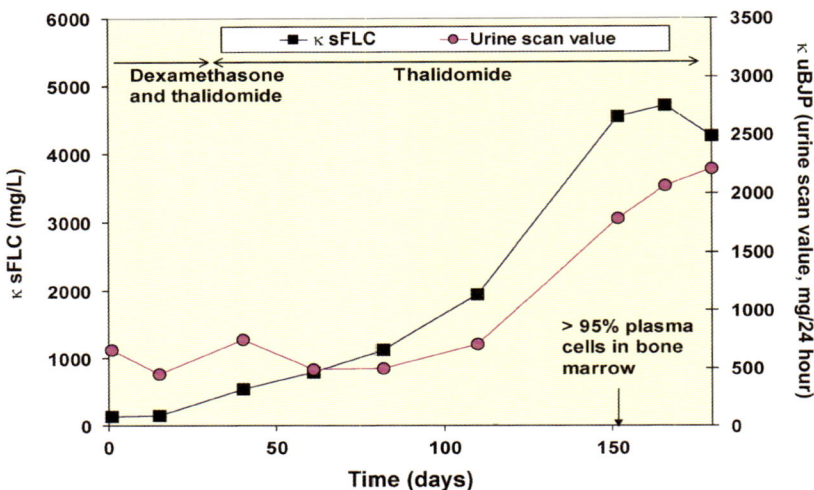

Figure 24.4. Serum and urine FLCs in a patient with LCMM. *Disease relapse can be identified 3 months earlier using serum rather than urine samples.*

24.4. Urine compliance

Urine provision remains an important issue in the serum versus urine debate; lack of urine with diagnostic serum samples has repeatedly been reported *(Section 23.5)*. Even once a diagnosis of monoclonal gammopathy has been confirmed, problems with urine provision continue. In a study of 496 newly diagnosed monoclonal gammopathy patients by Holding et al.[6], only 30% of serum samples had a matched urine sample provided within 7 days; this increased to 57% within 90 days. In a review of 55 multiple myeloma (MM) patients referred for autologous stem cell transplantation between 2006 and 2011, Fidler et al.[7] noted that 24-hour urine compliance was 55% and apparently falling, while sFLC compliance was slightly better (67%), and appeared to be rising over the same period.

Overall, the annual UK National Pathology Benchmarking Review for 2007/2008 reported that the number of UPE tests performed was much lower than serum protein electrophoresis (SPE), comprising only 14% of SPE requests (298,392)[6]. The authors of a screening study carried out at New Cross Hospital, Wolverhampton, UK, reported an extremely poor provision of matched urine samples (<5%) and concluded that "the debate over the relative merits of the sFLC assay versus uBJP analysis borders on the irrelevant"[8].

24.5. Urine FLC immunoassays

As an alternative to urine electrophoretic tests, FLC immunoassays can be used on urine samples *(Section 4.5.3)*. Although Van Hoeven et al.[9] reported that the sensitivity of urine FLC assays was greater than UPE for FLC measurement (75% vs. 44%; n=73), all data indicate that uIFE remains the most sensitive assay for the identification of monoclonal proteins in urine[10,11]. However, urinary FLC immunoassays do not solve any of the problems relating to renal threshold, urine collection and urine measurement indicated above. Furthermore, the diagnostic sensitivity of sFLC ratios is superior to urine FLC measurements[12]; this is a function of the proximal tubule absorption of FLCs and the much wider normal ranges for urinary FLC concentrations and the κ/λ FLC ratio *(Section 6.4)*[10].

The International Myeloma Working Group (IMWG) guidelines recommend sFLC assays in combination with SPE and serum IFE (sIFE) to screen for pathological monoclonal plasma cell proliferative disorders other than AL amyloidosis, which also requires a 24-hour uIFE[13]. The guidelines also state that "Measurement of urine FLC levels is not recommended" *(Chapter 25)*.

24.6. Clinical benefits of sFLC analysis

The improved sensitivity of serum over urine FLC measurements has had a major impact on the ease of diagnosis, monitoring and assessing risk of progression for many patients with the following diseases:

1. Light chain multiple myeloma (LCMM) *(Chapter 15)*.
2. Nonsecretory multiple myeloma (NSMM) *(Chapter 16)*.
3. Intact immunoglobulin multiple myeloma (IIMM) *(Chapters 17 and 18)*.
4. Smouldering multiple myeloma (SMM) *(Chapter 14)*.
5. Cast nephropathy *(Chapter 27)*.
6. Plasmacytoma *(Chapter 21)*.
7. AL amyloidosis *(Chapter 28)*.
8. Light chain deposition disease (LCDD) *(Chapter 29)*.
9. Monoclonal gammopathy of undetermined significance (MGUS) *(Chapter 13)*.

Figure 24.5 illustrates sFLC concentrations in patients with low monoclonal immunoglobulin production rates at the time of clinical diagnosis. Samples from patients with NSMM are shown as white circles which, by definition, have no detectable monoclonal proteins by both serum and urine electrophoretic tests. Hence, other patients with monoclonal sFLCs at or below these concentrations but with other types of plasma cell dyscrasias are difficult to identify by conventional tests. The figure also includes samples from many patients with AL amyloidosis and IIMM who were in remission by IFE.

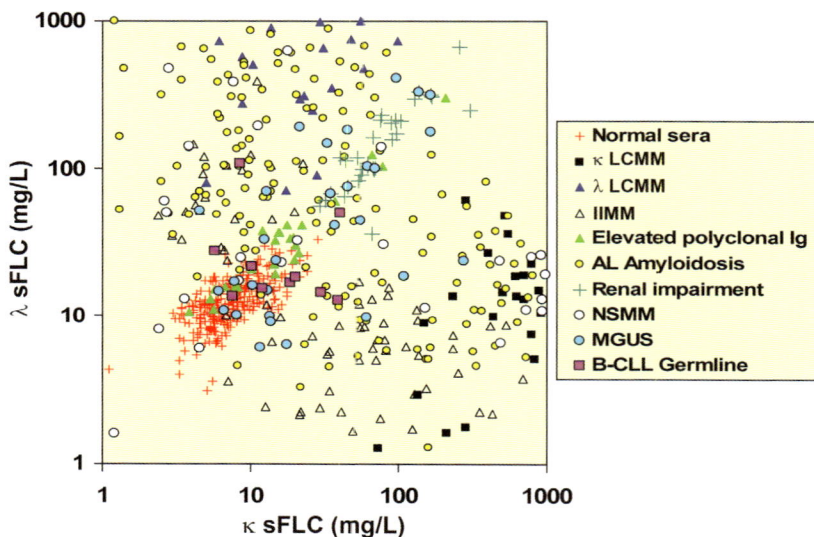

Figure 24.5. sFLCs in patients with low monoclonal immunoglobulin production rates. By electrophoretic tests, sFLCs are usually undetectable or unquantifiable in most of these patients. (See relevant chapters for details of the patient data).

24.7. Elimination of urine studies when screening for monoclonal gammopathies

A number of studies have now been published identifying the benefit of including sFLC analysis in screening protocols for lymphoproliferative disorders. In addition, two large diagnostic studies from the Mayo clinic[14,15] led to the conclusion that urine analysis could be eliminated, unless AL amyloidosis was suspected. These data are presented and discussed in Chapter 23 and the conclusions are now reflected in the IMWG guidelines *(Chapter 25)*.

24.8. Comparison of sFLCs and urinalysis for monitoring patients

Apart from the practical advantages of using serum samples rather than urine, the main advantage of monitoring patients with serum tests derives from their greater clinical sensitivity. The main studies are reported in detail in the relevant chapters, listed in Section 24.6, and monitoring examples are shown in Figure 24.1 and Section 15.2.

The relative sensitivity of the serum and urine tests was first highlighted more than a decade ago in a retrospective analysis of monitoring samples from 82 LCMM patients[1]. After treatment, 32% of patients achieved complete remission (CR) according to their urine results while only 11% achieved normalisation of their sFLC ratios; a percentage closely aligned to the 9.8% CR rate seen in patients monitored by their monoclonal intact immunoglobulin (and receiving the same treatment). Similar results were obtained by Avet-Loiseau et al.[16] in a large retrospective analysis of the IFM 2007-01 trial, comparing the utility of urine electrophoresis and sFLC measurements in monitoring MM. In 50% of uIFE-positive IIMM patients, uIFE became negative after two cycles of therapy compared with 5% by the κ/λ sFLC ratio. Similarly in LCMM, uIFE became negative in 50% of patients compared with 10% by sFLC. A further study from the same research group[17] compared sFLC and urine electrophoresis measurements for monitoring 25 LCMM patients; they found that sFLC was always more sensitive for the detection of residual disease and showed a better correlation with sIFE results. A further large comparison of sFLC analysis and urine electrophoresis included 700 patients (115 LCMM) from a 2009 French MM trial[18]. As previously, sFLC analysis was found to be more sensitive than urinalysis and showed better agreement with assessments in the IIMM patients, leading the authors to propose that the guidelines for response assessment in LCMM should incorporate sFLC measurement (see below). Katzmann et al.[19] assessed the monitoring potential of sFLCs and urinary monoclonal proteins (utilising UPE) in patients with clinically stable monoclonal gammopathy. The authors concluded that sFLCs were measurable in more patients than were urinary monoclonal proteins, and that sFLC measurements exhibited a lower total coefficient of variation (see also *Section 7.2.6*).

The correlation between serial measurements of sFLCs and urine monoclonal protein (by UPE) is insufficient to consider the tests interchangeable[20]. Consequently, international guidelines from 2009[13] recommended monitoring MM patients with sFLCs in the following situations: 1) in all MM patients who do not have sufficient concentrations of measurable serum or urine intact immunoglobulin monoclonal proteins (serum monoclonal protein <10 g/L or a urine monoclonal protein <200 mg/24 hours); and 2) in all MM patients to look for a "stringent complete response" *(Chapter 25)*. It seems probable that, as experience and confidence in the sFLC assays grows, they will increasingly replace the measurement of FLCs in urine for monitoring patients.

24.9. Discrepant serum and urine results

As demonstrated above, sFLC analysis is generally more sensitive than urine electrophoresis for indicating the presence of monoclonal FLCs. However, this advantage is dependent upon efficient renal reabsorption of FLCs *(Section 3.5)*. The renal metabolism of filtered FLCs combined with the analytical sensitivity and specificity of sFLC analysis over conventional urine tests makes sFLC analysis superior for the diagnosis and monitoring of monoclonal gammopathies associated with FLC production.

Occasionally, patients are reported to have "positive" urine when sFLC results are normal. This may be due to a number a reasons: 1) serum and urine samples collected at different time points; 2) false positive urine results (caused by the staining of intact immunoglobulin in urine); or 3) true positive urine results (when proximal tubule reabsorption is impaired). Such discrepant results and other scenarios are further discussed in Section 7.6.

24.10. Organisational cost savings and other benefits of sFLC analysis

As well as improved clinical diagnosis, there are organisational cost savings and other benefits to introducing sFLC assays. The laboratory issues and costs were analysed in 2004 at the Christie Hospital in Manchester, UK[21]. Superior analytical performance of the serum assays, faster reporting times and reduced laboratory costs were identified *(Table 24.1)*. Cost benefits in relation to clinical outcomes were not analysed in this study but they may accrue from earlier diagnosis and by treatments that reduce morbidity. It is well known that a delay in the diagnosis of MM is associated with more complications and reduced disease-free survival[22].

Most comparisons of the relative cost/benefits of serum versus urine FLC analysis have been made in the context of screening studies and these are presented in Section 23.6.

	sFLCs	Urine electrophoresis
Sensitivity	1.5 mg/L	50 mg/L
Precision	5%	>15%
Analysis time	15 minutes	1 hour
Reporting turnaround	1 hour	1 week
Cost per year (700 requests)	£6,500	£4,500
Extra staff costs per year	£0	£1,000
24-hour urine bottle usage	Not relevant	£1,000
Storage needs	30 cm^3	10 m^3

Table 24.1. Analytical and cost/benefit study of sFLC and urine electrophoresis tests[21].

24.11. Conclusions

If a choice has to be made between serum or urine tests, then the use of serum is clearly preferable for the many reasons given above and summarised in Table 24.2[23]. When both serum and urine tests are available, it is clinically reassuring to have two separate tests. Clearly, samples do occasionally get incorrectly analysed, mislabelled or misplaced, so supporting evidence for making a diagnosis or changing treatment is always helpful. In the context of a stem cell transplant in MM patients, for example, the additional cost of performing both serum and urine tests is inconsequential.

Serum versus urine measurements	
sFLC	**Urine electrophoresis**
Easy to collect	Difficult to collect
κ/λ ratio less affected by renal function	Renal function affects levels
Easily analysed	Samples may need concentrating
Easily stored	More difficult to store
More frequently abnormal in NSMM and AL amyloidosis	Less frequently abnormal
More sensitive for monitoring patients	Less sensitive for monitoring patients

Table 24.2. Summary of clinical and analytical comparisons of sFLC and urine electrophoresis tests[23].

Test Questions

1. Is there any remaining role for urine FLC tests when screening for monoclonal gammopathies?
2. Why are patients with excess monoclonal κ sFLCs more likely to have positive urine results?
3. Which is the more sensitive for detection of residual disease, serum or urine FLC analysis?

References

1. Bradwell AR, Carr-Smith HD, Mead GP, Harvey TC, Drayson MT. Serum test for assessment of patients with Bence Jones myeloma. Lancet 2003;361:489-91

2. Alyanakian MA, Abbas A, Delarue R, Arnulf B, Aucouturier P. Free immunoglobulin light-chain serum levels in the follow-up of patients with monoclonal gammopathies: correlation with 24-hr urinary light-chain excretion. Am J Hematol 2004;75:246-8

3. Nowrousian MR, Brandhorst D, Sammet C, Kellert M, Daniels R, Schuett P et al. Serum free light chain analysis and urine immunofixation electrophoresis in patients with multiple myeloma. Clin Cancer Res 2005;11:8706-14

4. Abadie JM, van Hoeven KH, Wells JM. Are renal reference intervals required when screening for plasma cell disorders with serum free light chains and serum protein electrophoresis? Am J Clin Pathol 2009;131:166-71

5. Siegel DS, McBride L, Bilotti E, Lendvai N, Gonsky J, Berges T et al. Inaccuracies in 24-hour urine testing for monoclonal gammopathies. Lab Med 2009;40:341-4

6. Holding S, Spradbery D, Hoole R, Wilmot R, Shields ML, Levoguer AM, Dore PC. Use of serum free light chain analysis and urine protein electrophoresis for detection of monoclonal gammopathies. Clin Chem Lab Med 2011;49:83-8

7. Fidler CJ, Hussein AKA, Gandhi N, Karur V, Sharma M, Klumpp TR et al. Evaluating trends in diagnostic and prognostic testing for multiple myeloma. Blood 2011;118:2067a

8. Robson EJD, Taylor J, Beardsmore C, Basu S, Mead G, Lovatt T. Utility of serum free light chain analysis when screening for lymphoproliferative disorders. Lab Med 2009;40:325-9

9. van Hoeven KH, Bilotti E, McBride L, Berges T, McNeill A, Schillen D, Siegel D. Serum free light chain assays are more sensitive than urinary tests for light chain monoclonal proteins. Clin Chem 2009;55:C30a

10. Snyder MR, Clark R, Bryant SC, Katzmann JA. Quantification of urinary light chains. Clin Chem 2008;54:1744-6

11. Viedma JA, Garrigos N, Morales S. Comparison of the sensitivity of 2 automated immunoassays with immunofixation electrophoresis for detecting urine Bence Jones proteins. Clin Chem 2005;51:1505–7

12. Herzog W, Hofmann W. Detection of free kappa and lambda light chains in serum and urine in patients with monoclonal gammopathy. Blood 2003;102:5190a

13. Dispenzieri A, Kyle R, Merlini G, Miguel JS, Ludwig H, Hajek R, et al. International Myeloma Working Group guidelines for serum-free light chain analysis in multiple myeloma and related disorders. Leukemia 2009;23:215-24

14. Katzmann JA, Dispenzieri A, Kyle RA, Snyder MR, Plevak MF, Larson DR, et al. Elimination of the need for urine studies in the screening algorithm for monoclonal gammopathies by using serum immunofixation and free light chain assays. Mayo Clin Proc 2006;81:1575–8

15. Katzmann JA, Kyle RA, Benson J, Larson DR, Snyder MR, Lust JA, et al. Screening panels for detection of monoclonal gammopathies. Clin Chem 2009;55:1517-22

16. Avet-Loiseau H, Mirbahai L, Mathiot C, Attal M, Moreau P, Harousseau J et al. Comparison of serum free light chain ratios with standard urine analysis in diagnosis and monitoring of multiple myeloma. Haematologica 2011;96:P-075a

17. Avet-Loiseau H, Young P, Mathiot C, Attal M, Harousseau J, Bradwell AR, Mirbahai L. Nephelometric measurements of kFLC and lFLC for monitoring light chain myeloma patients. Haematologica 2011;96:0853a

18. Corre J, Dejoie T, Caillon H, Attal M, Avet-Loiseau H, Moreau P. Serum free light chains should be the target of response evaluation in light chain multiple myeloma rather than urines: results from the IFM/DFCI 2009 trial. Blood 2014;124:180a

19. Katzmann JA, Snyder MR, Rajkumar SV, Kyle RA, Therneau TM, Benson JT, Dispenzieri A. Long-term biologic variation of serum protein electrophoresis M-spike, urine M-spike, and monoclonal serum free light chain quantification: implications for monitoring monoclonal gammopathies. Clin Chem 2011;57:1687-92

20. Dispenzieri A, Zhang L, Katzmann JA, Snyder M, Blood E, Degoey R et al. Appraisal of immunoglobulin free light chain as a marker of response. Blood 2008;111:4908-15

21. Carr-Smith HD, Harland B, Anderson J, Overton J, Wieringa G, Bradwell AR. The effect on laboratory organisation of introducing serum free light chain assays. Clin Chem 2004;50:A76a

22. Kariyawasan CC, Hughes DA, Jayatillake MM, Mehta AB. Multiple myeloma: causes and consequences of delay in diagnosis. QJM 2007;100:635-40

23. Carr-Smith HD, Mead GP, Bradwell AR. Serum free light chain assays as a replacement for urine electrophoresis. Haematologica 2005;90:PO404a

Guidelines for multiple myeloma and related disorders

Summary:

• Freelite® assays are recommended by name in International Myeloma Working Group guidelines.

• An involved/uninvolved sFLC ratio of ≥100 (and an involved sFLC concentration of ≥100 mg/L) is one of the diagnostic criteria for multiple myeloma.

25.1. Introduction

National and international guidelines for identifying and managing patients with plasma cell dyscrasias are published and updated on a regular basis. These guidelines are widely adopted for assessing new patients and for patient entry into clinical trials. This chapter provides an overview of guidelines that include serum free light chain (sFLC) and/or immunoglobulin heavy/light chain (Hevylite®; HLC) analysis (identified in blue). This chapter contains the guidelines for multiple myleloma (MM) and some related disorders while guidelines for AL amyloidosis are covered in Chapter 28.

All guidelines and proposed clinical utilities relating to sFLCs have been based upon data generated using Freelite® kits manufactured by The Binding Site. In some countries, products intended for measurement of sFLC have been made available by other manufacturers (Chapter 8). Trials of such products have produced poor correlations with sFLC concentrations determined using Freelite. Therefore, it is unlikely that other products will have the same clinical utility or give compliance with current guidelines listed in this chapter.

25.2. International Myeloma Working Group updated criteria for the diagnosis of multiple myeloma

Comprehensive guidelines on the classification of multiple myeloma (MM) and smouldering MM (SMM) were published in 2014[1], and are outlined below. In contrast to earlier guidelines[2,3,4,5], the requirement for the presence of a monoclonal protein is no longer mandatory in the MM diagnostic criteria, to account for patients with nonsecretory MM (NSMM; Chapter 16). sFLC analysis is included and an involved/uninvolved Freelite sFLC ratio ≥100 is designated as a biomarker of malignancy (Table 25.1).

25.2.1. Definition of multiple myeloma

MM is defined by the presence of clonal bone marrow plasma cells (≥10%) or biopsy-proven bony or extramedullary plasmacytoma and any one or more of the following myeloma defining events (Table 25.1)[1]:

Myeloma defining events	Details
Evidence of end organ damage that can be attributed to the underlying plasma cell proliferative disorder	**CRAB criteria:** • **Hypercalcaemia:** serum calcium >0.25 mmol/L (>1 mg/dL) higher than the upper limit of normal or >2.75 mmol/L (>11 mg/dL) • **Renal insufficiency:** creatinine clearance <40 mL per min or serum creatinine >177 µmol/L (>2 mg/dL) • **Anaemia:** haemoglobin value of >2 g/dL below the lower limit of normal, or a haemoglobin value <100 g/L • **Bone lesions:** one or more osteolytic lesions on skeletal radiography, CT, or PET-CT
Any one or more of the following biomarkers of malignancy	• Clonal bone marrow plasma cell percentage ≥60% • An involved/uninvolved sFLC ratio ≥100* • >1 focal lesion on MRI studies

Table 25.1. Myeloma defining events[1]. *These values are based on the Freelite assay. The involved FLC must be ≥100 mg/L.*

25.2.2. Definition of smouldering multiple myeloma

The definition of SMM requires that both of the following criteria must be met[1]:

- Serum monoclonal protein (IgG or IgA) ≥30 g/L or urinary monoclonal protein ≥500 mg/24 hours and/or clonal bone marrow plasma cells 10 - 60%
- Absence of myeloma defining events or amyloidosis

25.2.3. Definition of monoclonal gammopathy of undetermined significance

The MM guidelines[1] also summarise the current definitions of monoclonal gammopathy of undetermined significance (MGUS) *(Chapter 13)* and these are listed below *(Table 25.2)*:

MGUS type	Definition (all criteria must be met)
Non-IgM MGUS	• Serum monoclonal protein (non-IgM type) <30 g/L • Clonal bone marrow plasma cells <10% • Absence of end-organ damage (such as hypercalcaemia, renal insufficiency, anaemia and bone lesions [CRAB features]) or amyloidosis that can be attributed to the plasma cell proliferative disorder
IgM MGUS	• Serum IgM monoclonal protein <30 g/L • Bone marrow lymphoplasmacytic infiltration <10% • No evidence of anaemia, constitutional symptoms, hyperviscosity, lymphadenopathy, hepatosplenomegaly, or other end-organ damage that can be attributed to the underlying lymphoproliferative disorder
Light chain MGUS	• Abnormal FLC ratio (<0.26 or >1.65) • Increased level of the appropriate involved light chain (increased κ sFLCs in patients with ratio >1.65, and increased λ sFLCs in patients with ratio <0.26) • No immunoglobulin heavy chain expression on immunofixation • Absence of end-organ damage (such as CRAB features) or amyloidosis that can be attributed to the plasma cell proliferative disorder • Clonal bone marrow plasma cells <10% • Urinary monoclonal protein <500 mg/24 hours

Table 25.2. Categories of MGUS[1]. CRAB: hypercalcaemia, renal insufficiency, anaemia, bone lesions.

25.3. International Myeloma Working Group guidelines

25.3.1. Guidelines for serum free light chain analysis in multiple myeloma and related disorders (2009)

These guidelines[6] discuss published data that provides evidence for the utility and application of sFLC assays for most plasma cell disorders, including symptomatic MM, NSMM, light chain MM (LCMM), SMM, MGUS, solitary plasmacytoma and AL amyloidosis. Furthermore, the guidelines highlight key recommendations for the use of sFLC assays in screening, prognosis and in the assessment of patient response to treatment. Specific emphasis is placed on distinguishing between proven utility and those potential utilities that remain under investigation.

Screening

sFLC assays are recommended for use in combination with serum protein electrophoresis (SPE) and serum immunofixation electrophoresis (sIFE) to screen for pathological monoclonal plasma cell proliferative disorders although if AL amyloidosis is suspected, a 24-hour urine, immunofixation electrophoresis (uIFE) should also be performed.

Prognosis

It is recommended that baseline sFLC assay results are obtained at diagnosis for all patients with MGUS, SMM or active MM, solitary plasmacytoma and AL amyloidosis. Highly abnormal results have prognostic value in virtually every plasma cell disorder. Notably, in MGUS, SMM and plasmacytoma, a highly abnormal sFLC ratio indicates a substantial risk of progression to systemic disease.

Monitoring and response assessment

sFLC assays are recommended for the quantitatitve monitoring of patients with oligosecretory plasma cell disorders, including patients with AL amyloidosis, oligosecretory myeloma, and in nearly two-thirds of patients previously classified as having NSMM. Furthermore, in the absence of urinary evaluations or FLC measurements, light chain escape can be missed and so these tests should be performed periodically. Baseline results of sFLC testing are required prior to initiating new chemotherapy regimens for all patients with MM to determine if a stringent complete response has been attained after a complete response has been achieved. Despite limited published data validating the use of sFLC assays in patients with light chain deposition disease, it is stated that the personal experience of the guideline authors confirms their utility in these cases.

25.3.2. Guidelines for monoclonal gammopathy of undetermined significance and smouldering multiple myeloma (2010)

For patients with MGUS, the size of the monoclonal protein, type of monoclonal protein, sFLC ratio, as well as the proportion of aberrant plasma cells within the bone marrow are helpful in identifying patients who are at increased risk of progression[7,8,9,10,11]. These International Myeloma Working Group (IMWG) guidelines[5] recommend that patients with MGUS should be risk stratified at diagnosis, to optimise counselling and follow-up, using a model incorporating the following risk factors: 1) serum monoclonal immunoglobulin ≥15 g/L; 2) serum monoclonal immunoglobulin type (IgA or IgM); and 3) abnormal κ/λ sFLC ratio *(Table 25.3 and Chapter 13)*. For patients with low-risk MGUS, a baseline bone marrow examination or skeletal radiography is not routinely indicated. For patients with intermediate- and high-risk MGUS a bone marrow aspirate and biopsy should be carried out at baseline to rule out any underlying plasma cell malignancy[5].

MGUS risk group	Criteria	Absolute risk* (%)	Recommended follow-up
Low	No risk factors present	2	6 months initially, and if stable, follow up every 2 - 3 years or when symptoms suggest a plasma cell malignancy
Low-intermediate	Any one risk factor present	10	6 months initially, then annually and upon any change in the patient's clinical condition
High-intermediate	Any two risk factors present	18	
High	All three risk factors present	27	

*of progression at 20 years accounting for death as a competing risk. Risk factors are defined as serum monoclonal immunoglobulin ≥15 g/L, serum monoclonal immunoglobulin type (IgA or IgM) and an abnormal sFLC κ/λ ratio.

Table 25.3. Summary of MGUS risk groups and recommended follow-up.

For patients with SMM, the guidelines[5] recommend SPE plus electrophoresis of a 24-hour urine, to confirm the diagnosis and full blood cell count plus serum calcium and creatinine measurements to rule out MM, at baseline and after 2 - 3 months. Baseline sFLC measurements are required for risk stratification and a baseline bone marrow biopsy and skeletal survey are mandatory. If the results are stable, the studies should be repeated every 4 - 6 months for the first year, and then, if remaining stable, the follow-up period can be lengthened to 6 - 12 months[5].

25.3.3. Guidelines for standard investigative work-up of patients with suspected multiple myeloma (2011)

sFLC analysis is recommended as part of the standard investigative work-up in all newly diagnosed patients with plasma cell dyscrasias[12]. It was noted that sFLC testing is particularly important in patients with NSMM and LCMM, as well as in other patients with oligosecretory myeloma. Measurement of urine FLC levels is not recommended.

25.3.4. Guidelines for risk stratification in multiple myeloma (2011)

Evaluation of prognostic factors and risk stratification in newly-diagnosed patients is important to define treatment strategies, compare outcome of therapeutic trials and predict survival from diagnosis. The 2011 IMWG guidelines for risk stratification[15] state that the International Staging System (ISS)[16], incorporating serum albumin and β_2-microglobulin (β_2M), is applicable as a prognostic system in the majority of settings (Section 20.1).

The guidelines state that other factors may play significant roles in risk stratification, including extramedullary or plasmablastic disease, plasma cell leukaemia, renal failure, lactate dehydrogenase (LDH), IgA, high sFLCs and an abnormal κ/λ sFLC ratio.

Earlier staging systems included concentrations of monoclonal immunoglobulins. It has now been realised that these have little relevance to MM outcome. For IgG MM this may be due to variable recycling by FcRn receptors (Chapter 3). By contrast, elevated sFLC concentrations and abnormal κ/λ sFLC ratios do relate to disease stage and outcome (Chapter 20). This may be due to their more consistant clearance, capacity to cause renal damage (Chapter 26), and their association with IgH translocations[15].

25.3.5. Consensus recommendations for the uniform reporting of clinical trials (2011)

The IMWG consensus recommendations for the uniform reporting of clinical trials summarise the current response criteria in MM (Table 25.4)[16]. It is proposed that all future clinical trials in MM should follow these guidelines when reporting results. The recommendations are largely based on the IMWG uniform response criteria[19], with additional clarifications[4,16]. Incorporation of sFLC assays into the response criteria has facilitated the inclusion and evaluation of patients with oligosecretory and nonsecretory disease, and has also provided stricter definitions of complete response[17].

Response subcategory	Response criteria
Complete response (CR)	• Negative IFE of serum and urine, *and* • Disappearance of any soft tissue plasmacytomas, *and* • <5% plasma cells in bone marrow • In patients in whom the only measurable disease is by sFLC levels, CR is defined as a normal FLC ratio (0.26-1.65) in addition to the CR criteria listed above
Stringent complete response (sCR)	CR as defined above plus • Normal FLC ratio, *and* • Absence of clonal plasma cells by immunohistochemistry or 2-4 colour flow cytometry
Immunophenotypic CR	sCR plus • absence of phenotypically aberrant plasma cells in bone marrow with a minimum of one million total bone marrow cells analyzed by multiparametric flow cytometry (with ≥4 colours)
Molecular CR	CR plus • Negative ASO-PCR, sensitivity 10^{-5}
Very good partial response (VGPR)	• Serum and urine M-protein detectable by IFE but not on electrophoresis, or • ≥90% reduction in serum M-protein plus urine M-protein <100 mg per 24 hours • In patients in whom the only measurable disease is by sFLC levels, VGPR is defined as a >90% decrease in the difference between involved and uninvolved sFLC levels
Partial response (PR)	• ≥50% reduction of serum M-protein and reduction in 24-hour urinary M-protein by ≥90% or to <200 mg per 24 hours • In patients in whom the only measurable disease is by sFLC levels, PR is defined as a ≥50% decrease in the difference between involved and uninvolved sFLC levels • If serum and urine M-protein are unmeasurable, and sFLCs are also unmeasurable, ≥50% reduction in bone marrow plasma cells is required in place of M-protein, provided baseline percentage was ≥30% • In addition to the above criteria, if present at baseline, ≥50% reduction in the size of soft tissue plasmacytomas is also required
Stable disease (SD)	Not meeting criteria for CR, VGPR, PR or progressive disease

Progressive disease (PD)	• Increase of 25% from lowest response value in any one or more of the following:
	  - Serum M-protein (absolute increase must be ≥5 g/L) and/or
	  - Urine M-protein (absolute increase must be ≥200 mg/24 hours) and/or
	  - In patients in whom the only measurable disease is by sFLC levels, the difference between involved and uninvolved sFLC levels (absolute increase must be >100 mg/L)
	  - If serum and urine M-protein are unmeasurable, and sFLCs are also unmeasurable, bone marrow plasma cell percentage (absolute % must be ≥10%)
	• Definite development of new bone lesions or soft tissue plasmacytomas or definite increase in the size of existing bone lesions or soft tissue plasmacytomas
	• Development of hypercalcaemia (corrected serum calcium >11.5 mg/dL) that can be attributed solely to the plasma cell proliferative disorder

Note that all response categories require two consecutive assessments made at any time before the institution of any new therapy. CR, PR and SD categories also require no known evidence of progressive or new bone lesions if radiographic studies were performed. VGPR and CR categories require serum and urine studies to be performed regardless of whether baseline disease was measurable by serum and/or urine electrophoretic techniques. Radiographic studies are not required to satisfy these response requirements. Bone marrow assessments need not be confirmed. For PD, serum M-protein increases of ≥10 g/L are sufficient to define relapse if baseline M-protein is ≥50 g/L. ASO-PCR: allele-specific oligonucleotide polymerase chain reaction.

Table 25.4. IMWG: uniform response criteria for MM[16].

It is recommended that patients undergoing therapy be tracked monthly for the first year of new therapy and every alternate month thereafter. Patients with measurable disease by SPE or UPE (defined as serum monoclonal protein ≥10 g/L; urine monoclonal protein ≥200 mg/24 hours), or both, will be assessed for response based only on these two tests, and not by FLC assays. In these patients, FLC assays are only required for assessment of stringent complete response[17].

In patients in whom the only measurable disease is by sFLC levels (defined as involved FLC ≥100 mg/L, provided that the FLC ratio is abnormal), the definition of partial or very good partial sFLC response requires subtraction of the tumour ("involved") FLC from the non-tumour ("uninvolved") FLC. This difference calculation provides an interpretable result even when the non-tumour FLC is below the detection limit or fluctuating widely (thereby making the sFLC ratio unreliable). It is also helpful when interpreting high concentrations of the alternate FLC, as observed in patients with impaired renal function *(Chapter 27)*.

25.3.6. Recommendations for global myeloma care (2013)

The IMWG recommendations for global myeloma care[18] outline the minimal requirements for the diagnosis and monitoring of patients with MM. The aim of this publication was to provide relevant information and recommendations for clinicians worldwide, taking into consideration the substantial differences in healthcare systems.

At diagnosis, all of the following tests should be performed: SPE, UPE of a 24-hour urine specimen, serum and urine IFE and sFLC analysis. It is also recommended that sFLC measurements are used to monitor disease course, particularly in patients with oligosecretory or nonsecretory MM.

25.4. European Society of Medical Oncology: clinical practice guidelines for diagnosis, treatment and follow-up of multiple myeloma (2013)

The European Society of Medical Oncology (ESMO) clinical practice guidelines[19] are intended to provide oncology professionals with a set of recommendations for the best standards of cancer care, based on the findings of evidence-based medicine. The ESMO guidelines are also endorsed by the Japanese Society of Medical Oncology (JSMO) and include the following recommendations for the use of sFLC measurements:

Diagnosis

sFLC analysis should be used in the initial diagnostic work-up of MM.

Response evaluation and follow-up

IMWG response criteria, which include sFLC analysis, should be used for response evaluation *(Section 25.3.5)*. Outside the context of a clinical trial, it is recommended that serum and urine electrophoresis and/or sFLC determination should be carried out every 2 - 3 months.

25.5. UK Myeloma Forum and Nordic Myeloma Study Group: guidelines for the investigation of newly detected monoclonal proteins and management of monoclonal gammopathy of undetermined significance (2009)

These 2009 guidelines[23] recommend screening for monoclonal proteins in patients where there is clinical suspicion of plasma cell dyscrasia or B-cell malignancy. Screening should also be performed when the results of other laboratory tests raise the possibility of the presence of a monoclonal protein (such as raised erythrocyte sedimentation rate [ESR >30 mm/h], anaemia, renal failure, hypercalcaemia). SPE and UPE should be performed initially, and if the clinical suspicion of an underlying plasma cell dyscrasia is strong despite the absence of a detectable monoclonal protein, then IFE should be requested. sFLC analysis is required to detect NSMM and some cases of AL amyloidosis, and LCMM when urine is not available. sFLC analysis is also advised where serum immunoglobulin levels are low and no serum monoclonal protein is identified. Alternatively, a urine sample may be requested for IFE.

The guidelines also discuss the MGUS risk-stratification model published by Rajkumar et al.[10] and the value of the κ/λ sFLC ratio, along with monoclonal protein level and immunoglobulin type, in differentiating patients at low to high risk of malignant transformation. According to these guidelines[23], the frequency of monitoring MGUS patients considered to be at low-risk, particularly those with low paraprotein concentrations, could be reduced if actual life expectancy is low and all lymphoproliferative diseases other than MGUS have been excluded. This is in agreement with the IMWG guidelines *(Section 25.3.2)*[5]. For those patients with longer life expectancies, higher monoclonal protein levels, and non-IgG subtypes, monitoring every 3 - 4 months within the first year was advised and thereafter once or twice yearly in the absence of symptoms of progression. It is additionally noted that for MGUS patients with an abnormal baseline κ/λ sFLC ratio or significant Bence Jones proteinuria, the risk of renal failure and disease progression is increased. These patients should be considered for more frequent monitoring and be advised to maintain high fluid intake.

25.6. British Committee for Standards in Haematology Guidelines (2014)

British guidelines on the diagnosis and management of MM published in 2011[21,22] have been updated in 2013[23] and 2014[24]. These guidelines include the following uses of sFLC and Hevylite measurements:

Investigation and diagnosis

The guidelines recommend that the IMWG diagnostic criteria are used *(Section 25.2)*. Assessment of sFLCs is recommended as part of the diagnostic work-up of patients where there is a strong suspicion of myeloma but in whom routine SPE is negative. sFLC analysis is particularly useful in the initial investigation of patients with LCMM, NSMM and oligosecretory disease, and in cases where urine has not been supplied to the laboratory *(Chapters 23 and 24)*.

Prognostic factors in symptomatic myeloma

The guidelines recommend that the International Staging System (based on serum albumin and β_2-microglobulin) be used, and that fluorescent in situ hybridisation (FISH) studies are used for all patients at diagnosis. The guidelines recognise that newer techniques for prognostic assessment should continue to be utilised in the context of clinical trials to evaluate future incorporation into routine clinical practice, and highlight that baseline sFLC concentrations and the immunoglobulin heavy/light chain (Hevylite®) ratio, both at diagnosis and following treatment, may provide useful prognostic information *(Chapter 20)*.

Measuring response to therapy

The guidelines recommend that response to therapy is defined according to the IMWG uniform response criteria *(Section 25.3.5)* but that the stringent complete response (sCR) category is necessary only in the context of a clinical trial. sFLC assays should be used to routinely assess response in all patients with LCMM, NSMM and oligosecretory disease. It is also recommended that sFLC analysis is performed as part of the initial management of patients with renal failure.

Monitoring SMM

Monitoring patients with SMM should include regular clinical assessment and monoclonal protein measurement, including sFLC analysis when indicated.

25.7. National Comprehensive Cancer Network Clinical Practice Guidelines in Oncology (NCCN Guidelines®) for Multiple Myeloma V.1.2015

These guidelines developed by the National Comprehensive Cancer Network® (NCCN®) address diagnosis, treatment, follow-up and response assessment for patients with MM[25]. The most recent version of the NCCN Guidelines for Multiple Myeloma (V.2.2015) is available at www.nccn.org[26]. These guidelines include the following uses of sFLC measurements:

Initial diagnostic workup

sFLC analysis is recommended in the initial diagnostic work-up of all patients with suspected MM and related plasma cell disorders. Use of the sFLC assays, along with SPE and sIFE, yields high diagnostic sensitivity when screening for MM and related plasma cell disorders. These guidelines also note the prognostic value of sFLC assays in plasma cell disorders including MGUS, SMM, AL amyloidosis and solitary plasmacytoma.

Follow-up surveillance

The NCCN Guidelines recommend sFLC analysis for monitoring cases of active MM following primary and additional treatments, as clinically indicated. sFLC analysis is also recommended for monitoring solitary plasmacytoma after primary treatment and for monitoring SMM, as clinically indicated.

Response criteria

The NCCN Guidelines recommend use of the IMWG uniform response criteria in future clinical trials. These response criteria include sFLC analysis, and are described in Section 25.3.5.

25.8. Management of multiple myeloma in Asia: resource-stratified guidelines

In this review, Tan et al.[27] provide guidelines that have been developed specifically for the management of MM in Asia. These recommendations take into consideration differing health care resource and expertise across Asian countries.

Diagnostic work-up

These guidelines state that IFE and sFLC assessment are essential, especially in patients suspected of having myeloma but who have negative SPE results. Where these tests are not routinely available, physicians are advised to consider sending blood specimens to high-level centres for testing if a diagnosis of LCMM, oligosecretory MM or NSMM is suspected.

Disease monitoring

In patients with LCMM, oligosecretory MM or NSMM, sFLC analysis should be used for the assessment of response and subsequent progression. Treatment response should be defined according to the IMWG uniform response criteria *(Section 25.3.5)*. The sCR category may be applicable only in centres where sFLC testing is available, and may be more relevant in a clinical trial setting.

Test Questions

1. What algorithm do current guidelines recommend for the screening of suspected monoclonal gammopathies?

Answers

1. sFLC assays are recommended for use in combination with serum protein electrophoresis (SPE) and serum immunofixation electrophoresis (sIFE). However, if AL amyloidosis is suspected a 24-hour urine should also be requested. *(Section 25.3.1)*

References

1. Rajkumar SV, Dimopolous MA, Palumbo A, Blade J, Merlini G, Mateos MV et al. International Myeloma Working Group updated criteria for the diagnosis of multiple myeloma. Lancet Oncology 2014;15:e538-e548

2. Kyle R, Child JA, Anderson K, Barlogie B, Bataille R, Bensinger W, et al. Criteria for the classification of monoclonal gammopathies, multiple myeloma and related disorders: a report of the International Myeloma Working Group. Br J Haematol 2003;121:749-57

3. Durie BG, Harousseau JL, Miguel JS, Blade J, Barlogie B, Anderson K, et al. International uniform response criteria for multiple myeloma. Leukemia 2006;20:1467-73

4. Kyle RA, Rajkumar SV. Criteria for diagnosis, staging risk stratification and response assessment of multiple myeloma. Leukemia 2009;23:3-9

5. Kyle RA, Durie BG, Rajkumar SV, Landgren O, Blade J, Merlini G, et al. Monoclonal gammopathy of undetermined significance (MGUS) and smoldering (asymptomatic) multiple myeloma: IMWG consensus perspectives risk factors for progression and guidelines for monitoring and management. Leukemia 2010;24:1121-7

6. Dispenzieri A, Kyle R, Merlini G, Miguel JS, Ludwig H, Hajek R, et al. International Myeloma Working Group guidelines for serum-free light chain analysis in multiple myeloma and related disorders. Leukemia 2009;23:215-24

7. Kyle RA, Therneau TM, Rajkumar SV, Remstein ED, Offord JR, Larson DR et al. Long-term follow-up of IgM monoclonal gammopathy of undetermined significance. Blood 2003;102:3759-64

8. Blade J, Lopez-Guillermo A, Rozman C, Cervantes F, Salgado C, Aguilar JL et al. Malignant transformation and life expectancy in monoclonal gammopathy of undetermined significance. Br J Haematol 1992;81:391-4

9. Cesana C, Klersy C, Barbarano L, Nosari AM, Crugnola M, Pungolino E et al. Prognostic factors for malignant transformation in monoclonal gammopathy of undetermined significance and smoldering multiple myeloma. J Clin Oncol 2002;20:1625-34

10. Rajkumar SV, Kyle RA, Therneau TM, Melton LJ, III, Bradwell AR, Clark RJ et al. Serum free light chain ratio is an independent risk factor for progression in monoclonal gammopathy of undetermined significance. Blood 2005;106:812-7

11. Perez-Persona E, Vidriales MB, Mateo G, Garcia-Sanz R, Mateos MV, de Coca AG et al. New criteria to identify risk of progression in monoclonal gammopathy of uncertain significance and smoldering multiple myeloma based on multiparameter flow cytometry analysis of bone marrow plasma cells. Blood 2007;110:2586-92

12. Dimopoulos M, Kyle R, Fermand JP, Rajkumar SV, San MJ, Chanan-Khan A et al. Consensus recommendations for standard investigative workup: report of the International Myeloma Workshop Consensus Panel 3. Blood 2011;117:4701-5

13. Munshi NC, Anderson KC, Bergsagel PL, Shaughnessy J, Palumbo A, Durie B et al. Consensus recommendations for risk stratification in multiple myeloma: report of the International Myeloma Workshop Consensus Panel 2. Blood 2011;117:4696-700

14. Greipp PR, San Miguel J, Durie BG, Crowley JJ, Barlogie B, Blade J et al. International staging system for multiple myeloma. J Clin Oncol 2005;23:3412-20

15. Kumar S, Zhang L, Dispenzieri A, Van WS, Katzmann JA, Snyder M et al. Relationship between elevated immunoglobulin free light chain and the presence of IgH translocations in multiple myeloma. Leukemia 2010;24:1498-505

16. Rajkumar SV, Harousseau JL, Durie B, Anderson KC, Dimopoulos M, Kyle R et al. Consensus recommendations for the uniform reporting of clinical trials: report of the International Myeloma Workshop Consensus Panel 1. Blood 2011;117:4691-5

17. Durie BG, Harousseau JL, Miguel JS, Blade J, Barlogie B, Anderson K, et al. International uniform response criteria for multiple myeloma. Leukemia 2006;20:1467-73

18. Ludwig H, Miguel JS, Dimopoulos MA, Palumbo A, Garcia SR, Powles R et al. International Myeloma Working Group recommendations for global myeloma care. Leukemia 2013;28:981-92

19. Moreau P, San MJ, Ludwig H, Schouten H, Mohty M, Dimopoulos M, Dreyling M. Multiple myeloma: ESMO Clinical Practice Guidelines for diagnosis, treatment and follow-up. Ann Oncol 2013;24 Suppl 6:vi133-vi137

20. Bird J, Behrens J, Westin J, Turesson I, Drayson M, Beetham R, et al. UK Myeloma Forum (UKMF) and Nordic Myeloma Study Group (NMSG): guidelines for the investigation of newly detected M-proteins and the management of monoclonal gammopathy of undetermined significance (MGUS). Br J Haematol 2009;147:22-42

21. Bird JM, Owen RG, D'sa S, Snowden JA, Pratt G, Ashcroft J et al. Guidelines for the diagnosis and management of multiple myeloma 2011. Br J Haematol 2011;154:32-75

22. Snowden JA, Ahmedzai SH, Ashcroft J, D'sa S, Littlewood T, Low E et al. Guidelines for supportive care in multiple myeloma 2011. Br J Haematol 2011;154:76-103

23. Bird JM, Owen, RG, D'sa S, Snowden JA, Pratt G, Ashcroft J et al. Guidelines for the diagnosis and management of multiple myeloma 2013. BCSH guideline available online at www.bcshguidelines.com

24. Bird J, Owen R, D'Sa S, Snowden J, Ashcroft J, Yong K et al. Guidelines for the diagnosis and management of multiple myeloma 2014. BCSH guideline available online at www.bcshguidelines.com

25. Anderson KC, Alsina M, Bensinger W, Biermann JS, Chanan-Khan A, Cohen AD et al. Multiple myeloma. J Natl Compr Canc Netw 2011;9:1146-83

26. Referenced with permission from The NCCN Clinical Practice Guidelines in Oncology® for Multiple Myeloma V.2.2015. © National Comprehensive Cancer Network, Inc 2011. All rights reserved. Accessed December 9th, 2014. To view the most recent and complete version of the guideline, go online to www.nccn.org. NATIONAL COMPREHENSIVE CANCER NETWORK®, NCCN®, NCCN GUIDELINES®, and all other NCCN Content are trademarks owned by the National Comprehensive Cancer Network, Inc.

27. Tan D, Chng WJ, Chou T, Nawarawong W, Hwang SY, Chim CS et al. Management of multiple myeloma in Asia: resource-stratified guidelines. Lancet Oncol 2013;14:e571-e581

An overview of the kidney and monoclonal free light chains

26.1. Introduction

This chapter covers the normal renal handling of free light chains (FLCs) and the role of monoclonal FLCs in a range of renal pathologies including cast nephropathy, AL amyloidosis and light chain deposition disease (LCDD).

26.2. Renal clearance of FLCs

FLCs are present in similar concentrations in the vascular and extravascular compartments[1]. As a consequence, the vascular compartment may contain only 15-20% of the total amount of FLCs in the body. The serum concentrations of κ and λ FLCs are dependent upon the balance between production and clearance *(Chapter 3)*. Although κ FLCs are normally produced at a rate approximately twice that of λ FLCs, the renal clearance of monomeric κ FLCs is faster than dimeric λ FLCs. This accounts for the observed differences in their serum half-lives (κ sFLCs: approximately 2 hours; λ sFLCs: 4 - 6 hours) and their serum concentrations *(Chapter 3 and Section 6.1)*[2,3]. The molecular weight cut-off for glomerular filtration of circulating macromolecules is around 60 kDa. Therefore, whilst sFLCs are rapidly cleared from the blood by the kidneys, larger serum proteins such as albumin (66 kDa) and transferrin (81 kDa) are only filtered to a limited extent[4] and their serum concentrations are not dependent upon kidney function.

After filtration by the glomeruli, FLCs and other proteins enter the proximal tubules and bind to brush border membranes via low-affinity, high-capacity receptors called cubulin and megalin[4]. Binding results in internalisation of the bound proteins followed by proteolysis within the tubular epithelial cells. Subsequently, the constituent amino acids are returned to the circulation across the basolateral membrane[4]. Reabsorption of FLCs by the proximal tubule is highly efficient and a normal 24-hour urine collection will only contain around 10 mg of polyclonal FLCs[5].

Whilst the concentration of serum creatinine is a useful guide to kidney function, the glomerular filtration rate (GFR) is a more accurate measure. Estimated GFR (eGFR) values can be derived from various different calculations. Currently, the most widely used calculation is the one proposed by the Modification of Diet in Renal Disease (MDRD) study group, which incorporates serum creatinine along with age, sex, and ethnicity in the equation to produce an eGFR[6]. More recent calculations may be more accurate than the MDRD equation for kidney function measurement; in particular the CKD-EPI equation may replace MDRD in routine clinical practice in the near future[7].

26.3. Renal impairment and FLCs

Renal impairment is characterised by the reduced ability of the kidneys to excrete waste and maintain the electrolyte balance. This encompasses both acute kidney injury (AKI) and chronic kidney disease (CKD). CKD is very common, with 8.5% of the population having baseline impairment of kidney function (stage 3 - 5 chronic kidney disease, defined by an eGFR of <60 ml/min/1.73m^2)[9]. This has usually occurred over a period of years and is associated with diseases such as hypertension, cardiovascular disorders or diabetes[10]. AKI affects between 13 and 18% of all people admitted to hospital and the severity of the AKI is defined according to the amount by which serum creatinine has increased within a 48-hour period[11]. It is usually reversible but is associated with a major increased mortality risk in those affected[12]. In patients who present with AKI of unknown cause the underlying pathology may be multiple myeloma (MM) and they should be rapidly screened for monoclonal gammopathy *(Section 27.2)*.

In patients with renal impairment, the reticuloendothelial system becomes the dominant mechanism for the clearance of FLCs and other proteins from the blood. With decreased renal clearance, the relative concentrations of κ and λ sFLCs become increasingly influenced by production rates, leading to minor increases in the sFLC ratio in the absence of monoclonal gammopathy[13]. Application of a modified renal reference interval for patients with renal impairment may increase the specificity of the κ/λ sFLC ratio for detecting monoclonal FLC production *(Section 6.3)*. If there is complete renal failure, the serum half-life of κ and λ FLCs will be the same and may be prolonged to 2 - 3 days, resulting in significant increases in serum concentration for both light chains.

26.4. Nephrotoxicity of monoclonal FLCs

Plasma cell dyscrasias are often associated with kidney disease *(Figure 26.1)*. In many cases, this is caused by the nephrotoxicity of the individual monoclonal FLCs produced by a B-cell clone. The pattern of renal injury varies considerably, and is influenced by structural properties of the individual monoclonal FLC, particularly the variable domain, as well as environmental factors such as pH or local proteolysis[14].

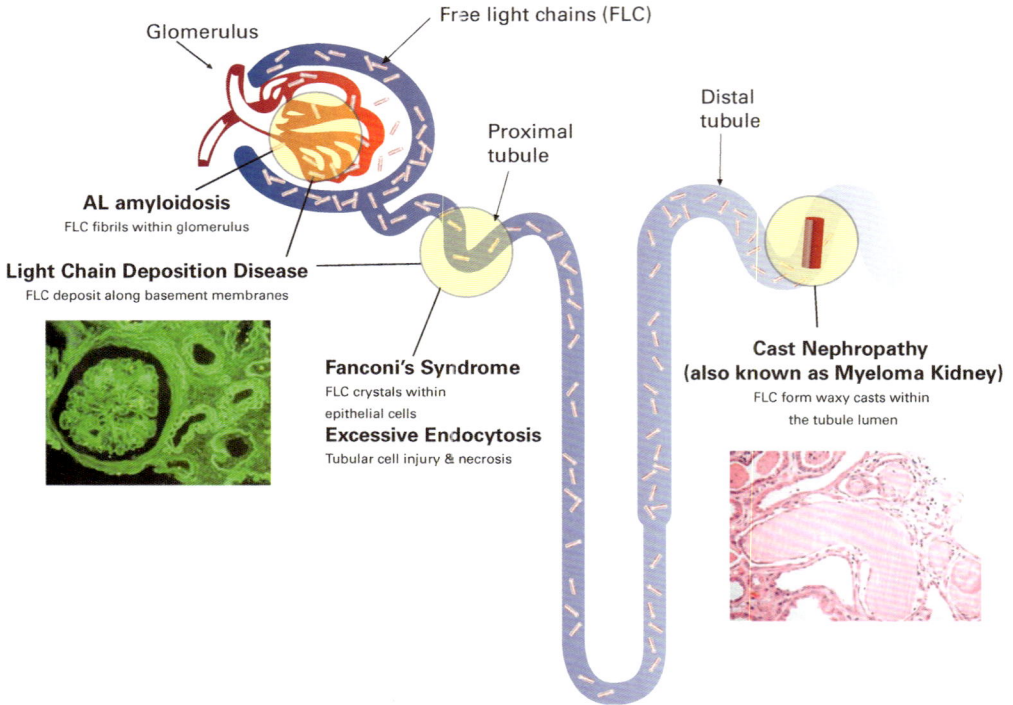

Figure 26.1. Renal injury caused by FLCs. *LCDD immunofluorescence magnification x150. (Copyright © 2007 Karger Publishers, Basel, Switzerland®).*

Renal disorders that are associated with plasma cell dyscrasias may be classified into two major groups according to the predominant type of injury: glomerular or tubulo-interstitial *(Table 26.1)*.

Tubulo-interstitial disorders include cast nephropathy, acute tubular necrosis and Fanconi syndrome. Cast nephropathy is the most frequent cause of severe AKI in MM patients, causing up to 90% of cases[16]. This pathology is discussed in detail in Chapter 27 along with issues relating to diagnosis and preservation of renal function in MM patients. A less common cause of AKI in MM is acute tubular necrosis[17]. In this condition, proximal tubular injury is associated with an acute ischaemic or toxic event. In some MM patients, endocytosis of nephrotoxic FLCs may directly cause proximal tubular cell injury and necrosis[18]. Fanconi syndrome may be due to proximal tubule dysfunction secondary to reabsorption of FLCs that are resistant to proteolysis and crystallise within epithelial cell lysosomes. This dysfunction leads to a loss of solutes, including phosphate, glucose, amino acids and bicarbonate and is characterised by renal tubular acidosis[19]. Interestingly, this is nearly always associated with FLCs of the Vκ1 subgroup, derived specifically from only two germline genes: IGKV1-39 and IGKV1-33[17]. Leung and Behrens[20] recently published a comprehensive review of myeloma-related kidney disease.

	Renal disease	Monoclonal immunoglobulin deposits	Ultrastructural appearance of deposits	Renal presentation
Tubulo-interstitial disorders	Cast nephropathy	FLC	Homogenous, proteinaceous, "waxy" casts (in distal tubule lumen)	AKI
	Fanconi syndrome	FLC (κ>λ)	Crystals (within proximal tubule epithelium)	CKD, proximal tubule dysfunction, osteomalacia
Glomerular disorders	AL amyloidosis *(Chapter 28)*	FLC (λ>κ)	Fibrils (Congo red positive)	Proteinuria, nephrotoxic syndrome, CKD
	Cryoglobulinaemia	Type I: often IgM Type II: IgM + polyclonal IgG	Microtubules (or rarely crystalline)	Hypertension, proteinuria, nephrotic syndrome, haematuria, CKD, acute nephrotic syndrome
	Monoclonal immunoglobulin deposition diseases *(Chapter 29)*	LCDD: FLC HCDD: truncated HC (α most common) LHCDD: FLC +truncated HC	Nodular glomerulosclerosis, linear amorphous deposits along tubular basement membranes	Hypertension, proteinuria, nephrotic syndrome, haematuria, CKD

AKI: acute kidney injury; HC: heavy chain; CKD: chronic kidney disease; HCDD: heavy-chain deposition disease; LHCDD: light- and heavy-chain deposition disease

Table 26.1. Main renal disorders related to monoclonal immunoglobulin deposition or precipitation. Table adapted from[15].

AL amyloidosis and LCDD are often associated with glomerular damage, albuminuria and progressive renal impairment. Whilst LCDD is frequently associated with MM (65%), AL amyloidosis is less frequently observed (10 - 20%)[8]. The kidney is the organ most affected in LCDD, with severe renal impairment evident in the majority of cases at presentation. The kidneys are adversely affected in approximately 75% of AL amyloidosis patients, the majority of whom present with heavy proteinuria, often with a nephrotic syndrome[8]. AL amyloidosis and LCDD are considered in more detail in Chapters 28 and 29 respectively.

Finally, it is important to note that more than one histological pattern can exist in the same kidney. The most common combinations are cast nephropathy with acute tubular necrosis, and cast nephropathy with LCDD[21].

26.4.1. Monoclonal gammopathy of renal significance

A new term, "monoclonal gammopathy of renal significance (MGRS)" was proposed by Leung and colleagues[22] to describe a group of haematological disorders associated with kidney disease that fail to meet the standard definitions for MM or lymphoma. In such cases, the renal impairment is often linked to the underlying haematological disorder. Their definition included AL amyloidosis *(Chapter 28)*, type I and II cryoglobulinaemias *(Section 34.2)*, monoclonal immunoglobulin deposition disease (MIDD; *Chapter 29)* and Fanconi syndrome[23]. The intention was to make a clear distinction between MGUS *(Chapter 13)*, a benign asymptomatic condition, and MGRS, which may be associated with significant morbidity and mortality. Supportive information was published by Johnson et al.[24]; after reviewing data from 425 patients with MGUS, it was found that an abnormal sFLC ratio and elevated involved sFLC concentrations were predictive of increased risk of developing renal disease. Yadav et al.[25] recommended the use of sFLC analysis when screening for MGRS.

References

1. Takagi K, Kin K, Itoh Y, Enomoto H, Kawai T. Human a pha 1-microglobulin levels in various body fluids. J Clin Pathol 1980;33:786-91

2. Miettinen TA, Kekki M. Effect of impaired hepatic and renal function on [131I] Bence Jones protein catabolism in human subjects. Clin Chim Acta 1967;18:395-407

3. Wochner RD, Strober W, Waldmann TA. The role of the kidney in the catabolism of Bence Jones proteins and immunoglobulin fragments. J Exp Med 1967;126:207-21

4. Christensen EI, Birn H, Storm T, Weyer K, Nielsen R. Endocytic receptors in the renal proximal tubule. Physiology (Bethesda) 2012;27:223-36

5. Bradwell AR, Carr-Smith HD, Mead GP, Tang LX, Showell PJ, Drayson MT, Drew R. Highly sensitive, automated immunoassay for immunoglobulin free light chains in serum and urine. Clin Chem 2001;47:673-80

6. Levey AS, Bosch JP, Lewis JB, Greene T, Rogers N, Roth D. A more accurate method to estimate glomerular filtration rate from serum creatinine: a new prediction equation. Modification of Diet in Renal Disease Study Group. Ann Intern Med 1999;130:461-70

7. Carter JL, Stevens PE, Irving JE, Lamb EJ. Estimating glomerular filtration rate: comparison of the CKD-EPI and MDRD equations in a large UK cohort with particular emphasis on the effect of age. QJM 2011;104:839-47

8. Merlini G, Pozzi C. Mechanisms of renal damage in plasma cell dyscrasias: an overview. Contrib Nephrol 2007;153:66-86

9. Stevens PE, O'Donoghue DJ, de LS, Van VJ, Klebe B, Middleton R et al. Chronic kidney disease management in the United Kingdom: NEOERICA project results. Kidney Int 2007;72:92-9

10. Stevens PE, Levin A. Evaluation and management of chronic kidney disease: synopsis of the kidney disease: improving global outcomes 2012 clinical practice guideline. Ann Intern Med 2013;158:825-30

11. Kidney disease: improving global outcomes (KDIGO) acute kidney injury work group. KDIGO clinical practice guideline for acute kidney injury. Kidney Int Suppl 2012;2:1-138

12. Srisawat N, Kellum JA. Acute kidney injury: definition, epidemiology, and outcome. Curr Opin Crit Care 2011;17:548-55

13. Hutchison CA, Harding S, Hewins P, Mead GP, Townsend J, Bradwell AR, Cockwell P. Quantitative assessment of serum and urinary polyclonal free light chains in patients with chronic kidney disease. Clin J Am Soc Nephrol 2008;3:1684-90

14. Hutchison CA, Blade J, Cockwell P, Cook M, Drayson M, Fermand JP et al. Novel approaches for reducing free light chains in patients with myeloma kidney. Nat Rev Nephrol 2012;8 234-43

15. Bridoux F, Fermand JP. Optimizing treatment strategies in myeloma cast nephropathy: rationale for a randomized prospective trial. Adv Chronic Kidney Dis 2012;19:333-41

16. Dimopoulos MA, Terpos E. Renal insufficiency and failure. Hematology Am Soc Hematol Educ Program 2010;2010:431-6

17. Hutchison CA, Batuman V, Behrens J, Bridoux F, Sirac C, Dispenzieri A et al. The pathogenesis and diagnosis of acute kidney injury in multiple myeloma. Nat Rev Nephrol 2011;8:43-51

18. Sanders PW. Mechanisms of light chain injury along the tubular nephron. J Am Soc Nephrol 2012;23:1777-81

19. Leung N, Behrens J. Current approach to diagnosis and management of acute renal failure in myeloma patients. Adv Chronic Kidney Dis 2012;19:297-302

20. Leung N, Gertz MA, Zeldenrust SR, Rajkumar SV, Dispenzieri A, Fervenza FC et al. Improvement of cast nephropathy with plasma exchange depends on the diagnosis and on reduction of serum free light chains. Kidney Int 2008;73:1282-8

21. Leung N, Bridoux F, Hutchison CA, Nasr SH, Cockwell P, Fermand JP et al. Monoclonal gammopathy of renal significance (MGRS): when MGUS is no longer undetermined or insignificant. Blood 2012;120:4292-5

22. Fermand JP, Bridoux F, Kyle RA, Kastritis E, Weiss BM, Cook MA et al. How I treat monoclonal gammopathy of renal significance (MGRS). Blood 2013;21:3583-90

23. Johnson L, Miller G, Stout S. Serum free light chains identify patients with monoclonal gammopathy at increased risk of developing renal disease. Blood 2013;122:1876a

24. Yadav P, Leung N, Sanders PW, Cockwell P. The use of immunoglobulin light chain assays in the diagnosis of paraprotein-related kidney disease. Kidney Int 2014 *In press*

Cast nephropathy in multiple myeloma

Cast nephropathy:

- Is the principal cause of severe acute kidney injury in multiple myeloma.
- Is the most likely diagnosis if patients present with acute kidney injury and sFLCs ≥500 mg/L.
- Is characterised by obstruction of the distal tubules by monoclonal FLCs in association with Tamm-Horsfall protein (uromodulin).
- Therapy can be monitored with sFLCs.
- Renal recovery and patient survival is improved with sustained reductions in sFLCs.

27.1. Renal impairment in multiple myeloma

Renal impairment (defined as an estimated glomerular filtration rate [eGFR] of <60 ml/min/1.73 m^2) is a common and potentially serious finding in multiple myeloma (MM). It is present in up to 40% of patients at diagnosis and affects up to 50% of patients at some time during their disease[1,2]. In most cases renal impairment is reversible, being caused by treatable factors such as dehydration, hypercalcaemia or nephrotoxic drugs. However, up to 10% of MM patients present with severe acute kidney injury (AKI), which requires dialysis. For up to 90% of such patients, the underlying cause is cast nephropathy[2].

Severe AKI is a significant problem: MM patients account for 2% of the dialysis population, with approximately 5,000 new cases worldwide per year[3,4]. A 2010 review of the data collected from a large European registry showed that renal morbidity was a considerable burden. Of the 159,367 patients on renal replacement therapy, the median survival was 0.91 years in MM and light chain deposition disease (LCDD) (n=2,453) versus 4.46 years in non-MM patients[4]. MM patients are associated with low rates of recovery of kidney function with the majority remaining on dialysis until death[5]. Early recovery of renal function should be a therapeutic aim as median survival is increased several-fold if this is achieved[6,7].

In this chapter, algorithms for screening for MM in patients presenting with AKI are reviewed together with serum free light chain (sFLC) measurements for monitoring light chain removal strategies such as plasma exchange, haemodialysis and adsorption techniques. Finally, there is some data concerning how renal recovery and patient survival can be predicted by sustained reductions in free light chains (FLCs)[8].

27.2. Screening for multiple myeloma in patients with unexplained AKI

Patients presenting with severe AKI of unknown cause should be screened for monoclonal gammopathy as part of their initial diagnostic workup. The window of opportunity for reversing renal impairment due to cast nephropathy is limited so early diagnosis and prompt treatment is important[9].

The International Myeloma Working Group (IMWG) recommends screening for monoclonal gammopathy using serum protein electrophoresis (SPE) and sFLC analysis *(Chapter 25)*. This algorithm allows the rapid detection of both FLC and intact immunoglobulin monoclonal proteins. For patients in whom a diagnosis of AL amyloidosis is suspected, the IMWG guidelines recommend a combination of sFLC analysis and immunofixation of serum and urine (sIFE and uIFE) *(Section 28.3)*[10].

A health economics model has been developed by Cook et al.[11], which compared the IMWG recommended pathway using SPE + sFLC against SPE alone, SPE + urine protein electrophoresis (UPE), and SPE + UPE + serum/urine IFE in parallel. The SPE + sFLC tests were the most cost effective, with cost savings and quality-adjusted life-year (QALY) gains in the diagnostic and treatment stages of the disease.

The recently formed International Kidney and Monoclonal Gammopathy Research Group (IKMGRG) also recommended the use of SPE and sFLC analysis to screen for monoclonal disease in patients presenting with AKI *(Figure 27.1)*[9]. The authors suggested that a concentration of monoclonal sFLCs ≥500 mg/L in patients with AKI, was indicative of tubular interstitial pathology, particularly cast nephropathy. It is of note that the ≥500 mg/L cut-off was based on data generated using Freelite® sFLC assays. In the only study performed so far using the Siemens N Latex FLC assays in the context of AKI, the authors concluded that the IKMGRG recommendations cannot be applied *(Chapter 8)*[12].

Application of a modified renal reference interval for the κ/λ sFLC ratio when screening patients with renal impairment may increase the diagnostic specificity with no loss of sensitivity *(Section 6.3)*[13]. Application of the renal reference interval and screening pathways for patients with AKI were reviewed in 2014 by Yadav et al.[14].

```
                           ┌──────────────────┐
                           │     New AKI       │
                           └──────────────────┘
                                    │
                                    ▼
                      ┌────────────────────────────┐
                      │  Exclude myeloma kidney      │
                      │  Assessment for FLC clone*   │
                      └────────────────────────────┘
```

Figure flowchart:

- **New AKI**
  - → **Exclude myeloma kidney Assessment for FLC clone***
    - → **FLC clone**
      - → **Clonal FLC ≥500 mg/L**
        - → **Probable FLC tubular interstitial pathology**
          - → ■ Requires hematology work-up ■ Initiation of disease-specific treatment to reduce serum FLC levels‡
      - → **Clonal FLC <500 mg/L**
        - **Either**
          - → **Alternative monoclonal FLC pathology**
          - → **Incidental MGUS**
            - → ■ Requires renal biopsy ■ Consider hematology work-up
    - → **No FLC clone**
      - → **AKI of another cause**

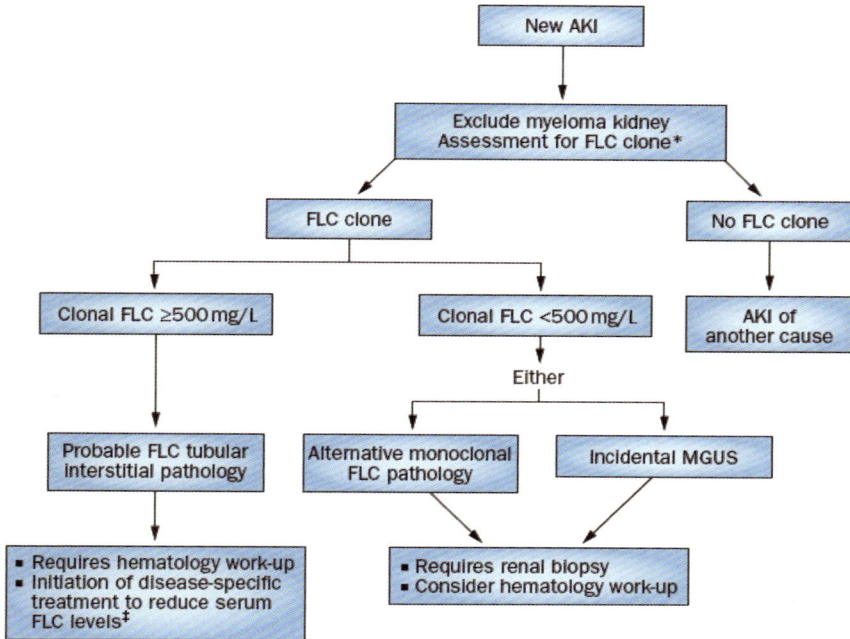

Figure 27.1. Screening algorithm for monoclonal disease in AKI. *To exclude the presence of an intact monoclonal immunoglobin, sFLC assays should be combined with SPE. For the assessment of AL amyloidosis and LCDD, urinary assessment is required. ‡Treatment based on high-dose dexamethasone. MGUS: monoclonal gammopathy of undetermined significance. (Reprinted by permission from Macmillan Publishers Ltd: Nature Reviews Nephrology[9], copyright 2011).*

27.3. Cast nephropathy

Cast nephropathy, also known as myeloma kidney, is the principal cause of AKI in MM[2]. In this condition, large quantities of monoclonal FLCs are produced by the tumour, and are filtered by the glomeruli, overwhelming the resorptive capacity of the proximal tubules. This leads to proximal tubule injury as a result of excessive endocytosis and large quantities of FLCs entering the distal tubules. In an analysis of 19 MM patients with dialysis-dependent AKI, Besemer et al.[15] noted that their median sFLC concentration was 8580 mg/L (range 1590 - 66100 mg/L).

FLCs entering distal tubules co-precipitate with Tamm-Horsfall protein (THP, also known as uromodulin) to form waxy casts within the tubule lumen *(Figure 27.2A and B)*. THP is a 105 kDa glycophosphatidylinositol (GPI)-anchored glycoprotein expressed in the thick ascending limb of the loop of Henle. Protease cleavage releases THP into normal urine, where it is found as the dominant high-molecular-weight protein polymer. THP is thought to be important in preventing ascending urinary infections and may have a protective role in AKI[16]. Interestingly, it contains a short peptide motif that has a high affinity for FLCs[17].

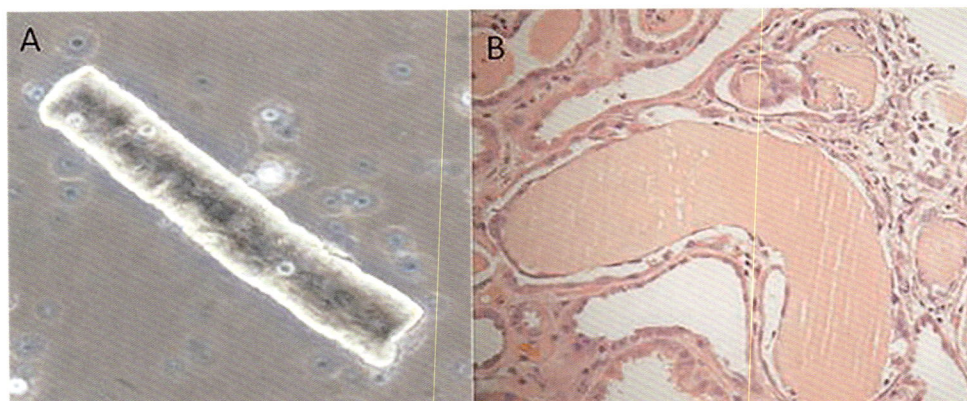

Figure 27.2. (A) Waxy cast from the urine of a patient with MM. (This figure was published in Investigation of renal disease: Urinalysis. Fogazzi GB. In: Johnson RJ, Feehally J, eds. Comprehensive clinical nephrology, Mosby: Page 41, Fig 4.3B © Elseivier [2003]). *(B) Classic casts in the distal tubules of a patient with light chain MM.* (Courtesy of C Hutchison).

The waxy casts in the distal tubules obstruct the tubular flow, resulting in leakage into the interstitium with subsequent inflammation and fibrosis[2]. Increasing concentrations of sFLCs are filtered by the remaining functioning nephrons which in turn become blocked, leading to a vicious cycle of further increases in sFLC concentrations and progressive renal damage. This may explain why some MM patients, without apparent pre-existing renal impairment suddenly develop catastrophic and irreversible renal failure. The process can be aggravated by factors that lower the threshold for cast precipitation such as dehydration, diuretics, hypercalcaemia, infections and nephrotoxic drugs[9].

Until a few years ago only 20% of patients with dialysis-dependent cast nephropathy ever recovered independent kidney function[2]. As early renal recovery has been shown to improve patient survival, attention has focused on providing a rapid diagnosis and ensuring early commencement of therapy directed at light chain reduction[18,19].

27.4. Light chain removal strategies in cast nephropathy

For patients with severe renal impairment, whilst effective chemotherapy can rapidly reduce FLC production, the half-life of the sFLCs will be prolonged and chemotherapy alone may not lead to an immediate reduction in sFLC concentrations. In such patients, it is tempting to think that strategies for direct removal of FLC will accelerate renal recovery. Plasma exchange, high-cut-off haemodialysis and adsorption have all been trialled as mechanisms for FLC removal; the results are discussed below.

27.4.1. Plasma exchange

In the largest randomised control trial of plasma exchange that included 107 patients with severe AKI associated with MM, Clark et al.[21] failed to demonstrate any benefit of plasma exchange for either renal recovery or overall patient survival. However, renal biopsy information was not available for all patients in the trial (so a diagnosis of cast nephropathy was not established) and sFLCs were not measured. Regarding the lack of sFLC measurement, a subsequent editorial in the Journal of the American Society of Nephrology[22] commented "This resembles anti-hypertensive treatment without measuring blood pressure." Clearly, the efficiency of plasma exchange for FLC removal could not be judged.

In a small study of 18 patients with biopsy-proven cast nephropathy, who were treated with bortezomib and plasma exchange, Leung et al.[19] concluded that patients were more likely to recover renal function if a 50% reduction in sFLC concentrations was achieved. For patients with pathologies other than cast nephropathy, the recovery of renal function did not depend on sFLC reduction, emphasising the necessity for biopsy confirmation of cast nephropathy when interpreting trial data.

In order to understand the efficiency of plasma exchange for FLC removal, Hutchison et al.[23] developed a compartmental mathematical model that was applicable to patients being treated for MM and renal failure. The following parameters were included: 1) sFLC concentrations at clinical presentation; 2) monomeric κ and dimeric λ clearance rates with and without renal failure; 3) partition of sFLCs between vascular and extravascular compartments (including oedema fluid); 4) flow of FLCs between compartments; 5) half-life of sFLCs in renal failure; 6) sFLC production rates; and 7) tumour killing rates with chemotherapy. Figure 27.3 displays the calculated clearance of κ FLCs in a light chain MM (LCMM) patient with renal failure treated with chemotherapy (assuming 10% tumour kill per day, Line 2). Addition of 6 plasma exchange treatments over 12 days is shown *(Figure 27.3, Line 3)*, and the rapid reductions in sFLC concentrations during the procedure and their subsequent re-entry from the extra-vascular to the intra-vascular compartment can be observed. Plasma exchange increased removal rates by approximately 25% but concentrations were not reduced below toxic levels (500 mg/L) at 4 weeks. Therefore, the lack of success of plasma exchange may be explained by the limited duration and frequency of this procedure, combined with on-going high production rates due to ineffective chemotherapy and re-entry of FLCs from extravascular compartments.

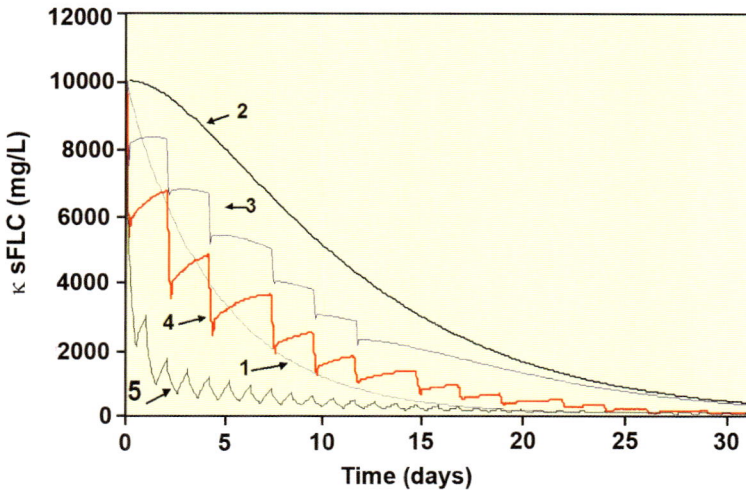

Figure 27.3. Calculated reduction of κ sFLCs in a patient with LCMM and renal failure by chemotherapy. Model assumes either 100% (immediate) tumour killing (1) or 10% per day (2). The effect of 6 x 3.5 litre plasma exchanges over 12 days is indicated (3) based on 10% kill per day (2) plus the addition of haemodialyis for 4 hours, x 3 per week (4) and 8 hours/day (5).

In 2010, an IMWG consensus statement acknowledged that "The role of plasma exchange in patients with suspected light chain cast nephropathy and renal impairment is controversial"[3]. A 2011 report of 14 patients with biopsy-proven or high probability cast nephropathy (defined as sFLC >2000 mg/L), treated with a combination of bortezomib-based chemotherapy plus a median of 8 plasma exchanges, described good patient outcomes. A partial renal response (PRR) or better was achieved in 86% of patients (a PRR was defined as a >50% reduction in serum creatinine from the maximum value, or freedom from haemodialysis within 6 months among patients who were initially undergoing haemodialyisis)[20]. The median time to the discontinuation of plasma exchange was 8 days (range 4 to 23) during which time the mean reduction in sFLCs was 74.6% (range 36.6 to 96.3%), and 6 patients had complete recovery of renal function within 6 months (Figure 27.4). However, this study did not include a control group so it was not possible to separate the efficacy of the chemotherapy from that of the plasma exchange.

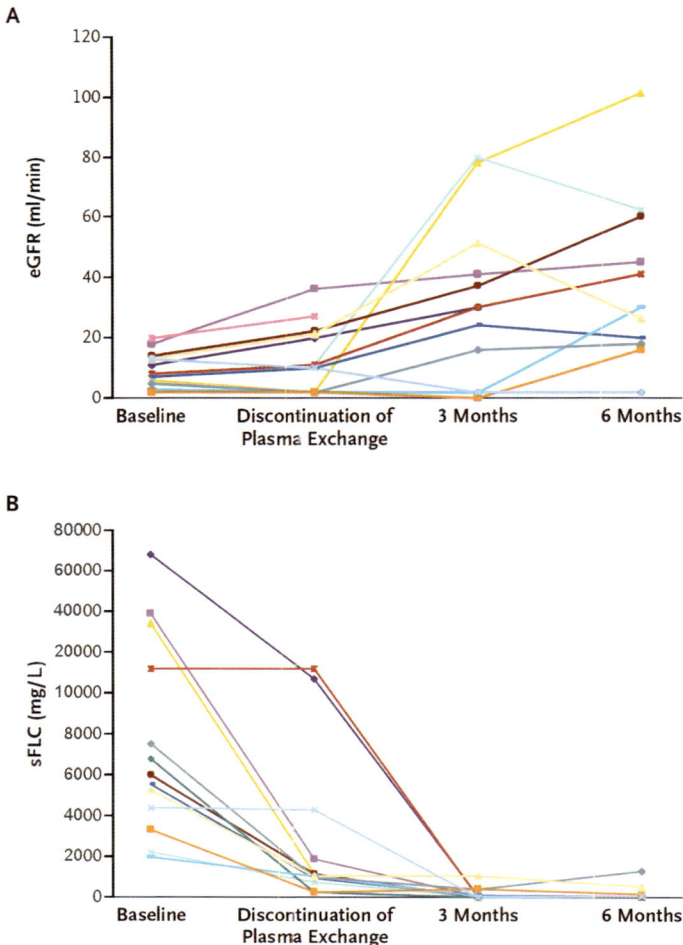

Figure 27.4. Changes in (A) eGFR and (B) sFLCs in 14 patients with MM receiving bortezomib plus plasma exchange. Data for patients in the two panels are identified by lines of the same colour. (From[20] Copyright © 2011 Massachusetts Medical Society. Reprinted with permission from Massachusetts Medical Society).

27.4.2. High cut-off haemodialysis

As an alternative to plasma exchange, sFLCs can be removed more effectively by haemodialysis. Conventional high-flux dialysers have a molecular weight cut-off around 15 - 20kDa so the filtration efficiency for FLCs is very low. However, a new generation of high cut-off (HCO) membranes have been designed to remove larger molecules *(Figure 27.5)*[24]. With high permeability for substances in the molecular weight range of 15 – 45 kDa, such membranes can effectively clear both κ and λ FLCs. Moreover, the duration of haemodialysis can be safely extended allowing further reductions in sFLCs.

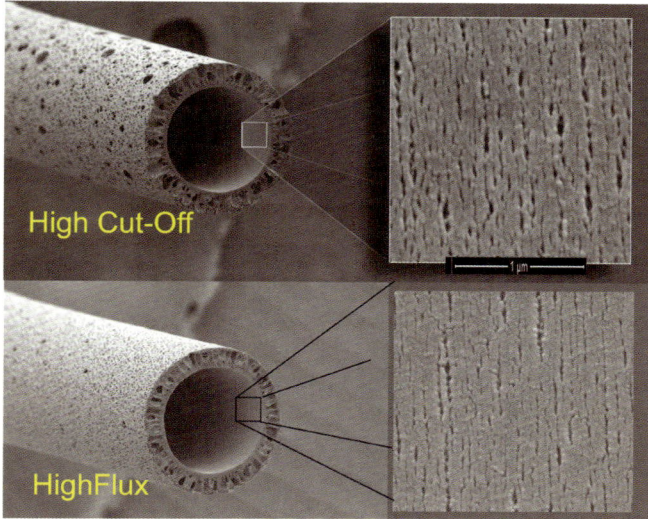

Figure 27.5. Photomicrograph of pores in a Gambro high cut-off membrane and a high-flux membrane (Polyflux™). *(Courtesy of M. Storr, Gambro Dialysatoren GmbH).*

Hutchison et al.[23] reported calculations from their mathematical model indicating that the prolonged daily use of HCO dialysers could rapidly reduce κ sFLC concentrations to less than 0.5 g/L in 2 - 3 days, equating to removal of around 95% of the total mass of sFLCs *(Figure 27.3; Line 5)*. This preliminary publication also reported results from treating 5 newly-diagnosed MM patients with dialysis-dependent cast nephropathy[23]. Figure 27.6 shows the rapid removal of λ FLCs in a patient with MM using the Gambro HCO 1100 dialysis membrane over a 6-hour period. Also shown are the large amounts of FLCs in the dialysate fluid. A total of nearly 40 grams of FLCs were removed in the single dialysis session. Sustained reductions in sFLC concentrations were observed in 3 patients who became independent of dialysis. Treatment examples are shown in Figures 27.7 and 27.8. The first of the figures shows good FLC reductions with recovery *(Figure 27.7)*. In the second, the patient failed to achieve renal recovery *(Figure 27.8)*. This patient developed sepsis and chemotherapy was stopped. Despite prolonged periods of haemodialysis and removal of 1.7 kg of FLCs, there was no recovery of renal function. It should be emphasised that for renal recovery to occur, patients needed both effective chemotherapy (to switch off FLC production) and rapid reduction of sFLCs. This is illustrated in Figure 27.9, in which a patient treated with HCO haemodialysis failed to respond to the initial chemotherapy but responded to bortezomib and subsequently recovered renal function.

A subsequent publication by Hutchison et al.[25] studied the effect of using two HCO 1100 dialysers in series, dialyser change, and haemodiafiltration on the efficiency of FLC removal. Based on the finding that the clearance rates of κ and λ FLCs increased when using two HCO 1100 dialysers in series, a new membrane, termed Theralite™, with a larger effective membrane area (2.1 m²) was developed.

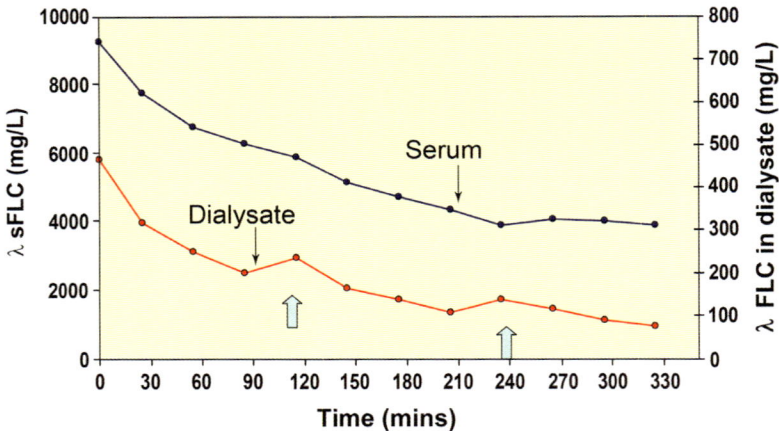

Figure 27.6. Concentrations of λ FLCs in serum and dialysate fluid of a patient with ARF due to LCMM undergoing dialysis with the Gambro high cut-off dialyser. The dialyser was renewed (arrows) as FLC leakage slowed.

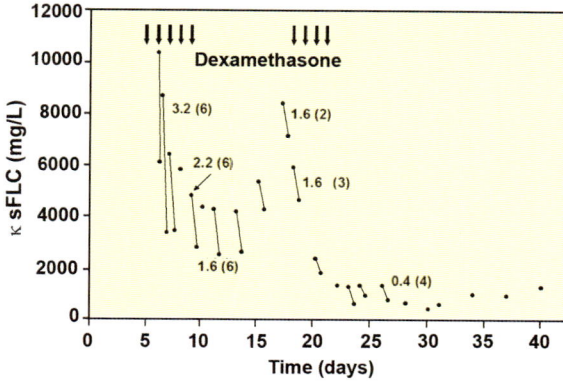

Figure 27.7. sFLCs in a patient presenting with MM and AKI who responded to haemodialysis with renal recovery. Pre- and post-dialysis concentrations are shown. Numbers indicate grams of FLCs removed (and hours of dialysis) per session. Dialysis was over 22 days leading to renal recovery that was maintained for over 2 years.

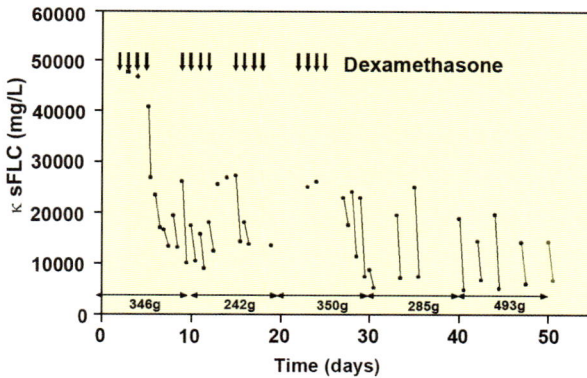

Figure 27.8. sFLCs in a patient presenting with relapsing MM and renal failure who remained on dialysis because of inadequate chemotherapy, despite removing 1.7 kg of FLCs (shown per 10 day period).

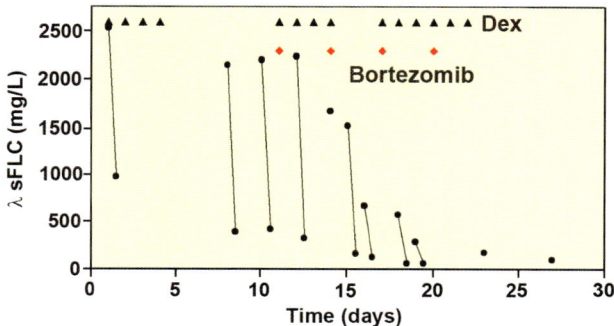

Figure 27.9. sFLC in a patient presenting with relapsing MM and AKI who recovered with chemotherapy and haemodialysis. Pre- and post-dialysis sFLC measurements are shown. The patient received dialysis over 20 days then had renal recovery with GFR rising to 50 ml/min/1.73m². At 1 year the patient remained in complete MM remission. Dex: dexamethasone.

HCO haemodialysis was further evaluated by the same research group in a series of 19 patients with dialysis-dependent acute renal failure who were receiving a standardised dialysis protocol using two HCO 1100 in series with conventional chemotherapy[18]. Six patients had early infective complications, resulting in their chemotherapy being withheld. These patients did not achieve an early sFLC reduction, and only one subsequently became independent of dialysis *(Figure 27.10A)*. The remaining 13 patients had successful chemotherapy plus dialysis, and all had an early reduction in sFLCs *(Figure 27.10A, shaded boxes)* with subsequent renal recovery at a median of 27 days *(Figure 27.10B)*. Patients who recovered renal function had a significantly improved survival (p<0.012; *Figure 27.10C)*.

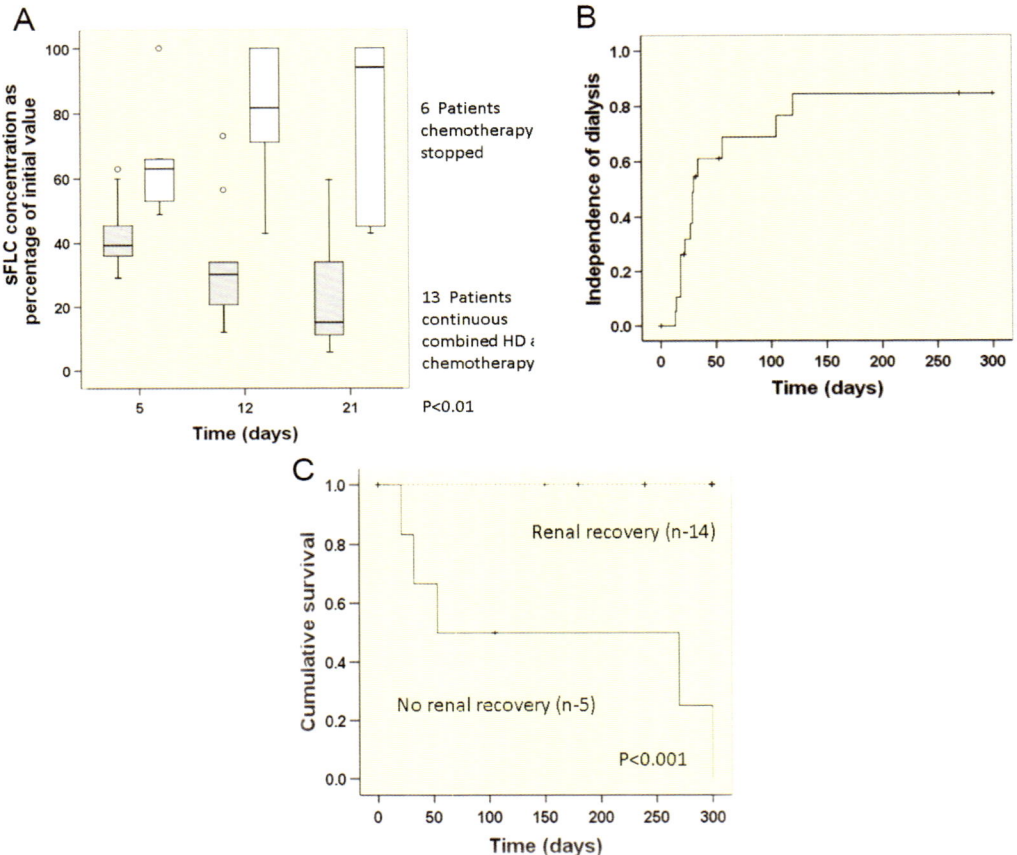

Figure 27.10. *(A) Reductions in sFLC concentrations at 5, 12, and 21 days. Results presented as patients who completed FLC removal HD with (clear boxes, n=6) and without (shaded boxes, n=13) a break in their chemotherapy. (B) Renal recovery rates of patients who received chemotherapy and FLC removal hemodialysis. (C) Kaplan-Meier survival analysis of patients treated with chemotherapy and FLC removal HD. Patients who developed complications requiring early interruption of chemotherapy (solid line, n=6) had a significantly reduced survival compared with patients who received uninterrupted chemotherapy (broken line, n=13); p<0.001. (Republished with permission of Clinical Journal of the American Society of Nephrology[18]; permission conveyed through Copyright Clearance Center, Inc.).*

An international, multi-centre, retrospective review of 67 patients with dialysis-dependent renal failure secondary to MM reported that 63% of patients became dialysis-independent following treatment with HCO haemodialysis and chemotherapy[26]. The probability of achieving dialysis independence increased linearly with increasing levels of reduction in sFLC concentrations by day 12 *(Figure 27.11)*. In a linear regression model, factors that predicted independence of dialysis were the degree of sFLC reduction at days 12 (p=0.002) and 21 (p=0.005) and the time from clinical presentation to the start of haemodialysis (p=0.006). In addition, patients treated in experienced centres (>3 patients) were more likely to become dialysis-independent. Analysis of treatment practices revealed that such centres had a shorter delay between the presentation with renal failure and the initiation of dialysis.

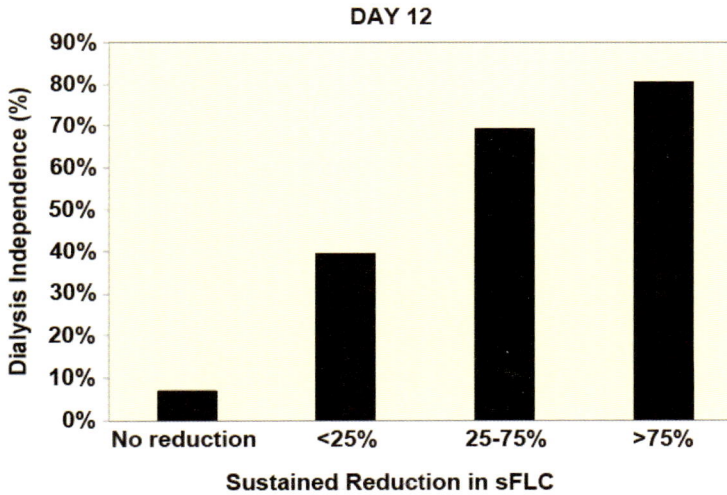

Figure 27.11. Relationship of dialysis independence with sustained reduction in sFLCs. Percentage of patients achieving dialysis independence according to sFLC reduction at day 12, p<0.01. (Reproduced by permission of Oxford University Press [26]).

Results from HCO haemodialysis trials have also been reported by other research groups. Khalafallah et al.[27] reported a series of four patients treated in Tasmania; the three de novo MM patients recovered renal function whilst the patient with relapsed disease did not. Five patients treated in Spain were the subject of a publication by Borrego-Hinojosa et al.[28]. Four of the five became dialysis independent and from consideration of their results the authors suggested that early initiation of treatment could be a determining factor for the response. Tan et al.[29] reported a case series of six patients treated in New Zealand, of whom only three became dialysis independent and the authors concluded that the benefit of HCO dialysis was unproven.

Haemodialysis may not be effective if the patients' plasma contains monoclonal FLCs that form large aggregates *(Section 7.5)*. Harding et al.[30] described two patients with renal failure and MM for whom HCO haemodialysis was not effective in removing monoclonal sFLCs. Size exclusion chromatography demonstrated that a significant proportion of the tumour-produced sFLCs were in the form of large polymers. Such aggregates were too large to pass through the dialysis membrane. Two large multicentre, prospective, randomised controlled trials, EuLITE and MYRE, are currently in progress to determine whether HCO haemodialysis improves patient outcomes[31,32].

Clinical case history

Resolution of cast nephropathy following FLC removal by haemodialysis.[33]

A 61-year-old Caucasian woman, having previously been fit and well, presented to her general practitioner complaining of feeling tired and weak. Initial investigations showed AKI, with a serum creatinine of 872 µmol/L (reference range: 60 - 110 µmol/L), serum urea of 31.5 mmol/L (reference range: 2.5 - 7.8 mmol/L) and haemoglobin 7.8 g/dL (reference range: 12.0 - 16.0 g/dL). Urine output was approximately 2 liters/day. Serum immunofixation electrophoresis (sIFE) identified a monoclonal κ FLC band, which was confirmed by sFLC analysis: κ sFLC 15,700 mg/L (reference range: 3.3 - 19.4 mg/L); λ sFLC 22.4 mg/L (reference range: 5.7 - 26.3 mg/L) and κ/λ sFLC ratio 701 (reference range: 0.26 - 1.65). A skeletal survey identified lytic lesions and a bone marrow examination showed 90% plasma cell infiltration. A renal biopsy confirmed a diagnosis of MM cast nephropathy. Casts affected approximately 30% of the distal tubules and collecting ducts with moderate diffuse interstitial fibrosis and tubular atrophy (Figure 27.12A).

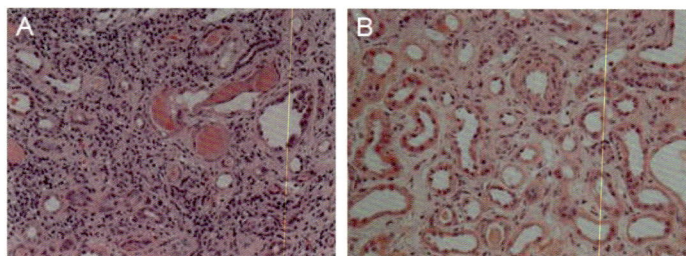

Figure 27.12. Renal biopsy of a patient with cast nephropathy. (A) At presentation and **(B)** 6 weeks after HCO haemodialysis, showing resolution of FLC casts in the distal tubules. (Courtesy of K. Basnayake).

The patient was initially treated with intravenous rehydration over 4 weeks, during which time a 40% reduction in sFLCs was observed, although renal function remained severely impaired (eGFR <10 ml/min/1.73 m²). Chemotherapy was commenced with high-dose dexamethasone and thalidomide, and κ sFLC concentrations were reduced to 1990 mg/L within 5 days of initiating the first cycle. Haemodialysis was initiated with two HCO 1100 dialysers in series for 3 hours, then for 6 - 8 hours daily for 5 days, 8 hours on alternate days for the next 7 days, and then 4 - 6 hours 3 times per week. After 16 haemodialysis sessions, κ sFLC concentrations had fallen to <500 mg/L and were subsequently maintained below this level (Figure 27.13). Despite this, the patient remained dialysis-dependent and a repeat renal biopsy was performed. The biopsy demonstrated resolution of waxy casts and partial resolution of the inflammatory infiltrate, but interstitial fibrosis and tubular atrophy was unchanged (Figure 27.12B). After a further six dialysis sessions the patient was switched to a standard high-flux schedule. After a further 5 days the haemodialysis was discontinued in accordance with the patient's wishes. Creatinine was 650 µm/L. One year on, the patient remains clinically well, with a maintained urine output and no uraemic symptoms despite having an eGFR of 8 ml/min/1.73 m². The patient's MM remains in remission.

In summary, this case illustrates how the sFLC assay can effectively monitor reductions in FLCs following treatment with chemotherapy and HCO haemodialysis. It also provides histological evidence that such reductions may be accompanied by resolution of intratubular casts.

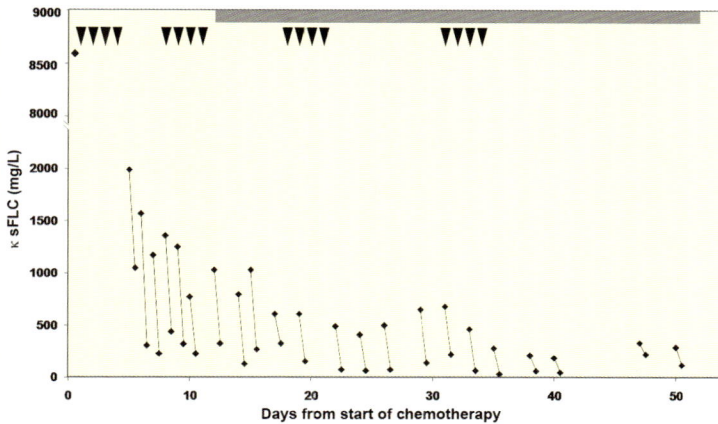

Figure 27.13. sFLC concentrations in a case of cast nephropathy treated with chemotherapy and HCO haemodialysis. Pre-dialysis and post-dialysis values are connected by lines. The concentration at the start of the first pulse of dexamethasone is also shown. The arrowheads represent daily doses of dexamethasone. Daily thalidomide is indicated by the solid line at the top of the chart. (Reproduced from[31] with permission from the Journal of Medical Case Reports).

27.4.3. Adsorption

As an alternative to removal of sFLCs by HCO haemodialysis, alternative strategies have been proposed that employ FLC adsorption or a combination of haemodialysis and adsorption. Polymethylmethacrylate (PMMA) membranes are routinely used to perform standard haemodialysis, but until recently their adsorption capacity for FLCs had not been well characterised. Fabbrini et al.[32] treated 10 patients with dialysis-dependent renal failure and high levels of monoclonal sFLCs (>500 mg/L) with at least one standard 4-hour dialysis session with a Toray BK 2.1 m^2 PMMA membrane. The study concluded that PMMA haemodialysis reduced κ and λ sFLCs to a similar extent (concentrations were reduced by 22.3% and 21.0%, respectively), but that the process was limited by membrane saturation. Dialyser replacement after 2 hours (termed "enhanced adsorption dialysis") increased the overall adsorption efficiency, particularly for λ FLCs[34]. Santoro et al.[35] reported similar findings using two PMMA membranes in sequence (termed the "DELETE system"). An illustrative case is shown in Figure 27.14.

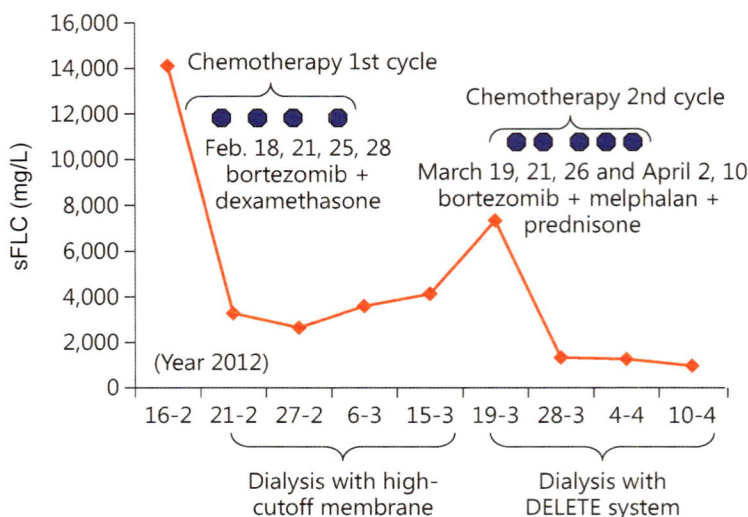

Figure 27.14. sFLC concentrations in a 77-year-old woman with MM treated with chemotherapy and dialysis[35]. *Dialysis was initially performed with HCO dialysers, and subsequently with a PMMA double-filter circuit. (Copyright © 2013 Karger Publishers, Basel, Switzerland).*

A different strategy for FLC removal employed a plasma filter followed by a sorbent cartridge. This technique, known as coupled plasma-filtration adsorption (CPFA), has been used in the extracorporeal treatment of sepsis. In an *in vitro* study of FLC removal by CPFA using a number of different resins, the MDR3 resin demonstrated the best adsorptive capacity[36]. For patients treated with at least six, 4-hour CPFA sessions using MDR3, sFLC concentrations progressively decreased (p=0.05), although the dialysis protocol remains to be optimised.

Another adsorption strategy has used "SUPRA HFR", a form of haemodiafiltration with separated convection, diffusion and adsorption stages that avoids the albumin losses seen with other HCO haemodialysis protocols. The filter comprised an HCO membrane (Synclear 0.2), followed by a low-flux polyphenylene membrane in a second diffusive stage, and a sorbent cartridge with a high affinity for FLCs. Three patients with dialysis-dependent renal failure due to biopsy-proven cast nephropathy were successfully treated with SUPRA HFR[37]. All patients showed a significant reduction of sFLCs and a complete recovery of renal function after 30, 50 and 90 days, respectively[37]. Pasquali et al.[38] reported four further patients treated with this protocol, of whom three recovered renal function.

27.5. Renal recovery is associated with reductions in FLCs

Hutchison et al.[39] demonstrated that irrespective of the treatment modality, recovery of renal function depended on early reduction of sFLCs. In their analysis, a total of 39 patients with biopsy-proven cast nephropathy were included, the majority of whom had severe renal failure at presentation (median eGFR 9 ml/min/1.73 m²). All patients received a combination of chemotherapy plus direct FLC removal by either plasma exchange (n=20) or extended HCO dialysis (n=19). Following treatment, two-thirds of the patients had some degree of renal recovery. While there was no significant difference in the overall renal recovery rate between the two treatment modalities, the rate of recovery was higher in those treated with HCO dialysis. Importantly, there was a linear relationship between the reduction in sFLCs and renal recovery. Multivariate analysis identified that a 60% reduction in sFLC by day 21 was associated with recovery of renal function in 80% of the study population (Figure 27.15A). The authors also concluded that the survival of patients with cast nephropathy was closely linked to renal recovery. The median survival of patients who recovered renal function was 42.7 months, compared with 7.8 months in those who did not (p<0.02; Figure 27.15B).

The findings of Hutchison et al. are supported by others who highlight the importance of monitoring light chain removal therapy with sFLC measurements. All agreed that sustained reductions in sFLCs consistently predicted renal recovery and improved survival in MM patients with cast nephropathy[18,19,40].

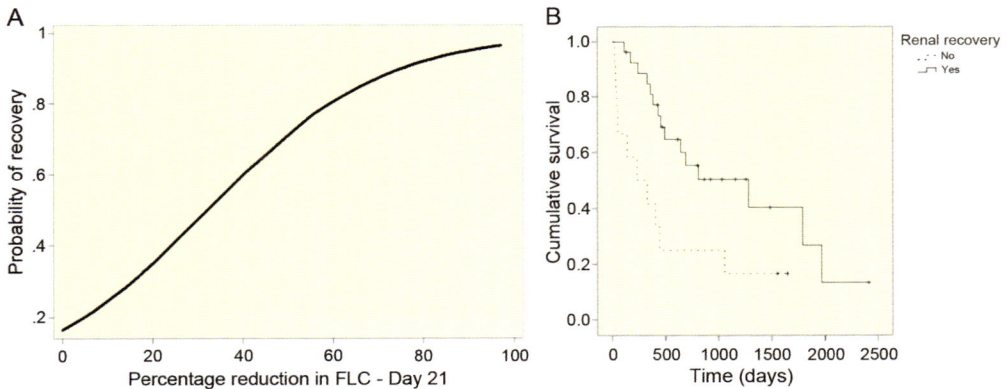

Figure 27.15. (A) Probability plot of renal recovery in relation to sFLC reductions at day 21. (B) Kaplan Meier survival curves for patients with cast nephropathy. (Republished with permission of Journal of the American Society of Nephrology[37] permission conveyed through Copyright Clearance Center, Inc.).

Test Questions

1. What percentage of MM patients have renal impairment at presentation?
2. What protein binds FLCs in the distal tubules?
3. Is renal recovery possible after cast nephropathy?

References

1. Bird JM, Owen RG, D'sa S, Snowden JA, Pratt G, Ashcroft J et al. Guidelines for the diagnosis and management of multiple myeloma 2011. Br J Haematol 2011;154:32-75

2. Hutchison CA, Blade J, Cockwell P, Cook M, Drayson M, Fermand JP et al. Novel approaches for reducing free light chains in patients with myeloma kidney. Nat Rev Nephrol 2012;8:234-43

3. Dimopoulos MA, Terpos E, Chanan-Khan A, Leung N, Ludwig H, Jagannath S et al. Renal impairment in patients with multiple myeloma: a consensus statement on behalf of the International Myeloma Working Group. J Clin Oncol 2010;28:4976-84

4. Tsakiris DJ, Stel VS, Finne P, Fraser E, Heaf J, de MJ et al. Incidence and outcome of patients starting renal replacement therapy for end-stage renal disease due to multiple myeloma or light-chain deposit disease: an ERA-EDTA Registry study. Nephrol Dial Transplant 2010;25:1200-6

5. Haynes RJ, Read S, Collins GP, Darby SC, Winearls CG. Presentation and survival of patients with severe acute kidney injury and multiple myeloma: a 20-year experience from a single centre. Nephrol Dial Transplant 2010;25:419-26

6. Bladé J, Fernández-Llama P, Bosch F, Montolíu J, Lens XM, Montoto S et al. Renal failure in multiple myeloma: presenting features and predictors of outcome in 94 patients from a single institution. Arch Intern Med 1998;158:1889-93

7. Knudsen LM, Hjorth M, Hippe E. Renal failure in multiple myeloma: reversibility and impact on the prognosis. Nordic Myeloma Study Group. Eur J Haematol 2000;65:175-81

8. Dimopoulos MA, Delimpasi S, Katodritou E, Vassou A, Kyrtsonis MC, Repousis P et al. Significant improvement in the survival of patients with multiple myeloma presenting with severe renal impairment after the introduction of novel agents. Ann Oncol 2014;25:195-200

9. Hutchison CA, Batuman V, Behrens J, Bridoux F, Sirac C, Dispenzieri A et al. The pathogenesis and diagnosis of acute kidney injury in multiple myeloma. Nat Rev Nephrol 2011;8:43-51

10. Dispenzieri A, Kyle R, Merlini G, Miguel JS, Ludwig H, Hajek R et al. International Myeloma Working Group guidelines for serum-free light chain analysis in multiple myeloma and related disorders. Leukemia 2009;23:215-24

11. Cook M, Cockwell P, Almond C, Cranmer H, Harding S, Hughes R et al. Serum free light chain assays in the early detection of cast nephropathy in patients presenting with unexplained acute kidney injury (AKI): Results from a pharmacoeconomic evaluation. Blood 2014;124:2612a

12. Hutchison CA, Cockwell P, Cook M. Diagnostic accuracy of monoclonal antibody based serum immunoglobulin free light chain immunoassays in myeloma cast nephropathy. BMC Clin Pathol 2012;12:12

13. Park JW, Kim YK, Bae EH, Ma SK, Kim SW. Combined analysis using extended renal reference range of serum free light chain ratio and serum protein electrophoresis improves the diagnostic accuracy of multiple myeloma in renal insufficiency. Clin Biochem 2012;45:740-4

14. Yadav P, Leung N, Sanders PW, Cockwell P. The use of immunoglobulin light chain assays in the diagnosis of paraprotein-related kidney disease. Kidney Int 2014 *In press*

15. Besemer B, Guthoff M, Kanz L, Heyne N, Weisel K. High-cut off dialysis in multiple myeloma patients with dialysis dependent acute renal failure shows durable renal recovery: a long-term follow up analysis. Blood 2013;122:3199a

16. El-Achkar TM, Wu XR. Uromodulin in kidney injury: an instigator, bystander, or protector? Am J Kidney Dis 2012;59:452-61

17. Huang ZQ, Sanders PW. Localization of a single binding site for immunoglobulin light chains on human Tamm-Horsfall glycoprotein. J Clin Invest 1997;99:732-6

18. Hutchison CA, Bradwell AR, Cook M, Basnayake K, Basu S, Harding S et al. Treatment of acute renal failure secondary to multiple myeloma with chemotherapy and extended high cut-off hemodialysis. Clin J Am Soc Nephrol 2009;4:745-54

19. Leung N, Gertz MA, Zeldenrust SR, Rajkumar SV, Dispenzieri A, Fervenza FC et al. Improvement of cast nephropathy with plasma exchange depends on the diagnosis and on reduction of serum free light chains. Kidney Int 2008;73:1282-8

20. Burnette BL, Leung N, Rajkumar SV. Renal improvement in myeloma with bortezomib plus plasma exchange. N Engl J Med 2011;364:2365-6

21. Clark WF, Stewart AK, Rock GA, Sternbach M, Sutton DM, Barrett BJ et al. Plasma exchange when myeloma presents as acute renal failure: a randomized, controlled trial. Ann Intern Med 2005;143:777-84

22. Ritz E. Nephrology beyond JASN: Plasma exchange for acute renal failure of myeloma - logical, yet ineffective. J Am Soc Nephrol 2006;17:914–6

23. Hutchison CA, Cockwell P, Reid S, Chandler K, Mead GP, Harrison J et al. Efficient removal of immunoglobulin free light chains by hemodialysis in multiple myeloma: in vitro and in vivo studies. J Am Soc Nephrol 2007;18:886-95

24. Gondouin B, Hutchison CA. High cut-off dialysis membranes: current uses and future potential. Adv Chronic Kidney Dis 2011;18:180-7

25. Hutchison CA, Harding S, Mead G, Goehl H, Storr M, Bradwell A, Cockwell P. Serum free-light chain removal by high cutoff hemodialysis: optimizing removal and supportive care. Artif Organs 2008;32:910-7

26. Hutchison CA, Heyne N, Airia P, Schindler R, Zickler D, Cook M et al. Immunoglobulin free light chain levels and recovery from myeloma kidney on treatment with chemotherapy and high cut-off haemodialysis. Nephrol Dial Transplant 2012;27:3823-8

27. Khalafallah AA, Loi SW, Love S, Mohamed M, Mace R, Khalil R et al. Early application of high cut-off haemodialysis for de-novo myeloma nephropathy is associated with long-term dialysis-independency and renal recovery. Mediterr J Hematol Infect Dis 2013;5:e2013007

28. Borrego-Hinojosa J, Perez-Del Barrio MP, Biechy-Baldan MD, Merino-Garcia E, Sanchez-Perales MC, Garcia-Cortes MJ et al. Treatment by long haemodialysis sessions with high cut-off filters in myeloma cast nephropathy: our experience. Nefrologia 2013;33:515-23

29. Tan J, Lam-Po-Tang M, Hutchison CA, de Zoysa JR. Extended high cut-off haemodialysis for myeloma cast nephropathy in Auckland, 2008-2012. Nephrology (Carlton) 2014;19:432-5

30. Harding S, Provot F, Beuscart JB, Cook M, Bradwell AR, Stringer S et al. Aggregated serum free light chains may prevent adequate removal by high cut-off haemodialysis. Nephrol Dial Transplant 2011;26:1438-40

31. Bridoux F, Fermand JP. Optimizing treatment strategies in myeloma cast nephropathy: rationale for a randomized prospective trial. Adv Chronic Kidney Dis 2012;19:333-41

32. Hutchison CA, Cook M, Heyne N, Weisel K, Billingham L, Bradwell AR, Cockwell P. European trial of free light chain removal by extended haemodialysis in cast nephropathy (EuLITE): a randomised control trial. Trials 2008;9:55

33. Basnayake K, Hutchison C, Kamel D, Sheaff M, Ashman N, Cook M et al. Resolution of cast nephropathy following free light chain removal by haemodialysis in a patient with multiple myeloma: a case report. J Med Case Reports 2008;2:380

34. Fabbrini P, Sirtori S, Casiraghi E, Pieruzzi F, Genovesi S, Corti D et al. Polymethylmethacrylate membrane and serum free light chain removal: enhancing adsorption properties. Blood purif 2013;35 Suppl 2:52-8

35. Santoro A, Grazia M, Mancini E. The Double Polymethylmethacrylate Filter (DELETE System) in the Removal of Light Chains in Chronic Dialysis Patients with Multiple Myeloma. Blood purif 2013;35 Suppl 2:5-13

36. Mancini E, Facchini M, Ricci D, Chiocchini A, Palladino G, Santoro A. Light chain removal by means of adsorption in the extracorpeal treatment of myeloma-induced cast nephropathy. World Congress of Nephrology 2013;SA393a

37. Pasquali S, Corradini M, Iannuzzella F, Mattei S, Bovino A, Stefani A et al. Extracorporeal free light chains removal in association with chemotherapy in myeloma acute kidney injury: New therapeutic options and old prognostic factors. Online 2013;SA394a

38. Pasquali S, Iannuzzella F, Corradini M, Mattei S, Bovino A, Stefani A et al. A novel option for reducing free light chains in myeloma kidney: supra-hemodiafiltration with endogenous reinfusion (HFR). J Nephrol 2014 In press

39. Hutchison CA, Cockwell P, Stringer S, Bradwell A, Cook M, Gertz MA et al. Early reduction of serum-free light chains associates with renal recovery in myeloma kidney. J Am Soc Nephrol 2011;22:1129-36

40. Roussou M, Kastritis E, Migkou M, Psimenou E, Grapsa I, Matsouka C et al. Treatment of patients with multiple myeloma complicated by renal failure with bortezomib-based regimens. Leuk Lymphoma 2008;49:890-5

AL amyloidosis

Summary:

- sFLC analysis provides an efficient diagnostic screen in combination with immunofixation of serum and urine.

- Baseline sFLC measurements provide important prognostic information.

- sFLCs are usually the most effective marker for evaluating the early effects of chemotherapy.

- sFLC concentrations during follow-up provide prognostic information on overall survival and organ responses.

- sFLCs increase during renal failure, independently of light chain synthesis.

28.1. Introduction

Primary systemic, or light-chain amyloidosis (AL) is a protein conformation disorder characterised by the accumulation of monoclonal free light chains (FLCs) or their fragments, as extracellular, insoluble amyloid fibrils that cause functional and structural organ damage *(Figure 28.1A)*[1]. Typically, a slowly growing clone of plasma cells secrete the monoclonal FLCs, which are more often of the λ subtype (κ to λ frequency: 1:3)[1,2].

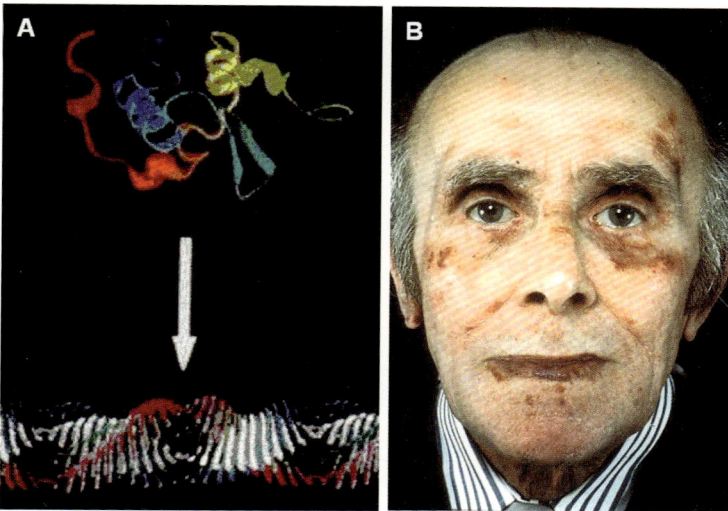

Figure 28.1. (A) AL amyloidosis showing formation of amyloid fibrils from FLC domains. (B) Classic facial features with periorbital purpura. (Courtesy of P. Hawkins).

As amyloid deposits can be formed by a range of proteins other than immunoglobulin light chains, the diagnosis of amyloidosis should be based initially on tissue biopsy, followed by confirmation of the amyloid type and extent of organ involvement[3]. Amyloid deposits in tissue biopsies stain with Congo red and produce pathognomonic red-green birefringence under polarised light. Immunohistochemical staining of tissue biopsies is frequently not diagnostic in AL amyloidosis, but is useful in confirming or excluding other amyloid types, such as the AA type (characterised by deposition of serum amyloid A protein)[1]. DNA analysis can also be used to distinguish AL amyloidosis from hereditary forms of amyloid, which may coexist with monoclonal gammopathy of undetermined significance (MGUS)[3]. The critical importance of identifying the amyloid type and the analytical tools available are described in a recent review of amyloid diagnosis[4].

AL amyloid fibrils are formed from the N-terminal fragment of a monoclonal FLC, and comprise the variable region and part of the constant region. The ability to form amyloid fibrils appears to be related to the structural characteristics of a particular variable region, with an over-representation of VκI and VκIV, and Vλ6a and Vλ3r gene segments, in κ and λ AL amyloidosis, respectively[1].

AL amyloidosis affects multiple organs, most frequently the kidney (74%), heart (60%), liver (27%), peripheral nervous system (22%) and autonomic nervous system (18%), although other organs may also be involved *(Figures 28.1B, 28.2A and 28.2B)*[1]. The monoclonal FLC type influences the spectrum of organ involvement: κ-type AL typically affects the gastrointestinal tract and liver, whereas nephrotic-range proteinuria is observed in a higher proportion of λ-type AL patients[2]. The tissue distribution may be related to structural characteristics of individual FLCs. It is of interest that λ FLCs derived from the Vλ6a gene segment are preferentially associated with kidney involvement[5].

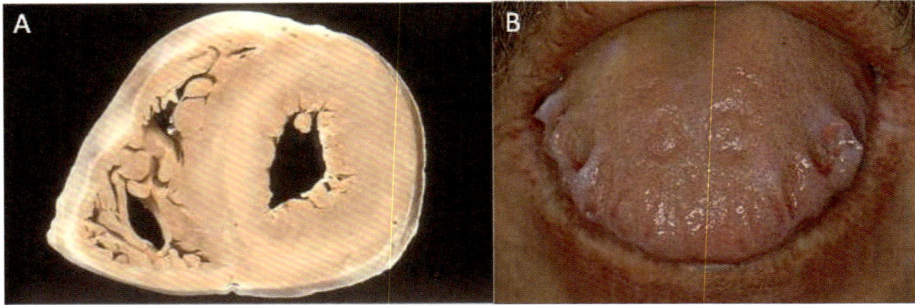

Figure 28.2. (A) AL amyloidosis in the heart showing thickening of the left ventricular walls leading to heart failure. (B) AL amyloidosis showing macroglossia that occurs in 20% of patients. (Courtesy of P. Hawkins).

The median survival of patients with AL amyloidosis is similar for κ and λ patients, and ranges from 12 to 18 months in different published series[6,7]. It is largely dependent on the number of organs involved and the degree to which their function is compromised. Whilst survival in AL amyloidosis has improved over the past decade with the introduction of several new therapeutic options, the 1-year mortality remains high at 43%[6].

AL amyloidosis is 5 times less common than multiple myeloma (MM). The age-adjusted incidence of AL amyloidosis in the United States is estimated to be between 5.1 and 12.8 per million per year[8], which is equivalent to approximately 600 new cases per year in the UK[9]. In an audit of 800 UK patients with AL amyloidosis, 66% were aged between 50 and 70 years of age at diagnosis, and 4% were aged less than 40 years[9]. There is an equal proportion of male to female patients. AL amyloidosis co-exists with MM in approximately 10 - 15% of patients, and more rarely with Waldenström's macroglobulinaemia and other lymphoid malignancies *(Chapters 32 and 31)*[9]. In a recent review of 1255 AL amyloidosis patients[10], the presence of CRAB criteria (hypercalcaemia, renal failure, anaemia and lytic bone lesions) or >10% bone marrow plasma cell infiltration was found to identify patients with a similarly poor prognosis. The authors suggested that both these patient groups should be considered together as having AL amyloidosis with MM.

As for MM, MGUS is a precursor condition for AL amyloidosis *(Section 13.3)*. In a study of archived sera from 20 American military personnel who went on to develop AL amyloidosis, 100% of pre-diagnostic sera had a detectable monoclonal gammopathy 4 years prior to diagnosis and serum FLC (sFLC) levels were also observed to rise in the years before diagnosis of AL amyloidosis[11].

28.2. Diagnosis of AL amyloidosis

Early diagnosis of AL amyloidosis is critical, to facilitate swift access to effective chemotherapy, and therefore suppress the production of amyloidogenic FLCs before irreversible organ damage occurs. Whilst the detection of a monoclonal protein does not provide a definitive diagnosis of AL amyloidosis, it does provide supportive evidence of an underlying plasma cell dyscrasia. Guidelines recommend that immunofixation of serum and urine in combination with sFLC analysis provides an efficient diagnostic screen for AL amyloidosis *(Section 28.3)*.

By electrophoretic techiques, a serum monoclonal protein is detected in approximately 80% of patients, and a urine monoclonal protein is detected in approximately 70%[4]. However, the underlying monoclonal gammopathy can be subtle and monoclonal proteins are undetectable in between 5 and 20% of patients, depending upon the sensitivity of the electrophoretic method used *(Chapter 4)*. Figure 28.3 shows a typical serum protein electrophoresis (SPE) result from a patient with AL amyloidosis; it demonstrates a nephrotic pattern (low albumin, elevated $\alpha2$ and low γ fraction) with no obvious monoclonal protein. Serum immunofixation electrophoresis (sIFE), however, reveals some polyclonal immunoglobulin in the γ region and a monoclonal λ FLC band in the β/γ region. This band is too small to be quantified by scanning densitometry of the SPE gel since it is undetectable against the background proteins. Figure 28.4 shows the urine protein electrophoresis (UPE) from the same patient. It contains a considerable amount of protein, particularly albumin, and there is a small monoclonal spike. Urine immunofixation electrophoresis (uIFE) indicates a monoclonal λ protein against a background of polyclonal κ and λ FLCs. As with the serum protein, the urine monoclonal band is difficult to quantify (by UPE) and is of modest utility for the purpose of disease monitoring.

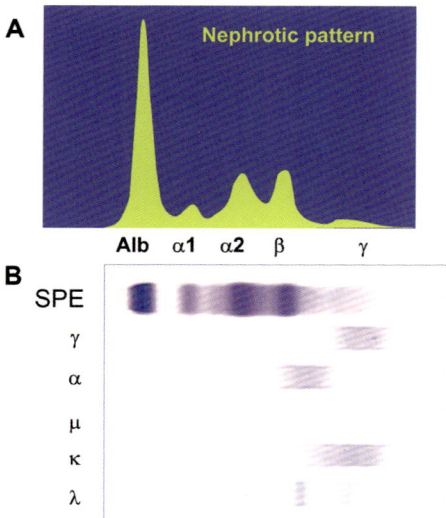

Figure 28.3. (A) Serum from a patient with AL amyloidosis showing a nephrotic pattern on SPE. (B) sIFE reveals a small (nonquantifiable) monoclonal λ protein in the β/γ region. (Courtesy of R. Kyle and J. Katzmann).

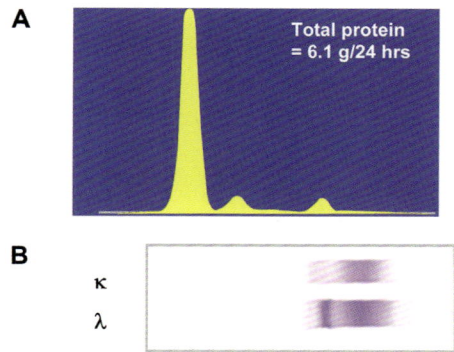

Figure 28.4. (A) UPE; and (B) uIFE from the same patient as in Figure 15.3, showing a monoclonal λ protein band. (Courtesy of R. Kyle and J. Katzmann).

There are now numerous published studies comparing the diagnostic performance of sFLC and electrophoretic assays in screening for AL amyloidosis *(Chapter 23)*. Katzmann et al.[12] compared diagnostic screening panels for identifying monoclonal gammopathy in patients suspected of having MM, AL amyloidosis and related monoclonal gammopathies. Focussing on the amyloid patients within this study, there were 581 with a confirmed diagnosis of AL amyloidosis and for these, the diagnostic sensitivity of the sFLC assays was 88.3%, which increased to 97.1% with the inclusion of sIFE *(Figure 28.5)*. Importantly, addition of uIFE to the serum panel increased the sensitivity to 98.1% (representing an additional 6/581 patients), confirming that in only a minority of AL amyloidosis patients, monoclonal FLCs may be detected by urine studies alone *(Section 7.6.1)*.

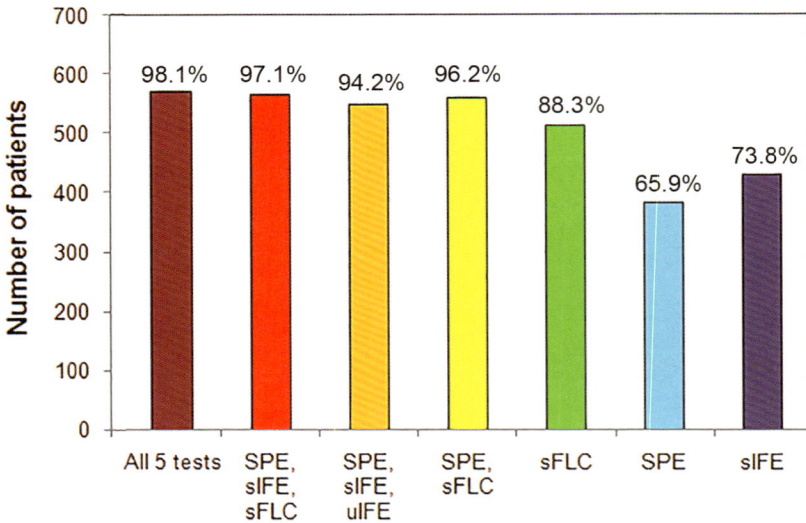

Figure 28.5. Comparison of the diagnostic sensitivity of screening panels in 581 patients with confirmed AL amyloidosis.

In a separate prospective study of 121 patients with biopsy-proven AL amyloidosis by Palladini et al.[13], the diagnostic sensitivity of the κ/λ sFLC ratio was 76%. By comparison, the diagnostic sensitivity of sIFE and uIFE was 96%. When AL amyloidosis patients were grouped according to monoclonal FLC type, the diagnostic sensitivity of the κ/λ sFLC ratio was significantly higher for κ clones than λ clones (97 vs. 69% respectively), whereas the diagnostic sensitivity of sIFE was lower for κ clones than λ clones (60 vs. 87%). The authors commented that this difference may be due to the formation of monoclonal κ FLC aggregates of variable size and electrophoretic mobility, resulting in the absence of a detectable monoclonal protein band by serum electrophoresis. They concluded that the diagnosis of AL amyloidosis should not rely on a single test, and that a screening algorithm comprising serum and urine IFE in combination with the κ/λ sFLC ratio had 100% diagnostic sensitivity for AL amyloidosis.

Previous studies on the diagnostic performance of the κ/λ sFLC ratio in AL amyloidosis reported a diagnostic sensitivity ranging from 75% to 98%[14,15,16,17,2,18]. In the first published study of 262 AL amyloidosis patients at the National Amyloidosis Centre, London, the κ/λ sFLC ratio was associated with a greater diagnostic sensitivity than the combination of serum and urine IFE (98% vs. 79%) *(Figure 28.6)*[14]. In all published studies to date, sFLC analysis has proven to be an important complementary technique to IFE for screening for monoclonal gammopathy in patients with suspected AL amyloidosis.

In a study by Kumar et al.[2], patients with AL amyloidosis had median concentrations of involved κ and λ FLCs of 314 mg/L and 194 mg/L, respectively, which is considerably lower than those concentrations seen in MM[19]. The generally lower sFLC concentrations seen in AL amyloidosis contribute to a small proportion of patients with discordant sFLC and electrophoresis results. For example, occasionally, patients may have positive uIFE results (for monoclonal FLC) but normal sFLC ratios. This may be due to the timing of serum/urine sample collections or the loss of albumin through the renal glomeruli overloading the renal capacity for protein reabsorption. This and other apparently

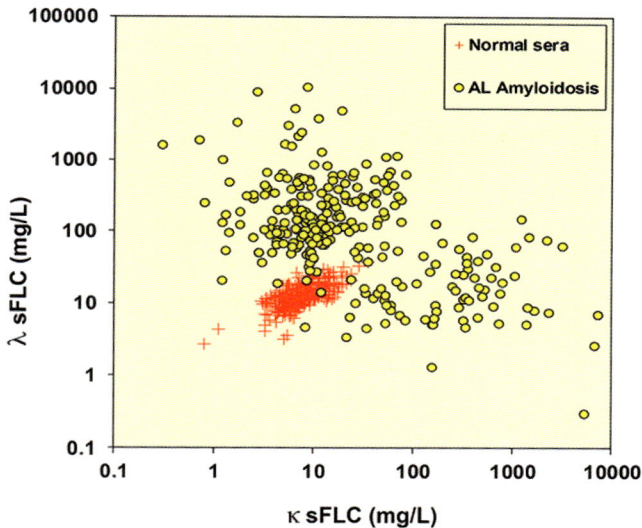

Figure 28.6. sFLCs in 262 patients with AL amyloidosis at diagnosis, compared with 282 normal serum samples.

discordant results are discussed in Section 7.6. Rare patients with AL amyloidosis may be negative by all serum and urine tests, but this is more frequent for patients with localised AL amyloidosis *(Section 28.2.1)*.

With the advent of alternative assays for sFLC measurement, discrepant sFLC quantitations can also occur. Comparisons of Freelite® with the Siemens N Latex FLC assays have highlighted significant variation in results for AL amyloidosis patients, confirming that data from the two assay formats is not interchangeable[20,21]. These results are presented in more detail in Chapter 8.

28.2.1 Localised amyloid disease

Rather than being a systemic disease, AL amyloidosis may also present as a localised disease, where amyloid deposition is limited to a single organ. The specific area of the body affected depends upon the biochemical nature of the amyloid fibril protein and, as in systemic AL amyloidosis, light chain fragments may be involved. Localised AL amyloidosis may first be suspected on the basis of its location. Typical sites associated with localised AL amyloidosis include the brain, bladder, skin, urinary tract, conjunctiva, larynx and the tracheobronchial tree in the absence of systemic visceral dysfunction[22,23]. For patients with localised AL amyloidosis, localised therapy and life-long monitoring are necessary, although these patients have been shown to have a normal life expectancy[23]. The frequent association of multinuclear giant cells with localized amyloid deposits and the equal prevalence of κ and λ type deposits has led to the suggestion that the pathogenesis may differ from that of systemic amyloidosis[24].

Serum free light chains (sFLCs) have been evaluated in patients with localised amyloid disease attending the UK National Amyloidosis Centre, as presented in Table 28.1. An enlarged series of 235 cases, was reported by the same group in 2005[25]. Of the 162/235 patients with tissue biopsy data available, the fibril type was classified as AL in 100 cases (27% κ, 73% λ). The study concluded that localised AL amyloidosis is associated with a generally excellent prognosis.

Overall, elevated levels of sFLCs are less commonly observed in localised amyloidosis than in systemic AL amyloidosis and, even when present, the concentrations are lower. sFLC concentrations may therefore assist in distinguishing the different types of amyloid disease and also systemic from localised light chain amyloid disease.

Site of amyloid deposits	Number of patients	Monoclonal proteins*	Abnormal κ/λ sFLC ratios
Bone	7	3 (43%)	6 (88%)
Bladder	25	1 (4%)	3 (12%)
Bowel	10	4 (40%)	3 (30%)
Bronchial	13	2 (15%)	1 (8%)
Nodular pulmonary	13	3 (23%)	3 (23%)
Laryngeal	22	0	1 (4.5%)
Nasopharynx	16	1 (6%)	2 (13%)
Skin	18	2 (11%)	2 (11%)
Ocular	10	2 (20%)	2 (20%)
Lymph node	16	3 (19%)	5 (31%)
Miscellaneous	6	0	1 (17%)

Table 28.1. Frequency of monoclonal proteins in patients with localised amyloid disease. *Serum monoclonal proteins or light chain proteinuria identified by electrophoretic tests[25]. (Courtesy of P. Hawkins).*

28.3. Guidelines for the diagnosis of AL amyloidosis

28.3.1. International Myeloma Working Group (2009)

In the guidelines for sFLC analysis in MM and related disorders, the International Myeloma Working Group (IMWG) recommend a combination of sFLC analysis and immunofixation of serum and urine to screen for AL amyloidosis[26]. The guidelines also recommend that baseline sFLC measurements are obtained for all AL amyloidosis patients, as highly abnormal results have prognostic value *(Section 28.4)*.

28.3.2. British Committee for Standards in Haematology (2015)

The British Committee for Standards in Haematology guidelines on the diagnosis and investigation of AL amyloidosis state that immunofixation of blood and urine and sFLCs should be measured in all patients with suspected AL amyloidosis[27]. They also recognise that Freelite sFLC assays are well established, whilst FLC assays from other manufacturers have not been validated *(Chapter 8)*.

Clinical case history 1

AL amyloidosis identified by FLC analysis when electrophoretic tests were doubtful[28].

A 40-year-old woman, with spontaneous bruises, asthenia, abdominal pains and possible cardiomyopathy, was investigated for suspicion of AL amyloidosis. Abdominal fat biopsy showed Congo red positivity. SPE showed hypogammaglobulinaemia but no monoclonal proteins.

IFE showed a weak λ band without a corresponding intact immunoglobulin *(Figure 28.7)*. Quantitative immunoglobulin measurements were: IgG 4.9 g/L; IgA 1.02 g/L and IgM 0.32 g/L indicating hypogammaglobulinaemia. sFLC analysis showed: κ 7.8 mg/L; λ 210 mg/L and κ/λ ratio of 0.04. This supported a diagnosis of AL amyloidosis.

Nephelometric sFLC quantification was clearly abnormal and provided a measurable parameter for subsequent disease monitoring. In contrast, FLCs were barely detectable by conventional electrophoretic assays.

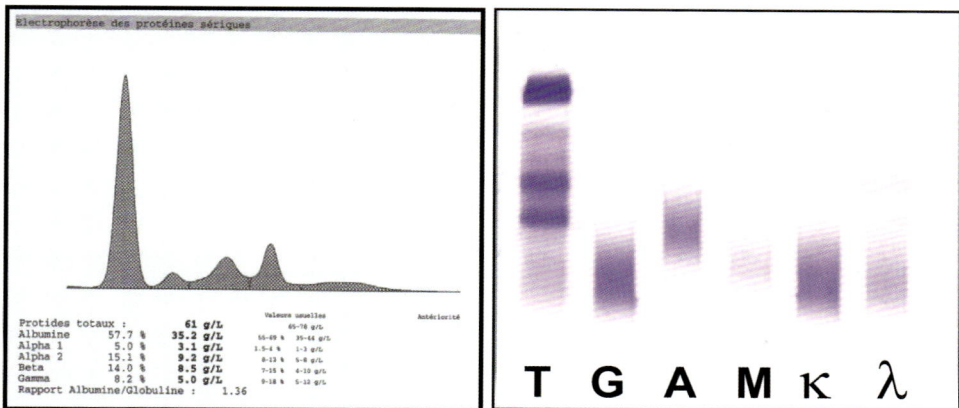

Figure 28.7. SPE and IFE results. A weak λ band is visible. (Courtesy of Dr Lucile Musset).

28.4. Prognostic value of sFLCs at diagnosis

In addition to assessing the degree of organ involvement[6,23], evaluation of sFLCs at baseline provides important prognostic information in AL amyloidosis, and is recommended in IMWG guidelines[26]. In a study of 730 patients, median overall survival was shorter among those with an abnormal sFLC ratio at baseline (16.2 months, n=644) than in those with a normal ratio (63.6 months, n = 86) *(Figure 28.8A)*[2]. When the analysis was repeated grouping patients according to sFLC burden (defined as the difference between involved and uninvolved FLC [dFLC]) above or below the median value (196 mg/L), the overall survival for patients with high dFLC was 10.9 months compared with 37.1 months for those with low dFLC (p<0.001) *(Figure 28.8B)*[2]. High baseline FLC levels have also been shown to be associated with poor outcome in AL amyloidosis patients undergoing stem cell transplant[29,30].

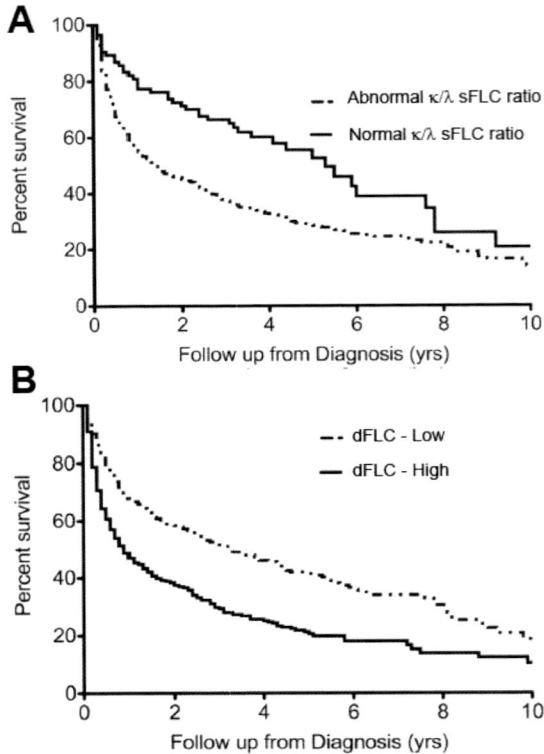

Figure 28.8. Relationship between overall survival outcome and sFLC measurements at diagnosis. (A) AL amyloidosis patients grouped according to sFLC ratio at baseline (normal versus abnormal). (B) AL amyloidosis patients grouped according to baseline dFLC (high: >196 mg/L vs. low: <196 mg/L). (This research was originally published in Blood[2] © the American Society of Hematology).

Kumar et al.[2] noted that AL amyloidosis patients had a worse survival if there was no intact monoclonal immunoglobulin detectable (12.6 months vs. 29.3 months, p=0.02). The patients without monoclonal heavy chain had a higher dFLC value (255 vs 153 mg/L, p<0.001) but on multivariate analysis both dFLC and the presence/absence of heavy chain were independently prognostic for survival. Kumar et al.[2] also reported that AL amyloidosis patients with high sFLC burden (dFLC >196 mg/L), had more frequent and severe cardiac involvement, with higher levels of cardiac biomarkers troponin T (cTnT) and pro-B-type natriuretic peptide (NT-ProBNP). However, in a multivariate analysis that included a variety of markers, baseline dFLC remained an independent predictor of survival. In a subsequent publication from the same centre[30], a revised staging system for AL amyloidosis was proposed incorporating dFLC alongside the cardiac biomarkers cTnT and NT-ProBNP. Patients were assigned a score of 1 for each of the following: 1) dFLC ≥180 mg/L; 2) cTnT ≥0.025 ng/mL or, 3) NT-ProBNP ≥1800pg/mL, to give stages I to IV (for 0 - 3 points, respectively). The staging system was derived from 810 patients with newly diagnosed AL amyloidosis and tested on two further populations (n=303 and n=103). The authors concluded that this revised Mayo staging system (based on sFLC measurements and cardiac biomarkers) allowed better discrimination of patient outcomes in AL amyloidosis than a staging system based on cardiac biomarkers alone, and should be incorporated into future clinical trials[30].

Wassef et al.[20] used the above staging system when comparing sFLC results produced by Freelite with another manufacturer's monoclonal antibody-based FLC assays. The quantitative results and stage allocation differed for the two immunoassays, indicating that the staging system cannot be extended to different assays without separate validation *(Chapter 8)*.

28.5. Monitoring patients with AL amyloidosis

"The introduction of the serum immunoglobulin free light chain assay has revolutionized our ability to assess hematological responses in patients with low tumor burden......."
Dispenzieri A, Gertz MA, Kyle RA. Blood 2004[32].

"The Freelite serum free light chain assay represents a landmark advance in the management of AL amyloidosis....."
Wechalekar AD, Hawkins PN, Gillmore JD. Br J Haem 2008[33].

The aim of therapy in AL amyloidosis is to suppress the monoclonal plasma cell clone that produces the amyloidogenic FLC, and to support and preserve organ function. Treatment regimens for AL amyloidosis have essentially been modified from those developed in MM. Patients must be monitored closely, since the toxicity of chemotherapy may be substantially greater than in MM due to reduced organ function and poor performance status.

Amyloid deposits exist in a state of dynamic turnover. When the supply of amyloid-forming protein is reduced by effective chemotherapy, the balance between amyloid deposition and clearance may be favourably altered. Although complete suppression of clonal plasma cells is desirable, reduction in the amyloidogenic sFLC concentrations is often sufficient to stabilise or reduce amyloid deposits[9].

Traditionally, haematological response assessment in AL amyloidosis followed the same guidelines as MM, i.e., using serial measurement of monoclonal protein, with measurable disease defined as >10 g/L[34]. However, this approach has limited utility in AL amyloidosis as the proportion of patients with measurable monoclonal immunoglobulin is very low; typically between 15 and 20%[7]. In contrast, nearly 90% of patients have measurable disease as assessed by sFLCs (defined as dFLC >50 mg/L at diagnosis, *Section 28.6.2)*[7,35].

Due to their short serum half-life, sFLCs are usually the most effective marker for evaluating the early effects of chemotherapy in AL amyloidosis *(Chapter 3)*. In a study evaluating the combination of bortezomib and dexamethasone treatment in patients with AL amyloidosis, sFLCs were assessed before each cycle of therapy[31]. Rapid haematological responses were observed, with a 50% reduction in the involved sFLC concentration in all responding patients within two courses of treatment *(Figure 28.9)*. The authors concluded that therapy may be discontinued after two cycles if there is no sFLC response and that an alternative treatment could be considered.

28.6. Guidelines for monitoring AL amyloidosis
28.6.1. International Myeloma Working Group (2009)

In the guidelines for sFLC analysis in MM and related disorders *(Section 25.3.1)*, the IMWG recommend sFLC assays for the quantitative monitoring of patients with oligosecretory plasma cell disorders, including patients with AL amyloidosis[26].

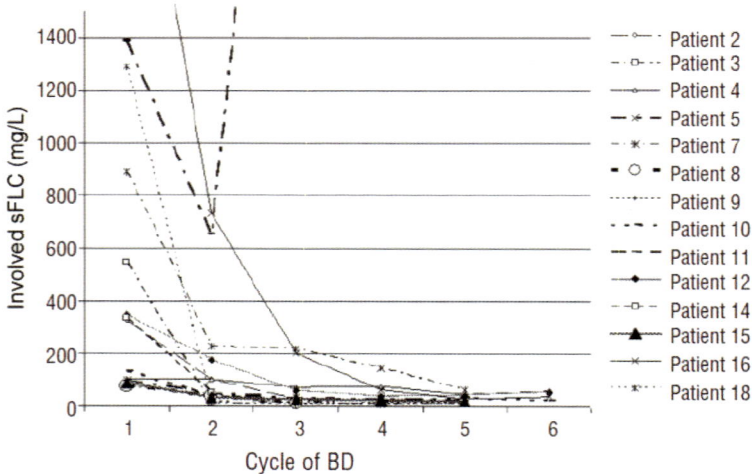

Figure 28.9. Monitoring response to bortezomib/dexamethasone with sFLCs[31]. Analysis of sFLCs was performed before each cycle of treatment. (Obtained from Haematologica Journal website: haematologica.org).

28.6.2. Consensus guidelines for the conduct and reporting of clinical trials in systemic light-chain amyloidosis (2012)

In 2012, Comenzo et al.[36] published consensus guidelines for the definition of organ involvement and response to treatment in AL amyloidosis. The guidelines are based on data from an international cohort of 816 patients from seven referral centres, for which haematological responses were assessed 3 and/or 6 months after initiation of first-line therapy. Haematological response categories were defined, as detailed in Table 28.2. There was a strong correlation between the haematological response category at 3 or 6 months and overall survival (Section 28.7). The haematological response criteria were subsequently validated in a prospective study of 374 patients[37], and have now been widely adopted and incorporated into national guidelines[38,39].

Haematologic response category	Definition
Complete response	Normalisation of sFLC levels and ratio, negative serum and urine immunofixation
Very good partial response	A reduction in the dFLC to <40 mg/L
Partial response	A >50% reduction in the dFLC
No response	Less than a PR
Progression	**From CR:** any detectable monoclonal protein or abnormal FLC ratio (light chain must double)
	From PR: 50% increase in serum monoclonal protein to >5 g/L, or 50% increase in urine monoclonal protein to >200 mg/day (a visible peak must be present) or FLC increase of 50% to >100 mg/L

Table 28.2. Haematologic response and progression criteria[36].

The definition of measurable disease by sFLC analysis was defined as a dFLC of >50 mg/L, and covers approximately 85% of newly diagnosed patients. For the 15% of patients with unmeasurable sFLCs at baseline, standard criteria for response in MM are available (a monoclonal intact immunoglobulin concentration of >5 g/L is considered assessable for response, *Chapter 25*).

28.6.3. British Committee for Standards in Haematology (2015)

The British Committee for Standards in Haematology guidelines on the management of AL amyloidosis[38] define haematological response criteria according to the international consensus guideline, described in Section 28.6.2[36]. The guidelines recommend monitoring response to treatment with sFLCs or monoclonal protein measurements after each cycle of chemotherapy and every 1 - 3 months thereafter, with the aim of switching to an alternative regimen as soon as the current one is proving ineffectual, which may be assessed after three cycles of therapy or earlier in cardiac patients. The guidelines also recognise that Freelite sFLC assays are well established for monitoring response in AL amyloidosis, whilst FLC assays from other manufacturers have not been validated *(Chapter 8)*.

28.7. Prognostic value of sFLC response

Kumar et al.[7] studied the prognostic significance of dFLC reductions in 347 patients undergoing an autologous stem cell transplant (SCT). A 50% decrease in dFLC provided poor clinical discriminatory value in predicting survival as 96% of patients in the study achieved this reduction *(Figure 28.10A)*. In contrast, a 90% reduction in dFLC was observed in 38% of patients, providing a more useful clinical separation. Furthermore, the median overall survival post-SCT, among those patients who achieved a 90% reduction in dFLC, was not reached, compared with the 37.4 months achieved in the remaining patients (p<0.001) *(Figure 28.10B)*. The prognostic value of achieving a 90% reduction in dFLC was confirmed in a separate cohort of 96 patients treated with melphalan and dexamethasone *(Figure 28.10C,D)*[7]. The authors concluded that assessment of the dFLC response allows clinicians to modify therapy in those patients failing to achieve a 90% reduction in dFLC. These results are supported by the findings of several other earlier studies[14,40,41,42,43]. The relative contribution of changes in monoclonal intact immunoglobulin protein and dFLC in predicting overall survival was also analysed by Kumar et al.[7]. Reductions in dFLC were shown to be superior to changes in intact immunoglobulins for predicting overall survival.

More recently, in the study used to derive the consensus agreement for response criteria *(Section 28.6.2)*, there was a strong correlation between the haematological response category at 3 or 6 months and overall survival *(Figure 28.11)*. Girnius and colleagues[44] noted that the studies used to produce the response criteria contained very few patients treated with high-dose melphalan and autologous stem cell transplant (HDM/ASCT). However, Girnius et al. were able to provide data indicating that the criteria did have prognostic value for 140 patients whose response was assessed 1 year after HDM/ASCT. Cordes et al.[45] analysed survival data for 74 patients who had received HDM/ASCT and concluded that the lowest post-treatment sFLC concentration provided the best indication of those patients who were more likely to survive for >10 years.

Palladini et al.[21] compared response to treatment as assessed by Freelite and the Siemens N Latex FLC assays. Although the results produced by both assays were prognostic, percentage reductions in FLC concentration were quite different, leading the authors to conclude that amended response criteria would be needed for the N Latex FLC assays *(Chapter 8)*.

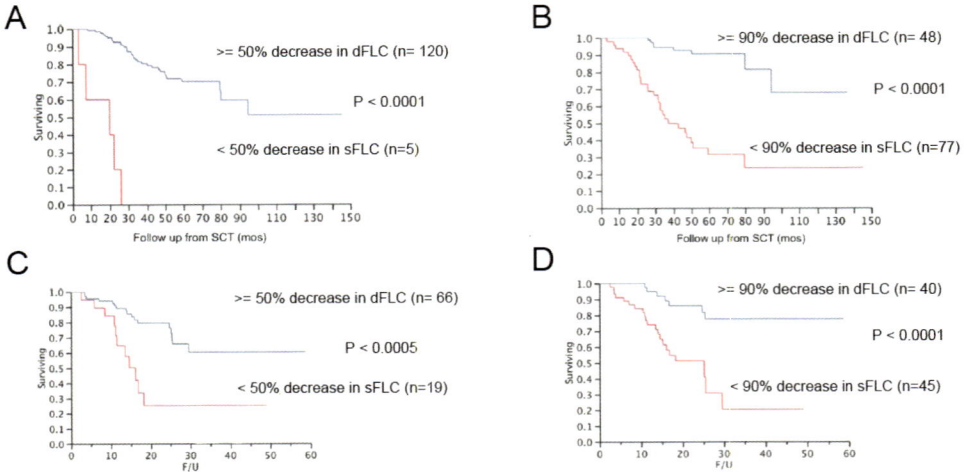

Figure 28.10. Prognostic value of reductions in sFLCs. (A,B) Kaplan Meier survival analysis of AL amyloidosis patients with a baseline dFLC ≥100 mg/L who survived at least 100 days post SCT. The median OS among those with a ≥90% reduction in dFLC (n=77) was not reached compared with 37.4 months for the remaining patients (n=48), p<0.001. **(C,D)** Kaplan Meier survival analysis of AL amyloidosis patients with a baseline dFLC >100 mg/L who survived three cycles of therapy with melphalan and dexamethasone. The median OS among those with a ≥50 % decrease in dFLC was not reached compared with 12.2 months for the remaining patients. The median OS among those patients with a ≥90% decrease in dFLC was not reached compared with 15.3 months for the remaining patients. (Reproduced with permission from the American Journal of Hematology[7] and John Wiley and Sons).

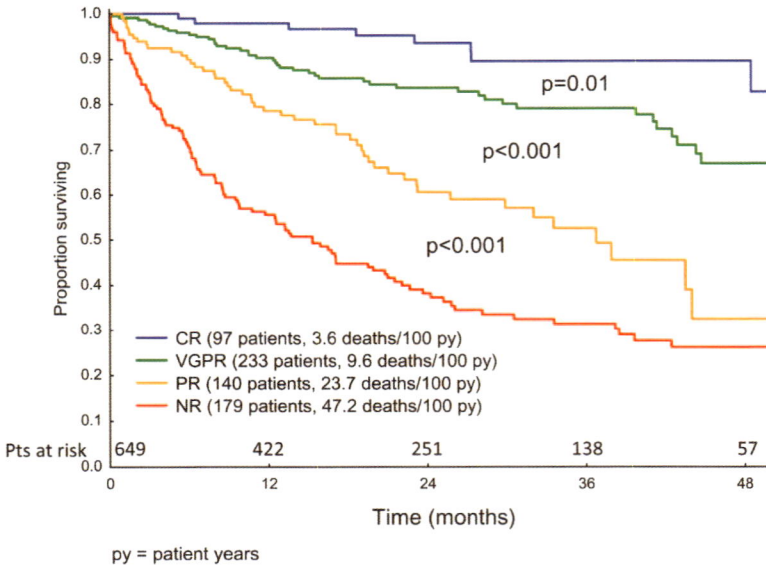

py = patient years

Figure 28.11. Prognostic relevance of haematological response assessed 6 months after the initiation of treatment. International case series of 649 patients treated with melphalan and dexamethasone (MDex, 43.6%), stem cell transplant (SCT, 11.4%), immunomodulatory drug-based therapy (IMiD-based, 22%) or bortezomib and dexamethasone (3%). py: patient years. (Republished with permission of American Society of Hematology, from[3]; permission conveyed through Copyright Clearance Center, Inc.).

28.7.1. sFLC response predicting cardiac outcome

Organ responses are typically slow to appear in patients with AL amyloidosis and are usually dependent on an adequate haematological response. The presence of cardiac amyloidosis is the major prognostic determinant in AL amyloidosis. Although cardiac involvement is present in only approximately half of patients at diagnosis, virtually all AL amyloidosis patients will die from cardiac-related sequelae[46]. Measurement of cardiac biomarkers, namely troponin T and B-type natriuretic peptide (NT-proBNP) are useful in defining prognosis at diagnosis *(Section 28.4)*, and should be monitored to assess response to therapy, in parallel with the assessment of haematological response[23,35,36].

The important link between improving cardiac function in AL amyloidosis and falling sFLC concentrations was first observed by Palladini and colleagues[47]. Fifty-one AL amyloidosis patients with symptomatic myocardial involvement were given chemotherapy and monitored with sFLCs and NT-proBNP. During treatment, 22 patients had a reduction of sFLCs by more than 50%, including nine patients who had disappearance of monoclonal immunoglobulins as assessed by IFE; a corresponding reduction of NT-proBNP levels was also observed (p<0.001). Survival was superior in responders than in non-responders (p<0.001). This finding was supported by a subsequent study by Kastritis et al.[48], which confirmed by multivariate analysis that a cardiac response was associated with a haematological response (46% vs. 0% in non-haematological responders; p<0.001).

Further studies have demonstrated a direct cardiotoxic effect of amyloidogenic FLCs[49,50], and support the clinical observation that a reduction in circulating monoclonal FLCs translates into a rapid improvement in cardiac function. Therefore, it is important to reduce the concentrations of cardiotoxic FLCs promptly in AL patients with cardiomyopathy.

28.7.2. sFLC response and renal outcome

Pinney et al.[51] assessed the value of the sFLC response in predicting long-term renal outcome in 923 patients with renal AL amyloidosis. Patients who achieved a greater sFLC response after chemotherapy demonstrated prolonged survival and superior renal outcomes. Patients who achieved more than a 90% FLC response at 6 months had an almost four-fold increase in the chance of renal response (p<0.001) and a lower rate of renal progression (p<0.001) compared with those achieving a FLC response of 0 - 50%. Among 752 patients with a baseline estimated glomerular filtration rate (eGFR) of ≥15 mL/min, those who achieved a 50 to 90% reduction or more than a 90% reduction in dFLC were less likely to experience renal progression requiring dialysis than patients achieving a <50% reduction in dFLC.

It should be noted that in cases of renal insufficiency, use of a modified renal reference interval for the κ/λ sFLC ratio may be appropriate. Application of this reference interval has been demonstrated to improve the diagnostic specificity of the sFLC ratio without affecting diagnostic sensitivity in patients with renal impairment *(Section 6.3)*.

28.8. SAP scintigraphy and sFLCs

I[123]-labelled serum amyloid P (SAP) scintigraphy was developed at the National Amyloidosis Centre in the UK for the diagnosis and quantitative monitoring of amyloid deposits[52]. I[123]-labelled SAP localises rapidly and specifically to amyloid deposits in proportion to the quantity of amyloid present. Whole body SAP scintigraphy (a SAP scan) allows the identification and quantification of amyloid deposits in affected organs, which varies greatly between patients. Furthermore, serial measurements demonstrate that amyloid deposits exist in a state of dynamic turnover, with variations in SAP uptake mirroring clinical status. This is seen in patients during treatment with chemotherapy and is compared with the concentrations of sFLCs in Figure 28.12.

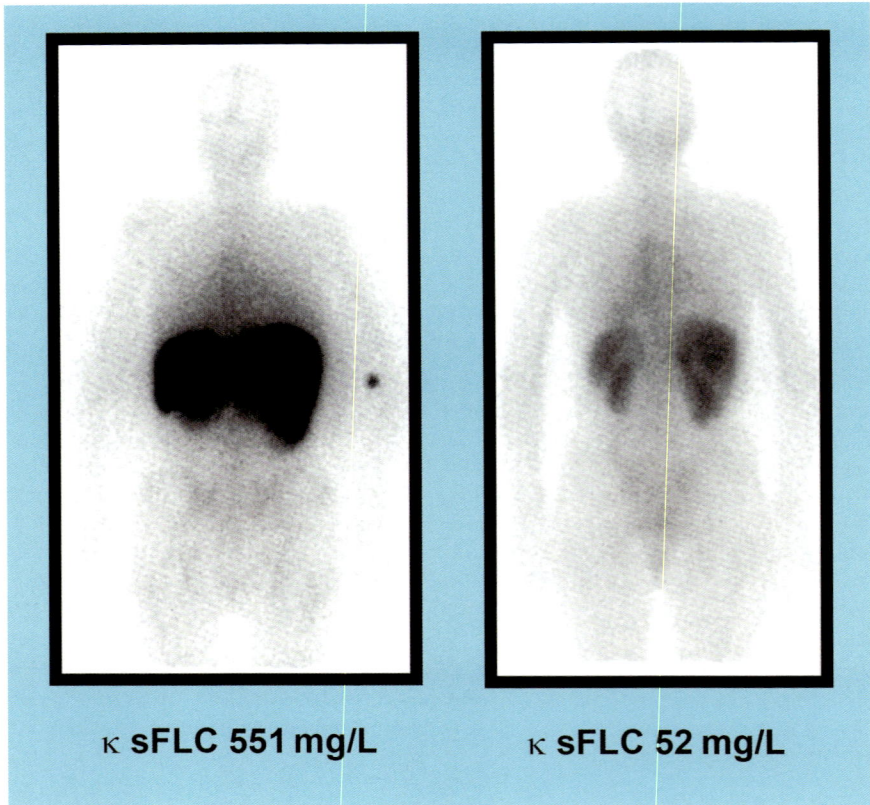

κ sFLC 551 mg/L   κ sFLC 52 mg/L

Figure 28.12. I[123] labelled serum amyloid P scans in a 52-year-old woman, viewed posteriorly. Reduction of AL deposits in the liver and spleen after one year of chemotherapy can be seen. κ sFLCs reduced from 551 mg/L to 52 mg/L over the same period. (Courtesy of P. Hawkins).

Investigations by Lachmann et al.[14] in 137 patients with AL amyloidosis confirmed the important relationship between amyloid deposits, as seen on SAP scans, and sFLC concentrations. Patients were divided into three groups dependent upon whether the SAP scans of the amyloid deposits showed regression, no change, or progression following chemotherapy. A good correlation with changes in sFLC concentrations was observed during the same period, indicating that sFLC measurments provided a simple measure of changes in disease status in patients with AL amyloidosis *(Figure 28.13).*

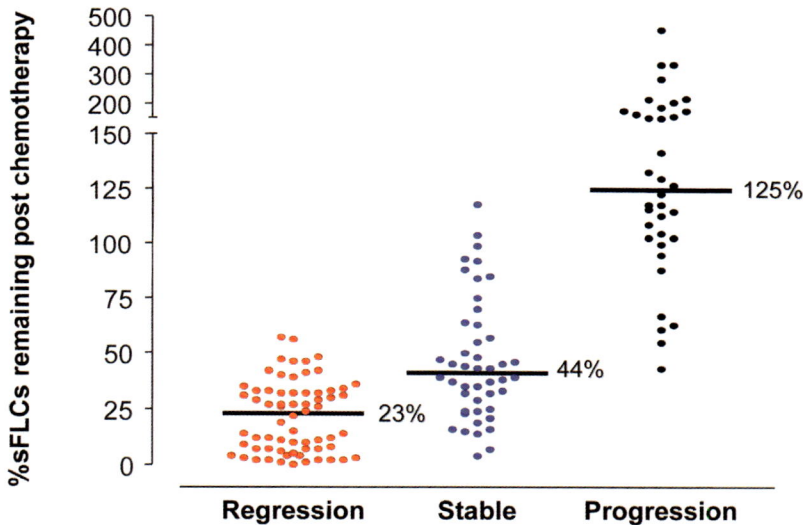

Figure 28.13. Comparison of disease status from serum amyloid P scans and sFLCs in 127 patients with AL amyloidosis before and 12 months after commencing chemotherapy. *The mean percentage of remaining sFLCs in each group are indicated (Kruskal-Wallis test: p<0.0001). (Courtesy of P. Hawkins).*

28.9. Hevylite in AL amyloidosis

The recent availability of assays that quantitatively measure immunoglobulin heavy/light chain (Hevylite®, HLC) pairs *(Chapter 9)* may provide an extra test for the diagnosis, prognosis and monitoring of AL amyloidosis[53,54].

Test Questions

1. What is the frequency of an abnormal κ/λ sFLC ratio in AL amyloidosis?

2. How frequently should sFLCs be assessed in patients undergoing treatment for AL amyloidosis?

3. What are the major prognostic factors for AL amyloidosis outcome?

Answers

1. An abnormal κ/λ sFLC ratio is found in 75 - 98% of patients (Section 28.2).

2. sFLCs are usually assessed prior to every cycle of chemotherapy. British guidelines recommend monitoring response to treatment with sFLCs after each cycle of chemotherapy and every 1 - 3 months thereafter, with the aim of switching to an alternative regimen as soon as the current one is proving ineffectual, which may be assessed after three cycles of therapy or earlier in cardiac patients (Section 28.6.3)

3. Cardiac involvement and response to therapy (Sections 28.4 and 28.7).

References

1. Merlini G, Stone MJ. Dangerous small B-cell clones. Blood 2006;108:2520-30

2. Kumar S, Dispenzieri A, Katzmann JA, Larson DR, Colby CL, Lacy MQ et al. Serum immunoglobulin free light chain measurement in AL amyloidosis: prognostic value and correlations with clinical features. Blood 2010;116:5126-9

3. Cohen AD, Comenzo RL. Systemic light-chain amyloidosis: advances in diagnosis, prognosis, and therapy. Hematology Am Soc Hematol Educ Program 2010;2010:287-94

4. Mollee P, Renaut P, Gottlieb D, Goodman H. How to diagnose amyloidosis. Intern Med J 2014;44:7-17

5. Comenzo RL, Wally J, Kica G, Murray J, Ericsson T, Skinner M, Zhang Y. Clonal immunoglobulin light chain variable region germline gene use in AL amyloidosis: association with dominant amyloid-related organ involvement and survival after stem cell transplantation. Br J Haematol 1999;106:744-51

6. Kumar SK, Gertz MA, Lacy MQ, Dingli D, Hayman SR, Buadi FK et al. Recent improvements in survival in primary systemic amyloidosis and the importance of an early mortality risk score. Mayo Clin Proc 2011;86:12-8

7. Kumar SK, Dispenzieri A, Lacy MQ, Hayman SR, Buadi FK, Zeldenrust SR et al. Changes in serum-free light chain rather than intact monoclonal immunoglobulin levels predicts outcome following therapy in primary amyloidosis. Am J Hematol 2011;86:251-5

8. Kyle RA, Linos A, Beard CM, Linke RP, Gertz MA, O'Fallon WM, Kurland LT. Incidence and natural history of primary systemic amyloidosis in Olmsted County, Minnesota, 1950 through 1989. Blood 1992;79:1817-22

9. Bird JM, Cavenagh J, Samson D, Mehta A, Hawkins P, Lachmann H. Guidelines on the diagnosis and management of AL amyloidosis. Br J Haematol 2004;125:681-700

10. Kourelis TV, Kumar SK, Gertz MA, Lacy MQ, Buadi FK, Hayman SR et al. Coexistent multiple myeloma or increased bone marrow plasma cells define equally high-risk populations in patients with immunoglobulin light chain amyloidosis. J Clin Oncol 2013;31:4319-24

11. Weiss BM, Hebreo J, Cordaro DV, Roschewski MJ, Baker TP, Abbott KC, Olson SW. Increased serum free light chains precede the presentation of immunoglobulin light chain amyloidosis. J Clin Oncol 2014;32:2699-2704

12. Katzmann JA, Kyle RA, Benson J, Larson DR, Snyder MR, Lust JA et al. Screening panels for detection of monoclonal gammopathies. Clin Chem 2009;55:1517-22

13. Palladini G, Russo P, Bosoni T, Verga L, Sarais G, Lavatelli F et al. Identification of amyloidogenic light chains requires the combination of serum-free light chain assay with immunofixation of serum and urine. Clin Chem 2009;55:499-504

14. Lachmann HJ, Gallimore R, Gillmore JD, Carr-Smith HD, Bradwell AR, Pepys MB, Hawkins PN. Outcome in systemic AL amyloidosis in relation to changes in concentration of circulating free immunoglobulin light chains following chemotherapy. Br J Haematol 2003;122:78-84

15. Abraham RS, Katzmann JA, Clark RJ, Bradwell AR, Kyle RA, Gertz MA. Quantitative analysis of serum free light chains. A new marker for the diagnostic evaluation of primary systemic amyloidosis. Am J Clin Pathol 2003;119:274-8

16. Katzmann JA, Abraham RS, Dispenzieri A, Lust JA, Kyle RA. Diagnostic performance of quantitative kappa and lambda free light chain assays in clinical practice. Clin Chem 2005;51:878-81

17. Bochtler T, Hegenbart U, Heiss C, Benner A, Cremer F, Volkmann M et al. Evaluation of the serum-free light chain test in untreated patients with AL amyloidosis. Haematologica 2008;93:459-62

18. Akar H, Seldin DC, Magnani B, O'Hara C, Berk JL, Schoonmaker C et al. Quantitative serum free light chain assay in the diagnostic evaluation of AL amyloidosis. Amyloid 2005;12:210-5

19. Snozek CL, Katzmann JA, Kyle RA, Dispenzieri A, Larson DR, Therneau TM et al. Prognostic value of the serum free light chain ratio in newly diagnosed myeloma: proposed incorporation into the international staging system. Leukemia 2008;22:1933-7

20. Wassef N, Berlanga O, Mahmood S, Lachmann H, Gillmore J, Hawkins P et al. Clinical comparison of polyclonal and monoclonal antibody based FLC assays for staging disease in systemic AL amyloidosis. Presented at XIV International Symposium on Amyloidosis 2014;PB-39a

21. Palladini G, Jaccard A, Milani P, Lavergne D, Foli A, Bender S et al. Comparison of the N-Latex and Freelite® assays for serum free light chain: clinical performance in AL amyloidosis. Presented at XIV International Symposium on Amyloidosis 2014;OP-35a

22. Biewend ML, Menke DM, Calamia KT. The spectrum of localized amyloidosis: a case series of 20 patients and review of the literature. Amyloid 2006;13:135-42

23. Gertz MA. How to manage primary amyloidosis. Leukemia 2012;26:191-8

24. Westermark P. Localized AL amyloidosis: a suicidal neoplasm? Ups J Med Sci 2012;117:244-50

25. Goodman HJ, Bridoux F, Lachmann HJ, Gilbertson JA, Gallimore R, Joshi J, et al. Localised amyloidosis: Clinical features and outcomes in 235 cases. Haematologica 2005;90:1413a

26. Dispenzieri A, Kyle R, Merlini G, Miguel JS, Ludwig H, Hajek R et al. International Myeloma Working Group guidelines for serum-free light chain analysis in multiple myeloma and related disorders. Leukemia 2009;23:215-24

27. Gillmore JD, Wechalekar A, Bird J, Cavenagh J, Hawkins S, Kazmi M et al. Guidelines on the diagnosis and investigation of AL amyloidosis. Br J Haematol 2015;168:207-18

28. Guis L, Diemert MC, Ghillani P, Choquet S, Leblond V, Vernant JP, Musset L. The quantitation of serum free light chains: Three case reports. Clin Chem 2004;50:F38a

29. Dispenzieri A, Lacy MQ, Katzmann JA, Rajkumar SV, Abraham RS, Hayman SR et al. Absolute values of immunoglobulin free light chains are prognostic in patients with primary systemic amyloidosis undergoing peripheral blood stem cell transplantation. Blood 2006;107:3378-83

30. Kumar S, Dispenzieri A, Lacy MQ, Hayman SR, Buadi FK, Colby C et al. Revised prognostic staging system for light chain amyloidosis incorporating cardiac biomarkers and serum free light chain measurements. J Clin Oncol 2012;30:989-95

31. Kastritis E, Anagnostopoulos A, Roussou M, Toumanidis S, Pamboukas C, Migkou M et al. Treatment of light chain (AL) amyloidosis with the combination of bortezomib and dexamethasone. Haematologica 2007;92:1351-8

32. Dispenzieri A, Gertz MA, Kyle RA. To the editor: Determining appropriate treatment options for patients with primary systemic amyloidosis. Blood 2004;104:2992-3

33. Wechalekar AD, Hawkins PN, Gillmore JD. Perspectives in treatment of AL amyloidosis. Br J Haematol 2008;140:365–77

34. Durie BG, Harousseau JL, Miguel JS, Blade J, Barlogie B, Anderson K et al. International uniform response criteria for multiple myeloma. Leukemia 2006;20:1467-73

35. Gertz MA, Merlini G. Definition of organ involvement and response to treatment in AL amyloidosis: an updated consensus opinion. Amyloid 2010;17:CP-Ba

36. Comenzo RL, Reece D, Palladini G, Seldin D, Sanchorawala V, Landau H et al. Consensus guidelines for the conduct and reporting of clinical trials in systemic light-chain (AL) amyloidosis. Leukemia 2012;26:2317-25

37. Palladini G, Dispenzieri A, Gertz MA, Kumar S, Wechalekar A, Hawkins PN et al. New criteria for response to treatment in immunoglobulin light chain amyloidosis based on free light chain measurement and cardiac biomarkers: impact on survival outcomes. J Clin Oncol 2012;30:4541-9

38. Wechalekar AD, Gillmore JD, Bird J, Cavenagh J, Hawkins S, Kazmi M et al. Guidelines on the management of AL amyloidosis. Br J Haematol 2015;168:186-206

39. Weber N, Mollee P, Augustson B, Brown R, Catley L, Gibson J et al. Management of systemic light chain (AL) amyloidosis: recommendations of the Myeloma Foundation of Australia Medical and Scientific Advisory Group. Intern Med J 2014 In press

40. Goodman HJB, Wechalekar AD, Lachmann HJ, Bradwell AR, Hawkins PN. Clonal disease response and clinical outcome in 229 patients with AL amyloidosis treated with VAD-like chemotherapy. Haematologica 2005;90:PO1408a

41. Tan TS, Dispenzieri A, Lacy MQ, Hayman SR, Buadi FK, Zeldenrust SR et al. Melphalan and dexamethasone is an effective therapy for primary systemic amyloidosis. Blood 2007;110:3608a

42. Wechalekar AD, Goodman HJB, Lachmann HJ, Offer M, Hawkins PN, Gillmore JD. Safety and efficacy of risk-adapted cyclophosphamide, thalidomide, and dexamethasone in systemic AL amyloidosis. Blood 2007;109:457-64

43. Sanchorawala V, Seldin DC, Magnani B, Skinner M, Wright DG. Serum free light-chain responses after high-dose intravenous melphalan and autologous stem cell transplantation for AL (primary) amyloidosis. Bone Marrow Transplant 2005;36:597-600

44. Girnius S, Seldin DC, Cibeira MT, Sanchorawala V. New hematologic response criteria predict survival in patients with immunoglobulin light chain amyloidosis treated with high-dose melphalan and autologous stem-cell transplantation. J Clin Oncol 2013;31:2749-50

45. Cordes S, Dispenzieri A, Lacy MQ, Hayman SR, Buadi FK, Dingli D et al. Ten-year survival after autologous stem cell transplantation for immunoglobulin light chain amyloidosis. Cancer 2012;118:6105-9

46. Dubrey SW, Cha K, Anderson J, Chamarthi B, Reisinger J, Skinner M, Falk RH. The clinical features of immunoglobulin light-chain (AL) amyloidosis with heart involvement. QJM 1998;91:141-57

47. Palladini G, Lavatelli F, Russo P, Perlini S, Perfetti V, Bosoni T et al. Circulating amyloidogenic free light chains and serum N-terminal natriuretic peptide type B decrease simultaneously in association with improvement of survival in AL. Blood 2006;107:3854-8

48. Kastritis E, Wechalekar AD, Dimopoulos MA, Merlini G, Hawkins PN, Perfetti V et al. Bortezomib with or without dexamethasone in primary systemic (light chain) amyloidosis. J Clin Oncol 2010;28:1031-7

49. Liao R, Jain M, Teller P, Connors LH, Ngoy S, Skinner M et al. Infusion of light chains from patients with cardiac amyloidosis causes diastolic dysfunction in isolated mouse hearts. Circulation 2001;104:1594-7

50. Mishra S, Guan J, Plovie E, Seldin DC, Connors LH, Merlini G et al. Human amyloidogenic light chain proteins result in cardiac dysfunction, cell death, and early mortality in zebrafish. Am J Physiol Heart Circ Physiol 2013;305:H95-103

51. Pinney JH, Lachmann HJ, Bansi L, Wechalekar AD, Gilbertson JA, Rowczenio D et al. Outcome in renal AL amyloidosis after chemotherapy. J Clin Oncol 2011;29:674-81

52. Hawkins PN. Serum amyloid P component scintigraphy for diagnosis and monitoring amyloidosis. Curr Opin Nephrol Hypertens 2002;11:649-55

53. Wechalekar AD, Young P, Wassef N, Gillmore JD, Gibbs SDJ, Pinney JH et al. Normal heavy/light chain (HLC) and free light chain (FLC) ratios are associated with prolonged survival in patients with systemic AL amyloidosis. Presented at XIII International Symposium on Amyloidosis 2012;PB30a

54. Sachchithanantham S, Berlanga O, Harding S, Wassef N, Mahmood S, Sayeed R et al. Heavy/light chain-pair suppression as a novel marker of poor outcomes in systemic AL amyloidosis. Presented at XIV International Symposium on Amyloidosis 2014;PB-34a

Light chain deposition disease

In light chain deposition disease:

- Renal impairment or nephrotic syndrome is often a presenting feature.
- Approximately two-thirds of patients have an underlying lymphoplasmacytic proliferative disorder, such as multiple myeloma.
- An abnormal κ/λ sFLC ratio is present in around 90% of patients at diagnosis.
- sFLCs are useful for monitoring disease, and are recommended in International Myeloma Working Group guidelines.

29.1. Introduction

The rare monoclonal immunoglobulin deposition diseases (MIDD) comprise light chain deposition disease (LCDD), light- and heavy-chain deposition disease (LHCDD) and heavy-chain deposition disease (HCDD)[1]. In LCDD, which comprises 80% of the cases of MIDD[2], monoclonal serum free light chains (sFLCs) are precipitated on basement membranes in the kidneys and less frequently, the heart, liver and other organs. Deposits can be visualised by staining of biopsy samples *(Figure 29.1)*. As with AL amyloidosis, the disease is progressive and leads to failure of the affected organs, and has a poor prognosis[1,3,4]. However, LCDD differs from AL amyloidosis in a number of ways: 1) it is more frequent in younger women (aged 30 - 50 years); 2) renal failure is a common presenting feature; 3) the predominant light chain type is κ (typically Vκ1 and Vκ4), rather than λ; and 4) light chain deposits do not contain serum amyloid P component (SAP, a protein that typically localises in areas of amyloid) and are congo red negative.

Approximately two-thirds of patients with LCDD have an underlying lymphoplasmacytic proliferative disorder: A study by Pozzi et al.[5] reported that out of 63 patients with LCDD, MM was diagnosed in 65% of cases, whilst chronic lymphocytic leukaemia was present in a further 3% of cases. The remaining 32% of patients did not have any detectable haematological disease. Whilst monoclonal proteins are detectable by serum or urine immunofixation electrophoresis in the majority of patients (76 or 90% of cases, respectively)[5], the concentrations may be low[6] and difficult to monitor.

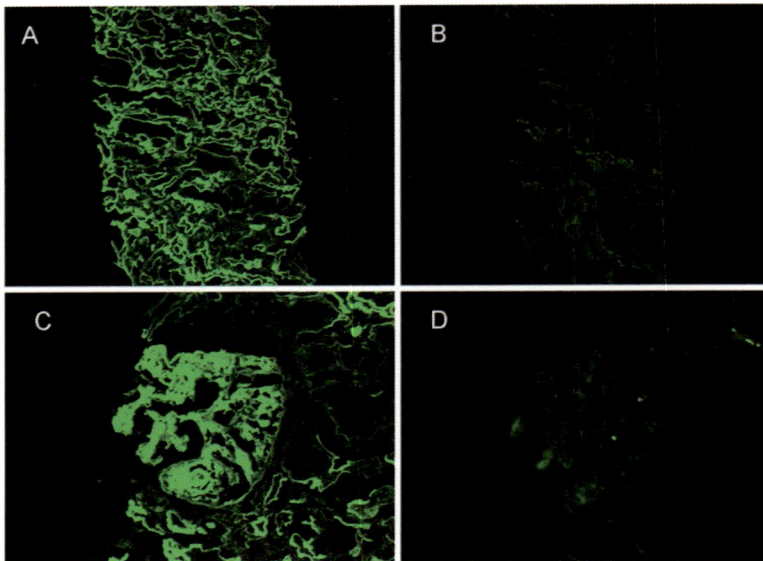

Figure 29.1. Immunofluorescence micrographs of a representative case of κ type light chain deposition disease. *There is diffuse linear staining of tubular basement membranes **(A)** and glomerular basement membranes **(C)** for κ light chains. Staining for λ light chains is negative along tubular **(B)** and glomerular **(D)** basement membranes. Magnification: x200 in A and B; x400 in C and D. (Republished with permission of Clinical Journal of the American Society of Nephrology[2]; permission conveyed through Copyright Clearance Center, Inc.).*

29.2. sFLC assays support a diagnosis of LCDD

A diagnosis of LCDD should be suspected in all cases of renal insufficiency of unknown origin. Whilst a definitive diagnosis of LCDD is based on renal biopsy with thorough histological examination and electron microscopy[5], sFLC analysis should be included in the initial laboratory testing algorithm as the majority of patients have monoclonal sFLCs. This was demonstrated by Katzmann et al.[7] for 18 LCDD patients who were included as part of a larger study aimed at evaluating different serum- and urine-based diagnostic algorithms. The analysis showed that sFLC testing alone, or a panel of serum protein electrophoresis (SPE) and sFLCs, were both as sensitive (14/18; 77.8%) for LCDD detection as a panel of SPE, serum immunofixation electrophoresis (sIFE) and urine IFE (uIFE). Guidelines published by the International Myeloma Working Group (IMWG)[8] recommend the use of sFLC analysis in combination with serum electrophoresis to screen for monoclonal gammopathies, with the exception of AL amyloidosis which additionally requires a 24-hour uIFE. Screening algorithms are discussed further in Chapter 23 and guidelines are detailed in Chapter 25.

The above study by Katzmann et al.[7] supports two previous studies by the same authors in which the diagnostic sensitivity of sFLC analysis in LCDD was evaluated. In one study[9], 89% (17/19) patients with LCDD had an abnormal κ/λ sFLC ratio, including 6/7 patients who were negative by sIFE *(Table 29.1)*. One sample was negative by sFLC analysis but positive by sIFE. In a subsequent publication, seven further patients were studied and all had abnormal κ/λ sFLC ratios[10].

Classification	Elevated sFLCs	Abnormal κ/λ sFLC ratio
sIFE κ +ve	8/9	8/9
sIFE λ +ve	3/3	3/3
sIFE -ve; uIFE κ +ve	4/4	4/4
sIFE and uIFE -ve. BMPCs κ +ve	1/3	2/3
Total abnormal for sFLCs	**16**	**17**

Table 29.1. Detection rates by sFLCs in 19 LCDD patients[9]. *BMPC: bone marrow plasma cells.*

The diagnostic sensitivity of sFLC analysis for LCDD demonstrated above by Katzmann et al. has similarly been shown by other researchers. In the largest single-centre series of renal MIDD published to date, Nasr et al.[2] reported that κ/λ sFLC ratios were abnormal in all patients tested (43/43 LCDD, 4/4HCDD and 4/4 LHCDD) and markedly abnormal (<0.125 or >8) in 78% of these. Cohen et al.[11] also reported abnormal sFLC ratios in 100% of patients (n=32). In a further study of 17 patients with biopsy-proven LCDD, Wechalekar et al.[12] found that 33% more patients with LCDD were identified by an abnormal κ/λ sFLC ratio than by standard electrophoretic methods, and concluded that sFLC analysis was a useful addition to electrophoretic tests when screening for LCDD. An early diagnosis can be clinically valuable as rapid treatment is fundamental for improving patient outcomes[13]. Clinical case history 1 illustrates the clinical sensitivity of the FLC tests compared with conventional serum and urine electrophoretic assays in a patient with LCDD and renal impairment.

Clinical case history 1

Light chain deposition disease undetectable by conventional electrophoretic assays[14].

A 66-year-old man suffering from asthenia and anaemia was investigated for serum protein abnormalities. SPE, sIFE and uIFE tests showed no evidence of monoclonal immunoglobulins *(Figure 29.2)*. Serum immunoglobulin concentrations were normal/low: IgG 8.5 g/L; IgA 0.4 g/L and IgM 0.2 g/L. However, sFLC concentrations were highly abnormal: κ 294 mg/L; λ 71.6 mg/L and κ/λ ratio 4.1. These results indicated a monoclonal gammopathy and renal impairment. In this patient, sFLC analysis allowed the detection of monoclonal FLCs and supported the clinical diagnosis of LCDD obtained by renal biopsy.

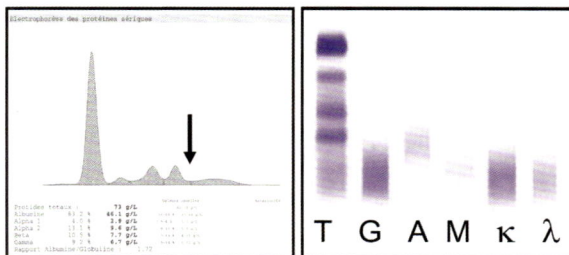

Figure 29.2. LCDD showing normal SPE (scanning densitometry) and IFE, but highly abnormal sFLCs (κ 294 mg/L, λ 71.6 mg/L and κ/λ ratio: 4.1). T: total protein stain. (Courtesy of L. Guis[14]*).*

29.3. Monitoring LCDD using sFLC assays

It is logical to monitor LCDD patients using sFLC assays. Although there is no published data formally validating the use of the sFLC assays for assessing haematological response in patients with LCDD, the personal experience of many authors confirms their utility[16,17,18] and international guidelines recommend sFLC analysis for monitoring LCDD[8] *(Chapter 25)*. Clinical case history 2 illustrates the benefit of sFLC analyses in a patient who was difficult to monitor by other methods[19].

Wechalekar et al.[12] monitored 10 LCDD patients receiving a range of systemic chemotherapy (and autologous stem cell transplant [ASCT] in in 2/10 cases). Eight patients had sFLC responses, with a median decrease of 63% (range 31 - 95%), compared with pre-treatment values. One patient, who had a normal sFLC ratio pre-treatment, had no change in sFLC levels but had a very good partial response of the monoclonal intact immunoglobulin post-treatment. Only two patients had complete normalisation of sFLC levels. The authors concluded that sFLC analysis was useful for monitoring responses to treatment.

Hassoun et al.[15] reported on five patients with LCDD, one with LHCDD and one with light chain proximal tubulopathy (a disease characterized by κ-restricted crystal deposits in the proximal tubule cytoplasm)[20]. All had abnormal sFLCs at diagnosis, whereas only one patient had a monoclonal band visible by SPE and two patients had IgGκ monoclonal proteins identified by sIFE. Patients were given high-dose melphalan and ASCT with good responses that could be monitored with sFLC assays *(Figure 29.3)*. Similarly, Jiminez-Zepeda et al.[6] found that measurement of sFLCs was useful in the follow-up of six patients with LCDD treated with bortezomib and ASCT. All six patients had elevated sFLCs at diagnosis whereas only two patients had serum monoclonal proteins >10 g/L. A decrease in the levels of involved sFLCs was associated with a significant reduction of proteinuria. Similarly, Minarik et al.[21] reported rapid and deep reductions in sFLC levels within two cycles of treatment with bortezomib-based induction regimens in three patients with LCDD.

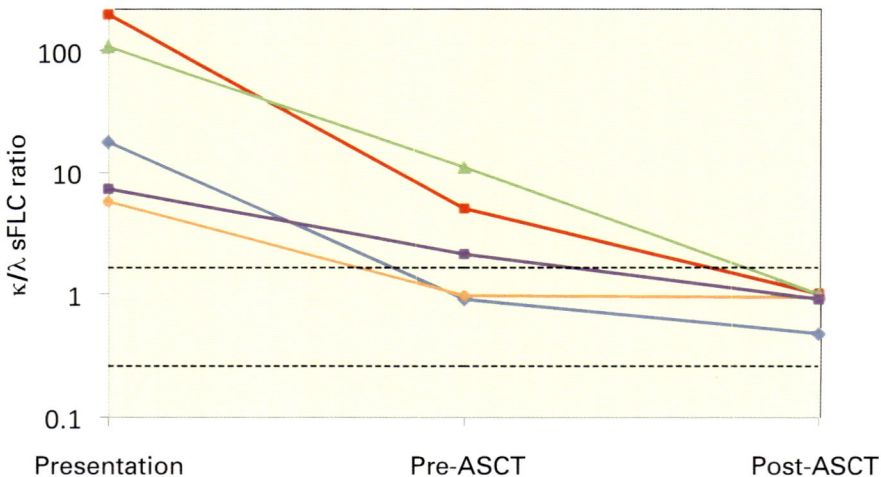

Figure 29.3. sFLC responses in 5 patients with κ light chain deposition disease. Patients received various induction therapies for MM before undergoing consolidation with high-dose melphalan and ASCT. All patients achieved a haematological complete response and normalised κ/λ sFLC ratio following ASCT. The reference interval for the κ/λ sFLC ratio (0.26 - 1.65) is indicated by the broken tramlines. (Graph plotted from data published in[15]).

Clinical case history 2

A patient with LCDD affecting the kidney, monitored with sFLC assays[19].

A 59-year-old Caucasian male presented to nephrologists with flu-like symptoms, hypertension and swelling of the face, hands and legs. Urinalysis revealed he had nephrotic range proteinuria (13.9 g/24 hours) and serum creatinine was elevated at 200 μmol/L. A renal biopsy showed nodular glomerulosclerosis with evidence of LCDD on electron microscopy (granular electron-dense material in the tubular basement membranes). Congo red staining was negative. Serum electrophoresis, immunoglobulin levels and urinary Bence Jones protein assays were all normal.

The patient was referred to the haematology department to rule out an underlying clonal B-cell disorder. A bone marrow aspirate and trephine revealed normal cellular marrow with no morphological or immunophenotypic evidence of MM. Congo red staining was, again, negative and a SAP scan also showed no evidence of amyloid deposition. Serum was tested for sFLCs with the following results: κ sFLC 526.0 mg/L (normal range 3.3 - 19.4 mg/L), λ sFLC 64.6 mg/L (normal range 5.7 - 26.3 mg/L) and κ/λ ratio 8.14 (normal range 0.26 - 1.65) *(Figure 29.4)*. The patient subsequently developed atrial fibrillation. A 24-hour tape showed irregularities in the atrial chamber and intermittent disruption of AV node conduction. A dual chamber pacemaker was fitted and cardiac biopsy performed, which showed no evidence of amyloid or light chain deposition.

His hypertension was treated with an angiotensin-converting enzyme inhibitor. However, within 12 months his renal function had deteriorated further (serum creatinine reached 300 μmol/L) and he continued to have heavy proteinuria. In order to prevent further progression of his renal disease, the patient was treated with 3 cycles of VAMP chemotherapy (vincristine 0.4 mg/day for 4 days, doxorubicin 9 mg/m^2/day for 4 days and methylprednisolone 1 g/m^2 for 5 days per cycle). Renal function subsequently improved (serum creatinine fell to ~200 μmol/L) and this was accompanied by decreasing sFLC levels and κ/λ ratio. Nine months after the chemotherapy, urinary protein excretion had fallen to 4.4 g/24 hours.

For the following year, renal function remained stable but subsequently, the κ/λ sFLC ratio and serum creatinine concentration began to increase again. The patient was treated with a further 3 cycles of VAMP and again, similar improvements in renal function and sFLC levels were seen. The authors concluded that this case was the first to demonstrate a direct relationship between the measurement of sFLCs and renal function in LCDD.

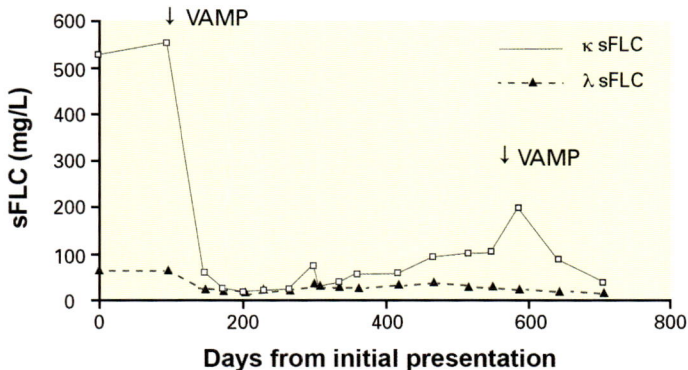

Figure 29.4. Monitoring a patient with LCDD using sFLC assays. (Reproduced by permission of Oxford University Press[19]).

Test Questions

1. What proportion of patients with LCDD have abnormal κ/λ sFLC ratios?

Answers

1. Between 78 and 100% in different series *(Section 29.2)*.

References

1. Buxbaum J, Gallo G. Nonamyloidotic monoclonal immunoglobulin deposition disease. Light-chain, heavy-chain, and light- and heavy-chain deposition diseases. Hematol Oncol Clin North Am 1999;13:1235-48

2. Nasr SH, Valeri AM, Cornell LD, Fidler ME, Sethi S, D'Agati VD, Leung N. Renal monoclonal immunoglobulin deposition disease: a report of 64 patients from a single institution. Clin J Am Soc Nephrol 2011;7:231-9

3. Buxbaum JN, Chuba JV, Hellman GC, Solomon A, Gallo GR. Monoclonal immunoglobulin deposition disease: light chain and light and heavy chain deposition diseases and their relation to light chain amyloidosis. Clinical features, immunopathology, and molecular analysis. Ann Intern Med 1990;112:455-64

4. Solomon A, Weiss DT, Herrera GA. Light-chain deposition disease. In: Mehta J, Singhal S, eds. Myeloma. Informa Healthcare, 2002:507-18

5. Pozzi C, D'Amico M, Fogazzi GB, Curioni S, Ferrario F, Pasquali S et al. Light chain deposition disease with renal involvement: clinical characteristics and prognostic factors. Am J Kidney Dis 2003;42:1154-63

6. Jimenez-Zepeda VH, Trudel S, Winter A, Reece DE, Chen C, Kukreti V. Autologous stem cell transplant for light chain deposition disease: incorporating bortezomib to the induction therapy. Am J Hematol 2012;87:822-3

7. Katzmann JA, Kyle RA, Benson J, Larson DR, Snyder MR, Lust JA et al. Screening panels for detection of monoclonal gammopathies. Clin Chem 2009;55:1517-22

8. Dispenzieri A, Kyle R, Merlini G, Miguel JS, Ludwig H, Hajek R et al. International Myeloma Working Group guidelines for serum-free light chain analysis in multiple myeloma and related disorders. Leukemia 2009;23:215-24

9. Katzmann JA, Clark RJ, Abraham RS, Bryant S, Lymp JF, Bradwell AR, Kyle RA. Serum reference intervals and diagnostic ranges for free kappa and free lambda immunoglobulin light chains: relative sensitivity for detection of monoclonal light chains. Clin Chem 2002;48:1437-44

10. Katzmann JA, Abraham RS, Dispenzieri A, Lust JA, Kyle RA. Diagnostic performance of quantitative kappa and lambda free light chain assays in clinical practice. Clin Chem 2005;51:878-81

11. Cohen C, Fermand J, Arnulf B, Knebelmann B, Bridoux F. Bortezomib is highly efficient in monoclonal immunoglobulin deposition disease. J Am Soc Nephrol 2013;24:TH-PO1048a

12. Wechalekar AD, Lachmann HJ, Goodman HJB, Bradwell AR, Hawkins PN. Role of serum free light chains in diagnosis and monitoring response to treatment in light chain deposition disease. Haematologica 2005;90:PO1414a

13. Econimo L, Gaggiotti M, Ravera S, Re A, Peli A, Tardanico R et al. Early treatment has a significant impact on renal survival in light chain deposition disease (LCDD). Presented at XIII International Symposium on Amyloidosis 2012

14. Guis L, Diemert MC, Ghillani P, Choquet S, Leblond V, Vernant JP, Musset L.; The quantitation of serum free light chains: Three case reports. Clin Chem 2004;50:F38a

15. Hassoun H, Flombaum C, D'Agati VD, Rafferty BT, Cohen A, Klimek VM et al. High-dose melphalan and auto-SCT in patients with monoclonal Ig deposition disease. Bone Marrow Transplant 2008;42:405-12

16. Kuypers DR, Lerut E, Claes K, Evenepoel P, Vanrenterghem Y. Recurrence of light chain deposit disease after renal allograft transplantation: potential role of rituximab? Transpl Int 2007;20:381-5

17. Lorenz EC, Sethi S, Poshusta TL, Ramirez-Alvarado M, Kumar S, Lager DJ et al. Renal failure due to combined cast nephropathy, amyloidosis and light-chain deposition disease. Nephrol Dial Transplant 2010;25:1340-3

18. Ronco P, Plaisier E, Aucouturier P. Monoclonal immunoglobulin light and heavy chain deposition diseases: molecular models of common renal diseases. Contrib Nephrol 2011;169:221-31

19. Brockhurst I, Harris KP, Chapman CS. Diagnosis and monitoring a case of light-chain deposition disease in the kidney using a new, sensitive immunoassay. Nephrol Dial Transplant 2005;20:1251-3

20. Larsen CP, Bell JM, Harris AA, Messias NC, Wang YH, Walker PD. The morphologic spectrum and clinical significance of light chain proximal tubulopathy with and without crystal formation. Mod Pathol 2011;24:1462-9

21. Minarik J, Scudla V, Tichy T, Pika T, Bacovsky J, Lochman P, Zadrazil J. Induction treatment of light chain deposition disease with bortezomib - rapid hematological response with persistence of renal involvement. Leuk Lymphoma 2012;53:330-1

An overview of other diseases with monoclonal or increased polyclonal immunoglobulins

30.1. Introduction

This chapter provides an overview of other diseases with monoclonal or increased polyclonal immunoglobulins. It covers the use of free light chain (FLC) and immunoglobulin heavy/light chain (Hevylite®, HLC) measurements in lymphoid malignances, plus autoimmune and infectious diseases. The role of serum FLCs (sFLCs) as a marker of mortality is also discussed.

30.2. sFLCs in lymphoid malignances

Although monoclonal proteins are a feature of plasma cell dyscrasias, they can also be detected in other B-cell malignances such as chronic lymphocytic leukaemia (CLL) and non-Hodgkin lymphoma (NHL)[1,2]. Consistent with this, many studies have demonstrated that inclusion of sFLC analysis in a screening panel alongside serum protein electrophoresis (SPE) identifies additional patients with CLL or lymphoma *(Chapter 23)*.

The incidence of sFLC abnormalities varies widely according to the lymphoid subtype *(Table 30.1)*. For example, an abnormal κ/λ sFLC ratio is found in approximately 5% of patients with Hodgkin lymphoma (HL; *Section 31.2)* but around 50% of patients with mantle cell lymphoma (MCL; *Section 31.4)*. sFLCs may be produced directly by the tumour (e.g. diffuse large B-cell lymphoma [DLBCL]; *Section 31.3)* or by B-cells in the surrounding microenvironment (e.g. HL; *Section 31.2)*.

There is a growing body of literature on the use of sFLCs as a prognostic marker in lymphoid malignances *(Table 30.1)*. For example, in DLBCL the absolute κ and λ sFLC levels were more predictive of outcome than the sFLC ratio *(Section 31.3.2)*, whereas in MCL the sFLC κ/λ ratio but not absolute levels were associated with overall survival *(Section 31.4)*. In CLL, both a monoclonal and a polyclonal sFLC elevation are associated with inferior outcome *(Section 33.3)*. It should be noted that polyclonal FLC elevation may be due to renal impairment or polyclonal stimulation *(Chapter 7)*.

Disease		Incidence of sFLC abnormalities		Prognosis		Monitoring
		Abnormal κ/λ sFLC ratio	Elevated concentration	Abnormal κ/λ sFLC ratio	Elevated concentration	
HL[3,4,5,6]		5 - 7%	~30% (κ and/or λ)	✗	✓	✓
NHL	DLBCL[7,8,9]	9 - 14%	19 - 32% (κ and/or λ)	✗	✓	✓
	FL[2]	4 - 8%	unknown	unknown	unknown	unknown
	MZL: MALToma[2]	16%	unknown	unknown	unknown	unknown
	MCL[2,10,11,12]	36 - 77%	40% (κ and/or λ)	✓	✗	✓
	BL[2]	12%	unknown	unknown	unknown	unknown
	WM[13,14,15]	77%	83% (iFLC)	unknown	✓	✓
CLL[16,17,18,19,20,21]		30 - 40%	32% (κ and/or λ)	✓	✓	✓

Table 30.1.Summary of the incidence of FLC abnormalities, and the role of sFLC measurements in HL, NHL and CLL. ✓: parameter shown to be of value; ✗: parameter shown not to be of value; iFLC: involved FLC; HL: Hodgkin lymphoma; NHL: non-Hodgkin lymphoma; DLBCL: diffuse large B-cell lymphoma; FL: follicular lymphoma; MZL: marginal zone lymphoma; MALT: lymphoma of mucosa-associated lymphoid tissue; MCL: mantle cell lymphoma; BL: Burkitt lymphoma; WM: Waldenström's macroglobulinaemia; CLL: chronic lymphocytic leukaemia.

sFLCs may be a useful marker for monitoring lymphoma. Their short serum half-life and the large clinical range provide a sensitive marker for assessment of response to treatment. The sFLC component indicating response may vary between the different lymphoma subtypes. For example, in Waldenström's macroglobulinaemia (WM), the involved FLC (iFLC) concentration was found to be a useful marker to monitor disease and may show response to treatment and progression earlier than IgM measurements *(Section 32.3.2)*. In MCL, both the κ/λ sFLC ratio and summated κ + λ FLC concentrations (ΣFLC) may be informative for monitoring *(Section 31.4)*. In cryoglobulinaemia, sFLCs could possibly serve as a useful tool for monitoring response, since direct measurement of cryoglobulins is technically difficult *(Section 34.2)*.

sFLC concentrations may also have prognostic value in predicting the risk of developing NHL in immunosuppressive states (e.g. HIV infection or recipients of solid organ transplants) and in conditions associated with chronic B-cell activation (e.g. primary Sjögren's syndrome and hepatits C virus infection). These are discussed in Chapter 35.

30.3. Hevylite in lymphoid malignancies

Preliminary findings suggest that abnormal HLC ratios are found in a significant percentage of lymphoma patients, particularly those with indolent types (follicular lymphoma [FL], marginal zone lymphoma [MZL] and WM). In a study of 145 patients with indolent and aggressive lymphomas, 64/145 (44%) had an abnormal HLC ratio *(Table 30.2 and Figure 30.1)*[22]. By comparison, a monoclonal protein was detected in the serum of 38/145 (26%) patients by SPE and 45/145 (31%) patients by immunofixation electrophoresis (IFE)[22]. This suggests that HLC assays provide a more sensitive means of detecting monoclonal protein production in lymphoproliferative malignancies than conventional electrophoretic techniques. HLC analysis may also be useful in situations where the monoclonal protein concentration is low and accurate quantitation by SPE is difficult *(Section*

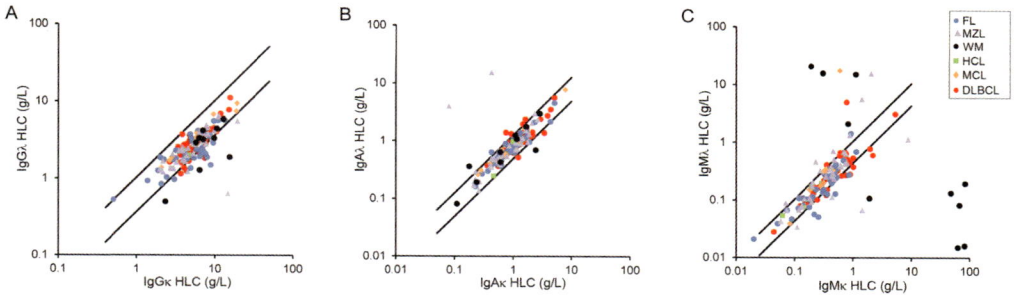

Figure 30.1. IgG, IgA and IgM HLC concentrations in NHL[22]. (A) *IgG HLC ratio was abnormal in 25/145 patients (12 FL, 3 MZL, 4 WM, 6 DLBCL).* **(B)** *IgA HLC ratio was abnormal in 14/145 patients (1 FL, 4 MZL, 2 WM and 7 DLBCL).* **(C)** *IgM HLC ratio was abnormal in 44/145 patients (8 FL, 13 MZL, 10 WM, 1 MCL, 12 DLBCL). Parallel lines indicate the normal range for the HLC ratio.* (Courtesy of G. Pratt).

Disease		HLC at diagnosis		Prognosis	Monitoring
		Abnormal HLC ratio	IFE positive		
HL		unknown	unknown	unknown	unknown
NHL	DLBCL [2,8,22]	24 - 44%	0 - 24%	IgMκ/IgMλ HLC ratio predicts PFS	unknown
	FL[2,22]	17%	8 - 24%	unknown	unknown
	MZL[2,22]	44%	36 - 37%	unknown	unknown
	MCL[2,22]	11%	20 - 22%	unknown	unknown
	BL[2]	unknown	12%	unknown	unknown
	WM [22,23,24]	97 - 100%	100%	Initial data supports use	Initial data supports use
CLL[18]		unknown	17%	unknown	unknown

Table 30.2. *Summary of the incidence of HLC and IFE abnormalities, and the role of HLC measurements in HL, NHL and CLL. PFS: progression-free survival; other abbreviations defined in Table 30.1.*

32.4.1). In addition, evidence suggests that HLC analysis is useful for monitoring WM *(Section 32.4.2)*.

In lymphoma patients, the most frequent HLC ratio abnormality was IgM, detected in approximately two-thirds of cases[22]. Approximately one quarter of patients had abnormal HLC ratios for more than one immunoglobulin class.

To date, only one study has investigated the prognostic value of HLC measurements in lymphoma. In a preliminary investigation following patients with DLBCL, multivariate analysis indicated that the IgMκ/IgMλ HLC ratio was predictive of progression-free survival *(Section 31.3.2)*[8].

The concentration of the uninvolved HLC-pair (e.g. IgGλ in a patient with monoclonal IgGκ) provides information on polyclonal immunosuppression. This is prognostic in a number of plasma cell disorders, including monoclonal gammopathy of undetermined significance (MGUS; *Chapter 13*) and multiple myeloma *(Chapter 20)*. Emerging evidence suggests that HLC-pair suppression may be present in a significant number of lymphoma patients. For example in WM, HLC-pair suppression was present in a quarter of individuals *(Section 32.4.3)*. Further studies on the prognostic utility of HLC-pair suppression in lymphoproliferative disorders are warranted.

Heavy chain disease (HCD) is characterised by the production of a monoclonal immunoglobulin heavy chain with no associated light chains *(Section 34.3)*. As HLC assays do not recognise the monoclonal heavy chain protein, they allow quantitation of the intact immunoglobulins and provide an indirect estimate of the heavy chain production (by subtraction of summated HLC values from total immunoglobulin measurements). In a study of 15 γ-HCD patients, Kaleta et al.[25] found that 20% of patients also had monoclonal sFLC production.

30.4. sFLCs as a biomarker of immune stimulation and inflammation

Measurement of polyclonal sFLCs provides an indication of total immunoglobulin synthesis that may serve as a biomarker of immune stimulation and inflammation *(Chapter 35)*[26].

In a number of autoimmune diseases, the concentrations of polyclonal sFLCs correlate with disease activity. These include systemic lupus erythematosus (SLE; *Section 35.4.1*), Sjögren's syndrome *(Section 35.4.2)*, and rheumatoid arthritis (RA; *Section 35.4.3*). Patients at risk of disease flare could be monitored with sFLCs, to allow early intervention and possibly reduce end-organ damage and mortality. Increased concentrations of polyclonal sFLCs have also been described in a number of inflammatory diseases. These include pneumonitis *(Section 35.8.1)*, rhinosinusitis *(Section 35.7)*, IgG4-related disease *(Section 35.8.5)*, viral infections e.g. hepatitis C virus *(Section 35.8.2)*, and HIV *(Section 35.6)*.

Hutchison and Landgren[26] speculated that sFLC measurement might complement the use of C-reactive protein (CRP) assays as a biomarker of inflammation. First, however, they suggested that a better understanding of the intra-patient variation in FLC measurements is required *(Section 7.2.6)*, alongside knowledge of whether it is advantageous to correct sFLC measurements for renal clearance or use unmodified measurements *(Section 6.3)*.

30.5. Cerebrospinal fluid FLCs and multiple sclerosis

The development of Freelite® assays that are validated for use in cerebrospinal fluid (CSF) provides an important tool to aid in the diagnosis of multiple sclerosis (MS). In this condition, κ FLC CSF concentrations are typically high, whilst λ FLC concentrations are only moderately elevated *(Chapter 36)*. An elevated κ FLC index supports a diagnosis of MS, with similar diagnostic accuracy to oligoclonal band detection *(Section 36.2)*.

30.6. sFLCs as a marker of mortality

General population studies have revealed an association between elevated polyclonal sFLCs and reduced survival, leading to the speculation that sFLC measurements could form a useful early investigation in a general health assessment. This is discussed further in Section 35.10.

30.7. The Combylite assay

Studies have reported the value of summated κ and λ sFLC concentrations in a number of conditions ranging from CLL *(Chapter 33)* and cardiovascular disease *(Section 35.3)* to HIV infection *(Section 35.6)*. Faint and colleagues[27] recently described the development of a new turbidimetric sFLC immunoassay that measures both κ and λ sFLCs simultaneously, producing a measurement of summated FLCs in a single assay (Combylite, cFLC). This should allow easier testing of sFLCs in a variety of inflammatory conditions.

References

1.   Charafeddine KM, Jabbour MN, Kadi RH, Daher RT. Extended use of serum free light chain as a biomarker in lymphoproliferative disorders: a comprehensive review. Am J Clin Pathol 2012;137:890-7

2.   Martin W, Abraham R, Shanafelt T, Clark RJ, Bone N, Geyer SM et al. Serum-free light chain-a new biomarker for patients with B-cell non-Hodgkin lymphoma and chronic lymphocytic leukemia. Transl Res 2007;149:231-5

3.   Pinto A, Iaccarino G, Russo F, Amoroso B, Morelli E, Riemma C, De Filippi R. Clinical and biological relevance of serum free light chains (sFLC) assessment in patients with Hodgkin's lymphoma. Hematology Reports 2010;2:p15

4.   Thompson CA, Maurer MJ, Cerhan JR, Katzmann JA, Ansell SM, Habermann TM et al. Elevated serum free light chains are associated with inferior event free and overall survival in Hodgkin lymphoma. Am J Hematol 2011;86:998-1000

5.   De Filippi R, Morabito F, Corazzelli G, Russo F, Calemma R, Iaccarino G et al. Use of the cumulative amount of serum-free light chains (sFLC) at diagnosis and PET2 for the early identification of high risk of treatment failure in Hodgkin lymphoma (cHL). J Clin Oncol 2012;30 suppl:8083a

6.   Corazzelli G, De Filippi R, Capobianco G, Frigeri F, De Rosa V, Iaccarino G et al. Tumor flare reactions and response to lenalidomide in patients with refractory classic Hodgkin lymphoma. Am J Hematol 2010;85:87-90

7.   Maurer MJ, Micallef IN, Cerhan JR, Katzmann JA, Link BK, Colgan JP et al. Elevated serum free light chains are associated with event-free and overall survival in two independent cohorts of patients with diffuse large B-cell lymphoma. J Clin Oncol 2011;29:1620-6

8.   Jardin F, Delfau-Larue MH, Molina TJ, Copie-Bergman C, Briere J, Petrella T et al. Immunoglobulin heavy chain/light chain pair measurment is associated with survival in diffuse large B-cell lymphoma. Leuk Lymphoma 2013;54:1898-907

9.   Witzig TE, Maurer MJ, Stenson MJ, Allmer C, Macon W, Link B et al. Elevated serum monoclonal and polyclonal free light chains and Interferon inducible protein-10 predicts inferior prognosis in untreated diffuse large B-cell lymphoma. Am J Hematol 2014;89:417-22

10. De Filippi R, Laccarino G, Frigeri F, Di Francia R, Amoroso B, Marchei A, Pinto A. The presence of serum free-immunoglobulin light chains and abnormal k/l ratios is a frequent finding in patients with Hodgkin's and B-cell non-Hodgkin's lymphoma. Hematology meeting reports 2008;2:C18a

11. Furtado M, Shah N, Levoguer A, Harding S, Rule S. Abnormal serum free light chain ratio predicts poor overall survival in mantle cell lymphoma. Br J Haematol 2013;160:63-9

12. Pinto A, De Filippi R, Iaccarino G, Di Francia R, Distinto M, Frigeri F et al. Abnormalities in serum free-immunoglobulin light chains show a high and differential frequency among WHO subtypes of B-cell non-Hodgkin's lymphoma (NHL) and may turn of value for therapeutic monitoring: A study of 354 newly diagnosed patients. Blood 2008;112:2813a

13. Leleu X, Moreau AS, Weller E, Roccaro AM, Coiteux V, Manning R et al. Serum immunoglobulin free light chain correlates with tumor burden markers in Waldenstrom macroglobulinemia. Leuk Lymphoma 2008;49:1104-7

14. Itzykson R, Le Garff-Tavernier M, Katsahian S, Diemert MC, Musset L, Leblond V. Serum-free light chain elevation is associated with a shorter time to treatment in Waldenstrom's macroglobulinemia. Haematologica 2008;93:793-4

15. Leleu X, Koulieris E, Maltezas D, Itzykson R, Xie W, Manier S et al. Novel M-component based biomarkers in Waldenstrom's macroglobulinemia. Clin Lymphoma Myeloma Leuk 2011;11:164-7

16. Pratt G, Harding S, Holder R, Fegan C, Pepper C, Oscier D et al. Abnormal serum free light chain ratios are associated with poor survival and may reflect biological subgroups in patients with chronic lymphocytic leukaemia. Br J Haematol 2009;144:217-22

17. Yegin ZA, Ozkurt ZN, Yagci M. Free light chain : a novel predictor of adverse outcome in chronic lymphocytic leukemia. Eur J Haematol 2010;84:406-11

18. Maurer MJ, Cerhan JR, Katzmann JA, Link BK, Allmer C, Zent CS et al. Monoclonal and polyclonal serum free light chains and clinical outcome in chronic lymphocytic leukemia. Blood 2011;118:2821-6

19. Morabito F, De FR, Laurenti L, Zirlik K, Recchia AG, Gentile M et al. The cumulative amount of serum free light chain is a strong prognosticator in chronic lymphocytic leukemia. Blood 2011;118:6353-61

20. Sarris K, Bartzis V, Maltezas D, Koulieris E, Tzenou T, Sachanas S et al. Significance of serum free light chains in chronic lymphocytic leukemia (CLL) prognosis. Blood 2012;120:4568a

21. Aue G, Farooqui M, Jones J, Valdez J, Martyr S, Soto S et al. In patients with chronic lymphocytic leukaemia (CLL) Ibrutinib effectively reduces clonal IgM paraproteins and serum free light chains while increasing normal IgM, IgA serum levels, suggesting a nascent recovery of humoral immunity. Blood 2013;122:4182a

22. Pratt G, Berlanga O, Lokare A, Randall K, Lee S, Harding S. Heavy/light chain characteristics of patients with indolent and aggressive lymphomas. Haematologica 2014;99:P454a

23. Koulieris E, Kyrtsonis MC, Maltezas D, Tzenou T, Mirbahai L, Mead G et al. Quantification of serum IgMk and IgMl in patients with Waldenström's macroglobulinaemia (WM): Clinical correlations. Hematology Reports 2010;2:F63a

24. Manier S, Lejeune J, Musset L, Boyle E, Dulery R, Debarri H et al. Hevylite, a novel M-component based biomarkers of response to therapy and survival in Waldenstrom macroglobulinemia. Blood 2011;118:2667a

25. Kaleta E, Kyle R, Clark R, Katzmann J. Analysis of patients with gamma-heavy chain disease by the heavy/light chain and free light chain assays. Clin Chem Lab Med 2014;52:665-9

26. Hutchison CA, Landgren O. Polyclonal immunoglobulin free light chains as a potential biomarker of immune stimulation and inflammation. Clin Chem 2011;57:1387-9

27. Faint JM, Basu S, Sutton D, Showell PJ, Kalra PA, Gunson BK et al. Quantification of polyclonal free light chains in clinical samples using a single turbidimetric immunoassay. Clin Chem Lab Med 2014;52:1605-13

Lymphoma

Summary:

- In patients with lymphoma, FLCs may be produced directly by the tumour or by B-cells in the surrounding microenvironment.

- In diffuse large B-cell lymphoma and Hodgkin lymphoma, elevated sFLCs are associated with inferior event-free survival and overall survival.

- IgM Hevylite® is a novel prognostic marker in diffuse large B-cell lymphoma, predicting inferior outcomes in patients with abnormal IgMκ/IgMλ ratios.

- In mantle cell lymphoma, an abnormal sFLC ratio at disease relapse is associated with significantly worse overall survival.

31.1. Introduction

Lymphoma is a type of cancer that originates in the lymphatic system. There are two main types: Hodgkin lymphoma (HL) and non-Hodgkin lymphoma (NHL)[1]. HL is less common and tends to affect the lymph nodes in the head and neck. It is distinguished from other types of lymphoma by the presence of Reed-Sternberg tumour cells[2]. NHL constitutes approximately 90% of lymphoma cases, and can affect any lymph node or related tissue in the body[1]. NHL is the sixth most common cancer in the UK, accounting for 4% of all new cases[3]. NHL is not a single disease, but comprises more than 60 subtypes that have distinct morphology, immunophenotype, genetic, molecular, and clinical features[1]. NHL is broadly divided into two major groups: B-cell lymphomas and T-cell lymphomas. B-cell NHLs account for approximately 85% of all NHLs and are discussed further below. Diffuse large B-cell lymphoma (DLBCL) is the most common form of NHL, accounting for up to one-third of cases. The frequencies of the other major NHL subtypes are summarised in Figure 31.1.

This chapter discusses the role of serum free light chain (sFLC) and immunoglobulin heavy/light chain (Hevylite, HLC) analysis in HL and NHL, with the exception of Waldenström's macroglobulinaemia, which is discussed in Chapter 32, and chronic lymphocytic leukaemia (considered part of a disease continuum with small lymphocytic lymphoma), which is discussed in Chapter 33. Conditions associated with increased lymphoma risk, such as solid organ transplantation and HIV infection, are covered in Chapter 35.

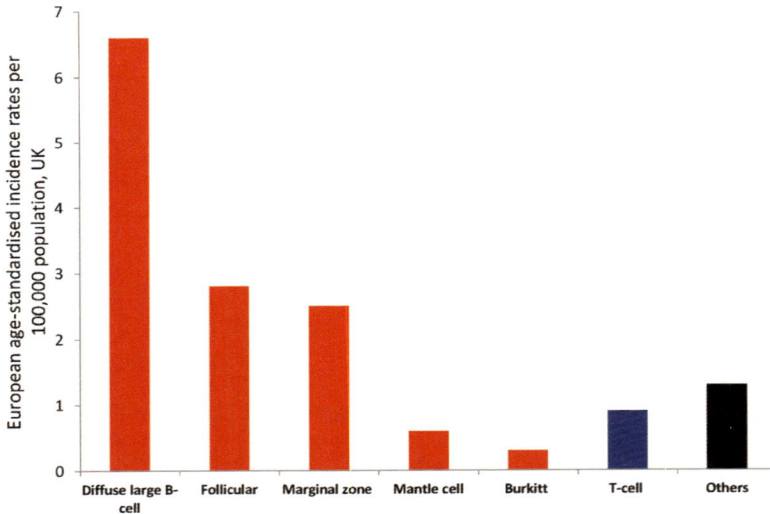

Figure 31.1. Frequencies of NHL subtypes in the UK. Red: B-cell NHL; Blue: T-cell NHL; others: Lymphoproliferative disorders not otherwise specified. Figure based on Haematological Malignancy Research Network (HMRN) data for 2004-2011[3]. (Produced with permission from Cancer Research UK).

31.2. Hodgkin lymphoma

The tumour cells of HL (Reed-Sternberg cells) derive from germinal centre B-cells that have lost the expression of most B-cell specific genes, including those for immunoglobulin proteins[2]. These cells account for only approximately 1% of cells in the tumour tissue. The remaining tumour bulk consists of non-malignant reactive cells, including B- and T-cells, plasma cells, eosinophils, neutrophils and mast cells. These non-malignant cells are recruited and/or induced to proliferate by the tumour cells[2]. In turn, they provide survival/proliferation signals to the tumour.

Since the Reed-Sternberg cells do not produce immunoglobulins, they would not be expected to produce FLCs[5,6]. However, B-cells account for between 2 and 50% of the infiltrating cells in HL lesions, and are likely to be a source of FLCs in HL tissue[7]. In fact, approximately 30% of newly diagnosed HL patients have an elevated κ and/or λ sFLC concentration at diagnosis[4,8]. The majority of HL patients have polyclonal sFLCs, with an abnormal κ/λ sFLC ratio present in only 5 - 7% of cases[4,8].

Thompson et al.[4] examined the prognostic significance of pre-treatment concentrations of sFLCs in 100 HL patients with a median follow-up of 48 months. Patients with elevated sFLCs had inferior event-free survival (EFS) and overall survival (OS) compared with patients with normal sFLCs *(Figure 31.2)*. Elevated sFLCs remained associated with inferior EFS after adjusting for both the International Prognostic Score (IPS, p=0.05) and glomerular filtration rate (GFR, p=0.004). An abnormal κ/λ sFLC ratio (without elevated FLCs) was not associated with outcome. The prognostic significance of elevated sFLCs was confirmed by Pinto et al.[8].

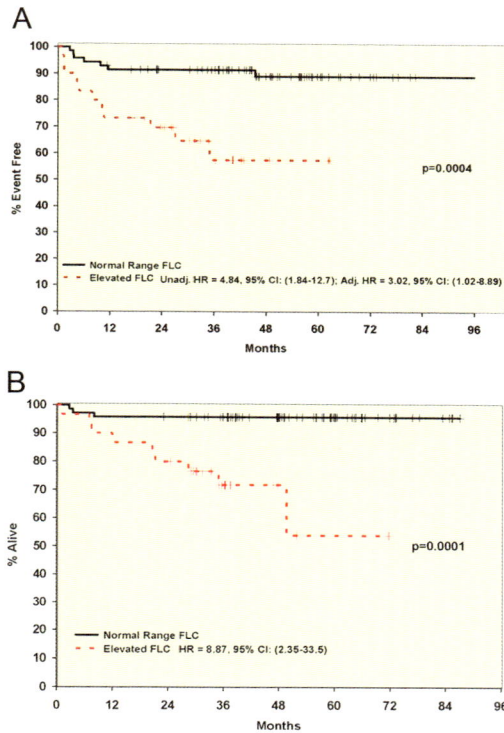

Figure 31.2. Kaplan-Meier survival curves for 100 HL patients. (A) *Event-free survival and* **(B)** *overall survival. Hazard ratios are unadjusted Cox models and Cox models adjusted for International Prognostic Score. (Reproduced with permission from the American Journal of Hematology[4] and John Wiley and Sons).*

De Filippi et al.[7] studied the prognostic value of $\kappa + \lambda$ sFLCs (ΣFLC) in a cohort of 248 untreated HL patients. Receiver operating characteristic (ROC) analysis defined 57.1 mg/L as the best threshold with which to discriminate outcomes. The proportion of patients achieving a complete response (CR) was significantly higher in those with ΣFLC <57.1 mg/L than in those with ΣFLC >57.1 mg/L (96% vs. 67% respectively; p<0.0001). In a multivariate model, only ΣFLC and positron emission tomography (PET) imaging remained independent predictors of outcome. The outcome for patients with both risk factors (elevated ΣFLC concentrations and PET positivity) was significantly worse than for those with one or neither of these factors (8-year EFS: <10% versus 36% or 93%; p<0.0001).

Pinto et al.[8] observed a statistically significant difference in κ and λ sFLC concentrations in newly diagnosed or relapsed patients compared with patients in complete remission. This suggests that sFLC measurements may have use in monitoring HL. In support of this, increased concentrations of sFLCs were associated with a lenalidomide-induced HL tumour flare reaction[9]. This is discussed in the case study below.

Clinical case history

A case of Hodgkin lymphoma tumour flare reaction monitored with sFLCs[9].

A 22-year-old male with biopsy-proven refractory HL (stage IVB) was one of three initial patients enrolled into a program of lenalidomide therapy. At baseline, ^{18}F-FDG-PET imaging demonstrated widespread lesions in nodal and extranodal (lungs, sternal ribs) sites *(Figure 31.3A)*. His spleen was enlarged with multiple nodulations. He had thrombocytopaenia, anaemia, and suffered from cough, exertion dyspnoea and persistent fever requiring methylprednisone.

The patient received 3 cycles of lenalidomide. Five days after starting the second course, the patient developed an acute inflammatory reaction characterised by the painful swelling of left inguinal lymph nodes and chest bone pain (exacerbated by finger pressure and breathing). A Grade 3 tumour flare reaction was diagnosed and the lenalidomide dose was reduced from 25 to 15 mg/day. Following the third course of lenalidomide (at 15 mg/day), the patient achieved a partial remission. This was associated with a reduction in the number and size of tumour lesions at all disease sites *(Figure 31.3B)*, and a stable recovery of platelets and haemoglobin.

sFLCs were measured at baseline and during therapy. Following lenalidomide therapy, sFLC concentrations increased, which is consistent with the observed tumour flare reaction. One month after the third course of lenalidomide sFLCs were markedly reduced, consistent with the response to treatment *(Figure 31.3C)*.

Tumour flare reactions were observed in a further two patients in this study[9]. In all three cases, flares were associated with the transient elevation of sFLC concentrations with a normal κ/λ sFLC ratio. Such findings are consistent with lenalidomide-induced activation of polyclonal B-cells within the tumour tissue. With continuing treatment, polyclonal sFLC concentrations decreased to normal concentrations.

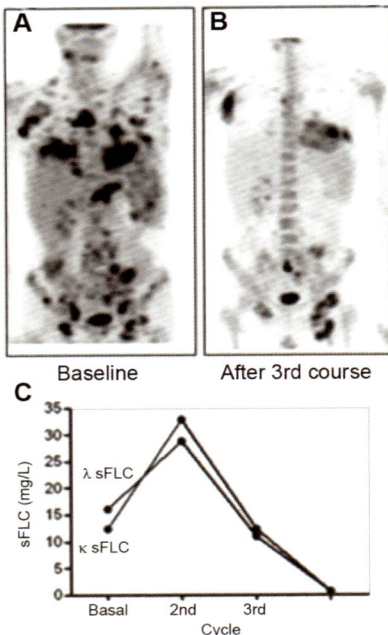

Figure 31.3. Response to lenalidomide therapy in a case of Hodgkin lymphoma. ^{18}F-FDG-PET imaging at *(A)* baseline and *(B)* after the 3rd course of therapy. *(C)* Changes in sFLC levels during therapy. (Reproduced with permission from the American Journal of Hematology[9] and John Wiley and Sons).

31.3. Non-Hodgkin lymphoma: diffuse large B-cell lymphoma

DLBCL is an aggressive B-cell lymphoma, and is the most common NHL, accounting for a third of all cases[1]. DLBCL is clinically, pathologically, and genetically diverse. Two principal DLBCL molecular subtypes have been defined by gene expression profiling: germinal centre B-cell (GCB) and activated B-cell (ABC). Each subtype is associated with a distinct clinical prognosis[11]. Tumour classification using immunohistochemistry algorithms (e.g. Hans, Choi and Tally) have been proposed as surrogates of gene expression profiling, but are not in routine clinical use[12].

DLBCL can be cured in more than 50% of cases[13]. The International Prognostic Index (IPI) is a clinical prognostic score for aggressive NHL including DLBCL[14]. However, there is a need for additional prognostic markers in DLBCL to identify patients likely to relapse after immunotherapy or fail to achieve remission.

31.3.1. sFLCs and HLCs in DLBCL

Although most cases of DLBCL are light chain restricted, only a minority of patients have sFLC abnormalities. Between 9 and 14% of DLBCL patients have an abnormal κ/λ sFLC ratio and between 19 and 32% have elevated κ and/or λ sFLCs[15,10]. Of the patients with elevated sFLCs, approximately 25% have monoclonal sFLCs (with an abnormal κ/λ sFLC ratio) while the remainder have polyclonal sFLCs (with a normal κ/λ sFLC ratio)[16].

Jardin et al.[10] characterised serum IgM, IgG and IgA HLC in DLBCL. An abnormal IgMκ/IgMλ, IgGκ/IgGλ or IgAκ/IgAλ HLC ratio was observed in the sera of 19.1%, 6.4% and 2.9% of patients, respectively[10]. This is consistent with the relative frequencies of B-cell receptor isotype expression by DLBCL cells[17]. The most frequent HLC abnormalities were reduced serum concentrations, observed in 11.2% (IgMκ) to 21% (IgGκ) of patients. There was little overlap between patients with sFLC and IgM HLC abnormalities (Figure 31.4).

Patients with an abnormal IgMκ/IgMλ HLC ratio had an increase in Cμ mRNA expression and a higher rate of IgM positive cases by immunohistochemistry compared with patients with normal HLC ratios[10]. Therefore, in the absence of any coexistent monoclonal gammopathies (e.g. monoclonal gammopathy of undetermined significance, Chapter 13), the source of a monoclonal protein in DLBCL is likely to be the tumour.

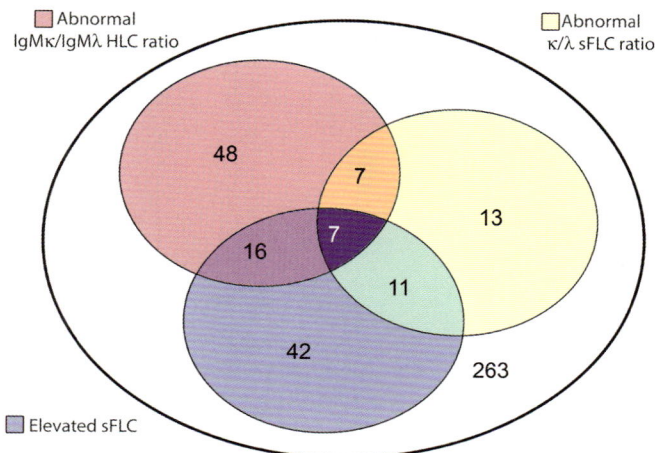

Figure 31.4. Venn diagram indicating the distribution of DLBCL patients according to κ/λ sFLC ratio, sFLC concentration and IgMκ/IgMλ HLC ratio. Chart generated using published data[10].

31.3.2. Prognostic value of sFLCs and HLCs in DLBCL

Maurer et al.[15] evaluated the prognostic utility of sFLC measurements in two large independent cohorts of untreated DLBCL patients (N0489: n=76 and MER: n=219). sFLC measurements were similar in the two cohorts *(Figure 31.5)*. Patients with elevated sFLCs (i.e. a κ and/or λ sFLC concentration above the normal range) had inferior EFS and OS compared to patients with normal sFLCs (both cohorts p<0.02) *(Figure 31.6)*[15]. The prognostic significance of elevated sFLCs persisted for a total of 6 years of follow-up[16]. Elevated sFLCs remained significantly associated with reduced OS and EFS after adjusting for the International Prognostic Index in both the N0489 (both p<0.02) and MER (both p<0.001) cohorts[15]. The prognostic utility of elevated sFLCs has been confirmed in other studies[10,18].

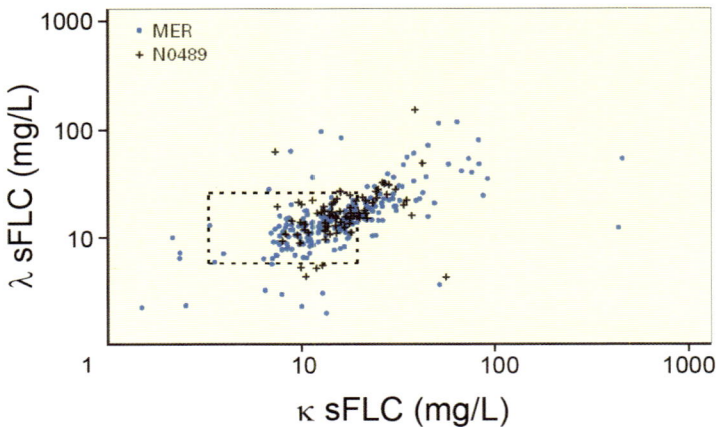

Figure 31.5. sFLC concentrations in two cohorts of DLBCL patients (MER and N0489). Dashed box indicates normal range. (Originally published by the American Society of Clinical Oncology[15]).

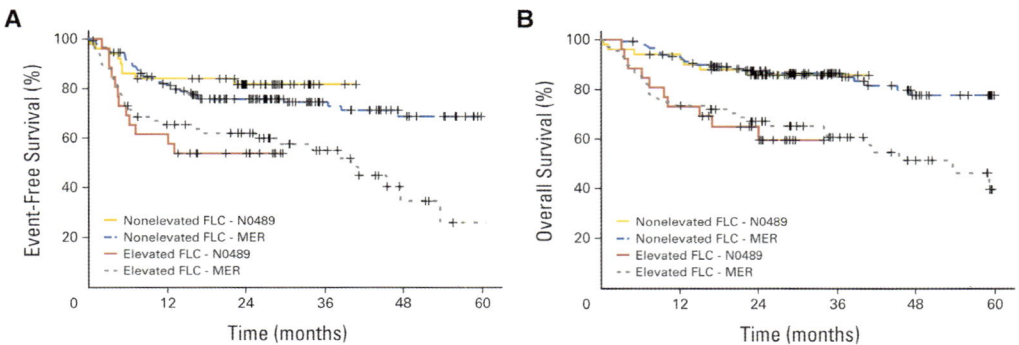

Figure 31.6. Kaplan-Meier survival curves for two cohorts of patients with untreated DLBCL (MER and N0489). (Originally published by the American Society of Clinical Oncology[15]).

Witzig et al.[16] reported that although DLBCL patients with monoclonal sFLC elevations tended to have poorer prognosis compared with that of patients with polyclonal sFLC elevations, this did not reach statistical significance. Moreover, monoclonal sFLCs predicted for ABC-type DLBCL: in all, 73% of patients with monoclonal sFLC elevations were of ABC-type (by the Hans algorithm) compared with 33% of patients with normal sFLCs[16]. By contrast, polyclonal elevations or normal sFLCs were not associated with a particular molecular subtype.

Elevated sFLCs were more common in patients with elevated serum creatinine (58%) than in patients with normal creatinine (29%)[15]. Interestingly, the association of elevated sFLCs and poor outcome was strengthened in the subset of patients with normal creatinine (n=241, OS Hazard ratio 4.09, p<0.001), while there was no association of elevated creatinine with outcome (n=40, OS Hazard ratio 1.00 p>0.60). This suggests that the association of sFLCs with outcome was not related to renal impairment.

Jardin et al.[10] studied the prognostic utility of HLC analysis in a cohort of 409 DLBCL patients enrolled on the LNH03-B clinical trial program of the French GELA study. Abnormal IgMκ/IgMλ HLC ratios and IgGκ/IgGλ HLC ratios or elevated IgMκ or IgMλ were each associated with significantly unfavourable outcomes. For example, patients with abnormal IgMκ/IgMλ HLC ratios had a 5-year OS of 50.8% compared with 78.1% for patients with normal IgM HLC ratios (p=0.0003) *(Figure 31.7)*. In multivariate analysis, which included six sFLC and HLC variables identified in univariate analysis, only an abnormal IgMκ/IgMλ HLC ratio remained predictive of progression-free survival (PFS) and OS. In a separate multivariate model, including IgMκ/IgMλ HLC ratio and IPI score, the IgMκ/IgMλ HLC ratio remained predictive of PFS (p=0.03).

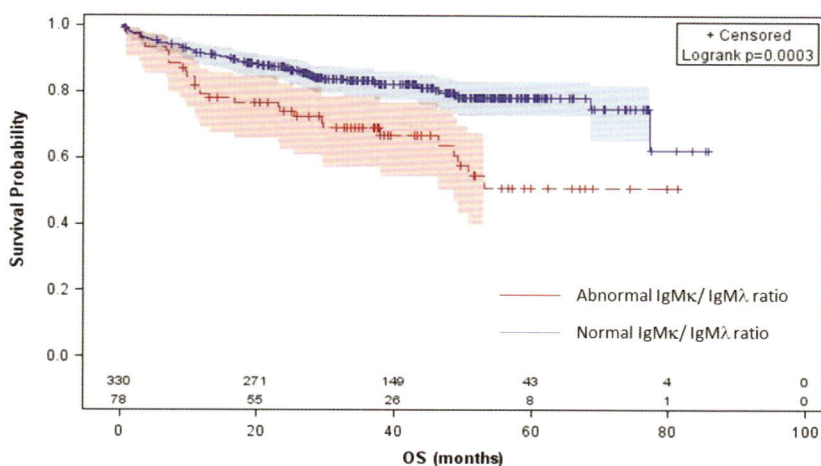

Figure 31.7. Overall survival according to IgMκ/IgMλ HLC ratio. (Reproduced with permission from Leukemia & lymphoma and Informa Healthcare[10]).

31.3.3. Use of sFLCs for monitoring DLBCL

Maurer et al.[15] evaluated the use of sFLCs for monitoring DLBCL in the N0489 trial. Pre- and post-treatment (cycle 6) sFLC measurements were available for 11 patients with κ- or λ-restricted tumours. Analysis of these samples revealed that, post-treatment, a greater reduction in the involved sFLC concentration was observed compared with the uninvolved sFLC (p=0.03). Serial monitoring samples were available for one λ-restricted DLBCL patient *(Figure 31.8)*[15]. The pre-treatment levels of λ sFLCs were highly elevated, with normal levels of κ sFLCs. λ sFLCs normalised after two cycles of treatment and the patient achieved a PET-negative complete response after six cycles. However, at 9 months post-treatment, λ sFLCs had increased, and tumour imaging and biopsy confirmed disease relapse. κ sFLCs remained unchanged throughout. This case illustrates that changes in the DLBCL tumour itself may directly influence changes in the corresponding sFLC.

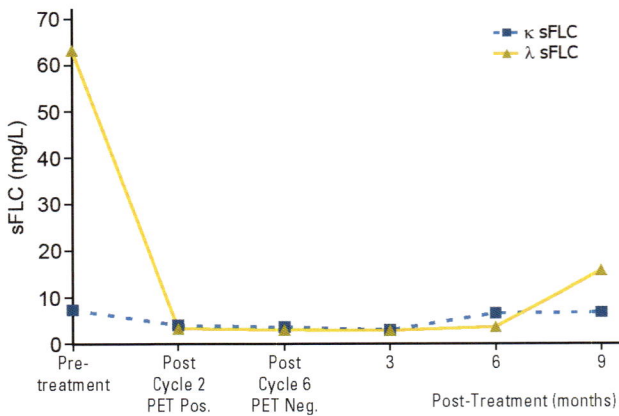

Figure 31.8. Serial sFLC measurements in a patient with λ-restricted DLBCL who relapsed 9 months after treatment. (Originally published by the American Society of Clinical Oncology[15]).

31.4. Non-Hodgkin lymphoma: mantle cell lymphoma

Mantle cell lymphoma (MCL) accounts for around 3 - 6 % of all NHL[20]. Although the disease demonstrates an initially encouraging response to treatment, its clinical course is usually marked by frequent relapses, with a median overall survival of only 4 - 5 years. Consequently, patients receive multiple lines of chemotherapy and are monitored closely for signs of disease relapse.

Several groups have reported a relatively high incidence of κ/λ sFLC ratio abnormalities ranging from 36 to 77%[21,22,19,23]. Furtado et al.[19] characterised sFLCs in a cohort of 20 relapsed/refractory MCL patients enrolled into a clinical trial of single agent oral lenalidomide. At disease relapse, 8 of 20 (40%) MCL patients had elevated sFLCs concentrations (classed as monoclonal [7/20] or polyclonal [1/20]). Overall survival was significantly shorter in patients with abnormal sFLC ratios than in those with normal sFLC ratios (p=0.001) *(Figure 31.9)*. For patients with an elevated sFLC ratio at trial entry, a 35% rise in the sFLC ratio correlated with disease progression. Summated κ + λ sFLCs (ΣFLC) did not correlate with disease outcome.

Furtado et al.[19] also recorded serial sFLC measurements following lenalidomide treatment. In five patients with monoclonal FLCs at disease relapse, normalisation of the sFLC ratio correlated with clinical improvement (reduction in lymph node size and/or resolution of 'B' symptoms). Of the patients with normal sFLC ratios at disease relapse, four individuals subsequently developed a polyclonal elevation of κ or λ sFLCs[19]. In such cases, the κ/λ sFLC ratio remained uninformative, but ΣFLC correlated with disease behaviour *(Figure 31.10)*. Use of the κ/λ sFLC ratio for monitoring response to treatment has been reported in other patients[23].

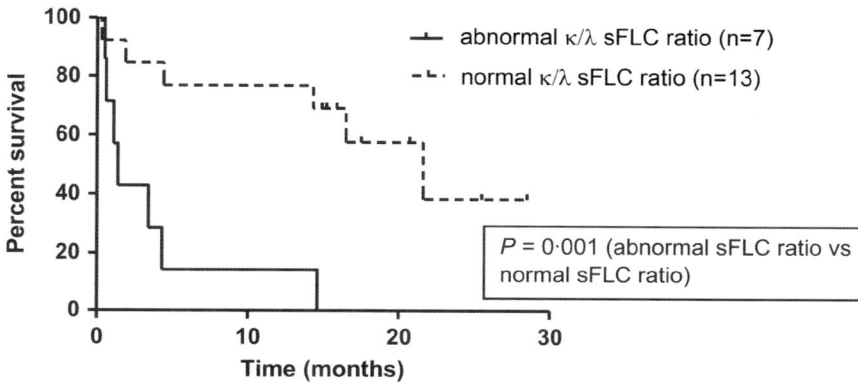

Figure 31.9. Overall survival stratified by κ/λ sFLC ratio. *(Reproduced with permission from the British Journal of Haematology[19] and John Wiley & Sons Ltd).*

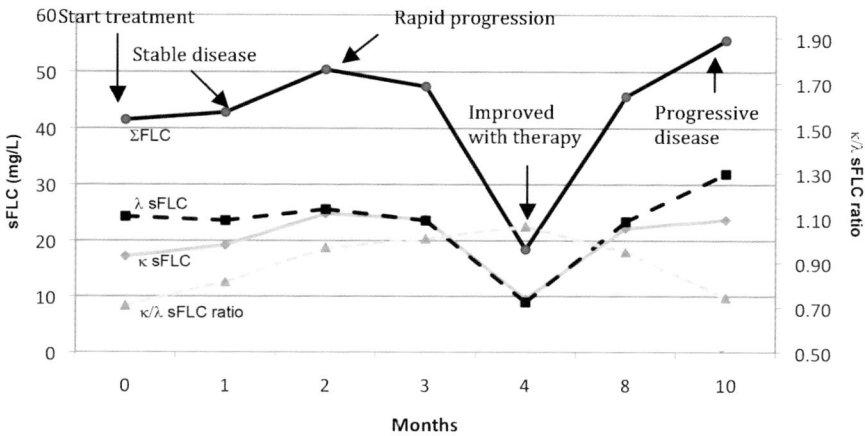

Figure 31.10. Serial sFLC measurements in a case of MCL. *(Reproduced with permission from the British Journal of Haematology[19] and John Wiley & Sons Ltd).*

Test Questions

1. What is the source of elevated polyclonal sFLCs in patients with lymphomas?

2. What type of lymphoma is associated with the highest incidence of κ/λ sFLC ratio abnormalities?

3. Why are sFLC measurements useful in DLBCL?

Answers

1. The immune response to the tumour, renal impairment, the systemic response to infection/inflammation or a combination of these factors.

2. Mantle cell lymphoma *(Section 31.4)*.

3. When elevated, sFLCs identify patients with inferior free event survival and overall survival. sFLCs may also be useful for monitoring some cases of DLBCL. *(Section 31.3)*.

References

1. Swerdlow SH, Campo E, Harris NL, Jaffe ES, Pileri SA, Stein H et al. WHO classification of tumours of haematopoietic and lymphoid tissues, Fourth ed. 2008

2. Kuppers R. The biology of Hodgkin's lymphoma. Nat Rev Cancer 2009;9:15-27

3. Non-Hodgkin lymphoma statistics. http://www.cancerresearchuk.org/cancer-info/cancerstats/types/nhl, accessed August 2014

4. Thompson CA, Maurer MJ, Cerhan JR, Katzmann JA, Ansell SM, Habermann TM et al. Elevated serum free light chains are associated with inferior event free and overall survival in Hodgkin lymphoma. Am J Hematol 2011;86:998-1000

5. Gladkowska-Dura MJ, Dura WT, Johnson WW. Light and immunoelectronmicroscopic study of Hodgkin's disease: evidence of immunoglobulin synthesis by tumor cells. Virchows Arch B Cell Pathol Incl Mol Pathol 1981;37:109-24

6. Marafioti T, Hummel M, Foss HD, Laumen H, Korbjuhn P, Anagnostopoulos I et al. Hodgkin and Reed-Sternberg cells represent an expansion of a single clone originating from a germinal center B-cell with functional immunoglobulin gene rearrangements but defective immunoglobulin transcription. Blood 2000;95:1443-50

7. De Filippi R, Morabito F, Corazzelli G, Russo F, Calemma R, Iaccarino G et al. Use of the cumulative amount of serum-free light chains (sFLC) at diagnosis and PET2 for the early identification of high risk of treatment failure in Hodgkin lymphoma (cHL). J Clin Oncol 2012;30 suppl:8083a

8. Pinto A, Iaccarino G, Russo F, Amoroso B, Morelli E, Riemma C, De Filippi R. Clinical and biological relevance of serum free light chains (sFLC) assessment in patients with Hodgkin's lymphoma. Hematology Reports 2010;2:p15

9. Corazzelli G, De Filippi R, Capobianco G, Frigeri F, De Rosa V, Iaccarino G et al. Tumor flare reactions and response to lenalidomide in patients with refractory classic Hodgkin lymphoma. Am J Hematol 2010;85:87-90

10. Jardin F, Delfau-Larue MH, Molina TJ, Copie-Bergman C, Briere J, Petrella T et al. Immunoglobulin heavy chain/light chain pair measurment is associated with survival in diffuse large B-cell lymphoma. Leuk Lymphoma 2013;54:1898-907

11. Rosenwald A, Wright G, Chan WC, Connors JM, Campo E, Fisher RI et al. The use of molecular profiling to predict survival after chemotherapy for diffuse large-B-cell lymphoma. N Engl J Med 2002;346:1937-47

12. Campo E, Swerdlow SH, Harris NL, Pileri S, Stein H, Jaffe ES. The 2008 WHO classification of lymphoid neoplasms and beyond: evolving concepts and practical applications. Blood 2011;117:5019-32

13. Armitage JO. My treatment approach to patients with diffuse large B-cell lymphoma. Mayo Clin Proc 2012;87:161-71

14. A predictive model for aggressive non-Hodgkin's lymphoma. The International Non-Hodgkin's Lymphoma Prognostic Factors Project. N Engl J Med 1993;329:987-94

15. Maurer MJ, Micallef IN, Cerhan JR, Katzmann JA, Link BK, Colgan JP et al. Elevated serum free light chains are associated with event-free and overall survival in two independent cohorts of patients with diffuse large B-cell lymphoma. J Clin Oncol 2011;29:1620-6

16. Witzig TE, Maurer MJ, Stenson MJ, Allmer C, Macon W, Link B et al. Elevated serum monoclonal and polyclonal free light chains and Interferon inducible protein-10 predicts inferior prognosis in untreated diffuse large B-cell lymphoma. Am J Hematol 2014;89:417-22

17. Ruminy P, Etancelin P, Couronne L, Parmentier F, Rainville V, Mareschal S et al. The isotype of the BCR as a surrogate for the GCB and ABC molecular subtypes in diffuse large B-cell lymphoma. Leukemia 2011;25:681-8

18. Kim YR, Kim SJ, Cheong JW, Kim Y, Jang JE, Lee JY et al. Monoclonal and polyclonal gammopathy measured by serum free light chain and immunofixation subdivide the clinical outcomes of diffuse large B-cell lymphoma according to molecular classification. Ann Hematol 2014;93:1867-77

19. Furtado M, Shah N, Levoguer A, Harding S, Rule S. Abnormal serum free light chain ratio predicts poor overall survival in mantle cell lymphoma. Br J Haematol 2013;160:63-9

20. Hitz F, Bargetzi M, Cogliatti S, Lohri A, Taverna C, Renner C, Mey U. Diagnosis and treatment of mantle cell lymphoma. Swiss Med Wkly 2013;143:w13868

21. Martin W, Abraham R, Shanafelt T, Clark RJ, Bone N, Geyer SM et al. Serum-free light chain-a new biomarker for patients with B-cell non-Hodgkin lymphoma and chronic lymphocytic leukemia. Transl Res 2007;149:231-5

22. De Filippi R, Laccarino G, Frigeri F, Di Francia R, Amoroso B, Marchei A, Pinto A. The presence of serum free-immunoglobulin light chains and abnormal k/l ratios is a frequent finding in patients with Hodgkin's and B-cell non-Hodgkin's lymphoma. Hematology meeting reports 2008;2:C18a

23. Pinto A, De Filippi R, Iaccarino G, Di Francia R, Distinto M, Frigeri F et al. Abnormalities in serum free-immunoglobulin light chains show a high and differential frequency among WHO subtypes of B-cell non-Hodgkin's lymphoma (NHL) and may turn of value for therapeutic monitoring: a study of 354 newly diagnosed patients. Blood 2008;112:2813a

Waldenström's macroglobulinaemia

Summary:

- Waldenström's macroglobulinaemia is a rare lymphoplasmacytic lymphoma associated with the production of monoclonal IgM.

- sFLC analysis is informative in the majority of patients at diagnosis.

- Elevated concentrations of sFLCs at baseline are associated with shorter time to treatment and reduced overall survival.

- The involved FLC concentration is a useful marker of response to treatment and may show responses and disease progression earlier than IgM.

- Quantification by IgM Hevylite® may be useful in cases where the monoclonal protein concentration is low, forms multimers or co-migrates with other serum protein peaks.

- IgM Hevylite may be useful for monitoring responses to treatment and identifying patients with inferior survival.

32.1. Introduction

Waldenström's macroglobulinaemia (WM) is a rare, low-grade, lymphoplasmacytic lymphoma characterised by the production of monoclonal IgM. The incidence rate of WM is approximately 5 cases per million persons per year, about 5 - 10% that of multiple myeloma (MM)[1]. The median age at diagnosis is 65 years, and up to 70% of patients are male[1,2]. Median survival is approximately 5 years (with 10% of patients still alive after 15 years); many die from unrelated causes[2]. The majority of patients diagnosed with WM do not require immediate therapy as they are detected before symptoms occur[3].

Infiltration of bone marrow and extramedullary sites by malignant B-cells, and elevated serum IgM concentrations are responsible for the majority of symptoms associated with WM[4]. Whilst the most common presenting symptom is fatigue related to anaemia, symptoms vary considerably among patients and may include night sweats, weight loss, bleeding tendency, polyneuropathy, lymphadenopathy, hepatosplenomegaly and symptoms relating to hyperviscosity (i.e. headaches, blurred vision, confusional episodes, epistaxis).

Cryoglobulinaemia (where monoclonal IgM reversibly precipitates at temperatures below 37 °C) affects up to 20% of patients, although <5% have symptoms *(Section 34.2)*[4]. The presence of cryoglobulins makes serum collection and laboratory quantification of IgM difficult, as they need to be performed at elevated temperatures.

Attempts to standardise diagnostic criteria have been made by the World Health Organisation (WHO) and the Mayo Clinic *(Table 32.1)*, but there are significant discrepancies between the two definitions[1].

Mayo Clinic WM diagnostic criteria:

• IgM monoclonal gammopathy (regardless of the size of the monoclonal protein).

• >10% bone marrow lymphoplasmacytic infiltration (usually inter-trabecular) by small lymphocytes that exhibit plasmacytoid or plasma cell differentiation.

• Tumour lymphocytes display a typical immunophenotype (surface IgM+, CD5-, CD10-, CD19+, CD20+, CD23-) that satisfactorily excludes other lymphoproliferative disorders, including chronic lymphocytic leukaemia and mantle cell lymphoma.

Table 32.1. Mayo Clinic WM diagnostic criteria[1,5]

32.2. IgM quantitation by routine laboratory tests

In WM, accurate determination of serum IgM is considered crucial both at diagnosis and to monitor response to therapy[7]. However, there are limitations to the routine laboratory methods used for IgM quantification.

Nephelometric total IgM assays may be unreliable due to an overestimation of IgM polymers, leading to a poor correlation with serum protein electrophoresis (SPE)[8]. Other disadvantages include the inability to distinguish between polyclonal IgM and disease-associated monoclonal IgM, especially at low monoclonal protein concentrations, when total IgM measurements may contain a significant proportion of polyclonal IgM. Nephelometric antisera may also react variably with monoclonal IgM from different patients[6].

Whilst monoclonal IgM quantitation by SPE has the advantage of separating monoclonal IgM from polyclonal background IgM, the method is more labour-intensive than nephelometric quantitation *(Chapter 4)*[6]. Other limitations of SPE include: inaccurate quantitation when the concentration of monoclonal IgM is low; cases of 'sticky IgM' (in which insoluble aggregates form that precipitate in the loading site); the presence of IgM multimers (which create 'overlapping peaks'); and comigration of monoclonal IgM in the β-region alongside other serum proteins *(Figure 32.1)*. In addition, the presence of cryoglobulins affects IgM measurements by all methods[9].

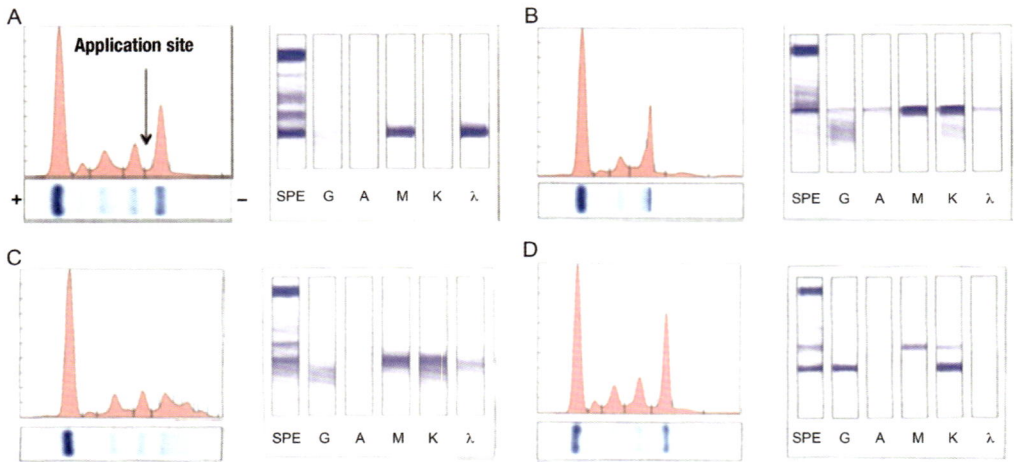

Figure 32.1. Serum electrophoresis of IgM monoclonal proteins. *Each example consists of the electropherogram (left) and the immunofixation gel (right). (A) IgMλ in the γ region with a straight forward quantitation. Position of anode (+) and cathode (−) are shown. (B) "Sticky" IgMκ showing precipitation at the application site and atypical peak shape on electropherogram. (C) IgMκ running as 3 peaks, most likely corresponding to higher order complexes. (D) Biclonal gammopathy (IgMκ and IgGκ). The IgMκ co-migrates with other serum proteins in the β-region. (Reproduced from Clinical Lymphoma, Myeloma & Leukemia[6], Copyright 2013, with permission from Elsevier).*

Immunoglobulin heavy/light chain immunoassays (Hevylite, HLC), may provide some benefits. HLC assays quantify the different light chain types of each immunoglobulin class (i.e. IgMκ and IgMλ), and the molecules are measured in pairs to produce HLC ratios (i.e. IgMκ/IgMλ) *(Chapter 9)*[10]. HLC analysis also allows the concentration of the uninvolved HLC-pair to be measured (e.g. IgMλ in an IgMκ patient). When the concentration of the HLC-pair is below the normal reference interval, this is termed "HLC-pair suppression" *(Section 11.2.2)*. In a WM patient with monoclonal IgMκ (for example), nephelometric measurement of IgMκ may provide a measure closer to the concentration of the monoclonal immunoglobulin than a total IgM assay. In addition, measurement of the HLC ratio, which is influenced by HLC pair suppression, has been found to be a sensitive marker of tumour activity in other diseases.

However, if a WM patient's tumour produces measurable quantities of monoclonal sFLCs, monitoring these concentrations could avoid most of the limitations encountered with monoclonal IgM quantitation (above).

32.3. sFLCs in Waldenström's macroglobulinaemia
32.3.1. sFLCs and WM diagnosis

FLC proteinuria occurs in up to 70% of WM patients. However, the amounts excreted are usually low and do not relate particularly well to changes in tumour burden[11]. In contrast, the sFLC assay is informative in the majority of patients *(Figure 32.2)*[7]. Importantly, sFLCs do not cryoprecipitate and are not affected by other factors that can make IgM measurements difficult[9].

Itzykson et al.[12] assessed sFLCs in 42 WM patients prior to treatment. The median involved FLC (iFLC) concentration was 48.6 mg/L (range 11.3 - 19400 mg/L), and was elevated above the normal range in 83% of patients. The iFLC and IgM monoclonal protein concentration were not related to each other (p=0.89), similar to findings in multiple myeloma patients *(Sections 11.2.5 and 17.2)*. Whilst guidelines state that sFLC analysis is not essential for the routine assessment of WM patients [4,7,13], in practice, it is routinely used by many clinicians in this context[3]. A recent survey of haematologists and oncologists in the Netherlands revealed that 43.4% currently measure sFLCs in the diagnostic work-up of patients with suspected WM[14].

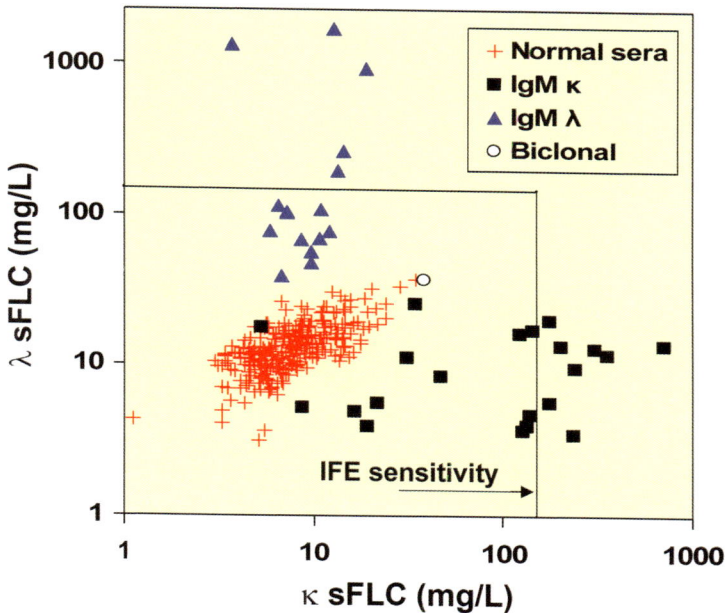

Figure 32.2. sFLC concentrations in normal sera and in 37 patients with WM at the time of plasma exchange for hyperviscosity syndrome.

32.3.2. Monitoring WM using sFLCs

sFLCs may be a useful additional marker to monitor WM. Their short serum half-life and the large clinical range provide a sensitive marker for assessment of response to treatment.

Leleu et al.[15] studied the use of sFLCs to monitor response to treatment in 48 WM patients (untreated [n=20] or relapse and/or refractory [n=28]), participating in a trial of bortezomib and rituximab treatment. The proportion of patients who demonstrated a response to therapy was higher using sFLC analysis (79%, defined as a ≥50% decrease in iFLC from baseline) than monoclonal protein quantification by SPE (60%). Similar results were obtained when the difference between the iFLC and uninvolved (uFLC) sFLC concentrations (dFLC) was used as an alternative measure of sFLC response (κ-statistic 0.89). In addition, the time to response was shorter when assessed using iFLC compared to the monoclonal protein response (2.1 vs 3.7 months, p=0.05)[15]. There was a significant correlation of progression as defined by iFLC or SPE criteria (a >25% increase from maximum response), with 81% of patients showing concordance of both markers (κ-statistic: 0.63). The median time to progression (TTP) was shorter as measured by iFLC than by following SPE criteria (13.7 vs. 18.9 months, respectively). The authors concluded that iFLC was a sensitive marker for the early determination of response and progression in WM.

An update of the consensus panel criteria for the assessment of clinical response in patients with WM stated that whilst there were insufficient data to incorporate sFLC assessments into the revised criteria, further prospective evaluation was encouraged[13]. Similarly, British guidelines also highlight the potential utility of sFLC measurements for the assessment of response in WM[7].

32.3.3. sFLCs and WM prognosis

Itzykson et al.[12] examined the prognostic utility of baseline sFLC measurements in 42 WM patients prior to treatment. iFLC concentrations were significantly increased in patients with adverse prognostic markers (elevated β_2-microglobulin >3 mg/L or low albumin <35 g/L; p<0.05). Furthermore, elevated iFLC concentrations (>80 mg/L) were independently associated with progressive disease and a shorter time to treatment (Figure 32.3). Similar findings were reported by Leleu et al.[16,26] who demonstrated that elevated concentrations of sFLC (>60 mg/L) were associated with adverse prognostic markers (elevated β_2-microglobulin or IgM, or low haemoglobin) and reduced overall survival. In a separate study, Leleu et al.[17] investigated the prognostic significance of a sFLC response in a prospective study of 72 WM patients. The 3-year probability of survival was significantly higher for those patients with sFLC concentrations <80 mg/L (96.8%) compared with those patients with values >80 mg/L (57.5%; p=0.05). The authors concluded that sFLC measurements should be included in future clinical WM trials to validate their results.

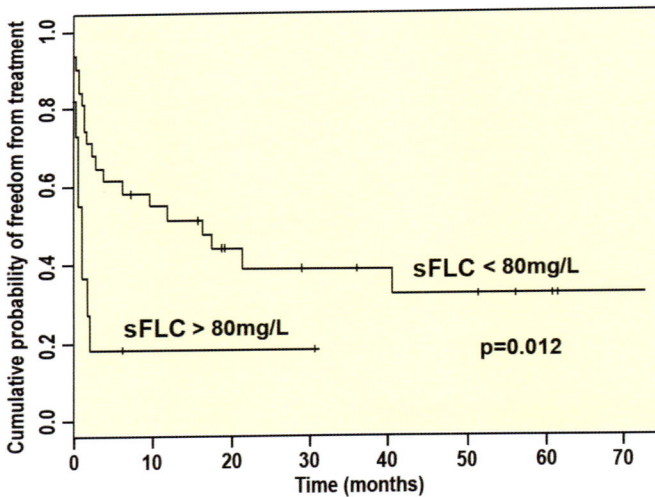

Figure 32.3. Time to treatment according to baseline involved FLC concentration.
(Republished with permission from Haematologica[12]).

Clinical case history

The value of sFLC analysis for monitoring in a case of Waldenström's macroglobulinemia with a type 1 cryoglobulin[9].

An 82-year-old male with chronic kidney disease (stage 3) and diabetes was referred to the haematology department by his general practitioner based on results of routine investigations. These revealed that he was anaemic (haemoglobin 8.9 g/dL) and had an elevated plasma viscosity (15 cp) with a serum total protein of 102 g/L.

SPE revealed a monoclonal protein which was typed as an IgMλ, but this could not be accurately quantified as it precipitated out in the gel *(Figure 32.4A)*. Furthermore, the serum sample appeared clotted after being stored at 4 °C, which was reversed once the sample was warmed to 37 °C, consistent with the presence of a cryoglobulin.

Haematological assessment highlighted symptoms which were consistent with hyperviscosity syndrome. These included dyspnoea, epistaxis, blurring of vision and sensory neuropathy, requiring plasma exchange. Although a diagnosis of WM was now expected, a rare case of IgM multiple myeloma could not be ruled out. A bone marrow aspirate was inconclusive but a trephine biopsy and immunohistochemistry confirmed the diagnosis of WM.

Cryoglobulin analysis confirmed the presence of a type 1 cryoglobulin *(Figure 32.4B)*. The patient started a course of chemotherapy, and serial measurements of sFLCs were used to assess response *(Figure 32.5)*.

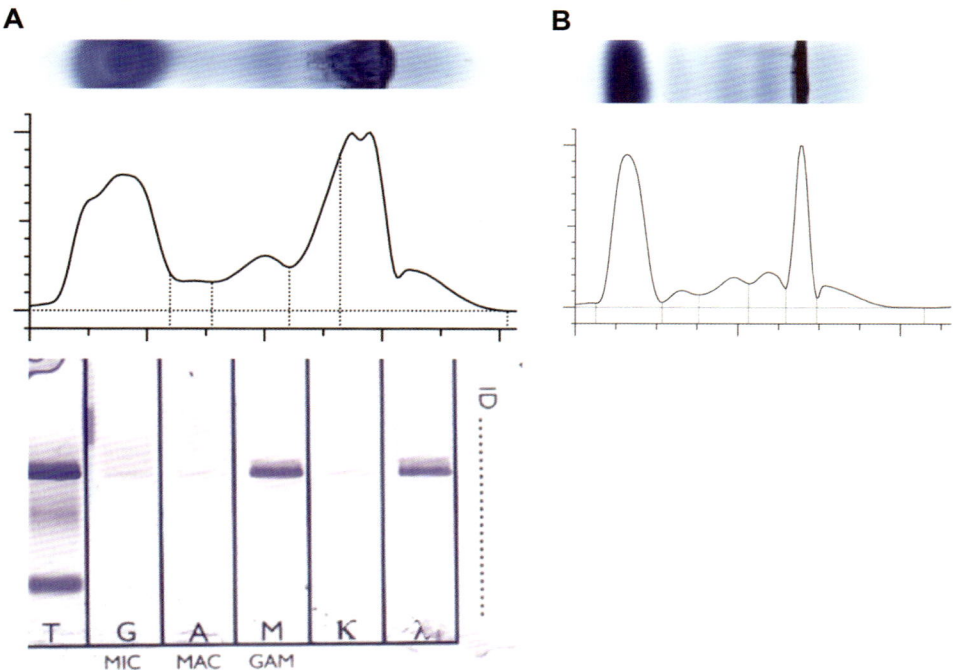

Figure 32.4. (A) SPE and serum immunofixation electrophoresis on samples at room temperature. (B) SPE on a sample at 37 °C. *(Reproduced by permission of SAGE Publications Ltd., London, Los Angeles, New Delhi, Singapore and Washington DC, from[9], © R.J. Pattenden, 2009).*

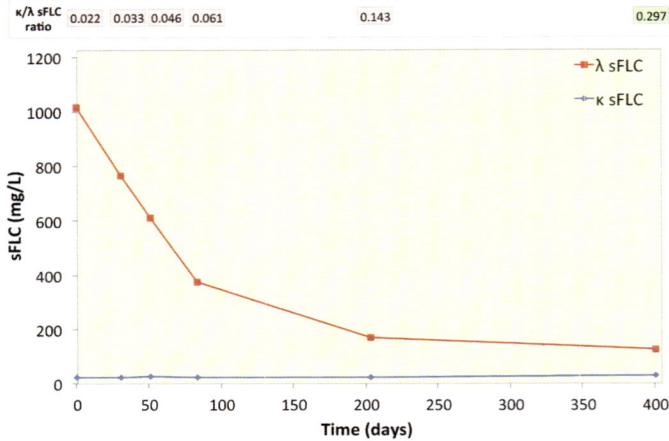

Figure 32.5. sFLC results at baseline and following initiation of chemotherapy. The κ/λ sFLC ratio had normalised by day 400[9].

32.4. IgM HLC in Waldenström's macroglobulinaemia

32.4.1. IgM HLC and WM diagnosis

When the monoclonal IgM concentration is low, accurate quantification by SPE or capillary zone electrophoresis (CZE) may be difficult. In such cases, IgM HLC may provide a more reliable quantitative assessment *(Figure 32.6)*[18,20]. Hevylite analysis may also be useful in cases where monoclonal proteins form multimers or co-migrate with other serum protein peaks (Section 17.4)[10].

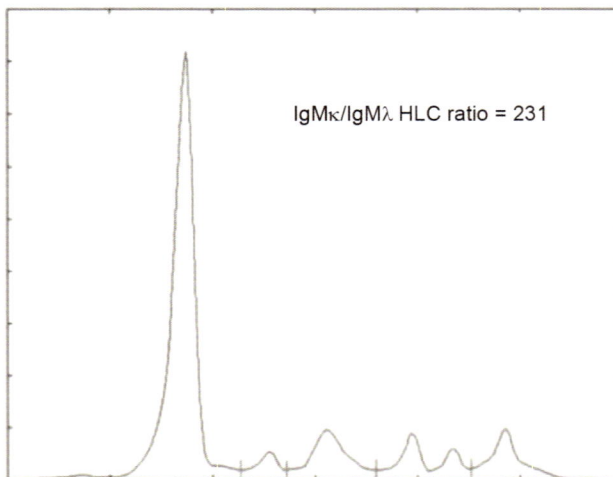

Figure 32.6. Serum electropherogram (capillary zone electrophoresis) and HLC results for a patient with WM. (Reproduced from Onkologie[18] with permission from S. Karger AG, Basel).

Koulieris et al.[21] assessed the diagnostic sensitivity of IgM HLC in 31 WM patients at presentation and showed that IgMκ/IgMλ HLC ratios were abnormal in 97% (30/31) of patients. Manier et al.[19] evaluated IgM HLC concentrations in 86 WM patients (71 at diagnosis, 15 at relapse). The involved IgM HLC values correlated well with the monoclonal protein quantified by SPE or total IgM assays *(Figure 32.7)*. The median (minimum – maximum) involved HLC concentration was 21.9 g/L (1.94 - 126 g/L), compared with 20.6 g/L (3.2 - 90 g/L) for monoclonal protein quantified by SPE, or 19.4 g/L (2.4 - 87g/L) for total IgM measured by nephelometry. In a recent report from Boyle et al.[22], 78/78 patients had abnormal HLC ratios at diagnosis despite the fact that 11/78 had "unquantifiable" SPE results and 4/78 had total IgM concentrations within the normal range.

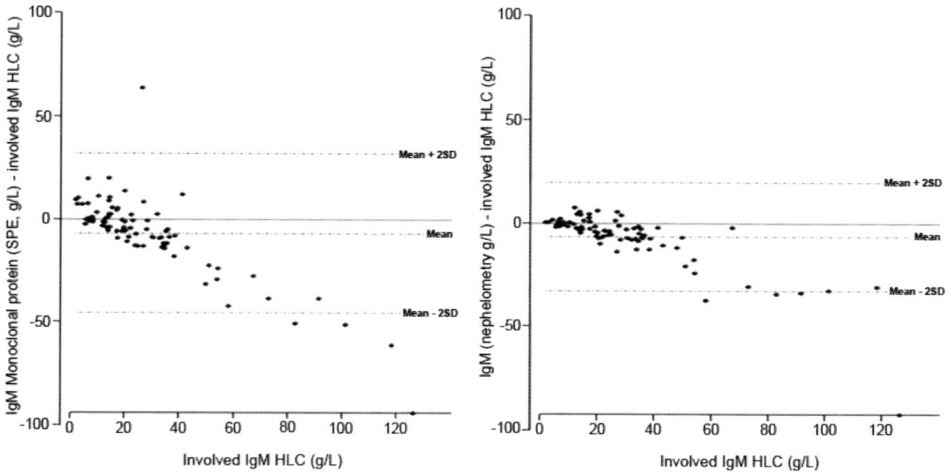

Figure 32.7. Bland-Altman plots showing the agreement between different methods used to quantify IgM. *(This research was originally published in Blood[19] © the American Society of Hematology).*

32.4.2. Monitoring WM using IgM HLC

Preliminary evidence suggests that IgM HLC may be useful for monitoring response to treatment in WM[19,23]. Manier et al.[19] compared the IgM response rate using SPE, IgM nephelometry and IgM HLC, for 10 WM patients who were treated as part of a Phase 3 trial. After 14 months, the proportion of patients achieving a partial response or better, vs. those who had stable disease, was similar across the three techniques. The median time to response and time to progression was also similar.

Koulieris et al.[23] monitored nine WM patients with IgM HLC. The involved HLC concentration and the IgMκ/IgMλ HLC ratio mostly followed disease fluctuations. During the study period patients only achieved a partial remission, and consistent with this, the IgM HLC ratio never normalised. Boyle et al.[22] compared HLC, SPE and total IgM results from 25 patients during follow-up. Although quantitative measurements of the monoclonal IgM were quite different for the three methods, a weighted kappa analysis confirmed that the assigned responses following treatment were very consistent. It was noted however, that when total IgM concentrations became normal in 7/25 patients, both the HLC ratio and sIFE remained positive and that the HLC ratio indicated residual disease in 5/25 patients who had a complete response by electrophoresis.

An update of the consensus panel criteria for the assessment of clinical response in WM stated that further prospective evaluation of the use of HLC to assess response in WM is encouraged[13].

32.4.3. IgM HLC and WM prognosis

Koulieris et al.[23] studied the prognostic significance of IgM HLC in 31 WM patients at diagnosis. The median involved/uninvolved IgM HLC ratio was significantly higher in WM patients requiring treatment (n=24) compared with patients not requiring treatment (n=7) (185.7 vs. 13.45; p=0.023). Leleu et al.[16] reported similar data: the median involved/uninvolved HLC ratio was significantly higher in progressing symptomatic patients compared with asymptomatic patients (p=0.014). Patients with a higher involved/uninvolved HLC ratio (>median) had a significantly shorter time to treatment than those patients with a lower HLC ratio *(Figure 32.8A)*.

Koulieris et al.[23] also reported a correlation between the IgM HLC ratio and bone marrow infiltration (p=0.029) and time to first treatment (p=0.003); they proposed a risk stratification model that identified 3 prognostic groups with respect to survival. This model comprised 3 risk factors: involved/uninvolved IgM HLC ratio (>median); β_2-microglobulin (>5.5 mg/L); and abnormal lactate dehydrogenase (LDH) *(Figure 32.8B)*.

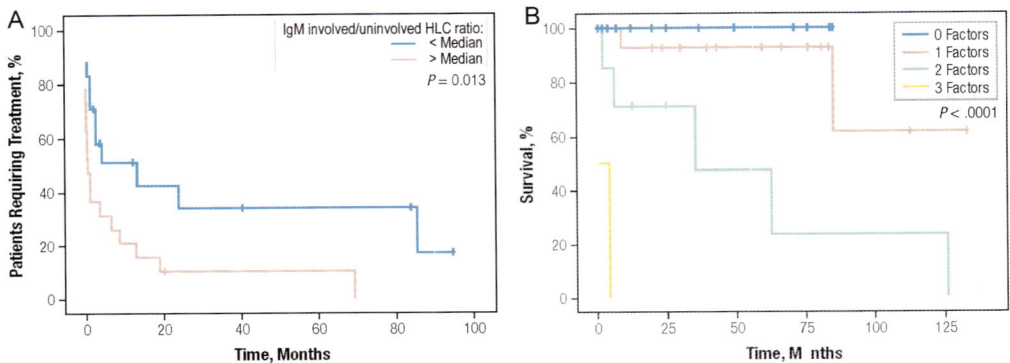

Figure 32.8. (A) Involved/uninvolved HLC ratio predicts time to treatment. (B) Kaplan-Meier overall survival plot according to presence of 0, 1, 2, or 3 risk factors. The risk factors were: 1) involved/uninvolved HLC ratio >median; 2) β_2-microglobulin >5.5 mg/L; and 3) abnormal LDH. (Reproduced from Clinical Lymphoma, Myeloma & Leukemia[16], Copyright 2011, with permission from Elsevier).

In a subsequent, larger study, Koulieris et al.[24] studied the prognostic significance of systemic hypogammaglobulinaemia and HLC-pair suppression in 70 WM patients at diagnosis. HLC-pair suppression was present in 26% (18/70) patients; whilst systemic hypogammaglobulinaemia (defined as IgG <7 g/L and/or IgA <0.7 g/L), was present in 49% (34/70) of patients. During follow-up (median 37 months), 48/70 patients were or became symptomatic and 16/70 died. Neither systemic hypogammaglobulinaemia nor HLC-pair suppression at diagnosis correlated with time to first treatment (p=0.358) or overall survival (p=0.874). Conversely, Murillo-Florez et al.[25] found that relapsed/refractory WM patients had a mean uninvolved HLC concentration that was lower than the patients who did not relapse (0.29 vs. 0.52 g/L; p=0.04). Therefore, the prognostic utility of HLC-pair measurement in WM has yet to be established.

32.5. Use of sFLC and HLC analysis to differentiate IgM MGUS and WM

Accurate diagnosis of WM is difficult in some cases, due to the ill-defined overlap of clinical features between WM and two related conditions i.e. IgM monoclonal gammopathy of undetermined significance (IgM MGUS), and asymptomatic WM[26]. New evidence suggests that FLC and HLC analysis may allow improved discrimination between these conditions.

Leleu et al.[26] compared involved sFLC concentrations in WM (n=98) and IgM MGUS (n=68). An abnormal κ/λ sFLC ratio was present in 76.5% and 23.5% of WM and IgM MGUS patients, respectively (p<0.001). Involved FLC concentrations were significantly higher in WM (median = 36 mg/L; range 16 - 140 mg/L) than in IgM MGUS (median 20 mg/L; range 16 - 33 mg/L): p<0.0003. Leleu and colleagues concluded that a sFLC cut-off of 60 mg/L separated WM from IgM MGUS with >95% specificity. Similar findings were also reported by Murillo-Florez et al.[27].

In a separate report, Murillo-Florez et al.[28] compared IgM HLC results from 29 WM patients with those of 21 IgM MGUS patients. The median involved/uninvolved HLC ratio was significantly higher in WM (381.8), than asymptomatic WM (75.84) or IgM MGUS (15.65; p=0.001) patients. Furthermore, the median uninvolved HLC concentration was significantly lower in WM than IgM MGUS (p=0.019). Further work is now required to study the combined use of FLC and HLC analysis to better discriminate WM and IgM MGUS.

Test Questions

1. Why are sFLCs useful for monitoring WM patients with cryoglobulinaemia?
2. Is sFLC and HLC analysis included in international WM guidelines?

Answers

1. Because sFLCs do not cryoprecipitate *(Section 32.3)*.
2. Yes, guidelines state that whilst they are not essential for the routine management of WM patients, further prospective evaluation is encouraged *(Sections 32.3.2, 32.4.1, and 32.4.2)*[13].

References

1. Ansell SM, Kyle RA, Reeder CB, Fonseca R, Mikhael JR, Morice WG et al. Diagnosis and management of Waldenström macroglobulinemia: Mayo stratification of macroglobulinemia and risk-adapted therapy (mSMART) guidelines. Mayo Clin Proc 2010;85:824-33

2. Morel P, Merlini G. Risk stratification in Waldenstrom macroglobulinemia. Expert Rev Hematol 2012;5:187-99

3. Gertz MA. Waldenstrom macroglobulinemia: 2013 update on diagnosis, risk stratification, and management. Am J Hematol 2013;88:703-11

4. Vos JM, Minnema MC, Wijermans PW, Croockewit S, Chamuleau ME, Pals ST et al. Guideline for diagnosis and treatment of Waldenstrom's macroglobulinaemia. Neth J Med 2013;71:54-62

5. Rajkumar SV, Dispenzieri A, Kyle RA. Monoclonal gammopathy of undetermined significance, Waldenstrom macroglobulinemia, AL amyloidosis, and related plasma cell disorders: diagnosis and treatment. Mayo Clin Proc 2006;81:693-703

6. Uljon SN, Treon SP, Tripsas CK, Lindeman NI. Challenges with serum protein electrophoresis in assessing progression and clinical response in patients with Waldenstrom macroglobulinemia. Clin Lymphoma Myeloma Leuk 2013;13:247-9

7. Owen RG, Pratt G, Auer RL, Flatley R, Kyriakou C, Lunn MP et al. Guidelines on the diagnosis and management of Waldenstrom macroglobulinaemia. Br J Haematol 2014;165:316-33

8. Murray DL, Ryu E, Snyder MR, Katzmann JA. Quantitation of serum monoclonal proteins: relationship between agarose gel electrophoresis and immunonephelometry. Clin Chem 2009;55:1523-9

9. Pattenden RJ, Davidson KL, Wenham PR. The value of serum free light chains in a case of Waldenstrom's macroglobulinaemia that produces a type I cryoglobulinaemia. Ann Clin Biochem 2009;46:531-2

10. Bradwell AR, Harding SJ, Fourrier NJ, Wallis GL, Drayson MT, Carr-Smith HD, Mead GP. Assessment of monoclonal gammopathies by nephelometric measurement of individual immunoglobulin kappa/lambda ratios. Clin Chem 2009;55:1646-55

11. Blade J, Montoto S, Rosinol L, Montserrat E. Appropriateness of applying the response criteria for multiple myeloma to Waldenstrom's macroglobulinemia? Semin Oncol 2003;30:329-31

12. Itzykson R, Le Garff-Tavernier M, Katsahian S, Diemert MC, Musset L, Leblond V. Serum-free light chain elevation is associated with a shorter time to treatment in Waldenstrom's macroglobulinemia. Haematologica 2008;93:793-4

13. Owen RG, Kyle RA, Stone MJ, Rawstron AC, Leblond V, Merlini G et al. Response assessment in Waldenstrom macroglobulinaemia: update from the VIth International Workshop. Br J Haematol 2013;160:171-6

14. Klodzinska S, Vos JM, Kersten MJ, Wijermans P, Minnema MC. A survey on diagnostic methods and treatment strategies used in patients with Waldenstrom's macroglobulinaemia in The Netherlands. Neth J Med 2013;71:90-6

15. Leleu XP, Xie W, Bagshaw M, Banwait R, Leduc R, Roper N et al. The role of serum immunoglobulin free light chain (sFLC) in response and progression in Waldenstrom macroglobulinemia (WM). Clin Cancer Res 2011;17:3013-8

16. Leleu X, Koulieris E, Maltezas D, Itzykson R, Xie W, Manier S et al. Novel M-component based biomarkers in Waldenstrom's macroglobulinemia. Clin Lymphoma Myeloma Leuk 2011;11:164-7

17. Leleu X, Leduc R, Rourke M, Chuma S, Sam A, Harris B et al. Serum immunoglobulin free light chain (sFLC) measurement as a new marker of response to therapy and survival in Waldenstrom macroglobulinemia (WM). Blood 2009;114:3952a

18. Gaiser F, Kleber M, Ihorst G, Greil C, Becherer U, Koch B et al. Hevylite assay (HLC) - an additional indispensible technique to the M-spike in MGUS, Multiple Myeloma(MM) and Waldenstroms macroglobulinemia (WM) patients (pts). Onkologie 2013;36:P529a

19. Manier S, Lejeune J, Musset L, Boyle E, Dulery R, Debarri H et al. Hevylite, a novel M-component based biomarkers of response to therapy and survival in Waldenstrom macroglobulinemia. Blood 2011;118:2667a

20. Eveillard J, Achour A, N'Go Sack F, Tempescul A, Calloc'h R, Dagorne A et al. Appraisal of IgM kappa/IgM lambda variations using Hevylite after Rituximab as consolidation therapy in patients with Waldenstroms macroglobulinemia. Blood 2012;120:4879a

21. Koulieris E, Kyrtsonis MC, Maltezas D, Tzenou T, Mirbahai L, Mead G et al. Quantification of serum IgMκ and IgMλ in patients with Waldenström's macroglobulinaemia (WM): Clinical correlations. Hematology Reports 2010;2:F63a

22. Boyle E, Lejeune J, Manier S, Musset L, Bories C, Dulery R et al. Comparison of Waldenstrom Macroglobulinemia responses using immunoglobulin heavy/light chain analysis and conventional electrophoresis techniques. Blood 2014;124:2978a

23. Koulieris E, Kyrtsonis M-C, Maltezas D, Tzenou T, Mirbahai L, Kafassi N et al. Quantification of serum IgMκ and IgMλ in patients with Waldenstrom's macroglobulinemia (WM) at diagnosis and during disease course; clinical correlations. Blood 2010;116:3004a

24. Koulieris E, Dimopolous MA, Harding S, Maltezas D, Tzenou T, Kastritis E et al. No correlation of systemic hypogammaglobulinemia and immunosuppression of the same immunoglobulin class with time to first treatment and overall survival in Waldenström's macroglobulinemia patients. Haematologica 2011;96:0875a

25. Murillo-Florez I, Montez-Limon A, Quintero-Gutierrez J, Andrade-Campos M, Colorado-Ledesma E, Grasa J, Giraldo P. Prognostic value of IgM heavy immunoglobulins chain analysis in IgM MGUS and Waldenstroms macroglobulinemia. Clinical Lymphoma, Myeloma & Leukaemia 2013;13:P-460a

26. Leleu X, Moreau AS, Weller E, Roccaro AM, Coiteux V, Manning R et al. Serum immunoglobulin free light chain correlates with tumor burden markers in Waldenstrom macroglobulinemia. Leuk Lymphoma 2008;49:1104-7

27. Murillo-Florez I, Andrade-Campos M, Montes A, Grasa-Ulrich J, Giraldo P. Are IgM Hevylite Immunoglobulin heavy chain/light chain analysis a useful tool to differentiate IgM-MGUS from Waldenstrom macroglobulinemia. Biochmica Clinica 2013;37:W272a

28. Murillo-Florez I, Montes-Limon A, Quintero-Gutierrez J, Andrade-Campos M, Grasa J, Giraldo P, Rubio D. Prognostic value of IgM heavy immunoglobulins chain analysis in IgM-MGUS and Waldenstrom Macroglobulinaemia. Haematologica 2013;98:B1509a

349

Chronic lymphocytic leukaemia

In chronic lymphocytic leukaemia:

- FLCs are the most commonly detected monoclonal proteins, with an abnormal sFLC ratio present in 30 - 40% of patients at diagnosis.

- Elevated polyclonal FLCs are present in a further 15% of patients at diagnosis.

- A monoclonal or polyclonal FLC elevation is associated with a shorter time to first treatment and reduced overall survival.

- Summated $\kappa + \lambda$ FLCs is an important new prognostic marker that identifies patients requiring early treatment.

33.1. Introduction

With an incidence of 4.2 per 100,000 per year, chronic lymphocytic leukaemia (CLL) is the most common type of leukaemia in the Western world[1]. The median age at presentation is 72 years and the incidence is higher in men than women[1]. CLL is a clinically heterogeneous disease. Approximately two-thirds of patients are asymptomatic at diagnosis, and CLL is frequently diagnosed incidentally, following a routine full blood count. Other patients present with lymphadenopathy, systemic symptoms (such as tiredness, night sweats and weight loss), or infection. The clinical outcome of CLL is variable. Some patients survive for decades without requiring treatment, whilst others experience an aggressive form of the disease and may die shortly after diagnosis, either of disease- or therapy-related complications[1].

The diagnosis of CLL is based on the presence of an absolute monoclonal B-cell count of >5 x 10^9/L in the peripheral blood (persisting for >3 months) with a characteristic immunophenotype and morphology[2]. Two related disorders—monoclonal B-cell lymphocytosis (MBL) and small lymphocytic lymphoma (SLL) —share many clinical and diagnostic features in common with CLL. A diagnosis of MBL requires a monoclonal B-cell count of <5 x 10^9/L, in the absence of lymphadenopathy or organomegaly, cytopenias or disease-related symptoms[2]. SLL is also characterised by a B-cell count of <5 x 10^9/L, with the addition of lymph node or other tissue infiltration by cells characteristic of CLL[2].

Two well-established CLL clinical staging systems (Rai and Binet) are in routine use. These are particularly useful for predicting outcome in patients presenting with lymphadenopathy, hepatosplenomegaly or bone marrow failure[1]. However, significant clinical heterogeneity exists within patients classified as early CLL (Binet stage A or Rai stage 0/1). Therefore, additional prognostic markers are required to identify patients at risk of clinical progression. A number of prognostic biomarkers have been shown to predict progression and survival in CLL. These include immunoglobulin heavy chain variable region gene (IGHV) mutation status, serum β_2-microglobulin, CD38/ZAP-70 expression, and cytogenetic abnormalities[3]. However, these techniques have several limitations. For example, assessment of IGHV mutation status is complex, expensive and is not widely available. Other techniques (e.g. ZAP-70 expression) are poorly standardised and suffer from significant inter-laboratory variation[4].

33.2. Monoclonal and polyclonal sFLCs in CLL

CLL is thought to originate from the expansion of an antigen-activated B-cell clone. Persistent immune stimulation and polyclonal B-cell activation/dysfunction may play an important role in its pathogenesis[5]. This is supported by research demonstrating that increased concentrations of both monoclonal and polyclonal free light chains (FLCs) exist up to 10 years prior to CLL diagnosis[6].

FLCs are the most commonly detected serum monoclonal proteins in CLL, with an abnormal sFLC ratio being reported in 30 - 40% of patients[7,8,9,10]. By comparison, Maurer et al.[9] reported 16% of patients with a monoclonal protein detected by serum protein electrophoresis. In several published plasma cell disease screening studies, addition of sFLC analysis to the testing panel has identified additional CLL patients *(Chapter 23)*[11,12,13]. Therefore, identification of abnormal sFLC ratios in screening samples should prompt the consideration of other lymphoproliferative disorders, particularly CLL, in addition to plasma cell dyscrasias.

Maurer et al.[9] characterised both monoclonal and polyclonal FLC abnormalities in 339 newly diagnosed, untreated CLL patients. They defined three different types of FLC abnormality: monoclonal FLC elevation, polyclonal FLC elevation and ratio-only abnormality *(Table 33.1)*.

Abnormality	κ and λ concentration	κ/λ sFLC ratio	Number of patients
Monoclonal sFLC elevation	Elevated κ and/or λ	Abnormal	57 (17%)
Polyclonal sFLC elevation	Elevated κ and/or λ	Normal	52 (15%)
Ratio-only abnormality	Normal κ and λ	Abnormal	54 (16%)
Any abnormality			**163 (48%)**

Table 33.1. sFLC abnormalities in newly diagnosed CLL patients[9].

In patients with an abnormal sFLC ratio (ratio-only abnormality or a monoclonal FLC elevation), the involved sFLC type matched the CLL B-cell light chain restriction in 92% and 96% of cases, respectively[9]. Such findings suggest that an abnormal sFLC ratio is disease-related in the majority of cases. Morabito et al.[10] studied the distribution of monoclonal and polyclonal FLC synthesis in the CLL tumour microenvironment by immunohistochemistry. Lymph node infiltrates comprised a prominent population of plasmacytoid lymphocytes expressing the involved FLC, along with a smaller number of lymphocytes expressing the corresponding uninvolved FLC. These lymphocytes populated the same infiltrates in the lymph node and bone marrow, and were associated with scattered FLC-producing plasma cells *(Figure 33.1)*.

Polyclonal B-cell activation found in CLL also underlies the pathogenesis of some inflammatory/autoimmune conditions *(Chapter 35)*. Interestingly, both CLL and inflammatory/autoimmune conditions may be associated with lymphomatous transformation. This occurs in approximately 5 - 15% of CLL patients, and histologically resembles diffuse large B-cell lymphoma or Hodgkin lymphoma *(Chapter 31)*[1].

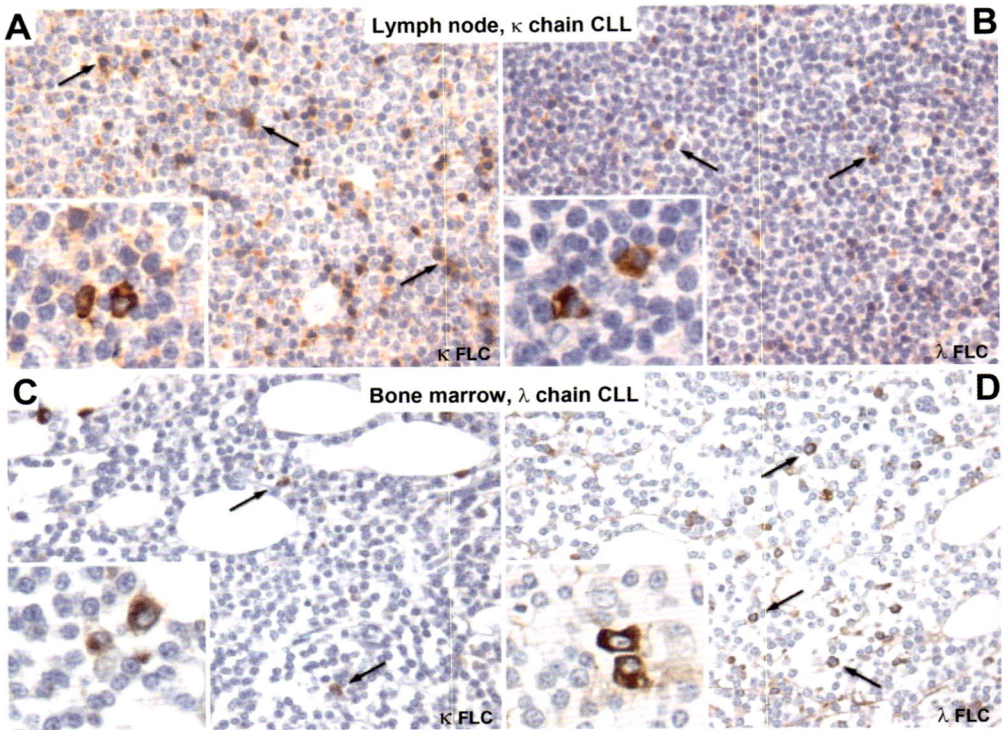

Figure 33.1. In situ immunohistochemical detection of κ and λ FLCs in the CLL microenvironment. (A-B) In lymph node infiltrates of a κ-chain CLL case, a prominent population of plasmacytoid lymphocytes expressing κ FLCs is detected along with a lower number of lymphocytes expressing the clone-unrelated λ FLCs, both populating the same microenvironment. Scattered plasma cells with either κ or λ FLC expression are also detected (panels A and B insets). *(C-D)* A similar picture is observed in bone marrow lymphoid infiltrates of a λ-chain CLL case. Immunohistochemistry performed by the labelled streptavidin-biotin method with 3-3'-diaminobenzidine as chromogen (brown signal). Original magnifications x200 for all panels, and x400 for insets. (This research was originally published in Blood[10] © the American Society of Hematology).

33.3. Prognostic value of sFLCs at baseline

The concentrations of sFLCs observed in CLL patients are typically much lower than those found in multiple myeloma *(Figure 33.2A)*, and are similar to patients with B-cell lymphomas *(Chapter 31)*.

In a retrospective study of 259 CLL patients comprising 181 untreated/pre-treatment and 78 treated individuals, an abnormal κ/λ sFLC ratio was associated with shorter time to first treatment; median 48 months vs. 117 months for a normal ratio (p=0.001) *(Figure 33.2B)*[7]. Patients were allocated to one of three groups based on their normal or abnormal κ/λ sFLC ratios (analysing abnormally high or low ratios separately). An abnormal sFLC ratio was prognostic for reduced overall survival (OS) from diagnosis *(Figure 33.2C)*. The sFLC ratio remained prognostic for OS when the groups of 181 untreated/pre-treatment patients were considered separately[7]. Similar findings have been reported by Morabito et al[10]. On multivariate analysis, four independent prognostic variables for OS were identified: 1) κ/λ sFLC ratio (p=0.024); 2) β_2-microglobulin concentration (p=0.01); 3) IGHV mutation status (p=0.017); and 4) ZAP-70 expression (p=0.0001)[7].

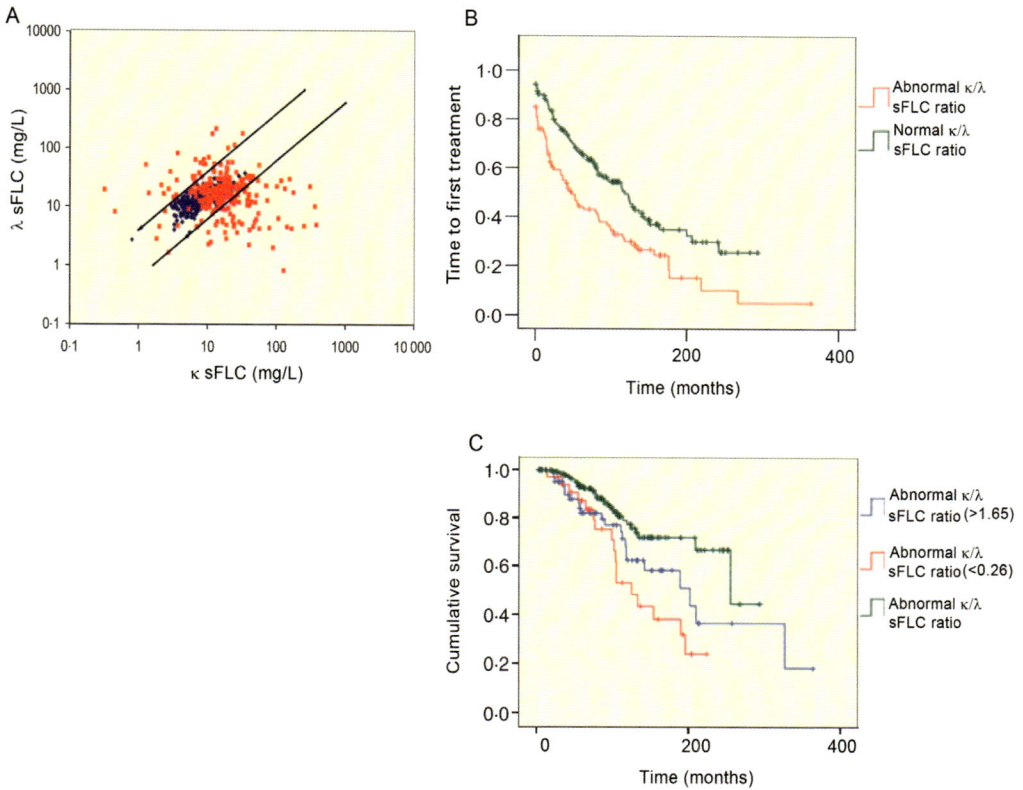

Figure 33.2. (A) sFLC concentrations in 259 CLL patients. Red squares: CLL cases; blue diamonds: normal controls. (B) Time to first treatment for 257 CLL patients based on normal (n=157) or abnormal (n=100) κ/λ sFLC ratios (p=0.001). (C) Kaplan-Meier survival curves for 259 CLL patients based on normal (n=159) or abnormal (>1.65, n=66; <0.26, n=34) κ/λ sFLC ratios (p=0.001). (Reproduced with permission from the British Journal of Haematology[7] and John Wiley & Sons Ltd).

Maurer et al.[9] studied the prognostic value of monoclonal sFLC elevation, polyclonal sFLC elevation and ratio-only abnormality in a cohort of 339 newly diagnosed, untreated CLL patients. After a median follow-up of 47 months, 26% had been treated and 10% had died. All three sFLC abnormalities were associated with a reduced time to first treatment (Figure 33.3A). A monoclonal or polyclonal sFLC elevation was also associated with poor overall survival, compared with patients with normal sFLC concentrations (Figure 33.3B). The group with monoclonal sFLC elevation had the worst prognosis, and was shown to have distinct clinical characteristics associated with more aggressive disease. These included a higher prevalence of high-risk biologic characteristics (CD38+, CD49d+, ZAP-70+, IGHV unmutated, and high-risk cytogenetic abnormalities) compared with patients with normal sFLC. Consistent with this finding, the most common cause of death in the monoclonal sFLC elevation group was progressive CLL. In contrast, most deaths in the polyclonal sFLC group were due to other causes, and the authors concluded that polyclonal FLC elevations may serve as a marker of host "fitness".

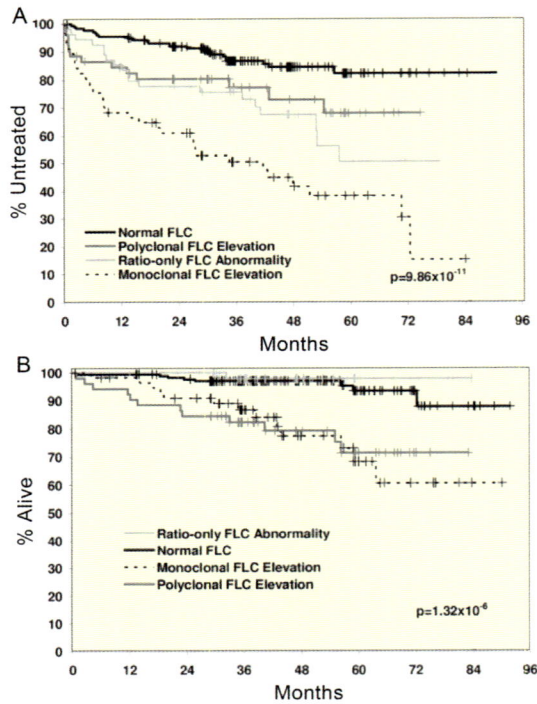

Figure 33.3. (A) Time to first treatment and (B) overall survival of 339 newly diagnosed, untreated CLL patients according to sFLC abnormality. (This research was originally published in Blood[9] © the American Society of Hematology).

33.4. Prognostic value of summated FLC measurements

Summated $\kappa + \lambda$ sFLCs (ΣFLC) is a measure of both monoclonal tumour cell and polyclonal "bystander" FLC production. Morabito et al.[10] studied the prognostic utility of ΣFLC in 449 untreated CLL patients. After a median follow-up of 3 years, 33% of patients had received treatment. Receiver operating characteristic (ROC) analysis defined an optimal cut-off of ΣFLC (60.6 mg/L) that identified patients with inferior outcome. The percentages of patients not requiring treatment at 3 years were 84.1% and 51.8% for patients with ΣFLC $\leq$60.6 mg/L or >60.6 mg/L, respectively *(Figure 33.4A)*. A further study by Sarris et al.[14] confirmed that baseline ΣFLC >60 mg/L were associated with shorter TTFT, and also demonstrated that ΣFLC >60 mg/L correlated with shorter OS. Morabito et al.[10] demonstrated that on multivariate analysis, ΣFLC >60.6 mg/L, ZAP-70 expression, cytogenetic abnormalities, and Binet stage B+C remained significantly associated with inferior TTFT. The prognostic significance of ΣFLC >60.6 mg/L was significantly higher than the sFLC κ/λ ratio, with a 3-fold higher risk of early treatment requirement for patients with ΣFLC >60 mg/L compared to those with an abnormal κ/λ sFLC ratio (hazard ratios of 3.5 [p<0.0001] versus 1.5 [p=0.015]).

A novel prognostic scoring system was proposed in which ΣFLC >60.6 mg/L, ZAP-70 expression, cytogenetic abnormalities and Binet stage were combined[10]. In this model, 1 point was assigned for each unfavourable marker present. The percentages of patients not requiring treatment at 3 years were 94.8%, 84.5%, 61.6% and 21.1% for patients scoring 0, 1, 2 or 3/4 respectively (p<0.0001) *(Figure 33.4B)*. The authors concluded that the cumulative amount of ΣFLC, irrespective of their clonality, represents a strong and independent prognostic predictor in CLL.

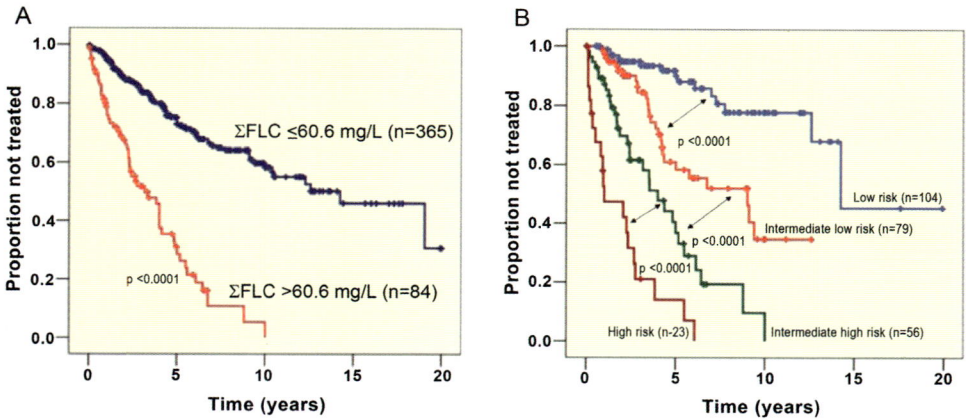

Figure 33.4. (A) Treatment-free survival for 449 untreated CLL patients according to ΣFLC concentrations. (B) Treatment-free survival of 262 CLL patients according to a prognostic scoring system. Unfavourable prognostic markers were ZAP-70 expression, FISH abnormalities, Binet stage and ΣFLC concentration >60.6 mg/L. Low risk: 0 markers; intermediate-low risk: 1 marker, intermediate-high risk: 2 markers; high risk: 3 or 4 markers. (This research was originally published in Blood[10] © the American Society of Hematology).

33.5. Monitoring CLL with sFLCs

An preliminary study by Aue et al.[15] highlighted the potential utility of sFLCs for monitoring CLL. Prior to treatment, a total of 8/11 patients with a κ CLL clone had κ sFLC concentrations above the normal range. After 6 months of ibrutinib therapy, there was a 76% reduction in κ sFLCs (p<0.01), and in 7/8 patients sFLC concentrations had normalised. By contrast, λ FLCs were initially low and then increased to normal levels following therapy. Similar findings were reported for 8 of 9 patients with a λ clone. The authors suggested that sFLC monitoring might provide an insight into both the killing of the tumour cells and the recovery of normal B-cell function.

Test Questions

1. What is the source of sFLCs in CLL?

Answers

1. FLCs may be produced by the tumour clone, polyclonal bystander lymphocytes and plasma cells in the tumour microenvironment *(Section 33.2)*.

References

1. Oscier D, Dearden C, Erem E, Fegan C, Follows G, Hillmen P et al. Guidelines on the diagnosis, investigation and management of chronic lymphocytic leukaemia. Br J Haematol 2012;159:541-64

2. Hallek M, Cheson BD, Catovsky D, Caligaris-Cappio F, Dighiero G, Dohner H et al. Guidelines for the diagnosis and treatment of chronic lymphocytic leukemia: a report from the International Workshop on Chronic Lymphocytic Leukemia updating the National Cancer Institute-Working Group 1996 guidelines. Blood 2008;111:5446-56

3. Zenz T, Frohling S, Mertens D, Dohner H, Stilgenbauer S. Moving from prognostic to predictive factors in chronic lymphocytic leukaemia (CLL). Best Pract Res Clin Haematol 2010;23:71-84

4. Letestu R, Rawstron A, Ghia P, Villamor N, Boeckx N, Boettcher S et al. Evaluation of ZAP-70 expression by flow cytometry in chronic lymphocytic leukemia: A multicentric international harmonization process. Cytometry B Clin Cytom 2006;70:309-14

5. Damle RN, Ghiotto F, Valetto A, Albesiano E, Fais F, Yan XJ et al. B-cell chronic lymphocytic leukemia cells express a surface membrane phenotype of activated, antigen-experienced B lymphocytes. Blood 2002;99:4087-93

6. Tsai HT, Caporaso NE, Kyle RA, Katzmann JA, Dispenzieri A, Hayes RB et al. Evidence of serum immunoglobulin abnormalities up to 9.8 years before diagnosis of chronic lymphocytic leukemia: a prospective study. Blood 2009;114:4928-32

7. Pratt G, Harding S, Holder R, Fegan C, Pepper C, Oscier D et al. Abnormal serum free light chain ratios are associated with poor survival and may reflect biological subgroups in patients with chronic lymphocytic leukaemia. Br J Haematol 2009;144:217-22

8. Yegin ZA, Ozkurt ZN, Yagci M. Free light chain: a novel predictor of adverse outcome in chronic lymphocytic leukemia. Eur J Haematol 2010;84:406-11

9. Maurer MJ, Cerhan JR, Katzmann JA, Link BK, Allmer C, Zent CS et al. Monoclonal and polyclonal serum free light chains and clinical outcome in chronic lymphocytic leukemia. Blood 2011;118:2821-6

10. Morabito F, De FR, Laurenti L, Zirlik K, Recchia AG, Gentile M et al. The cumulative amount of serum free light chain is a strong prognosticator in chronic lymphocytic leukemia. Blood 2011;118:6353-61

11. Bakshi NA, Gulbranson R, Garstka D, Bradwell AR, Keren DF. Serum free light chain (FLC) measurement can aid capillary zone electrophoresis in detecting subtle FLC-producing M proteins. Am J Clin Pathol 2005;124:214-8

12. Holding S, Spradbery D, Hoole R, Wilmot R, Shields ML, Levoguer AM, Dore PC. Use of serum free light chain analysis and urine protein electrophoresis for detection of monoclonal gammopathies. Clin Chem Lab Med 2011;49:83-8

13. Robson EJD, Taylor J, Beardsmore C, Basu S, Mead G, Lovatt T. Utility of serum free light chain analysis when screening for lymphoproliferative disorders. Lab Med 2009;40:325-9

14. Sarris K, Bartzis V, Maltezas D, Koulieris E, Tzenou T, Sachanas S et al. Significance of serum free light chains in chronic lymphocytic leukemia (CLL) prognosis. Blood 2012;120:4568a

15. Aue G, Farooqui M, Jones J, Valdez J, Martyr S, Soto S et al. In patients with chronic lymphocytic leukaemia (CLL) Ibrutinib effectively reduces clonal IgM paraproteins and serum free light chains while increasing normal IgM, IgA serum levels, suggesting a nascent recovery of humoral immunity. Blood 2013;122:4182a

Other diseases with abnormal immunoglobulin production

Summary:

- sFLC analysis may be of use in monitoring some patients with monoclonal cryoglobulinaemia.
- Monoclonal sFLCs are sometimes associated with heavy chain disease. Hevylite® antibodies do not recognize the solitary, truncated heavy chains produced.
- The plasma cell proliferations underlying POEMS syndrome are typically small and difficult to detect. sFLC concentrations are usually elevated but less than 20% of patients have abnormal sFLC ratios.

34.1. Introduction

The three disorders described in this chapter can all result from monoclonal plasma cell proliferations; for POEMS syndrome this is exclusively so, while heavy chain disease (HCD) may be a consequence of other B-cell lymphoproliferative disorders. Cryoglobulinaemia may likewise be associated with a lymphoproliferative malignancy but is most usually seen in association with hepatitis C virus (HCV) infections. A feature they share is the production of abnormal immunoglobulins. They have all been investigated using serum free light chain (sFLC) and/or immunoglobulin heavy/light chain (Hevylite, HLC) analysis.

34.2. Cryoglobulinaemia

Cryoglobulins are serum immunoglobulins that reversibly precipitate at temperatures below 37°C. Cryoglobulinaemia is classified according to the clonality and rheumatoid factor activity of the cryoglobulin[1]. It is associated with many illnesses, which can be broadly grouped into infections, autoimmune disorders, and malignancies. The most common cause is infection with HCV[2].

sFLC concentrations are elevated in many patients with monoclonal cryoglobulinaemia, and may serve as a useful tool for monitoring response to treatment since direct measurement of cryoglobulins is technically difficult. Pattenden et al.[3] described a case of Waldenström's macroglobulinaemia associated with a type 1 cryoglobulin. Serum protein electrophoresis (SPE) revealed the presence of an IgMλ monoclonal protein that could not be quantitated since it precipitated out of the gel. However, serial sFLC measurements were successfully used to monitor response to chemotherapy (*Chapter 32, clinical case history*). Besada et al.[4] report a case of type-1 (IgGκ) cryoglobulinaemic vasculitis (treated successfully with bortezomib after rituximab failure) that was effectively monitored with sFLCs.

34.3. Heavy chain diseases

HCDs are rare B-cell lymphoproliferative disorders characterised by the production of a monoclonal immunoglobulin heavy chain with no associated light chains. The heavy chain is typically truncated, and its small size results in low serum concentrations due to rapid renal clearance *(Chapter 3)*[6]. The three main types are α-, γ- and μ-HCD.

Since HLC assays target junctional epitopes that span the immunoglobulin heavy and light chains *(Chapter 9)*, the monoclonal protein associated with HCD is not recognised by HLC assays. However, in such cases, HLC assays allow quantitation of the polyclonal immunoglobulins.

Kaleta et al.[5] evaluated the use of IgG HLC assays in 15 patients with γ-HCD. By immunofixation electrophoresis, each patient's serum contained a discrete γ-heavy chain with no associated κ or λ light chains *(Figure 34.1A)*. The concentration of polyclonal IgG (determined by HLC analysis: IgGκ + IgGλ) accounted for 18% of the total IgG (as measured by a total IgG nephelometric assay). This indicated that 82% of the IgG did not have an associated light chain. Subtraction of IgGκ + IgGλ HLC concentrations from total IgG measurements was an indirect measure of the monoclonal heavy chain produced by the tumour[5]. The relationship between the heavy chain concentration determined by this indirect nephelometric measure was compared with that determined by SPE (using scanning densitometry) *(Figure 34.1B)*. The monoclonal protein concentration determined by nephelometry was approximately 2-fold higher than the value determined by SPE. This overestimation of total IgG may be due to the calibrator comparing poorly with the monoclonal heavy chain fragment.

Although no light chains are bound to monoclonal heavy chains, monoclonal sFLCs have been reported[5,6]. In a study of 15 patients with γ-HCD, 20% had monoclonal κ sFLCs[5]. This finding was supported by flow cytometry of tumour cells from a patient with γ-HCD plus monoclonal κ sFLCs where the tumour cells were positive for cytoplasmic IgG with κ restriction[7]. This indicated that the tumour was the source of both the monoclonal γ-heavy chain and κ sFLCs.

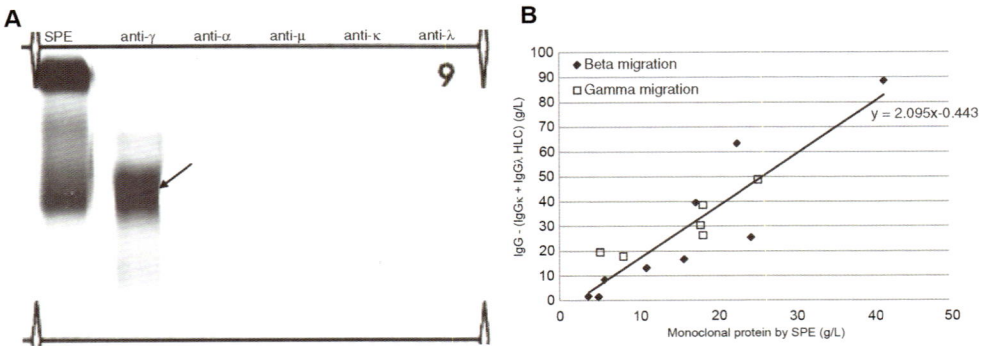

Figure 34.1. (A) Immunofixation electrophoresis of serum from a patient with γ-HCD. *The arrow indicates heavy chain reactivity. There is no corresponding light chain reactivity.* **(B) The relationship between the monoclonal protein concentration determined by SPE scanning densitometry and the calculated monoclonal IgG fragment.** *The monoclonal IgG fragment concentration was calculated indirectly using total IgG minus summated IgGκ and IgGλ. (Reproduced with permission from J. A. Katzmann)[5].*

34.4. POEMS syndrome

POEMS syndrome is a rare paraneoplastic syndrome related to an underlying plasma cell disorder (PCD) that is usually monoclonal λ-restricted[8,9]. The term POEMS is an acronym encompassing the features **P**olyneuropathy, **O**rganomegaly, **E**ndocrinopathy, **M**onoclonal PCD, and **S**kin changes. However, not all of these features are required to make a diagnosis, and there are other additional important clinical features not covered by the acronym (such as elevated vascular endothelial growth factor levels, sclerotic bone lesions, extravascular volume overload and Castleman disease)[10].

Whilst SPE and sFLC analysis constitute a simple and efficient diagnostic screen for the majority of monoclonal gammopathies *(Chapter 23)*, the diagnostic sensitivity of this algorithm is inadequate for POEMS syndrome, where the monoclonal protein production is often small. A large screening study by Katzmann et al.[11] concluded that serum immunofixation electrophoresis (sIFE) should be performed in addition to SPE and sFLC analysis when a diagnosis of POEMS syndrome is suspected.

Stankowski-Drengler et al.[8] studied sFLC measurements in 50 patients with newly diagnosed POEMS syndrome. In all cases the involved FLC type was λ. Forty-five patients (90%) had elevated λ sFLCs, 34 (68%) had elevated κ sFLCs, but only nine (18%) had abnormal sFLC ratios. Similar findings were reported by Wang et al.[9] who characterised sFLC measurements in a Chinese population comprising 83 newly diagnosed POEMS patients. Both studies concluded that polyclonal FLC elevations in POEMS syndrome may be due to renal impairment and/or polyclonal activation of B-cells *(Section 6.2)*[8,9]. In such conditions, elevated polyclonal κ sFLCs may neutralise the abnormal sFLC ratio induced by the subtle production of monoclonal λ sFLCs.

A preliminary study of the utility of HLC analysis in POEMS syndrome was performed by Wang et al.[9]. The cohort comprised 10 newly diagnosed POEMS patients with IgAλ or IgGλ monoclonal gammopathy. At diagnosis, 80% of IgAλ patients had elevated IgAλ HLC concentrations and 20% had HLC-pair suppression. A total of 80% of IgAλ patients had abnormal IgAκ/IgAλ HLC ratios. Similar findings were reported for the IgGλ patients: 80% of patients had elevated IgGλ HLC concentrations and 20% had HLC-pair suppression but all patients had abnormal IgGκ/IgGλ HLC ratios.

Test Questions

1. What are cryoglobulins?
2. Can Hevylite assays measure the monoclonal immunoglobulin in heavy chain disease?
3. Is sFLC analysis informative in POEMS syndrome?

1. Cryoglobulins are serum immunoglobulins that reversibly precipitate at temperatures below 37°C, this makes laboratory measurements problematic *(Section 34.2)*.

2. No, because the monoclonal heavy chain lacks the HLC epitopes. However, subtracting HLC measurements from total immunoglobulin concentrations will give an estimate of the monoclonal heavy chain *(Section 34.3)*.

3. Polyclonal elevations of sFLCs are present in most patients with POEMS syndrome but less than 20% have abnormal sFLC ratios *(Section 34.4)*.

References

1. Ramos-Casals M, Stone JH, Cid MC, Bosch X. The cryoglobulinaemias. Lancet 2012;379:348-60

2. Lauletta G, Russi S, Conteduca V, Sansonno L. Hepatitis C virus infection and mixed cryoglobulinemia. Clin Dev Immunol 2012;2012:502156

3. Pattenden RJ, Davidson KL, Wenham PR. The value of serum free light chains in a case of Waldenstrom's macroglobulinaemia that produces a type I cryoglobulinaemia. Ann Clin Biochem 2009;46:531-2

4. Besada E, Vik A, Koldingsnes W, Nossent JC. Successful treatment with bortezomib in type-1 cryoglobulinemic vasculitis patient after rituximab failure: a case report and literature review. Int J Hematol 2013;97:800-3

5. Kaleta E, Kyle R, Clark R, Katzmann J. Analysis of patients with gamma-heavy chain disease by the heavy/light chain and free light chain assays. Clin Chem Lab Med 2014;52:665-9

6. Lee MT, Parwani A, Humphrey R, Hamilton RG, Myers DI, Detrick B. Gamma heavy chain disease in a patient with diabetes and chronic renal insufficiency: diagnostic assessment of the heavy chain fragment. J Clin Lab Anal 2008;22:146-50

7. Lopez-Anglada L, Puig N, Diez-Campelo M, Alonso-Ralero L, Barrena S, Aparicio MA et al. Monoclonal free light chains can be found in heavy chain diseases. Ann Clin Biochem 2010;47:570-2

8. Stankowski-Drengler T, Gertz MA, Katzmann JA, Lacy MQ, Kumar S, Leung N et al. Serum immunoglobulin free light chain measurements and heavy chain isotype usage provide insight into disease biology in patients with POEMS syndrome. Am J Hematol 2010;85:431-4

9. Wang C, Su W, Zhang W, Di Q, Duan MH, Ji W et al. Serum immunoglobulin free light chain and heavy/light chain measurements in POEMS syndrome. Ann Hematol 2014;93:1201-6

10. Dispenzieri A. POEMS syndrome: 2014 Update on diagnosis, risk-stratification, and management. Am J Hematol 2014;89:213-23

11. Katzmann JA, Kyle RA, Benson J, Larson DR, Snyder MR, Lust JA et al. Screening panels for detection of monoclonal gammopathies. Clin Chem 2009;55:1517-22

Diseases with elevated polyclonal free light chains

Summary:

- Elevated polyclonal sFLC concentrations may result from decreased renal clearance and/or increased production.

- Increased polyclonal sFLCs may be a sensitive marker of B-cell stimulation.

- In patients with immune stimulation, polyclonal sFLC concentrations may increase 10- to 20-fold.

- In general population studies, elevated sFLCs are associated with increased mortality.

- In conditions associated with an increased risk of lymphoma (e.g. HIV infection), increased concentrations of sFLCs identify patients at highest risk.

35.1. Introduction

Elevated polyclonal serum free light chains (sFLCs) associated with normal/near-normal κ/λ ratios result from increased polyclonal production, reduced renal clearance or a combination of both mechanisms *(Section 3.5)*. Increased FLC production is due to proliferation of plasma cells and/or their progenitors. This is a common finding in diseases associated with immune stimulation and B-cell activation, such as infection, inflammation and autoimmune disease, and is often associated with high concentrations of polyclonal immunoglobulins.

When immunoglobulin synthesis is increased, sFLC concentrations would, likewise, be expected to be elevated. This relationship was demonstrated in patients with polyclonal hypergammaglobulinemia who were studied by Katzmann et al.[1] as a control group when establishing the reference intervals and diagnostic ranges for the sFLC assays *(Section 6.1)*. All 25 patients had elevated total immunoglobulins (18 - 39 g/L) but only a proportion had sFLC concentrations above the normal range, indicating a modest correlation between immunoglobulin and sFLC concentrations *(Figure 35.1)*. However, some individuals did have sFLC concentrations raised 10- to 20-fold. The κ/λ sFLC ratios in this study were all within the normal range, in contrast to patients with renal impairment *(Section 6.3)*.

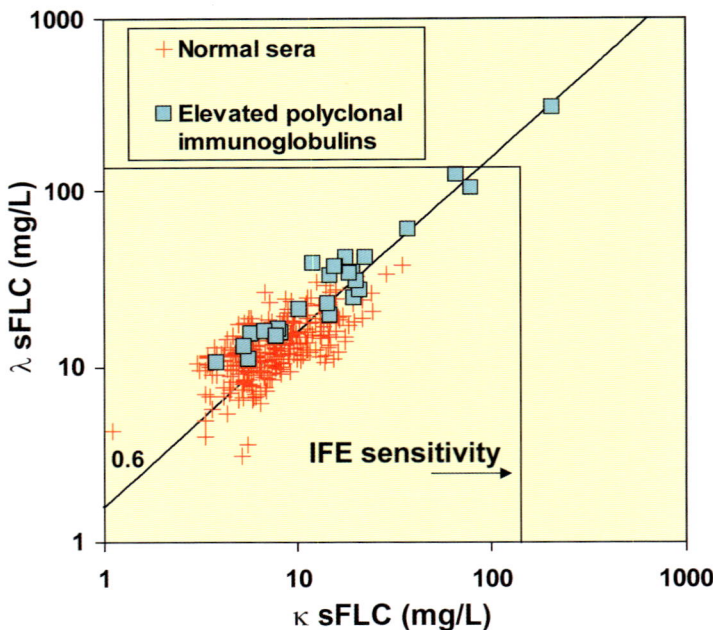

Figure 35.1. sFLCs in 25 patients with polyclonal hypergammaglobulinaemia (blue squares), compared with normal individuals (red crosses). (Courtesy of R.A. Kyle and J.A. Katzmann).

C-reactive protein (CRP) concentrations are widely used as a marker of both acute and chronic inflammation, yet comparisons of CRP and sFLC concentrations in different disease cohorts revealed only weak correlations, even after correction for renal clearance[2]. Burmeister et al.[2] concluded that polyclonal sFLCs and CRP provide independent information regarding immune stimulation/inflammatory status. Hutchison and Landgren[3] speculated that in the future, sFLC measurement might complement the use of CRP assays as a biomarker of inflammation.

Many studies have now been published detailing the polyclonal sFLC increases in patients with a variety of diseases and these are reviewed below. Although sFLC concentrations are significantly influenced by renal function, they are not subject to the variable catabolism that limits changes in IgG concentrations *(Section 3.5.3)* and may, therefore, have some advantage over immunoglobulin or autoantibody measurements for monitoring disease activity. Increases in polyclonal FLC have also been observed in patients with haematological neoplasms, notably B-cell chronic lymphocytic leukaemia and B-cell lymphomas. These data are presented in Chapters 31, 32 and 33 . More recently, general population studies have revealed an association between polyclonal sFLC elevations and reduced overall survival, leading to the speculation that sFLC measurements could form a useful early investigation in general health assessments[4]; these studies are discussed below *(Section 35.10)*.

35.2. Chronic kidney disease

Chronic kidney disease (CKD) is considered to be a major public health problem and it has been estimated that more than 10% of the adult population are affected to some degree[5]. Reduced clearance of sFLCs results from an impaired renal glomerular filtration rate (GFR) and is a frequent finding in CKD. This can be seen even in apparently healthy individuals who may have normal serum creatinine concentrations, but elevated polyclonal sFLCs from a slightly reduced GFR. This was first observed in elderly subjects when deriving the sFLC reference ranges *(Figure 6.2)*[1]. Reduced renal clearance of sFLCs leads to a preferential rise in κ sFLC (and hence the κ/λ sFLC ratio). The mechanisms of sFLC clearance are described in Section 3.5 and the derivation of a renal reference interval for the altered ratio is explained in Section 6.3.

Hutchison et al.[5] analysed sFLC concentrations in 688 patients with CKD of varying severity. Higher sFLC concentrations were associated with more advanced CKD *(Figure 6.3)*, and the concentrations of both FLCs were correlated with other measures of glomerular filtration *(Table 35.1)*. There was also a correlation between CKD stage and urinary FLC excretion.

Parameter	κ sFLCs	λ sFLCs
Creatinine	0.78	0.73
Cystatin C	0.80	0.79
eGFR	-0.72	-0.66

Table 35.1. Spearman correlation coefficients for polyclonal sFLCs with serum creatinine, estimated GFR (eGFR), and cystatin C in CKD[6]. eGFR calculated using the Cockcroft-Gault formula[7].

Hutchison et al.[8] subsequently showed that the sum of κ and λ sFLC concentrations (ΣFLC) was raised in 848 CKD patients and inversely correlated with estimated GFR (eGFR). Outcomes for these patients were monitored (median follow-up: 63 months) and elevated ΣFLC was a predictor of mortality within 1 year (p<0.001) independently of all other factors, including renal function and CRP concentrations *(Figure 35.2)*. Similar associations of ΣFLC with survival have been reported in preliminary publications from other studies[9,10]. Contrary to previous studies, Thilo et al.[11] reported that higher sFLC concentrations were associated with improved survival in 160 CKD patients. The most frequent cause of death in CKD patients is cardiovascular disease[12], which is independently associated with elevated sFLCs *(Section 35.3)* and could partially account for the relationship.

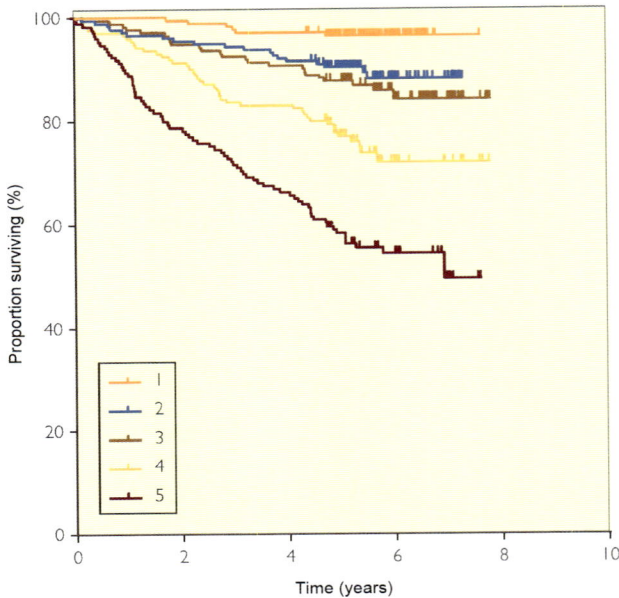

Figure 35.2. Survival by quintiles of ΣFLC levels, for 848 patients with chronic kidney disease.
(Reproduced from[8], with permission from Elsevier).

Whilst monoclonal FLC deposition in kidney tubules is frequently seen in multiple myeloma *(Chapter 27)*, AL amyloidosis *(Chapter 28)* and light chain deposition disease *(Chapter 29)*, polyclonal light chain deposition is rarely observed. However, Basnayake et al.[13] found polyclonal FLC deposition in renal parenchyma in CKD. Parasuraman et al.[14] investigated biopsies from 33 patients with renal disease (but no clonal FLC) and reported significant polyclonal FLC staining in proximal tubules and glomeruli. The FLC deposition was correlated with loss of the brush-border and interstitial fibrosis. Thus, it is possible that polyclonal FLC deposition may contribute to the progression and poor outcomes seen in patients with CKD.

35.3. Cardiovascular disease

Studies have looked exclusively at the relationship between cardiovascular diasease and sFLC concentrations. Kurt et al.[15] reported higher sFLC concentrations in patients with heart failure, and a reduction after treatment with a novel therapeutic (levosimendan), although no relationship was found with the degree of heart failure. Jackson et al.[16] used a novel assay, Combylite®, to measure combined concentrations of κ and λ sFLCs (cFLC) in patients hospitalised with decompensated heart failure (n=628). Individuals with cFLC concentrations within the upper quartile had a higher risk of death than those with concentrations in the lowest quartile (Hazard Ratio [HR] 2.3; p<0.0001); this remained significant after adjusting for 22 other established risk factors (HR 1.48; p=0.009).

35.4. Rheumatic diseases

Many rheumatic diseases feature polyclonal B-cell activation, high concentrations of autoimmune antibodies and polyclonal elevations of serum immunoglobulins. Earlier studies employing gel-diffusion and radio-immunoassay techniques have detected excess polyclonal FLCs in the serum and urine of patients with rheumatic diseases[17,18,19], hence it was speculated that their measurement might be useful for assessing disease activity.

Hoffman et al.[20] investigated the relationship between sFLCs and other markers of disease activity in patients with a number of rheumatic diseases. Patients with concurrent illnesses were excluded from the analysis to ensure that the changes were due exclusively to the disease under study. High polyclonal sFLC concentrations were found in rheumatoid arthritis (RA), systemic lupus erythematosus (SLE), Sjögren's syndrome, vasculitis and systemic sclerosis when compared with control groups (28 patients with fibromyalgia and 19 blood donors; p<0.05) (Figure 35.3). sFLC concentrations were more frequently elevated than intact immunoglobulins. As might be expected, there was a positive correlation between concentrations of sFLCs and serum creatinine in all patient groups.

A preliminary study analysing sera from patients with different forms of vasculitis revealed similar ΣFLC elevations[21]. The production of FLCs in certain rheumatic disorders has been studied in more detail, and the relevant publications are discussed below.

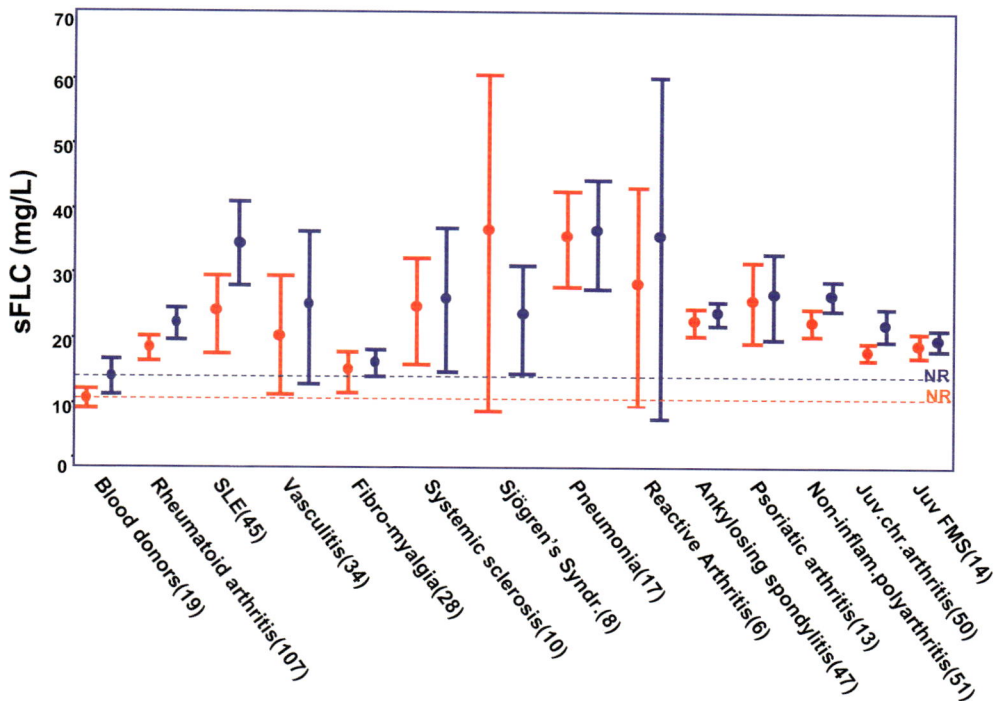

Figure 35.3. sFLCs in different diseases compared with blood donors. Bars show range and mean concentrations of κ (red) and λ (blue) sFLCs. Juv chr arthritis: juvenile chronic arthritis; Juv FMS: juvenile fibromyalgia syndrome. Number of patients in brackets. (Courtesy of U. Hoffmann).

35.4.1. Systemic lupus erythematosus

Hoffman et al.[20] studied 45 patients with SLE and showed that sFLC concentrations were approximately 3-fold greater than normal (Figure 35.3). Predictably, sFLC concentrations were higher in SLE patients with renal involvement than in those with normal renal function (Figure 35.4). Clinical scores of SLE correlated with sFLC levels, particularly when the disease was active. In a subsequent prospective study, the clinical scores (European Consensus Lupus Activity Measurement, ECLAM[22]) in eight patients were compared with a variety of laboratory parameters[23]. sFLC concentrations showed a strong correlation with disease activity that was not observed for CRP or erythrocyte sedimentation rate (ESR). A larger study with 75 SLE patients[24] also showed a strong association between ΣFLC concentrations and disease activity (as measured by the SLE Disease Activity Index, SLEDAI; $p<0.001$). The association of ΣFLC with disease activity was further corroborated in a study that employed a third disease activity scoring system (British Isles Lupus Assessment Group index, BILAG)[25]. Assessment of autoantibody production is included (directly or indirectly) in SLE disease scoring systems and ΣFLC have, unsurprisingly, been found to be higher in anti-DNA positive versus anti-DNA negative patients ($n=62$)[26]. However, in a group of 11 patients[27], falling concentrations of FLCs were monitored after B-cell depletion with rituximab and showed a significant correlation with total IgG but not with anti-DNA titres.

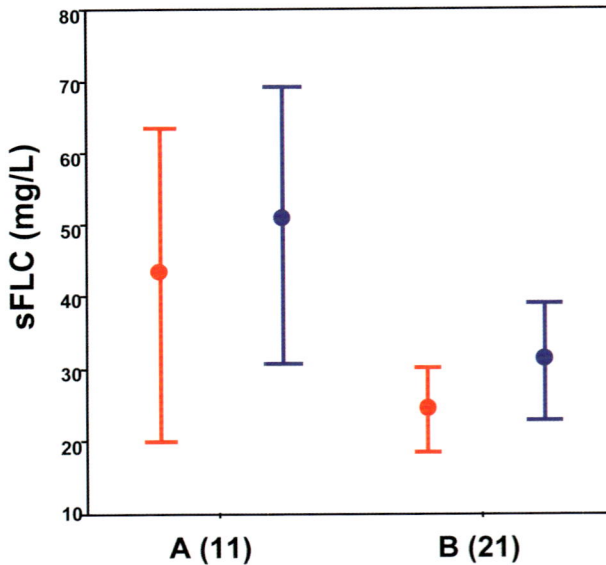

Figure 35.4. sFLCs in SLE (A) with and (B) without renal involvement. Number of patients in brackets. Bars show range and mean concentrations of κ (red) and λ (blue) sFLCs. (Courtesy of U. Hoffmann).

In addition to renal function, a further complicating factor when interpreting sFLC concentrations in SLE patients is the potential influence of immunosuppressant treatments. In a cross-sectional study of 77 SLE patients, Jolly et al.[28] found that the correlation of sFLC concentrations with disease activity (Physicians Global Assessment [PGA] and SLEDAI scoring) was stronger after controlling for steroid use. The authors concluded that sFLC measurement was potentially superior to anti-DNA antibody or IL-6 for disease monitoring.

35.4.2. Primary Sjögren's syndrome

Gottenberg et al.[29] evaluated sFLC measurements in 139 patients with primary Sjögren's syndrome (pSS), an autoimmune condition that typically affects lacrimal and salivary exocrine glands. A total of 22% of patients had raised sFLC concentrations, and mean levels were significantly higher than controls ($p<0.001$) *(Figure 35.5)*. sFLC concentrations were significantly correlated with IgG ($p<0.001$), rheumatoid factor ($p<0.005$), β_2-microglobulin ($p<0.001$) and B-cell activating factor (BAFF, $p<0.01$). Association of elevated sFLCs with β_2-microglobulin, gammaglobulin and lymphopenia was also reported for a mixed group of 22 patients with primary or secondary Sjögren's syndrome[30]. In Gottenberg's study[29], mean sFLC concentrations were higher in patients with autoantibodies, particularly when both anti-SSA and anti-SSB antibodies were present *(Figure 35.6)*. In addition, patients with extra-glandular involvement had higher levels of sFLCs than those with glandular involvement alone. These results suggest that extra-glandular involvement in pSS is associated with more intense stimulation of B-cells.

pSS is associated with an increased risk of non-Hodgkin lymphoma (particularly mucosa-associated lymphoid tissue (MALT) lymphoma) with an odds ratio of 12.9[31]. In a cohort of 395 patients enrolled into a 5-year prospective study (the ASSESS biobank), Gottenberg et al.[29] sought to discover whether sFLC measurements could identify pSS patients at increased risk of lymphoma. At enrolment, a total of 16/395 patients had a history of lymphoma; median serum concentrations of BAFF and β_2-microglobulin were significantly higher in these patients but sFLC concentrations and ratios were normal. Data from the follow-up of this cohort has yet to be released.

There has been increasing interest in the role of BAFF as a marker of disease activity and as a potential therapeutic target in pSS. In a phase 2 trial of belimumab (a monoclonal antibody against BAFF), in which sFLC measurements were included as part of the haematological assessment, significant reductions in sFLC concentrations were observed following treatment[32].

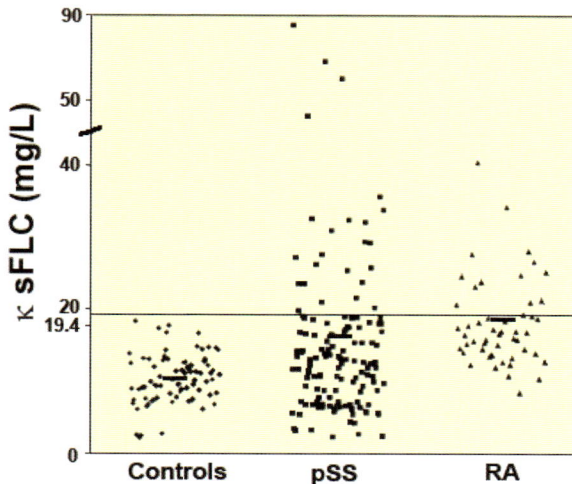

Figure 35.5. κ *sFLC concentrations (and mean values) in patients with primary Sjögren's syndrome (pSS), rheumatoid arthritis (RA) and healthy controls.* The line at 19.4mg/L κ sFLC indicates the upper end of the normal range. (Reproduced from[29], with permission from BMJ Publishing Group Ltd. © 2007).

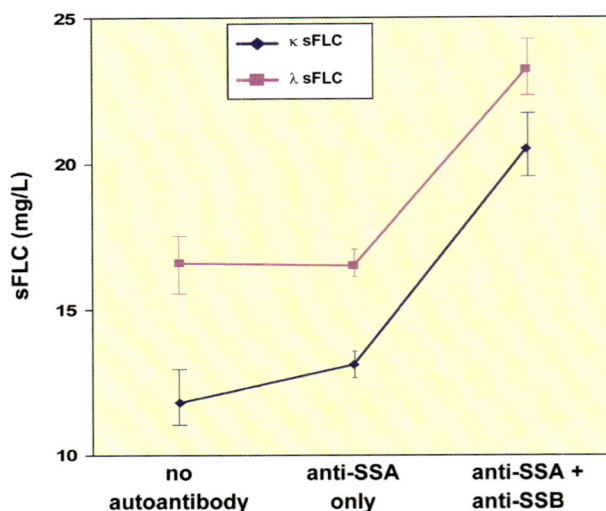

Figure 35.6. sFLC concentrations in relation to the presence of SSA and SSB antibodies in patients with Sjögren's syndrome. (Courtesy of X. Mariette).

35.4.3. Rheumatoid arthritis

Gottenberg et al.[29] studied 50 patients with RA: 36% had raised sFLCs with mean values significantly higher than controls (p<0.001) *(Figure 35.5)*, while κ/λ sFLC ratios were normal in all but three patients. sFLC concentrations were significantly correlated with IgG (p≤0.04), CRP (p≤0.04), and rheumatoid factor (for κ only; p=0.03), but not with anti-cyclic citrullinated peptide (CCP) antibodies. Significant correlations were observed between disease activity assessed by the Disease Activity Score 28 (DAS28) and both κ (p=0.0004; *Figure 35.7*) and λ sFLC concentrations (p=0.05; data not shown). Other studies by Ye et al.[34] and Djidjik et al.[35] have also identified a correlation between sFLC elevations and disease activity in RA. sFLC concentrations as determined by ELISA were greater in RA patients and correlated with disease activity, whilst the FLC concentrations in synovial fluid were increased, suggesting local production[36]. Further indication of local production was provided by synovial tissue cells staining positively for FLC and CD138 (Syndecan 1; a plasma cell marker) and these findings support the functional relationship between B-cells and disease activity. Interestingly, no correlation was observed between DAS28 and IgG[29]. This may be explained by the longer half-life of IgG (approximately 21 days) compared with sFLCs (2 to 6 hours, *Section 3.5*). The fast turnover of sFLCs might account for their observed correlation with disease activity.

In a further study including 710 patients with arthritis, Gottenburg et al.[37] found that polyclonal FLCs (and other markers of B-cell activation) were higher in early RA than in undifferentiated arthritis. The authors concluded that B-cell activation is an early pathogenic event in the disease. This was supported by data from the Mayo Clinic. A focused, further analysis of their general population cohort *(Section 35.10)* revealed increased ΣFLC concentrations in RA patients (n=270), which were not explained by any differences in eGFR, and elevations could be recognised 3 to 5 years before the clinical onset of RA *(Figure 35.8)*[33].

In addition to the studies investigating correlations between sFLCs and disease activity, others have assessed the utility of sFLC measurements in assessing response to treatment in RA. Kormelink et al.[36] measured sFLC concentrations at 3 and 6 months following treatment with rituximab (for depletion of CD20-positive cells) and found that they were reduced more significantly in clinical responders than in non-responders, and did not correlate well with intact immunoglobulin measurements. Sellam et al.[38] compared baseline concentrations of various markers in 208 RA patients and found that elevated IgG, presence of rheumatoid factor or anti-CCP antibodies were predictive of response to rituximab, whereas sFLC concentrations were not. Unfortunately, the changes in serum markers in response to treatment were not recorded. A further study of rituximab treatment in 28 RA patients indicated that monitoring changes in sFLC concentrations (and other serum markers) was the most informative way of assessing response to treatment and identifying relapse[39].

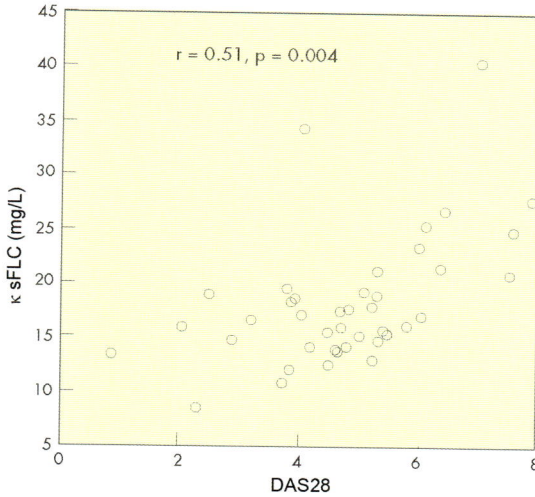

Figure 35.7. Correlation between κ sFLC concentrations and Disease Activity Score 28 (DAS28) in patients with RA. (Reproduced from[29], with permission from BMJ Publishing Group Ltd. © 2007).

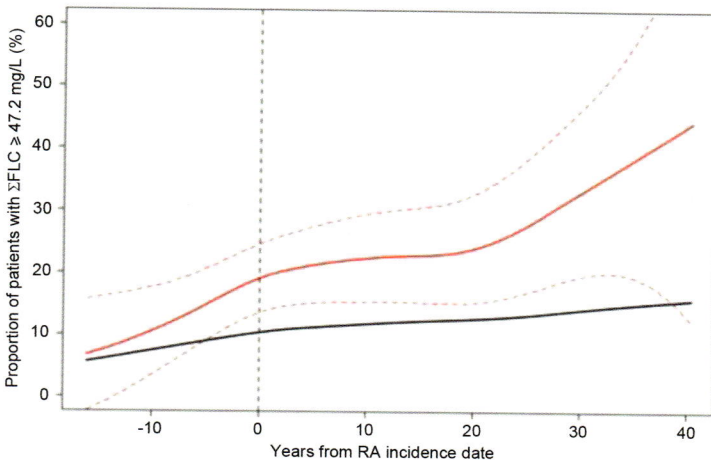

Figure 35.8. ΣFLC concentrations prior to clinical onset of RA and during follow-up. Red line = trend for RA patients with 95% confidence interval. Black line = trend for general population. (Reproduced with permission from the Journal of Rheumatology[33]).

35.5. Diabetes mellitus

Approximately 30 years ago it was noted that the urinary excretion of κ FLCs (and the κ FLC/albumin excretion ratio) was significantly higher in type 1 diabetes mellitus patients than in patients with non-diabetic proteinuria[41]. Subsequently, the same authors suggested that elevated FLC/albumin excretion ratios were an early indicator of diabetic nephropathy. They directly implicated a renal cause of the FLC leakage rather than excess production and their finding of normal sFLC concentrations supported this hypothesis[42]. Mechanistically, hyperfiltering glomeruli leak more albumin which competes with FLC removal in the proximal tubules thereby displacing it into the urine (Section 3.5.2). In a more recent investigation of urinary FLCs in obesity and diabetes, Thethi et al.[43] found higher urinary concentrations in obese (n=442) versus non-obese, type 2 diabetic patients (n=195). Higher concentrations were also found in obese patients with diabetes and hypertension compared with those without these conditions.

Hutchison et al.[44] studied FLC concentrations in both serum and urine of type 2 diabetic patients, to assess their utility as an early marker of diabetic kidney disease. It was clear that diabetic patients had raised serum and urine concentrations of polyclonal FLCs before overt renal impairment developed (p<0.001) (Figure 35.9). κ sFLC concentrations were higher than λ sFLC concentrations but only 1.9% of patients had a monoclonal gammopathy of undetermined significance (MGUS; Chapter 13). A good correlation existed between sFLC concentrations and various markers of GFR, including serum creatinine, cystatin-C and eGFR (Figure 35.10; λ sFLC data not shown). South-Asian diabetic patients had higher sFLCs than Caucasian diabetic patients, a finding that was independent of renal function and suggestive of underlying inflammation. In the same study[44], 68% of patients with normal urinary albumin/creatinine ratios (ACRs) had abnormal urinary FLC/creatinine ratios. Nevertheless, there was a degree of correlation between urine FLC concentrations and urinary ACR (κ FLCs: r=0.32; p<0.01 and λ FLCs: r=0.25; p<0.01). However, some patients had normal eGFR with high concentrations of sFLCs indicating increased production, and again, suggestive of generalised inflammation/vasculopathy. Perhaps retinopathy and nephropathy are the most readily observed clinical signs of a generalised inflammatory process that is correlated with raised FLC production.

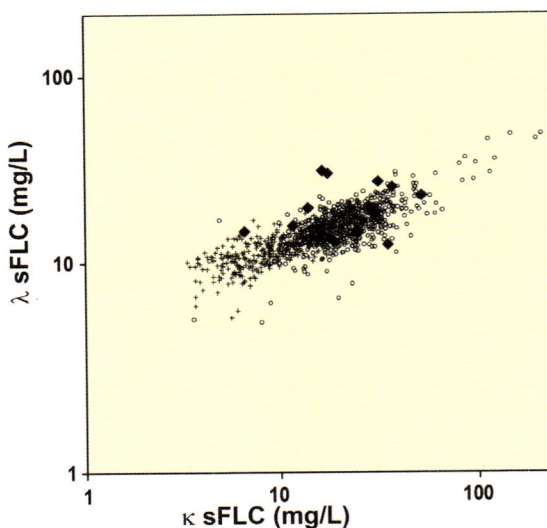

Figure 35.9. sFLC concentrations in 745 patients with early diabetes mellitus[44]. Circles: diabetic patients without MGUS; diamonds: diabetic patients with MGUS; crosses: normal controls. (© 2008, Informa Healthcare[40]. Reproduced with permission of Informa Healthcare).

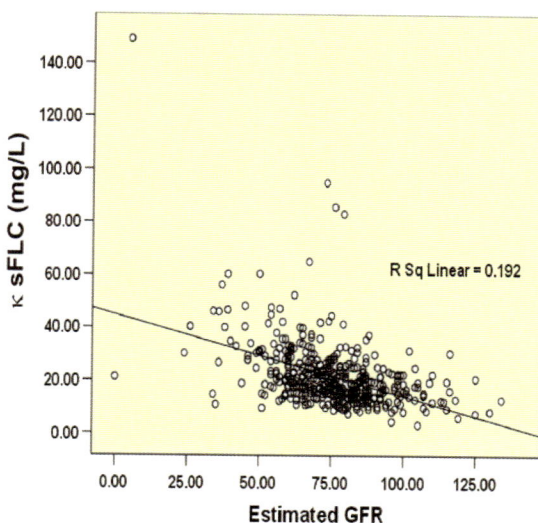

Figure 35.10. κ sFLCs in 745 patients with type 2 diabetes correlated with eGFR[44]. *eGFR was calculated using the Modification of Diet in Renal Disease formula*[40]*; (p<0.001). (© 2008, Informa Healthcare*[40]*. Reproduced with permission of Informa Healthcare).*

In a further investigation of the same type 2 diabetic population[45], higher ΣFLC concentrations were found in patients who experienced cardiovascular disease events within 2 years of follow-up. In multivariate analysis, a ΣFLC concentration of >57.2 mg/L remained significantly associated with cardiovascular events even after adjusting for age, albumin/creatinine ratio, diabetes duration or treatment[45]. Since polyclonal FLCs are potentially nephrotoxic, increased concentrations may contribute to progressive nephropathy. It has also been suggested that monoclonal FLCs may play a role in some patients' renal disease[46]. Indeed, mesangial monoclonal FLC deposits observed in renal biopsies of patients with renal impairment are sometimes similar in appearance to those found in diabetic glomerulosclerosis[47].

Thus, type 2 diabetic patients have significantly raised concentrations of serum and urinary polyclonal FLCs before overt renal disease occurs, and measurement of polyclonal FLCs could provide a useful tool in early diagnosis of diabetic kidney disease.

35.6. Human immunodeficiency virus

Human immunodeficiency virus (HIV) infection is associated with non-specific polyclonal activation of B-cells and, consequently, elevations in polyclonal IgG and sFLCs have been observed[48,49]. Bibas et al.[50] measured ΣFLCs in 182 patients with HIV infection but without co-morbidities known to raise FLC levels (e.g. MGUS, renal impairment or a concurrent malignancy) and found that median concentrations were above normal, indicating that FLC production was raised in response to the HIV infection. Elevated concentrations of ΣFLCs were associated with other adverse prognostic markers, including higher viral load, shorter duration of undetectable viraemia, greater patient age and lower CD4 T-cell count. ΣFLC was also noted to be higher in untreated patients and those positive for hepatitis C virus (HCV). Similar results were reported by Zemlin et al.[51] in sera collected from 369 HIV patients. Elevated sFLC concentrations correlated positively with viral load and negatively with CD4 cell counts, albumin concentration and anti-retroviral treatment. In both of the above studies it was confirmed that sFLC elevations were polyclonal, with normal κ/λ sFLC ratios. Shiels et al.[52] compared sFLC concentrations between HIV patients with (n=252) and without (n=252) clinical acquired immune deficiency syndrome (AIDS). Polyclonal sFLC elevation was associated with a 4-fold increase in the risk of AIDS, whilst a monoclonal elevation was not. The authors suggested that polyclonal B-cell dysfunction may contribute to HIV-related immune suppression and predispose patients to clinical AIDS events.

Emerging evidence suggests a prognostic role for sFLCs in predicting HIV-lymphoma risk[48,53]. Lymphoma is the leading cause of cancer-related death among HIV-infected patients (*Chapter 31*)[54,55]. Non-Hodgkin lymphoma (NHL) is one of the AIDS-defining malignancies, and HIV-infected individuals have a 60- to 200-fold higher risk of developing NHL compared with that of the general population[54,55]. Likewise, HIV-infected patients are at increased risk of developing Hodgkin lymphoma (HL), with a 5- to 15-fold higher risk compared with that of the general population (*Section 31.2*)[56].

There are conflicting data on the association between elevated total immunoglobulin levels and NHL risk in HIV-infected individuals[53,57]. However, emerging evidence suggests there is a prognostic role for sFLCs in predicting HIV-lymphoma risk. Landgren et al.[53] studied 4,635 HIV infected individuals, 66 of whom developed NHL. Elevated κ or λ sFLC concentrations were present 2 to 5 years prior to NHL diagnosis, and were significantly associated with an increased NHL risk. The risk of NHL was 3.8- or 8.1-fold greater in patients with elevated κ or λ sFLC concentrations.

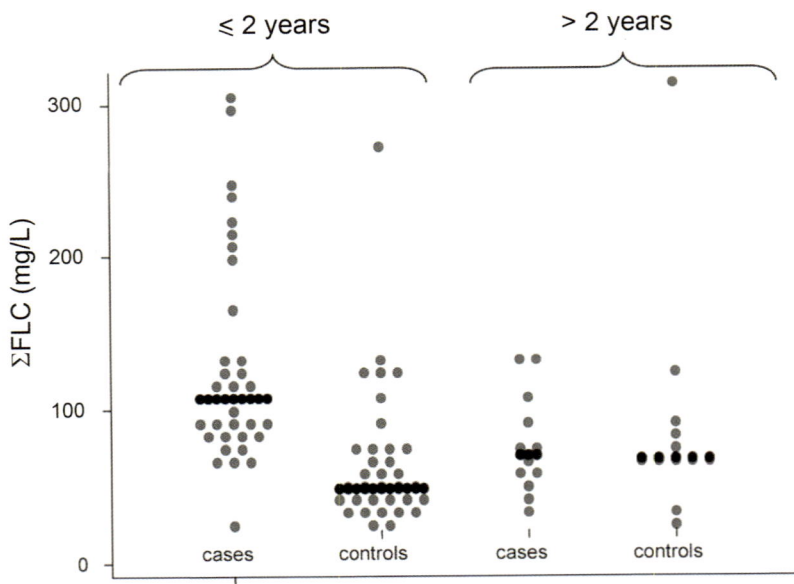

Figure 34.11. Summated κ and λ sFLC concentration in HIV-infected cases and controls according to time from sample. (Reproduced with permission from the American Journal of Hematology[48] and John Wiley and Sons).

The prognostic value of elevated sFLCs in predicting HIV-lymphoma was also shown by Bibas et al.[48]. Of 6513 participants studied, 86 developed lymphoma. After excluding patients with comorbidities that may have caused elevated sFLCs (e.g. renal impairment or autoimmune disease), the remaining cohort comprised 46 patients. Of these, 30 patients developed NHL and 16 developed HL. In patients who subsequently developed lymphoma, summated $\kappa + \lambda$ sFLC (ΣFLC) concentrations 2 years prior to lymphoma diagnosis were significantly higher than those of lymphoma-free HIV-infected controls (Figure 34.11). In multivariate analysis, elevated ΣFLCs (defined as >2-times the upper limit of normal) remained a significant predictor of lymphoma risk and was independent of CD4 T-cell count. The authors concluded that the measurement of polyclonal sFLCs merits consideration for introduction into routine clinical practice for HIV patients[48].

A further study highlighted a potential utility of sFLCs in monitoring HIV-related lymphoma patients[58]. The sFLC concentrations at lymphoma diagnosis (46 samples) were compared with sFLC concentrations at complete response (28 samples). Serum κ, λ and ΣFLC concentrations were significantly lower at complete response compared with those at lymphoma diagnosis, indicating that further study of the potential utility of sFLCs for monitoring is warranted.

35.7. Allergies

A research group based in Utrecht, in the Netherlands, has published a series of articles exploring the association and potential function of FLCs in allergic responses. The early studies (employing mouse models) reported that FLC molecules exhibiting antigen specificity could mediate mast cell-dependent hypersensitivity-like reactions[59]. Passive administration of FLCs was reported to cause mast cell activation and acute broncho-constriction, while use of a 9-mer peptide ("F991": sequence derived from Tamm-Horsfall protein) that binds to FLC, abrogated FLC-induced symptoms[60]. The authors of this latter study also measured sFLCs in adult humans and found higher κ (but not λ) sFLC concentrations in asthmatics (n=31). For patients with hypersensitivity pneumonitis and idiopathic pulmonary fibrosis, FLC concentrations were reported to be elevated in both serum and bronchoalveolar lavage fluid with histochemistry identifying FLC-positive B-cells and plasma cells in patients' lungs[61]. Similarly, in patients with chronic rhinosinusitis, elevated FLC concentrations were found in nasal secretions, particularly if nasal polyps were present, and histology identified FLC-positive cells in nasal polyp tissue. However, increases in sFLC concentrations were not statistically significant[62].

In a study performed by another research group, children with atopic dermatitis (n=73) were found to have significantly higher sFLC concentrations compared with controls[63]. ELISA measurement of sFLCs[64] indicated significant elevations of κ sFLC but not λ sFLC in infants with atopic dermatitis (n=25), while treatment with dietary oligosaccharides reduced concentrations of both light chains. sFLC concentrations have also been reported to be raised in infants with cows' milk allergy[65], while in casein-sensitised mice, serum levels were raised and symptoms could be reduced by the FLC binding peptide F991[65].

35.8. Other diseases

35.8.1. Respiratory disease

An early report by Sölling[66] documented modest increases in sFLCs in a small number of patients with tuberculosis and chronic bronchitis. Elevations in sFLCs were also found in patients with active sarcoidosis, at approximately twice the concentration found in normal individuals. A later study by Hoffman et al.[20] demonstrated elevated levels of polyclonal sFLCs in patients with acute pneumonia (Figure 35.12). Western blots and ELISAs were used to investigate FLCs in murine lung emphysema models, and amounts were found to be increased in serum and lymph node extracts after smoke exposure; sFLCs were also found to be elevated in patients with chronic obstructive pulmonary disease (COPD; n=6)[67]. Further experiments indicated the binding of FLCs to neutrophils and a potential role in the pathology of COPD[67]. An initial report from a study of ΣFLC concentrations in the sera of 294 patients with alpha-1-antitrypsin-related COPD described associations with mortality, chronic bronchitis and chronic colonisation of the lower respiratory tract, but concluded that any role for ΣFLC monitoring in these patients was yet to be determined[68].

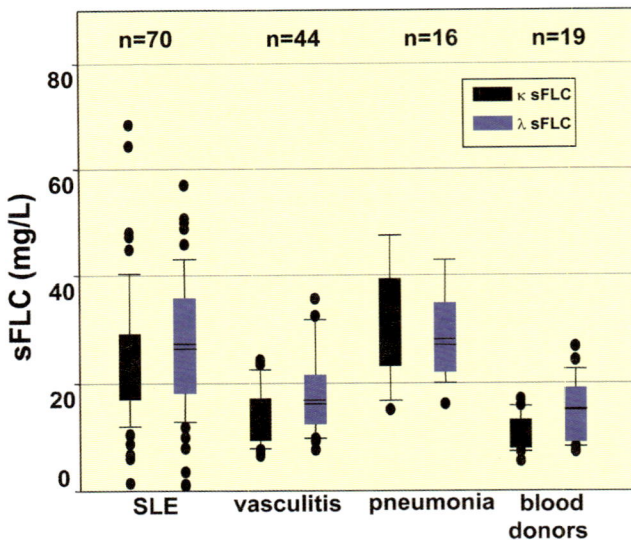

Figure 35.12. sFLCs in patients with pneumonia compared with other diseases. *The slight increase in κ (black) compared with λ sFLC concentrations (blue) may be related to renal impairment. (Courtesy of U. Hoffmann).*

35.8.2. Hepatitis C virus and liver disease

Chronic viral infection is a significant cause of elevated polyclonal immunoglobulins and sFLCs. Chronic hepatitis C virus (HCV) infection is also associated with the development of B-cell disorders including mixed cryoglobulinaemia (MC) and B-cell NHL[70]. Patients with HCV-related MC are at a 35-fold increased risk of lymphoproliferative disease compared with the general population[71].

Terrier et al.[72] studied 59 patients with HCV infections and MC. The results showed elevated sFLCs in nearly 50% of patients. Furthermore, mean polyclonal sFLC concentrations progressively increased with worsening disease category (p<0.001) and increasing cryoglobulin concentrations (p<0.0001). Ten patients had an abnormal κ/λ ratio at baseline, and changes in the ratio correlated with the virological response to HCV treatment. The authors speculated that following antiviral therapy, the κ/λ sFLC ratio was a surrogate marker of the control of HCV-related lymphoproliferation. A subsequent study by Terrier et al.[73] included 155 HCV-infected patients and compared sFLC and IgM Hevylite® (HLC) measurements in the following four groups: 1) no MC; 2) asymptomatic MC; 3) MC vasculitis; and 4) MC vasculitis with B-cell NHL. On univariate analysis, the κ/λ sFLC ratio and IgMκ/IgMλ HLC ratio were significantly different between the groups (both p<0.0001). However, in multiparametric analysis (including a total of 7 serum biomarkers), neither the sFLC ratio nor IgM HLC ratio remained significantly different between patients with and without overt B-cell NHL. No data on the FLC or HLC concentrations was provided.

Analysis of sera from 80 patients with chronic liver disease of mixed aetiology revealed higher than normal ΣFLC concentrations[69]. After correction for renal function, patients with alcoholic liver disease exhibited the most consistent elevations *(Figure 35.13)*, indicative of increased FLC production and also demonstrating the importance of accounting for renal function when interpreting FLC results *(Section 6.3)*. Developing this line of investigation further, Faint et al.[74] measured combined sFLC concentrations in sera from 340 patients with alcoholic liver disease using a new turbidimetric assay (Combylite, cFLC)[75]. Addition of cFLC to an accepted risk stratification calculation (Model for End-stage Liver Disease; MELD) improved the prediction of time to transplant *(Figure 35.14)*.

Teng et al.[76] determined that adding sFLC or albumin measurements to that of alpha-fetoprotein would improve the diagnosis of hepatocellular carcinoma. While albumin measurement would appear to be the simplest choice for diagnostic purposes, the authors considered that sFLC elevation probably reflected the developing B-cell response to viral infection and that further study was merited to investigate the role and potential utility of sFLC measurement.

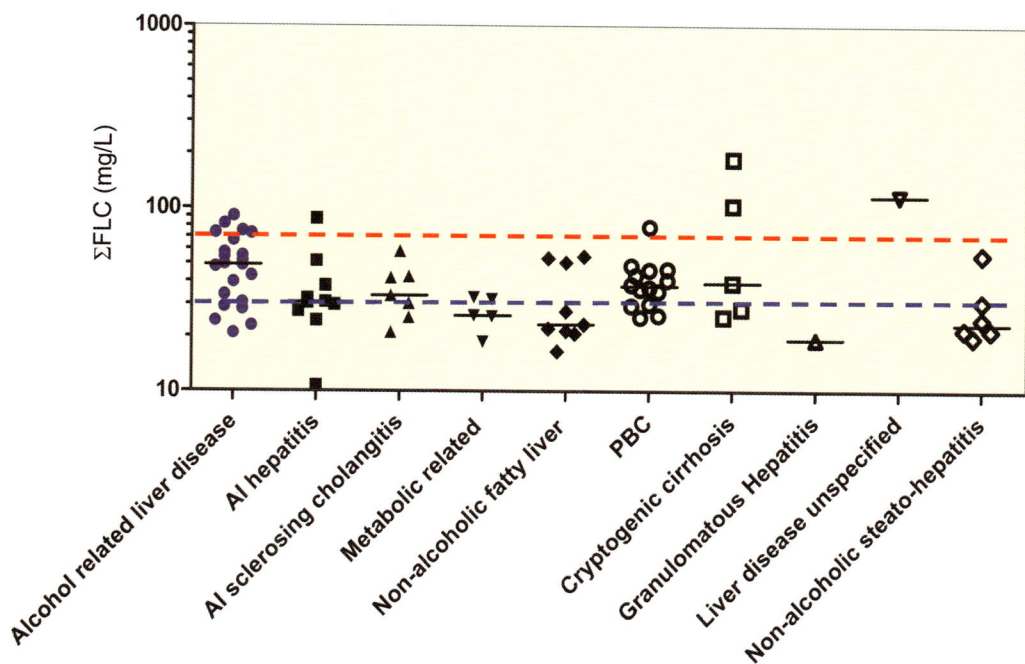

Figure 35.13. ΣFLC concentrations in various liver diseases, corrected for renal function (using cystatin C). Broken lines show values for non-liver disease patients with normal renal function (blue: median value; red: 95% upper limit). *(Reprinted from[69], with permission from EASL).*

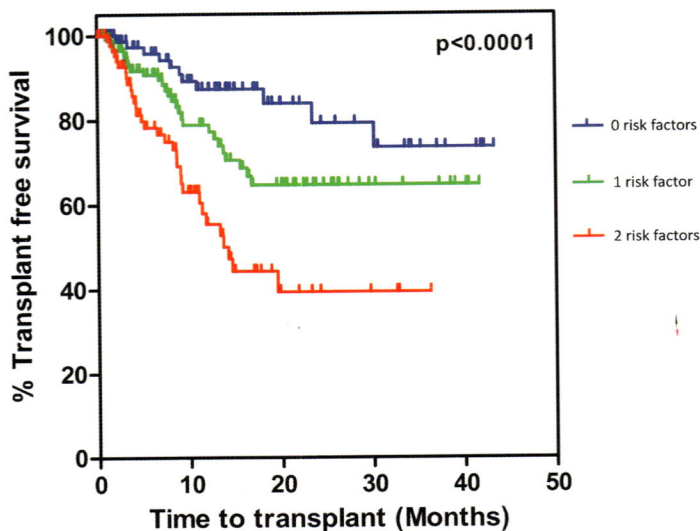

Figure 35.14. Alcoholic liver disease risk stratification model incorporating MELD and cFLC.
Risk factors were cFLC >50mg/L or MELD >11. (Courtesy of D. Adams).

35.8.3. Renal transplantation

Three preliminary reports have been published concerning FLCs in renal transplant recipients. Li et al.[77] found that, out of a number of urinary proteins measured, FLCs provided the best prediction of early allograft rejection (n=103). Shabir et al.[78] measured serum ΣFLCs in two transplant cohorts (n=399 and n=40) and found variations according to the type and level of immunosuppression. It was speculated that sFLC measurement might provide information useful for managing immunosuppressive regimes. Shabir et al.[79] quantified ΣFLCs in serial serum samples collected from 79 renal transplant recipients and corrected values for renal function to give a better estimate of FLC production (eFLC). eFLC was lower when more aggressive immunosuppression was being administered and low levels were predictive of increased risk of infection.

35.8.4. Post-transplant lymphoproliferative disorder

Post-transplant lymphoproliferative disorder (PTLD) can be a serious complication of solid organ transplantation and haematopoietic stem cell transplantation. It comprises a spectrum of B-cell hyperproliferative states ranging from benign lymphoid hyperplasia to malignant neoplasms (mostly NHL)[80]. Epstein-Barr virus (EBV) is present in the majority of PTLD tumours and plays a crucial role in the pathogenesis of these tumours. Whilst most PTLD patients have detectable EBV DNA in peripheral blood, this is a non-specific finding[81]. Therefore, there is a need for additional markers to identify transplant patients at risk of PTLD.

Engels et al.[80] studied the value of sFLCs to predict risk of PTLD in solid organ transplant patients. Pre-diagnostic serum samples were available (on average 3.5 months prior to diagnosis) from 29 transplant recipients with PTLD and 57 matched controls. A polyclonal sFLC elevation was found in a higher proportion of cases compared with controls (59% vs 37%), and was significantly associated with increased risk of early-onset and polymorphic PTLD. A stronger relationship between sFLCs and PTLD was observed among non-kidney transplant recipients. A subsequent study of PTLD in renal transplant patients found no association of elevated sFLC concentrations with PTLD risk[82]. This suggests that non-specific increases in sFLCs due to renal insufficiency *(Section 6.3)* reduce the utility of such rises for predicting PTLD.

In a second study by Engels and colleagues[83], plasma FLC concentrations from 36 paediatric transplant recipients were measured (18 allogeneic, haematopoietic stem cell transplants and 18 liver transplants). Polyclonal FLC elevations were seen in 26% of the patients and monoclonal elevations in 6%; all of the latter had PTLD. It was also noted that there was a tendency for FLC concentrations to change in parallel with measurements of EBV load. Monoclonal immunoglobulins were present in over 90% of the plasma samples but these did not always match the light chain clonality indicated by FLC ratios. The authors suggested this was because PTLD is an oligoclonal disorder rather than a truly monoclonal one. In a more recent, third report from Engels et al.[84], 43 allogeneic haematopoietic stem cell transplant recipients were enrolled and 11 with PTLD were compared with 32 without PTLD. Of the 11 patients with PTLD, only three had elevated FLC concentrations and none had abnormal ratios and there were more frequent FLC abnormalities amongst the controls, indicating that FLC concentrations were not associated with the risk of developing PTLD. In both cases and controls, elevations of κ FLC were more frequent than λ. However, the authors considered that the timing of their serum collection, soon after transplant, may have compromised the identification of PTLD (which tends to arise later) and concluded that further investigations were warrented to understand the biological implications of FLC abnormalities in transplant recipients.

35.8.5. IgG4-related disease

IgG4-related disease is a fibro-inflammatory condition often, but not always, associated with elevated serum IgG4 concentrations. Grados et al.[85] reported that sFLC concentrations were significantly higher in IgG4-related disease than normal, and 43% of patients had abnormally high κ/λ sFLC ratios. This was independent of renal function, and the authors concluded that there was a disproportionate increase in κ FLC production. Patient numbers were too small (n=16) to assess any relationship with disease activity or prognosis.

35.9. FLCs as bioactive molecules in inflammatory diseases

Although frequently regarded as merely a by-product of immunoglobulin synthesis *(Chapter 3)*, there have now been a number of reports indicating a bioactive role for soluble FLCs, distinct from the pathological roles of depositing and plaque-forming FLCs *(Figure 35.15)*. While this is still a relatively new area of inquiry, reports have been published by several independent research groups.

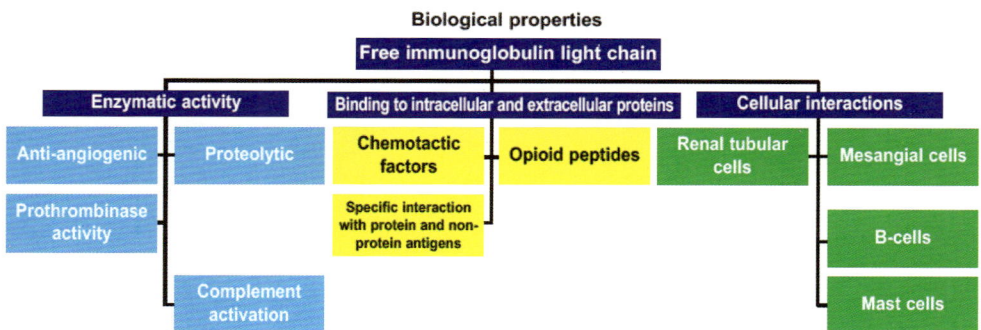

Figure 35.15. Biological actions of sFLCs include enzymatic activity, binding to tissue substrates and mast cells. (Reprinted from[86], Copyright 2008, with permission from Elsevier).

Van der Heijden et al.[87] and Thio et al.[86] reviewed relevant publications and, based upon their own studies of FLC-induced mast cell activation, proposed that FLCs could be an appropriate target for therapy of inflammatory diseases. This idea was explored further by Thio et al.[88], who concluded that FLCs mediated antigen-specific cellular activation and that FLC cross-linking was required to initiate a local allergic response (Section 35.7). A brief report by Hutchinson et al.[89] presented data indicating FLC binding to a number of different cell types, including lymphocytes and monocytes. Cohen and Horl[90] reviewed their research on the interaction of FLCs with neutrophils (which reduced migration, glucose uptake and apoptosis), and postulated that FLCs might interfere with the normal resolution of inflammation and contribute to the chronic inflammatory state found in patients with renal impairment. Also in the field of renal medicine, Wang and Sanders[91] and Basnayake et al.[92] published details of experiments demonstrating the generation of H_2O_2 following endocytosis of FLCs by renal, proximal tubular cells and the subsequent activation of the signal transduction molecule c-Src. In their experiments, monoclonal FLCs were used to challenge the cultured cells but the results might well be relevant to the raised polyclonal FLC concentrations observed in patients with CKD.

35.10. General population studies

In 2012, a population study was published by the Mayo Clinic (Rochester, Minnesota) that utilised sera collected between 1995 and 2003 from Olmsted County residents over the age of 50[93]. After excluding subjects with abnormal κ/λ sFLC ratios or other evidence of a monoclonal process, the population comprised >15,000 individuals, with a median follow-up of 12.7 years. In this population, the sum of κ and λ sFLC concentrations (ΣFLC) was found to be a significant predictor of reduced overall survival. This was particularly noticeable for subjects in the top decile (>47.2 mg/L) and remained so even after correction for age, sex and serum creatinine (Figure 35.16). Increased mortality was associated with many causes of death, with "Circulatory", "Neoplasms" and "Respiratory" being the most frequent. The authors concluded that their data added to the body of literature connecting inflammation, aging and chronic disease, but acknowledged that information on other inflammatory markers was lacking.

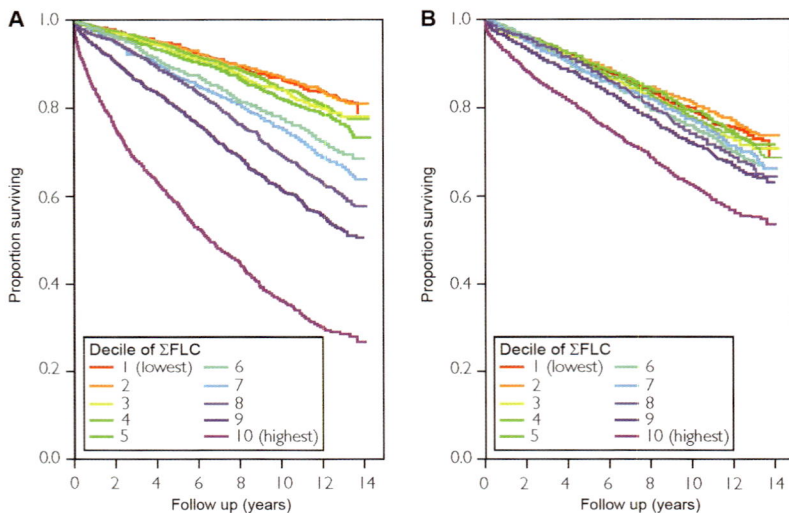

Figure 35.16. Risk of death according to ΣFLC concentration. (A) All patients, crude data. (B) All patients, corrected for age and creatinine level based on the overall distribution in the study. (Reproduced from[93], with permission from Elsevier).

Similar findings have been reported in another study, conducted in Germany, which analysed sera from 4350 subjects who had been monitored as part of an investigation of cardiac risk factors[94]. CRP data was also available for these patients, and elevated ΣFLC was found to be associated with increased mortality independently of sex, age, renal function and CRP concentrations. Further follow-up of this population is continuing.

Anandram and colleagues[95] analysed mortality in a population referred for haematological investigation. The population was smaller than those discussed above (n=723) but more diagnostic information was available. Again, elevated ΣFLCs was associated with increased mortality and this was independent of other risk factors, including decreased serum albumin, reduced renal function, increased erythrocyte sedimentation rate (ESR) and elevated CRP concentrations. This cohort forms the basis of a pilot study for a large prospective study, which is currently in progress[95].

35.11. Conclusions

The data demonstrating polyclonal FLC increases due to increased production in inflammatory conditions, or reduced clearance in renal disease, is now well established. However, the utility of measuring polyclonal sFLCs (or ΣFLC) for diagnosis, monitoring, or prognosis needs to be confirmed with suitably designed further studies. The same could be said regarding the potential role(s) of FLC in disease pathology, and the possibility of FLCs as therapeutic targets. Hutchison and Langren[3] reviewed the literature concerning polyclonal FLCs as biomarkers of immune stimulation and inflammation. They speculated that sFLC measurement might, in the future, complement the use of CRP assays as a biomarker of inflammation, but concluded that more information was required before this could be advocated. They suggested this should include a better understanding of the intra-patient variation in FLC measurements *(Section 7.2.6)*, of the relationship with CRP and other acute-phase proteins, and whether it is advantageous to correct sFLC measurements for renal clearance or use unmodified measurements *(Section 6.3)*.

Brebner and Stockley[96] also reviewed the recent investigations of polyclonal FLCs as disease markers, bioactive molecules and potential therapeutic targets. They noted that the increasing use of B-cell targeted therapies for treatment of autoimmune disease, highlighted the potential of sFLC measurement for risk-stratification and monitoring responses. They also emphasised the requirement for further research such as large prospective studies to define the role of FLCs as predictors of mortality and the importance of determining whether, and where, FLC receptors exist.

Thus, although the study of polyclonal FLC elevations is an area of considerable interest and with an increasing number of publications, many important questions remain unanswered. Faint and colleagues[75] recently described the development of a new turbidimetric sFLC immunoassay that measures both κ and λ sFLCs simultaneously: producing a measurement of ΣFLC from a single assay. Hopefully, this will facilitate and encourage the further studies that are needed.

Test Questions

1. Do conditions causing hypergammaglobulinaemia produce increases in sFLCs?

2. Why are sFLCs highly elevated in patients with SLE?

3. Suggest why measurement of FLCs may be useful in type 2 diabetes?

4. What percentage of hepatitis C-infected patients have abnormal sFLCs?

Answers

1. FLC production normally increases alongside increased production of the intact immunoglobulin molecules (Section 35.1).

2. Because of increased production and reduced renal clearance (Section 35.4.1).

3. Type 2 diabetic patients have significantly raised concentrations of serum and urinary polyclonal FLCs before overt renal disease occurs. Therefore, measurement of polyclonal FLCs could provide a useful tool in early diagnosis of diabetic kidney disease (Section 35.5).

4. Nearly 50% if there is associated cryoglobulinaemia (Section 35.8.2).

References

1. Katzmann JA, Clark RJ, Abraham RS, Bryant S, Lymp JF, Bradwell AR, Kyle RA. Serum reference intervals and diagnostic ranges for free kappa and free lambda immunoglobulin light chains: relative sensitivity for detection of monoclonal light chains. Clin Chem 2002;48:1437-44

2. Burmeister A, Assi LK, Ferro CJ, Hughes RG, Barnett AH, Bellary S et al. The relationship between high-sensitivity CRP and polyclonal free light chains as markers of inflammation in chronic disease. Int J Lab Hematol 2013;36:415-24

3. Hutchison CA, Landgren O. Polyclonal immunoglobulin free light chains as a potential biomarker of immune stimulation and inflammation. Clin Chem 2011;57:1387-9

4. Bradwell AR. Clinical importance of serum free light chain analysis. Personalized Medicine 2010;7:229-31

5. Coresh J, Selvin E, Stevens LA, Manzi J, Kusek JW, Eggers P et al. Prevalence of chronic kidney disease in the United States. JAMA 2007;298:2038-47

6. Hutchison CA, Harding S, Hewins P, Mead GP, Townsend J, Bradwell AR, Cockwell P. Quantitative assessment of serum and urinary polyclonal free light chains in patients with chronic kidney disease. Clin J Am Soc Nephrol 2008;3:1684-90

7. Cockcroft DW, Gault MH. Prediction of creatinine clearance from serum creatinine. Nephron 1976;16:31-41

8. Hutchison CA, Burmeister A, Harding SJ, Basnayake K, Church H, Jesky MD et al. Serum polyclonal immunoglobulin free light chain levels predict mortality in people with chronic kidney disease. Mayo Clin Proc 2014;89:615-22

9. Ritchie J, Bevins A, Assi L, Hoefield R, Cockwell P, Kalra P. High levels of combined serum free light chains are associated with poor outcomes in chronic kidney disease. NDT 2013;28:SO067a

10. Thilo F, Caspari C, Scholze A, Tepel M. Higher serum levels of free k plus l immunoglobulin light chains ameliorate survival of hemodialysis patients. Kidney Blood Press Res 2011;34:344-9

11. Thilo F, Caspari C, Scholze A, Tepel M. Higher serum levels of free k plus l immunoglobulin light chains ameliorate survival of hemodialysis patients. Kidney Blood Press Res 2011;34:344-9

12. Tonelli M, Wiebe N, Culleton B, House A, Rabbat C, Fok M et al. Chronic kidney disease and mortality risk: a systematic review. J Am Soc Nephrol 2006;17:2034-47

13. Basnayake K, Stringer SJ, Hutchison CA, Cockwell P. The biology of immunoglobulin free light chains and kidney injury. Kidney Int 2011;79:1289-301

14. Parasuraman R, Wolforth SC, Wiesend WN, Dumler F, Rooney MT, Li W, Zhang PL. Contribution of polyclonal free light chain deposition to tubular injury. Am J Nephrol 2013;38:465-74

15. Kurt IH, Yavuzer K, Batur MK. Short-term effect of levosimendan on free light chain kappa and lambda levels in patients with decompensated chronic heart failure. Heart Vessels 2010;25:392-9

16. Jackson C, Haig C, Welsh P, Mcconnaichie A, Faint J, Dalzell J et al. Combined free light chains: a novel predictor of prognosis in heart failure. European Journal of Heart Failure 2014;16:85a

17. Epstein WV, Tan M. Increase of L-chain proteins in the sera of patients with systemic lupus erythematosus and the synovial fluids of patients with peripheral rheumatoid arthritis. Arthritis Rheum 1966;9:713-9

18. Hopper JE, Sequeira W, Martellotto J, Papagiannes E, Perna L, Skosey JL. Clinical relapse in systemic lupus erythematosus: correlation with antecedent elevation of urinary free light-chain immunoglobulin. J Clin Immunol 1989;9:338-50

19. Hopper JE, Golbus J, Meyer C, Ferrer GA. Urine free light chains in SLE: clonal markers of B-cell activity and potential link to in vivo secreted Ig. J Clin Immunol 2000;20:123-37

20. Hoffman U, Opperman M, Kuchler S, Ventur Y, Teuber W, Michels H et al. Free immunoglobulin light chains in patients with rheumatic diseases. Zeitschrift für Rheumatologie 2003;62:Fr40a

21. Assi L, McClean A, Webb G, Harper L, Hutchison CA. Serum polyclonal free light chain levels in patients with vasculitis. J Am Soc Nephrol 2011;22:FR-PO1887a

22. Vitali C, Bencivelli W, Isenberg DA, Smolen JS, Snaith ML, Sciuto M et al. Disease activity in systemic lupus erythematosus: report of the Consensus Study Group of the European Workshop for Rheumatology Research. II. Identification of the variables indicative of disease activity and their use in the development of an activity score. The European Consensus Study Group for Disease Activity in SLE. Clin Exp Rheumatol 1992;10:541-7

23. Urban S, Oppermann M, Reucher SW, Schmolke M, Hoffmann U, Hiefinger-Schindlbeck R, Helmke KH. Free light chains (FLC) of immunoglobulins as parameter resembling disease activity in autoimmune rheumatic diseases. Ann Rheum Dis 2004;63:141a

24. Aggarwal R, Sequeira W, Kokebie R, Mikolaitis RA, Fogg L, Finnegan A et al. Serum free light chains as biomarkers for systemic lupus erythematosus disease activity. Arthritis Care Res 2011;63:891-8

25. Assi L, Lisnevskaia L, Ross E, Hughes R, Rahman A, Isenberg D. Elevated combined serum free light chains are associated with active disease in systemic lupus erythematosus. Arthritis & Rheumatism 2013;65:2531a

26. Jimenez JJ, Anton JA, Campos ML, de Carvalho NB, De Becerra JO, De Larramendi CH. Total sFLC correlation with SLE activity markers. Clinical Chemistry 2012;58:C-171a

27. Chiche L, Cournac JM, Mancini J, Bardin N, Thomas G, Jean R et al. Normalization of serum-free light chains in patients with systemic lupus erythematosus upon rituximab treatment and correlation with biological disease activity. Clin Rheumatol 2011;30:685-9

28. Jolly M, Francis S, Aggarwal R, Mikolaitis R, Niewold T, Chubinskaya S et al. Serum free light chains, interferon-alpha, and interleukins in systemic lupus erythematosus. Lupus 2014;23:881-888

29. Gottenberg JE, Aucouturier F, Goetz J, Sordet C, Jahn I, Busson M, et al. Serum immunoglobulin free light chain assessment in rheumatoid arthritis and primary Sjogren's syndrome. Ann Rheum Dis 2007;66:23-7

30. Maignan M, Driad A, Jacob C, Jay N, Dousset B, Vignaud JM, De Korwin JD. Sjögren's syndrome and serum free light chain analysis in newly diagnosed patients. Hematology Reports 2010;2:E47a

31. Ekstrom Smedby K, Vajdic CM, Falster M, Engels EA, Martinez-Maza O, Turner J et al. Autoimmune disorders and risk of non-Hodgkin lymphoma subtypes: a pooled analysis within the InterLymph Consortium. Blood 2008;111:4029-38

32. Mariette X, Quartuccio L, le Seror R, Salvin S, Desmoulins F, Fabris M et al. Results of the Beliss study, the first open phase 2 study of belimumab in primary Sjorgen's syndrome. Arthritis and Rheumatism 2012;64:2555a

33. Deng X, Crowson CS, Rajkumar SV, Dispenzieri A, Larson DR, Therneau TM et al. Elevation of serum immunoglobulin free light chains during the pre-clinical period of rheumatoid arthritis: impact on mortality. J Rheumatol 2015 *In press*

34. Ye Y, Li SL, Xie M, Jiang P, Liu KG, Li YJ. Judging disease activity in rheumatoid arthritis by serum free kappa and lambda light chain levels. Kaohsiung J Med Sci 2013;29:547-53

35. Djidjik R, Messaoudani N, Raaf N, Boudjella ML, Abdessmed A, Bahaz N et al. Are immunoglobulin free light chains levels reliable to assess disease activity in rheumatoid arthritis? Joint Bone Spine 2013;80:437-8

36. Kormelink TG, Tekstra J, Thurlings RM, Boumans MH, Vos K, Tak PP et al. Decrease in immunoglobulin free light chains in patients with rheumatoid arthritis upon rituximab (anti-CD20) treatment correlates with decrease in disease activity. Ann Rheum Dis 2010;69:2137-44

37. Gottenberg JE, Miceli-Richard C, Ducot B, Goupille P, Combe B, Mariette X. Markers of B-lymphocyte activation are elevated in patients with early rheumatoid arthritis and correlated with disease activity in the ESPOIR cohort. Arthritis Res Ther 2009;11:R114

38. Sellam J, Hendel-Chavez H, Rouanet S, Abbed K, Combe B, Loet XL et al. B-cell activation biomarkers as predictive factors of the response to rituximab in rheumatoid arthritis. Arthritis Rheum 2011;63:933-8

39. Cambridge G, Perry HC, Nogueira L, Serre G, Parsons HM, De LT, I et al. The effect of B-cell depletion therapy on serological evidence of B-cell and plasmablast activation in patients with rheumatoid arthritis over multiple cycles of rituximab treatment. J Autoimmun 2013;50:67-76

40. Hutchison CA, Cockwell P, Harding S, Mead GP, Bradwell AR, Barnett AH. Quantitative assessment of serum and urinary polyclonal free light chains in patients with type II diabetes: an early marker of diabetic kidney disease? Expert Opin Ther Targets 2008;12:667-76

41. Levey AS, Bosch JP, Lewis JB, Greene T, Rogers N, Roth D. A more accurate method to estimate glomerular filtration rate from serum creatinine: a new prediction equation. Modification of Diet in Renal Disease Study Group. Ann Intern Med 1999;130:461-70

42. Teppo AM, Groop L. Urinary excretion of plasma proteins in diabetic subjects. Increased excretion of kappa light chains in diabetic patients with and without proliferative retinopathy. Diabetes 1985;34:589-94

43. Groop L, Makipernaa A, Stenman S, DeFronzo RA, Teppo AM. Urinary excretion of kappa light chains in patients with diabetes mellitus. Kidney Int 1990;37:1120-5

44. Thethi T, Katalenich B, Liu S, Pasal R, Fonseca V, Batuman V. Urinary free light chain excretion in obesity and diabetes. J Am Soc Nephrol 2013;24:TH-PO428a

45. Bellary S, Faint JM, Assi LK, Hutchison CA, Harding SJ, Raymond NT, Barnett AH. Elevated serum free light chains predict cardiovascular events in type 2 diabetes. Diabetes Care 2014;37:2028-30

46. Dillon JJ, Sedmak DD, Cosio FG. Rapid-onset diabetic nephropathy in type II diabetes mellitus. Ren Fail 1997;19:819-22

47. Sanders PW, Herrera GA, Kirk KA, Old CW, Galla JH. Spectrum of glomerular and tubulointerstitial renal lesions associated with monotypical immunoglobulin light chain deposition. Lab Invest 1991;64:527-37

48. Bibas M, Trotta MP, Cozzi-Lepri A, Lorenzini P, Pinnetti C, Rizzardini G et al. Role of serum free light chains in predicting HIV-associated non-Hodgkin lymphoma and Hodgkin's lymphoma and its correlation with antiretroviral therapy. Am J Hematol 2012;87:749-53

49. Lane HC, Masur H, Edgar LC, Whalen G, Rook AH, Fauci AS. Abnormalities of B-cell activation and immunoregulation in patients with the acquired immunodeficiency syndrome. N Engl J Med 1983;309:453-8

50. Bibas M, Lorenzini P, Cozzi-Lepri A, Calcagno A, Di Giambenedetto S, Costantini A et al. Polyclonal serum free light chains elevation in HIV infected patients. AIDS 2012;26:2107-10

51. Zemlin AE, Ipp H, Germishuys JJ, Rensburg M, Esser M, Janse van Vuuren M. Serum free light chains in patients with HIV: their association with markers of disease stage and severity, and the effect of antiretroviral therapy. Haematologica 2012;97:0968a

52. Shiels MS, Landgren O, Costello R, Zingone A, Goedert JJ, Engels EA. Free light chains and the risk of AIDS-defining opportunistic infections in HIV-infected individuals. Clin Infect Dis 2012;55:e103-e108

53. Landgren O, Goedert JJ, Rabkin CS, Wilson WH, Dunleavy K, Kyle RA et al. Circulating serum free light chains as predictive markers of AIDS-related lymphoma. J Clin Oncol 2010;28:773-9

54. Gopal S, Patel MR, Yanik EL, Cole SR, Achenbach CJ, Napravnik S et al. Temporal trends in presentation and survival for HIV-associated lymphoma in the antiretroviral therapy era. J Natl Cancer Inst 2013;105:1221-9

55. Grogg KL, Miller RF, Dogan A. HIV infection and lymphoma. J Clin Pathol 2007;60:1365-72

56. Biggar RJ, Jaffe ES, Goedert JJ, Chaturvedi A, Pfeiffer R, Engels EA. Hodgkin lymphoma and immunodeficiency in persons with HIV/AIDS. Blood 2006;108:3786-91

57. Grulich AE, Wan X, Law MG, Milliken ST, Lewis CR, Garsia RJ et al. B-cell stimulation and prolonged immune deficiency are risk factors for non-Hodgkin's lymphoma in people with AIDS. AIDS 2000;14:133-40

58. Baptista M, Morgades M, Briega A, Tapia G, Moreno M, Sancho J et al. Serum free light chains levels in patients with HIV-related lymphoma are lower at complete response than at diagnosis. Haematologica 2013;98:B862a

59. Redegeld FA, van der Heijden MW, Kool M, Heijdra BM, Garssen J, Kraneveld AD et al. Immunoglobulin-free light chains elicit immediate hypersensitivity-like responses. Nat Med 2002;8:694-701

60. Kraneveld AD, Kool M, van Houwelingen AH, Roholl P, Solomon A, Postma DS et al. Elicitation of allergic asthma by immunoglobulin free light chains. Proc Natl Acad Sci U S A 2005;102:1578-83

61. Groot Kormelink T, Pardo A, Knipping K, Buendia-Roldan I, Garcia-de-Alba C, Blokhuis BR et al. Immunoglobulin free light chains are increased in hypersensitivity pneumonitis and idiopathic pulmonary fibrosis. PLoS ONE 2011;6:e25392

62. Groot KT, Calus L, de RN, Holtappels G, Bachert C, Redegeld FA, Gevaert P. Local free light chain expression is increased in chronic rhinosinusitis with nasal polyps. Allergy 2012;67:1165-72

63. Kayserova J, Capkova S, Skalicka A, Vernerova E, Polouckova A, Malinova V et al. Serum immunoglobulin free light chains in severe forms of atopic dermatitis. Scand J Immunol 2010;71:312-6

64. Schouten B, van Esch BC, Kormelink TG, Moro GE, Arslanoglu S, Boehm G et al. Non-digestible oligosaccharides reduce immunoglobulin free light-chain concentrations in infants at risk for allergy. Pediatr Allergy Immunol 2011;22:537-42

65. Schouten B, van Esch BC, van Thuijl AO, Blokhuis BR, Groot KT, Hofman GA et al. Contribution of IgE and immunoglobulin free light chain in the allergic reaction to cow's milk proteins. J Allergy Clin Immunol 2010;125:1308-14

66. Solling K, Solling J, Romer FK. Free light chains of immunoglobulins in serum from patients with rheumatoid arthritis, sarcoidosis, chronic infections and pulmonary cancer. Acta Med Scand 1981;209:473-7

67. Braber S, Thio M, Blokhuis BR, Henricks PA, Koelink PJ, Groot KT et al. An association between neutrophils and immunoglobulin free light chains in the pathogenesis of chronic obstructive pulmonary disease. Am J Respir Crit Care Med 2012;185:817-24

68. Brebner J, Turner A, Stockley R. Polyclonal free light chains: A potential biomarker for immune activation in alpha-1-antitrypsin deficiency (A1ATD) related chronic obstructive pulmonary disease. Thorax 2013;68:S62a

69. Assi LK, Hughes RG, Gunson B, Webb GM, Drayson MT, Bradwell AR, Adams DH. Abnormally elevated serum free light chains in patients with liver disease. Journal of Hepatology 2010;51:S440-S441

70. Sansonno L, Tucci FA, Sansonno S, Lauletta G, Troiani L, Sansonno D. B cells and HCV: an infection model of autoimmunity. Autoimmun Rev 2009;9:93-4

71. Monti G, Pioltelli P, Saccardo F, Campanini M, Candela M, Cavallero G et al. Incidence and characteristics of non-Hodgkin lymphomas in a multicenter case file of patients with hepatitis C virus-related symptomatic mixed cryoglobulinemias. Arch Intern Med 2005;165:101-5

72. Terrier B, Sene D, Saadoun D, Ghillani-Dalbin P, Thibault V, Delluc A et al. Serum-free light chain assessment in hepatitis C virus-related lymphoproliferative disorders. Ann Rheum Dis 2009;68:89-93

73. Terrier B, Chaara W, Dufat L, Geri G, Rosenzwajg M, Musset L et al. Serum biomarker signature identifies patients with B-cell non-Hodgkin lymphoma associated with cryoglobulinemia vasculitis in chronic HCV infection. Autoimmun Rev 2013;13:319-26

74. Faint J, Assi L, Gunson B, Darlow E, Adams D. Raised combined serum free light chains are associated with liver transplantation in alcoholic liver disease. Journal of Hepatology 2013;58:s216

75. Faint JM, Basu S, Sutton D, Showell PJ, Kalra PA, Gunson BK et al. Quantification of polyclonal free light chains in clinical samples using a single turbidimetric immunoassay. Clin Chem Lab Med 2014;52:1605-13

76. Teng M, Pirrie S, Ward DG, Assi LK, Hughes RG, Stocken D, Johnson PJ. Diagnostic and mechanistic implications of serum free light chains, albumin and alpha-fetoprotein in hepatocellular carcinoma. Br J Cancer 2014;110:2277-82

77. Li M, Chouhan KK, Gullo KE, Simon EE, Zhang R, Batuman V. Urinary free light chains predict acute rejection in patients with a kidney transplant. Presented at World Congress of Nephrology 2011;SU531a

78. Shabir S, Bevins A, Cockwell P, Borrow R, Hutchison CA. Polyclonal immunoglobulin free light chains provide a novel insight into immunosuppressant use in renal transplant recipients. J Am Soc Nephrol 2011;22:TH-PO1007a

79. Shabir S, Bevins A, Church HL, Borrows R, Hutchison C. Production rates of free light chains predict infections post-transplant. Nephrology 2012;17:47-75

80. Engels EA, Preiksaitis J, Zingone A, Landgren O. Circulating antibody free light chains and risk of posttransplant lymphoproliferative disorder. Am J Transplant 2012;12:1268-74

81. Allen U, Preiksaitis J. Epstein-barr virus and posttransplant lymphoproliferative disorder in solid organ transplant recipients. Am J Transplant 2009;9 Suppl 4:S87-S96

82. Fernando RC, Rizzatti EG, Braga WM, Santos MG, de Oliveira MB, Pestana JO et al. Serum free light chain and post-transplant lymphoproliferative disorder in patients with renal transplant. Leuk Lymphoma 2013;54:2177-80

83. Engels EA, Savoldo B, Pfeiffer RM, Costello R, Zingone A, Heslop HE, Landgren O. Plasma markers of B-cell activation and clonality in pediatric liver and hematopoietic stem cell transplant recipients. Transplantation 2013;95:519-26

84. Engels EA, Landgren O, Costello R, Burton D, Mailankody S, Storek J. Serum immunoglobulin free light chains and post-transplant lymphoproliferative disorder among allogeneic hematopoietic stem cell transplant recipients. Bone Marrow Transplant 2015;50:146-7

85. Grados A, Ebbo M, Boucraut J, Vely F, Aucouturier P, Rigolet A et al. Serum immunoglobulin free light chain assessment in IgG4-related disease. Int J Rheumatol 2013;2013:426759

86. Thio M, Blokhuis BR, Nijkamp FP, Redegeld FA. Free immunoglobulin light chains: a novel target in the therapy of inflammatory diseases. Trends Pharmacol Sci 2008;29:170–4

87. van der Heijden M, Kraneveld A, Redegeld F. Free immunoglobulin light chains as target in the treatment of chronic inflammatory diseases. Eur J Pharmacol 2006;533:319-26

88. Thio M, Groot KT, Fischer MJ, Blokhuis BR, Nijkamp FP, Redegeld FA. Antigen binding characteristics of immunoglobulin free light chains: crosslinking by antigen is essential to induce allergic inflammation. PLoS ONE 2012;7:e40986

89. Hutchinson AT, Jones DR, Raison RL. The ability to interact with cell membranes suggests possible biological roles for free light chain. Immunol Lett 2012;142:75-7

90. Cohen G, Horl WH. Free immunoglobulin light chains as a risk factor in renal and extrarenal complications. Semin Dial 2009;22:369-72

91. Wang PX, Sanders PW. Immunoglobulin light chains generate hydrogen peroxide. J Am Soc Nephrol 2007;18:1239-45

92. Basnayake K, Ying WZ, Wang PX, Sanders PW. Immunoglobulin light chains activate tubular epithelial cells through redox signaling. J Am Soc Nephrol 2010;21:1165-73

93. Dispenzieri A, Katzmann JA, Kyle RA, Larson DR, Therneau TM, Colby CL et al. Use of nonclonal serum immunoglobulin free light chains to predict overall survival in the general population. Mayo Clin Proc 2012;87:517-23

94. Eisele L, Durig J, Huttman A, Duhrsen U, Fuhrer A, Kieruzel S et al. Polyclonal free light chain elevation and mortality in the German Heinz Nixdorf Recall Study. Blood 2010;116:3903a

95. Anandram S, Assi LK, Lovatt T, Parkes J, Taylor J, MacWhannell A et al. Elevated, combined serum free light chain levels and increased mortality: a 5-year follow-up, UK study. J Clin Pathol 2012;65:1036-42

96. Brebner JA, Stockley RA. Polyclonal free light chains: a biomarker of inflammatory disease or treatment target? F1000 Med Rep 2013;5:4

Cerebrospinal fluid and free light chains

Summary:

- In patients with intrathecal immunoglobulin synthesis, κ FLC concentrations in cerebrospinal fluid are typically high, whilst λ FLC concentrations are only moderately elevated.
- It is preferable to calculate a κ FLC index by correcting for FLC diffusion into the CSF.
- An elevated κ FLC index can support a diagnosis of multiple sclerosis.
- An elevated κ FLC index has been found more diagnostically sensitive than oligoclonal band detection.

36.1. Introduction

Inflammation of the central nervous system (CNS) may be caused by infections (e.g. viral encephalitis, cerebral malaria) or autoimmune disorders such as Guillain-Barré syndrome or, notably, multiple sclerosis (MS). When inflammation of the CNS occurs, there is usually synthesis of intrathecal immunoglobulins[1]. Since the blood-brain barrier largely prevents their escape into the blood, the immunoglobulins gradually accumulate in the cerebrospinal fluid (CSF). They are then detectable as oligoclonal bands on electrophoretic gels or can be quantitated using protein assays.

When determining the clinical relevance of oligoclonal bands, CSF samples should always be assessed alongside paired serum samples to determine whether the immunoglobulin was synthesised locally within the CSF or has diffused from the blood[2]. The presence of oligoclonal bands in the CSF that are not present in the serum is consistent with intrathecal synthesis. However, if the patient's serum contains monoclonal immunoglobulins produced in the bone marrow, some will cross the blood-brain barrier, making interpretation of intrathecal production difficult[2]. Similarly, if there is inflammation of the meninges, serum proteins will enter the CSF more readily. The gold standard for detection of oligoclonal bands is isoelectric focusing (IEF), followed by immunoblotting[2]. However, this protocol is non-quantitative, time-consuming, and interpretation may be difficult; consequently, it is not always, routinely available.

Alternatively, quantitative IgG analysis may be used as a measure of intrathecal immunoglobulin synthesis. To ensure that measurements represent local (intrathecal) synthesis and not IgG which has diffused from the blood, values are corrected using albumin measurements. This serves as a marker of the blood-CSF barrier function because albumin is never synthesised within the CNS. For example, the IgG index is calculated as follows: [CSF IgG/serum IgG]/[CSF albumin/serum albumin]. Alternative, non-linear formulae improve the diagnostic accuracy of IgG measurements and are recommended[2]. However, in general, quantitative IgG analysis will only identify around 75% of oligoclonal-band positive patients[2].

Consequently, there is a need for alternative, sensitive tests to identify intrathecal immunoglobulin synthesis.

Immunoglobulin free light chains (FLCs) are typically secreted along with intact immunoglobulins from plasma cells *(Section 3.4)*. If they are produced intrathecally, they should accumulate locally and significant diffusion from the blood is unlikely as serum concentrations are low due to rapid renal clearance *(Section 3.5)*. For these reasons, the measurement of FLCs in CSF is a potentially sensitive marker of intrathecal immunoglobulin synthesis and it has been investigated a number of times using various assay techniques *(Section 36.2)*.

36.1.1. Multiple sclerosis and intrathecal immunoglobulin synthesis

The majority of the studies exploring the measurement of FLCs as an alternative marker of intrathecal immunoglobulin synthesis have focused on MS.

MS is an autoimmune inflammatory disease of the CNS, characterised by myelin loss, axonal pathology, and progressive neurologic dysfunction[3]. The majority of patients will first present with what is termed a clinically isolated syndrome (CIS). However, over a period of 20 years, about 60% of patients will suffer a second demyelinating event and progress to a diagnosis of clinically definite MS[4]. The diagnosis of MS is made primarily on the basis of medical history and physical examination, with Magnetic Resonance Imaging (MRI) used to identify neurological lesions[5]. Positive CSF findings (ie. 2 or more oligoclonal bands, or an elevated IgG index) can be important in supporting the inflammatory demyelinating nature of the condition, evaluating alternative diagnoses, and predicting clinically definite MS[5].

36.2. CSF FLCs as a marker of intrathecal immunoglobulin synthesis

A number of researchers have investigated FLCs in CSF as alternative markers of intrathecal inflammation[7,8,9,10,11]. The detection methods for CSF FLCs have included isoelectric focusing, quantitation by enzyme/radio-immunoassays and nephelometry but results have not led to routine incorporation of the test. However, the development of Freelite® turbidimetric and nephelometric assays provoked renewed interest in the measurement of FLCs in CSF. Indeed, CE-marked Freelite assays intended for the measurement of FLCs in CSF (in addition to serum and urine) are now available for Binding Site SPAPLUS® and Siemens BN™II instruments.

Fischer et al.[6] studied CSF/serum pairs from 95 patients who had been investigated for intrathecal immunoglobulin synthesis. Oligoclonal immunoglobulin synthesis was identified in 71/95 patients, including 49 with multiple sclerosis and 22 with other neurological diseases. The median κ FLC concentrations in the CSF from both groups of patients with neurological diseases were higher than non-diseased samples *(Figure 36.1)* but λ FLC concentrations were found to be uninformative. When samples with increased albumin leakage were excluded, there was no overlap between normal and disease groups (cut-off level of κ FLC concentrations: 0.5 mg/L). This indicated that determination of κ FLC concentrations in CSF provided information similar to that of oligoclonal band measurements. As an alternative strategy for eliminating the influence of impaired blood-CSF barrier function, a κ FLC index was constructed ([CSF κ FLC/serum κ FLC]/[CSF albumin/serum albumin]). An empirically defined, non-linear κ FLC index threshold line provided good separation of patients with and without intrathecal immunoglobulin synthesis; only two normal samples were misclassified *(Figure 36.2)*. The authors stated that a major advantage of the use of κ FLC CSF measurements in MS diagnosis was the availability of the Freelite assay on automated nephelometric analysers *(Chapter 37)*.

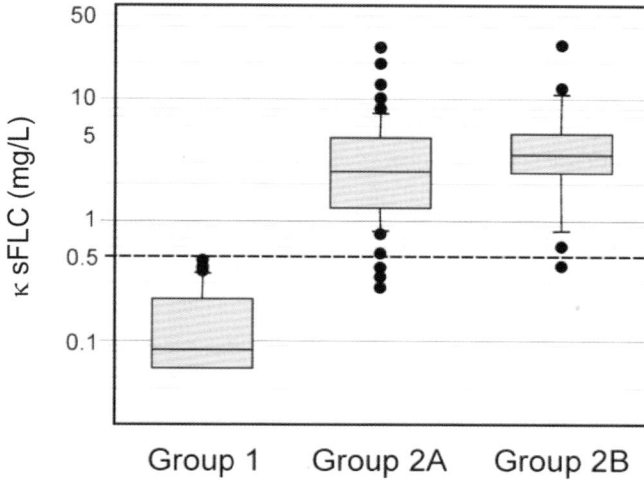

Figure 36.1. Box plot of κ FLC CSF concentrations in patients investigated for intrathecal immunoglobulin synthesis. *Group 1: no detectable intrathecal fraction and no oligoclonal bands; Group 2A: MS patients, oligoclonal band positive; Group 2B other neurologic diseases, oligoclonal band positive. The median and 25th and 75th percentiles (shaded boxes), the 10th and 90th percentiles (error bars), and the outliers (black dots) are indicated. The cutoff for κ FLC concentrations (0.5 mg/L) is indicated (dashed line). (Republished with permission of Clinical Chemistry[6]; permission conveyed through Copyright Clearance Center, Inc.).*

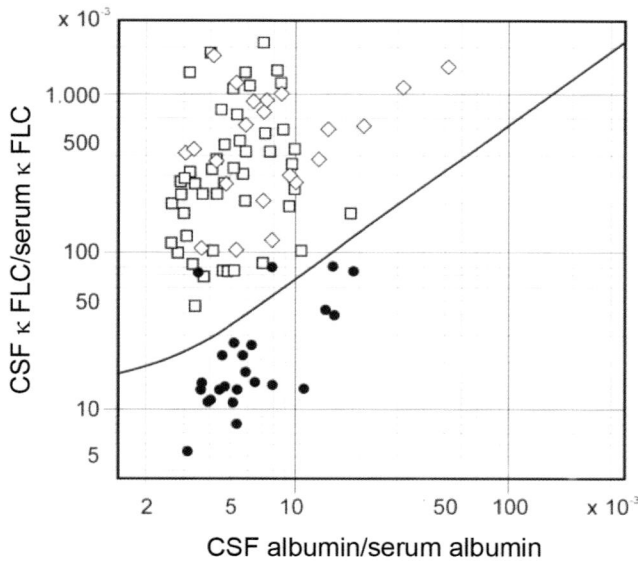

Figure 36.2. Quotients of κ FLC concentrations in CSF and serum plotted against the respective albumin quotients. *Samples are from patients in Figure 36.1: Group 1 (black dots), Group 2A (squares) and Group 2B (diamonds). (Republished with permission of Clinical Chemistry[6]; permission conveyed through Copyright Clearance Center, Inc.).*

A number of other groups have reported a strong correlation between elevated κ FLC CSF concentrations and positive oligoclonal bands and/or the diagnosis of MS[12,13]. Calculation of a κ FLC index (as above) has been shown to improve the diagnostic sensitivity and specificity[12,13,14]. Presslauer et al.[14] studied the use of a κ FLC index to diagnose MS in 438 subjects who underwent lumbar puncture. This included 41 patients with MS, and 29 patients with a CIS suggestive of MS. A control group (n=45) comprised individuals with normal pressure hydrocephalus, undefined dementia, or a primary suspected but unconfirmed subarachnoid bleed (and with no sign of inflammation). For the control group FLC CSF concentrations were low: κ FLC CSF median value 0.18 mg/L (range 0.13 - 0.22 mg/L); λ FLC CSF median value 0.16 mg/L (range 0.13 - 0.2 mg/L). Serum FLC (sFLC) concentrations were within the normal range, resulting in low κ and λ FLC indices (*Figure 36.3*, λ FLC index not shown).

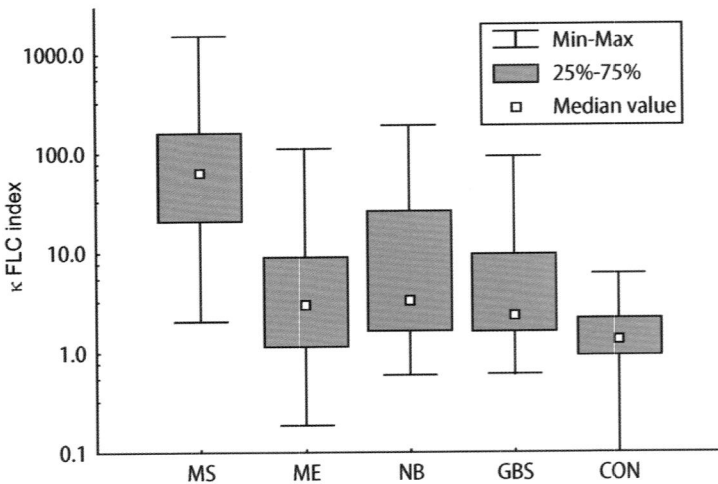

Figure 36.3. Median values and ranges of κFLC index in different subgroups. MS: multiple sclerosis; ME: meningitis/ encephalitis; NB: neuroborreliosis; GBS: Guillain-Barré syndrome; CON: control. (Reproduced with kind permission from Springer Science+Business Media:[14] Figure 1).

Conversely, in the MS group, κ FLC CSF concentrations were typically high (median 4.12 mg/L, range 1.4 – 8.77 mg/L), whilst λ FLC concentrations were only moderately elevated (median 0.67 mg/L, range 0.25 - 1.54 mg/L)[14]. Patients with other diseases associated with intrathecal infection (e.g. meningitis/encephalitis) or inflammation (e.g. Guillain-Barré syndrome), typically had only moderate increases in both κ and λ FLC CSF concentrations and indices *(Figure 36.3*, λ FLC index not shown). Similar findings were also reported by Arneth and Birklein[13].

Presslauer and colleagues also compared the diagnostic performances of the κ FLC index, κ FLC CSF concentration, λ FLC index and IgG index using receiver operating characteristic (ROC) analysis[14]. The test with the best performance (and highest area under the ROC curve) was the κ FLC index. Using a cut-off value of 5.9, the diagnostic sensitivity of the κ FLC index was 96%. Only 3 patients (1 MS and 2 CIS suggestive of MS) had a κ FLC index below this level (these patients were also negative for oligoclonal bands and had a normal IgG index). By comparison, the diagnostic sensitivity of oligoclonal bands and the IgG index (≥0.6) was 91% and 80%, respectively. The κ FLC index for the MS patients was significantly higher than those for the other disease groups (meningitis/encephalitis:

p=0.003; neuroborreliosis: p=0.001; and Guillain-Barré syndrome: p=0.009, *Figure 36.3*)[14]. Fifty patients without MS also had an elevated κ FLC index, resulting in a diagnostic specificity (for MS) of 86%; this was lower than the specificity of oligoclonal bands (92%), but distinctly higher than that of the IgG index (77%). Presslauer et al.[14] concluded that the κ FLC index should be interpreted alongside clinical findings together with other CSF analyses (including λ FLC concentrations and the λ FLC index).

The same research group refined their cut-off for the κ FLC index by expanding the number of samples included in defining the normal range[15]. CSF samples were collected from 861 patients who underwent lumbar puncture and after exclusion of patients with contaminated samples or possible inflammatory conditions, 420 control samples remained. κ FLC CSF measurements in controls were used to define the upper limit of normal for the κ FLC ratio (CSF κ FLC/serum κ FLC) under different blood-CSF barrier conditions[15]. Briefly, controls were divided into 23 subgroups based on blood-CSF barrier function (defined by the [CSF albumin/serum albumin] ratio). For each subgroup, the mean value of the κ FLC ratio + 3SD was plotted against the mean albumin ratio, to produce a κ FLC index threshold line *(Figure 36.4)*. The upper limit of the threshold line included 98% of control patients (i.e. the diagnostic specificity was 98%). Intrathecal immunoglobulin synthesis (defined by a κ FLC index above the threshold line) was detected in 97% of MS patients (n=65, *Figure 36.5A*) and 97% of CIS patients (n=69, *Figure 36.5B*)[15]. In both MS and CIS, the diagnostic sensitivity of the κ FLC index was superior to that of oligoclonal band detection or the IgG index *(Table 36.1)*. In the subgroup of MS or CIS patients who were negative for oligoclonal bands, 76% had elevated κ FLC index values *(Figure 36.5C)*. This suggests that the κ FLC index can detect very low plasma cell activity in the CSF, beyond the analytical sensitivity of IEF. Of the patients who were positive for oligoclonal bands, 98% had elevated κ FLC index values *(Figure 36.5D)*. The authors concluded that the measurement of κ FLCs in CSF should become a first-line screen in diagnostic algorithms for MS and CIS[15].

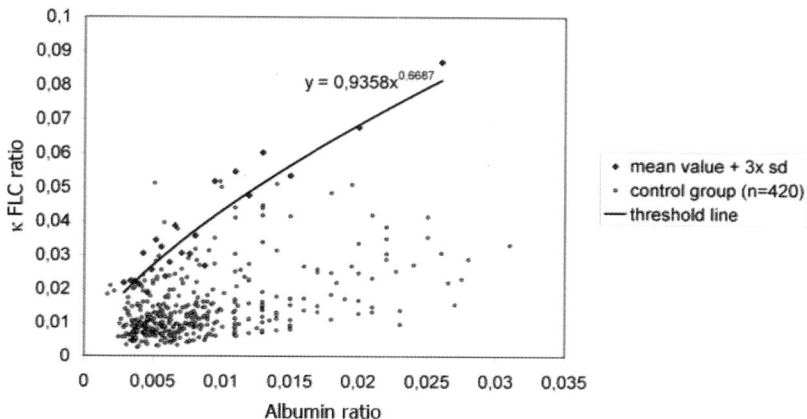

Figure 36.4. κ FLC index threshold line. *sd: standard deviation. (Reproduced from PLoS ONE[15]).*

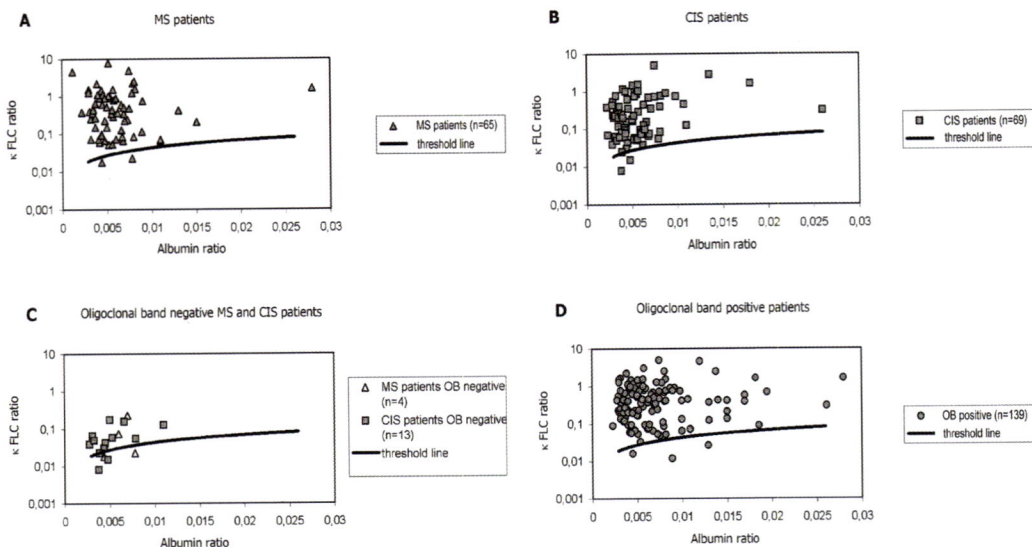

Figure 36.5. κ FLC threshold line in half-logarithmic diagrams with results of different patient groups. CIS: clinically isolated syndrome. (Reproduced from PLoS ONE[15]).

Disease	Oligoclonal bands	IgG index	κ FLC index (threshold value)
MS (n=65)	94%	85%	97%
CIS (n=69)	81%	74%	97%

Table 36.1. Diagnostic sensitivity of oligoclonal bands, IgG index and κ FLC index in MS and CIS[15].

36.3. Prognostic significance of CSF FLCs

Villar et al. investigated whether κ FLC CSF concentrations in patients with CIS were predictive of conversion to MS[16]. The study included 78 consecutive CIS patients and 25 controls (patients with non-inflammatory neurological diseases). A cut-off value of κ FLC CSF >0.53 mg/L (defined as the mean + 2 standard deviations for the control group) identified CIS patients with an increased probability of conversion to MS (p<0.0001). In a multivariate Cox regression analysis (adjusted for gender, age and basal MRI findings), the hazard ratio was 6.41 (p<0.003). Conversely, in a similar number of patients, Presslauer et al.[15] did not find a significant difference in the κ FLC index values between stable CIS patients and those who underwent conversion to MS. Therefore, the prognostic value of FLC CSF measurements remains to be established.

Test Questions

1. Why should a κ FLC index be used in preference to κ FLC concentrations to identify intrathecal immunoglobulin synthesis?

Answers

1. Because correcting CSF κ FLC values using albumin measurements provides an indicator of whether the FLCs were produced locally, or have diffused from the blood due to blood/brain barrier dysfunction (Section 36.1).

References

1. Hickey WF. Migration of hematogenous cells through the blood-brain barrier and the initiation of CNS inflammation. Brain Pathol 1991;1:97-105

2. Freedman MS, Thompson EJ, Deisenhammer F, Giovannoni G, Grimsley G, Keir G et al. Recommended standard of cerebrospinal fluid analysis in the diagnosis of multiple sclerosis: a consensus statement. Arch Neurol 2005;62:865-70

3. Nylander A, Hafler DA. Multiple sclerosis. J Clin Invest 2012;122:1180-8

4. Disanto G, Morahan JM, Barnett MH, Giovannoni G, Ramagopalan SV. The evidence for a role of B cells in multiple sclerosis. Neurology 2012;78:823-32

5. Polman CH, Reingold SC, Banwell B, Clanet M, Cohen JA, Filippi M et al. Diagnostic criteria for multiple sclerosis: 2010 revisions to the McDonald criteria. Ann Neurol 2011;69:292-302

6. Fischer C, Arneth B, Koehler J, Lotz J, Lackner KJ. Kappa free light chains in cerebrospinal fluid as markers of intrathecal immunoglobulin synthesis. Clin Chem 2004;50:1809-13

7. DeCarli C, Menegus MA, Rudick RA. Free light chains in multiple sclerosis and infections of the CNS. Neurology 1987;37:1334-8

8. Jenkins MA, Cheng L, Ratnaike S. Multiple sclerosis: use of light-chain typing to assist diagnosis. Ann Clin Biochem 2001;38:235-41

9. Khoury SJ, Weiner HL. Kappa light chains in spinal fluid for diagnosing multiple sclerosis. JAMA 1994;272:242-3

10. Krakauer M, Schaldemose Nielsen H, Jensen J, Sellebjerg F. Intrathecal synthesis of free immunoglobulin light chains in multiple sclerosis. Acta Neurol Scand 1998;98:161-5

11. Lamers KJ, de Jong JG, Jongen PJ, Kock-Jansen MJ, Teunesen MA, Prudon-Rosmulder EM. Cerebrospinal fluid free kappa light chains versus IgG findings in neurological disorders: qualitative and quantitative measurements. J Neuroimmunol 1995;62:19-25

12. Desplat-Jego S, Feuillet L, Pelletier J, Bernard D, Cherif AA, Boucraut J. Quantification of immunoglobulin free light chains in cerebrospinal fluid by nephelometry. J Clin Immunol 2005;25:338-45

13. Arneth B, Birklein F. High sensitivity of free lambda and free kappa light chains for detection of intrathecal immunoglobulin synthesis in cerebrospinal fluid. Acta Neurol Scand 2009;119:39-44

14. Presslauer S, Milosavljevic D, Brucke T, Bayer P, Hubl W. Elevated levels of kappa free light chains in CSF support the diagnosis of multiple sclerosis. J Neurol 2008;255:1508-14

15. Presslauer S, Milosavljevic D, Huebl W, Parigger S, Schneider-Koch G, Bruecke T. Kappa Free Light Chains: Diagnostic and Prognostic Relevance in MS and CIS. PLoS ONE 2014;9:e89945

16. Villar LM, Espino M, Costa-Frossard L, Muriel A, Jimenez J, Alvarez-Cermeno JC. High levels of cerebrospinal fluid free kappa chains predict conversion to multiple sclerosis. Clin Chim Acta 2012;413:1813-16

Freelite immunoassay instrumentation

Freelite® sFLC immunoassays:

- Are optimised for use on Binding Site analysers: SPAPLUS®, Optilite®, and MININEPHPLUS®, all of which have prozone parameters.
- Can also be used on the majority of other nephelometric and turbidimetric analysers.

37.1. Introduction

Freelite immunoassays for the measurement of free light chains (FLCs), are available for the majority of nephelometric and turbidimetric laboratory instruments. The assays all utilise latex enhancement to allow detection of FLCs at low concentrations. Turbidimeters and nephelometers have similar levels of sensitivity and precision, but instruments vary in their ability to handle samples, clean reaction cuvettes, identify antigen excess, etc.

37.2. Binding Site SPAPLUS

The Binding Site SPAPLUS is an automated, bench-top, batch mode turbidimeter with host interface capability, barcoded sample identification and reagent management systems *(Figure 37.1)*. Precision is maintained through a combination of acid/alkali cuvette washing and an innovative reaction cuvette mixing system *(Table 37.1)*. Air pressure is used in place of stirrers to mix the reaction mixture in a U-shaped cuvette. No physical contact is made with the reaction mixture, thereby removing any possibility of carry-over on a stirrer. Calibration curves are made from calibrator sets and validated by assay of control fluids supplied with the kits. Samples are initially measured at the standard programmed sample dilution and if out of range, the instrument automatically re-measures the samples at the appropriate alternative dilutions. All dilutions are made with the instrument's pipetting system, which is capable of dilutions between 1/10 and 1/100. The assays include prozone parameters *(Section 7.4)*. The instrument has a good overall performance compared with other analysers, and provides good throughput for patient samples in spite of its relatively small size.

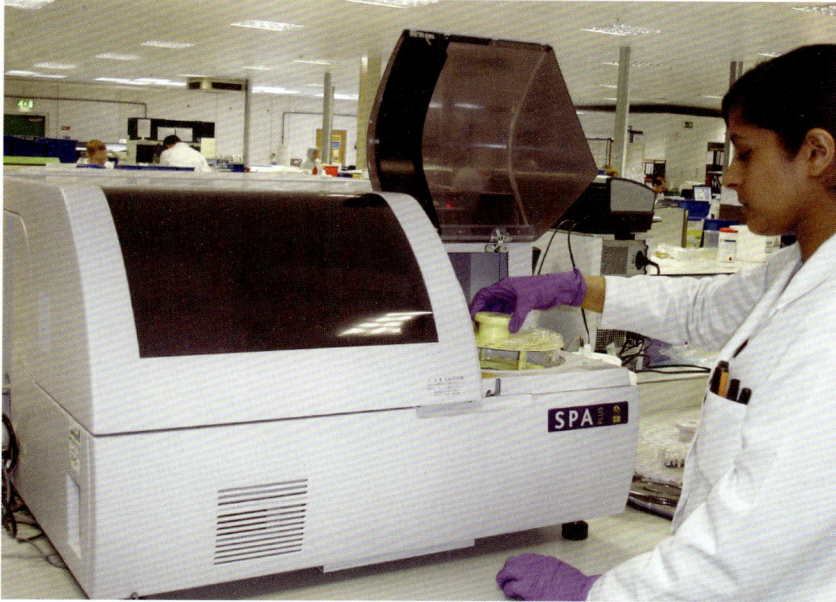

Figure 37.1. The Binding Site SPAPLUS.

	κ sFLC	λ sFLC
Range at 1/10	4.0 - 180.0 mg/L	4.5 - 165.0 mg/L
Sensitivity at 1/1	0.4 mg/L	0.5 mg/L
Assay time	15 min	15 min
Precision: within-run	3.3% at 7.2 mg/L	3.4% at 10.4 mg/L
	1.6% at 35.7 mg/L	2.4% at 35.1 mg/L
	1.8% at 123.8 mg/L	2.0% at 142.1 mg/L
Precision: between-run	4.2% at 7.2 mg/L	2.2% at 10.4 mg/L
	1.9% at 35.7 mg/L	0.0% at 35.1 mg/L
	2.3% at 123.8 mg/L	2.4% at 142.1 mg/L

Table 37.1. Freelite assay performance on the Binding Site SPAPLUS.

37.3. Binding Site Optilite

The Binding Site Optilite is an automated, bench-top, random access turbidimeter allowing host interface capability with barcoded parameter entry, sample identification and reagent management systems *(Figure 37.2)*. Precision is good due to the use of disposable cuvettes *(Table 37.2)*. Single vial calibrators are used that are diluted automatically by the instrument to generate the calibration curves. Starting sample dilutions are 1/10 for κ sFLC assays and 1/8 for λ sFLC assays. Samples reporting outside of the standard assay measuring range are automatically re-diluted, with one lower and three higher sample dilutions programmed within the assay parameters. Very high level samples may still require further off-line dilutions. The assays include prozone parameters, with a higher automatic re-dilution being performed for samples that prompt the "prozone detected" data flag.

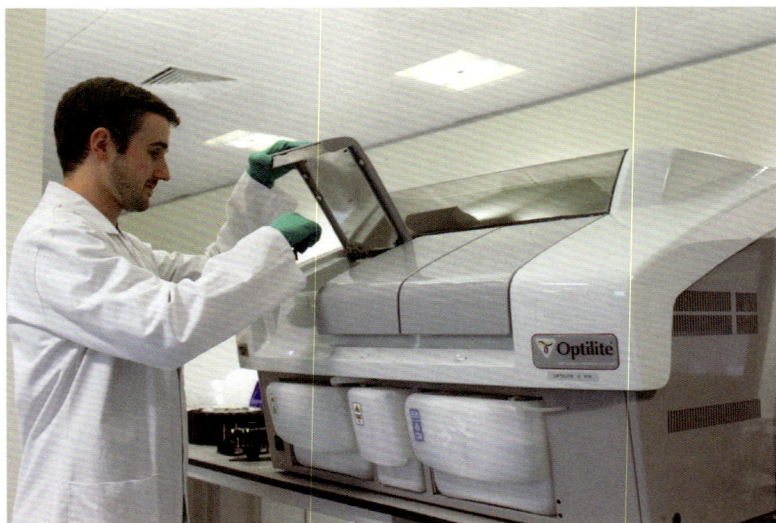

Figure 37.2. The Binding Site Optilite.

	κ sFLC	λ sFLC
Range 1/10 (κ); 1/8 (λ)	2.9 - 127.0 mg/L	5.2 - 139.0 mg/L
Sensitivity (undiluted)	0.6 mg/L	1.3 mg/L
Assay time	15 min	15 min
Precision: within-run	2.6% at 4.9 mg/L	2.1% at 4.7 mg/L
	1.5% at 23.2 mg/L	1.8% at 19.8 mg/L
	3.3% at 71.8 mg/L	1.8% at 71.1 mg/L
Precision: between-run	2.9% at 4.9 mg/L	3.2% at 4.7 mg/L
	1.8% at 23.2 mg/L	2.1% at 19.8 mg/L
	1.8% at 71.8 mg/L	2.4% at 71.1 mg/L

Table 37.2. Freelite assay performance on the Binding Site Optilite.

37.4. Binding Site MININEPHPLUS

The Binding Site MININEPHPLUS is a small, manual nephelometer designed for sFLC analysis *(Figure 37.3)*. The calibration curves are stored on magnetic swipe-cards. Once loaded into the instrument's memory, curve validity is confirmed by assaying control samples. Patient samples are analysed individually by semi-automated addition of reagents into cuvettes within the instrument. The assays show good precision and linearity, and include prozone parameters *(Table 37.3)*. The instrument may find use in laboratories with low workloads (<10 samples per day) or when the cost of a larger instrument cannot be justified.

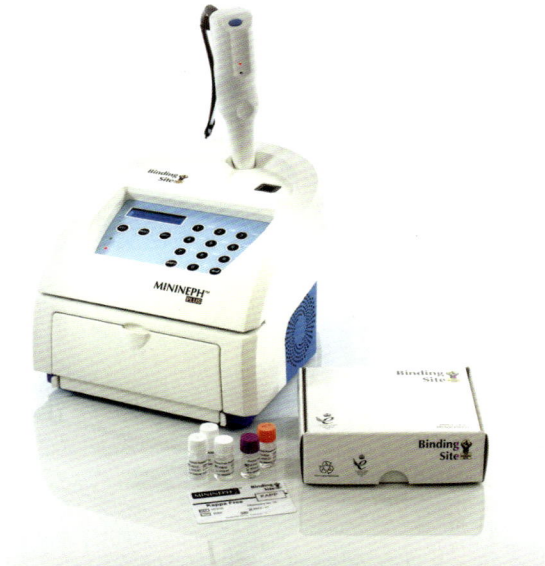

Figure 37.3. The Binding Site MININEPHPLUS.

	κ sFLC	λ sFLC
Range at 1/20	3.0 - 72.4 mg/L	4.9 - 98.3 mg/L
Sensitivity at 1/20	3.0 mg/L	4.9 mg/L
Assay time	5 min	5 min
Precision: within-run	7.3% at 55.9 mg/L	5.1% at 80.5 mg/L
	5.7% at 18.7 mg/L	3.9% at 29.4 mg/L
	4.9% at 4.8 mg/L	3.2% at 7.6 mg/L
Precision: between-run	8.9% at 55.8 mg/L	6.7% at 80.5 mg/L
	6.8% at 18.7 mg/L	3.8% at 29.4 mg/L
	5.0% at 4.8 mg/L	7.4% at 7.6 mg/L

Table 37.3. Freelite assay performance on the Binding Site MININEPHPLUS.

37.5. Other analytical platforms

In addition to the Binding Site instruments listed above, Freelite immunoassays are also available for the majority of nephelometric and turbidimetric laboratory instruments including: 1) Beckman Coulter AU™ (400, 640, 2700 and 5400); 2) Beckman Coulter IMMAGE™ and IMMAGE 800; 3) Roche Cobas™ c501, c502 and Integra™ (400,400 plus and 800); 4) Roche Hitachi 911/912/917 and Modular P; and 5) Siemens ADVIA™ (1650, 1800 and 2400), BN™II and BN ProSpec™.

Test Questions

1. Which Binding Site instrument provides random-access sample measurement?

Answers

1. The Optilite instrument offers random-access sample measurement *(Section 37.3)*.

396

Hevylite immunoassay instrumentation

Section	Page
38.1. Introduction	**397**
38.2. Binding Site SPAPLUS	**397**

Summary:
- Hevylite® assays can be run on the Binding Site SPAPLUS® and Siemens BN™II analysers.
- IgM Hevylite assays have in-built prozone parameters.

38.1. Introduction

Immunoglobulin heavy/light chain immunoassays (Hevylite®; HLC) assays are available for the Binding Site SPAPLUS and Siemens BNII analysers. Hevylite assays for the Binding Site Optilite® instrument are currently in development. General features of Binding Site instruments are discussed in Chapter 37. Whilst IgGκ, IgGλ, IgAκ and IgAλ Hevylite assays are antisera-based assays, IgMκ and IgMλ Hevylite assays are latex-enhanced immunoassays, with in-built prozone parameters. The development of Hevylite assays, normal ranges, and implementation and interpretation are covered in Chapters 9, 10 and 11, respectively.

38.2. Binding Site SPAPLUS

The Binding Site SPAPLUS is an automated, bench top, random-access turbidimeter. All Hevylite specificities are 15 minute assays. Hevylite calibration curves are made from a set of six calibrators, and are validated using two control fluids supplied with the kits. If a Hevylite result is outside the initial measuring range at the standard dilution (1/20 for IgG HLC assays and 1/10 for IgA and IgM assays), the sample is automatically re-diluted by the instrument. Assay parameters define one higher or one lower automatic re-dilution; very high level samples may require further offline dilutions.

Hevylite assays have good analytical sensitivity and within-run and between-run precision. Performance characteristics are summarised in Table 38.1. A particular advantage of the Binding Site SPAPLUS Hevylite assays is their wide measuring range. In comparison with the Siemens BNII, SPAPLUS assays require fewer dilutions to reach the upper limit of the reportable range. Measuring ranges are discussed further in Section 9.4.3.

	IgGκ	IgGλ	IgAκ	IgAλ	IgMκ	IgMλ
Range (at standard dilution)	1.9 - 40.0 g/L (1/20)	0.92 - 29.5 g/L (1/20)	0.18 - 11.2 g/L (1/10)	0.16 - 10.4 g/L (1/10)	0.2 - 5.0 g/L (1/10)	0.18 - 4.50 g/L (1/10)
Sensitivty (neat assay dilution)	0.094 g/L	0.046 g/L	0.018 g/L	0.016 g/L	0.02 g/L	0.018 g/L
Total reportable range	0.094 - 160 g/L	0.046 - 118 g/L	0.018 - 67.2 g/L	0.016 - 62.4 g/L	0.02 - 45.0 g/L	0.018 - 40.5 g/L
Assay time	15 min	15 min	15 min	15 min	15 min	15 min
Precision: within run	2.3% at 3.18 g/L	2.1% at 1.73 g/L	3.1% at 0.31 g/L	3.2% at 0.26 g/L	2.4% at 0.34 g/L	2.0% at 0.29 g/L
	1.2% at 9.69 g/L	1.4% at 5.33 g/L	2.4% at 2.09 g/L	2.1% at 1.99 g/L	1.5% at 1.80 g/L	2.0% at 0.96 g/L
	1.2% at 25.18 g/L	0.7% at 23.75 g/L	1.2% at 8.86 g/L	1.4% at 8.31 g/L	1.8% at 4.13 g/L	1.7% at 4.11 g/L
Precision: between run	4.1% at 3.18 g/L	4.7% at 1.73 g/L	4.1% at 0.31 g/L	2.2% at 0.26 g/L	3.3% at 0.34 g/L	2.1% at 0.29 g/L
	2.6% at 9.69 g/L	2.6% at 5.33 g/L	2.3% at 2.09 g/L	2.4% at 1.99 g/L	1.3% at 1.80 g/L	0.5% at 0.96 g/L
	2.0% at 25.18 g/L	2.5% at 23.75 g/L	2.7% at 8.86 g/L	2.3% at 8.31 g/L	1.8% at 4.13 g/L	1.5% at 4.11 g/L

Table 38.1. Hevylite assay performance on the Binding Site SPAPLUS analyser.

Antigen excess (prozone) parameters exist for IgMκ and IgMλ Hevylite SPAPLUS assays, and are discussed further in Section 11.4. Samples detected as being in antigen excess are automatically flagged by the instrument with a prozone (P) flag and the sample is automatically re-assayed at the higher re-dilution.

Test Questions

1. Which Hevylite assays have antigen excess (prozone) parameters?

Answers

1. The IgM Hevylite assays have prozone parameters on the Binding Site SPAPLUS and the Siemens BNII analysers (Section 38.1).

External quality assurance schemes for Freelite and Hevylite immunoassays

Summary:

- There are currently five external quality assurance schemes for sFLC analysis, and one scheme for Hevylite® analysis.
- The UK NEQAS scheme has the highest number of participants, with over 380 laboratories registered.
- When submitting sFLC results as part of an external quality assurance scheme it is important to treat the sample as routine (including antigen excess checks) and ensure that concentrations are reported using the correct units.

39.1. Introduction

It is important that all laboratories participate in external quality assurance (QA) schemes when performing monoclonal protein analysis. There are several national and international QA schemes for assessing serum free light chains (sFLC). Particular care should be taken when reporting sFLC results: in the USA mg/dL units are commonly used, while elsewhere, mg/L is the norm. Individual QA scheme results that are 10- or 100-fold different from the majority view can probably be attributed to errors in calculating or recording the sample concentration.

39.2. The Binding Site schemes

39.2.1. QA003

The Binding Site IMMPROVE™ serum paraprotein QA scheme (QA003) was the first scheme to include sFLC analysis. To date, there have been more than 70 distributions over 12 years, and over 300 laboratories worldwide currently participate in the scheme. Four serum samples are issued per year and results can be returned via the IMMPROVE website. Methodologies assessed include serum protein electrophoresis (SPE), serum immunofixation electrophoresis (sIFE) and sFLC assays *(Chapter 4)*. Laboratories are able to return quantitative results for IgG, IgA, IgM, β_2-microglobulin, κ sFLCs, λ sFLCs and the κ/λ sFLC ratio. A comprehensive report is returned to each laboratory in which sFLC results are categorised according to nephelometric/turbidimetric instrument type to allow user group comparisons to be made. The report also includes examples of electrophoresis gels and an interpretative comment regarding the sample and results.

Electrophoresis and sFLC results from a typical QA003 report (Distribution 129, August 2014) are shown in Figures 39.1, 39.2 and 39.3. Whilst 82% of laboratories reported that no monoclonal protein was visible by SPE or sIFE, the majority of participants reporting Freelite® results identified monoclonal κ FLCs of approximately 500 mg/L. A small sub-group of laboratories reported significantly lower κ sFLC concentrations. This sub-group primarily consisted of laboratories using another (non-Freelite) method for FLC measurement. This distribution illustrates that absolute FLC values reported by other FLC assays may be significantly different to those reported by Freelite *(Chapter 8)*.

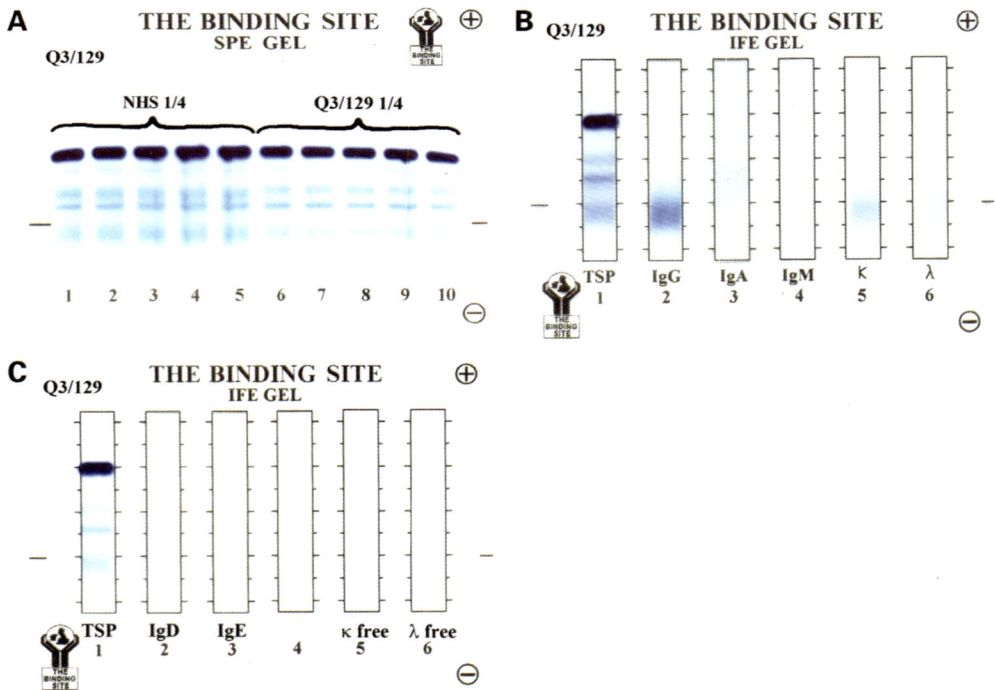

Figure 39.1. QA003 Distribution 129, August 2014. (A) SPE gel accompanying report. Lanes 1-5: normal human serum (NHS); Lanes 6-10; QA003 serum. (B) and (C) sIFE gels accompanying report. No obvious monoclonal protein is visible. This sample contained monoclonal κ FLC by sFLC analysis.

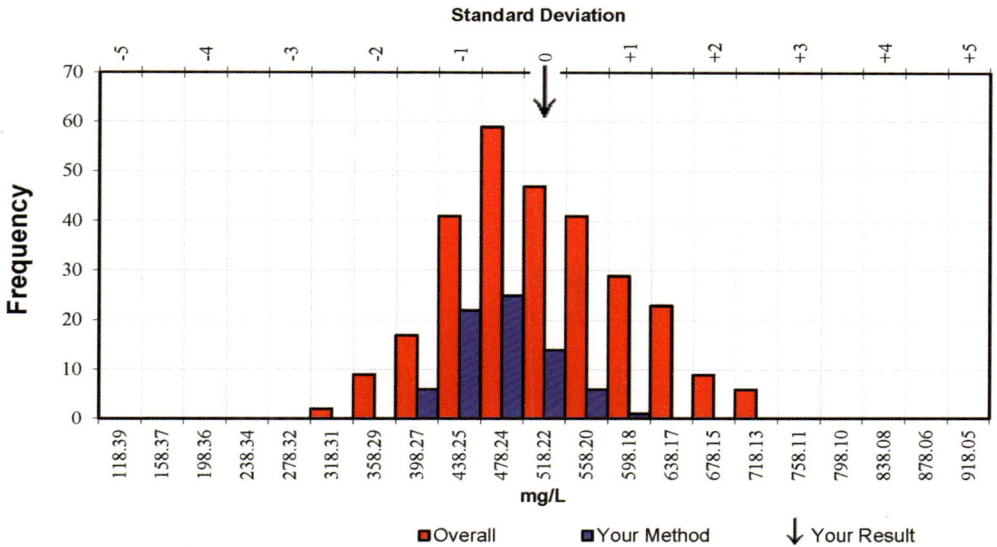

Figure 39.2. QA003 Distribution 129, August 2014. *Frequency distribution of reported κ sFLC results. Red histogram: all participants; blue histogram: Binding Site SPAPLUS® results. The result from the reporting laboratory is indicated by an arrow.*

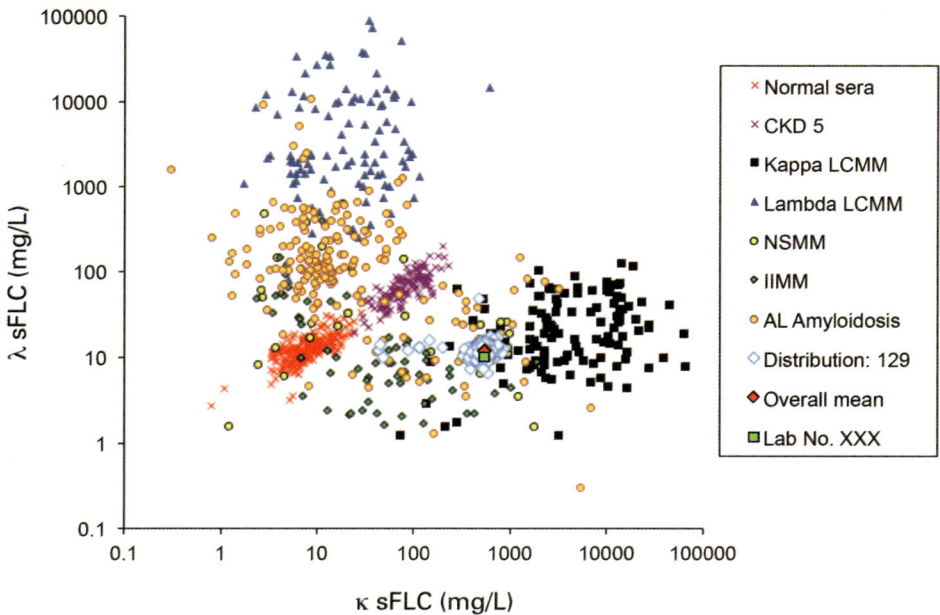

Figure 39.3. QA003 Distribution 129, August 2014. *sFLC results for normal sera and different patient groups represented on a dot plot. The result from the reporting laboratory and overall mean value are identified.*

39.2.2. QA003.H

In May 2013 the Binding Site launched a pilot quality assurance scheme for Hevylite analysis (QA003.H). Four samples are distributed each year and over 40 laboratories currently participate in the scheme. The scheme requires samples to be initially screened by SPE and sIFE, followed by Hevylite assays with the HLC pair selected as indicated by the immunofixation results. Participants receive a comprehensive report that includes analysis of qualitative results for SPE/sIFE and quantitative results for HLC assays that correspond with the monoclonal intact immunoglobulin type. Examples from a typical report are shown in Figures 39.4 and 39.5.

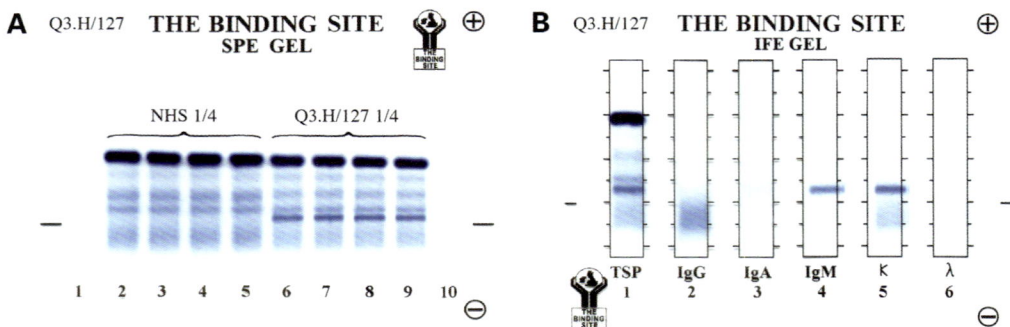

Figure 39.4. QA003.H Distribution 127, February 2014. (A) SPE gel accompanying report. Lanes 2-5: normal human serum *(NHS); Lanes 6-9; QA003.H serum. 94% of laboratories who returned SPE/CZE results reported the presence of a monoclonal protein. (B) sIFE gels accompanying report. This sample contained an IgMκ monoclonal protein which was correctly identified by all of the laboratories who returned IFE results.*

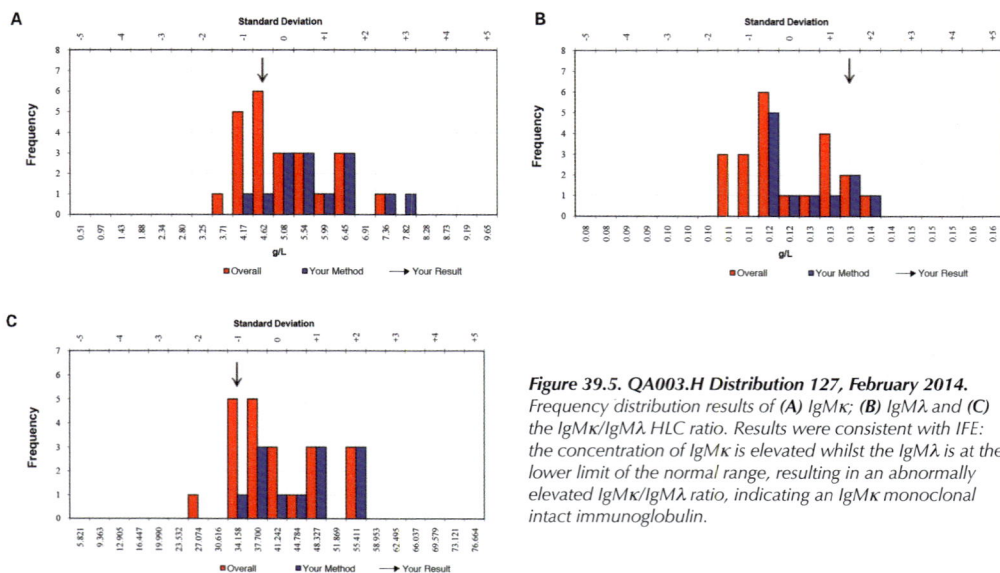

Figure 39.5. QA003.H Distribution 127, February 2014. Frequency distribution results of *(A)* IgMκ; *(B)* IgMλ and *(C)* the IgMκ/IgMλ HLC ratio. Results were consistent with IFE: the concentration of IgMκ is elevated whilst the IgMλ is at the lower limit of the normal range, resulting in an abnormally elevated IgMκ/IgMλ ratio, indicating an IgMκ monoclonal intact immunoglobulin.

39.3. United Kingdom National External Quality Assessment Service scheme

The United Kingdom National External Quality Assessment Service (UK NEQAS) for Immunology, Immunochemistry & Allergy (IIA) provides a Monoclonal Protein Identification scheme that is accredited by the United Kingdom Accreditation Service (UKAS). The scheme has incorporated sFLC analysis since 2005 and there are six distributions per year comprising unmatched serum and urine samples. Over 380 UK and international laboratories are registered for the scheme, and approximately 170 report quantitative sFLC results. Quantitative sFLC results are reported separately to other laboratory test results and are categorised by both instrument type and reagent manufacturer.

Past distributions have highlighted the need for all participants to be aware of sFLC assay technical issues. For example, the Dade Behring BN™II Freelite κ sFLC results for UK NEQAS Distribution 095 were bimodal: peaks were observed at 143 mg/L and 1001 mg/L *(Figure 39.6)*. It is likely that these two peaks corresponded to those participants who did not, and those who did, screen for sFLC antigen excess (following the dilution protocol in the product insert). The phenomenon of antigen excess is further discussed in Section 7.4.

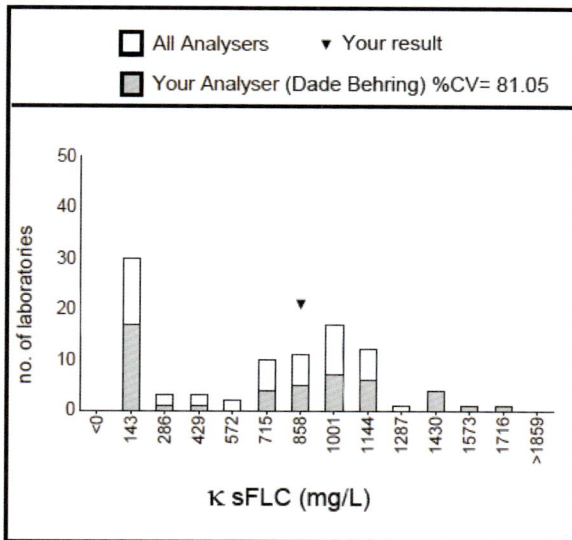

Figure 39.6. UK NEQAS IIA monoclonal protein identification scheme distribution 095. *κ Freelite results show bimodal distribution due to antigen excess. Some participants reported κ concentrations from initial sample dilution (falsely low due to antigen excess), others reported the true value. (Reproduced with permission from UK NEQAS).*

Since 2012, Siemens N Latex FLC assays have been reported as a separate user group. This has allowed the absolute values reported by Freelite and N Latex FLC assays to be compared. For example in Distribution 136, N Latex FLC results were significantly lower than those reported by Freelite *(Figure 39.7)*. The results indicate that the two assays do not compare well; this is discussed further in Section 8.5.3.

Specimen : 136-1	n	Mean	SD	CV(%)
All methods [ALTM]	164	316.51	115.63	36.5
Beckman - IMMAGE-BS	18	299.04	80.26	26.8
Beckman - Olympus-BS	4	294.21	193.81	65.9
Binding Site - SPA Plus-BS	32	414.25	41.43	10.0
Other	6	307.83	107.20	34.8
Roche - Cobas C-BS	12	340.47	15.58	4.6
Roche-Hitachi-BS	4	403.27	27.46	6.8
Roche-Integra-BS	7	349.99	12.62	3.6
SMS. Diag. - BNII-BS	35	351.47	51.18	14.6
SMS. Diag. - BNII-SMS	13	84.63	4.93	5.8
SMS.Diag-ProSpec-SMS	8	89.69	9.24	10.3
SMS.Diag.-ProSpec-BS	20	327.44	33.76	10.3

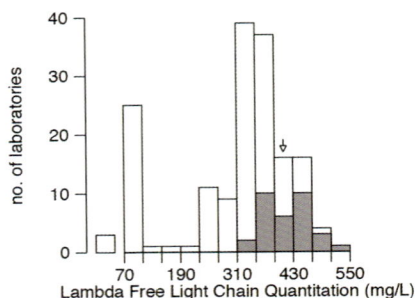

Figure 39.7. UK NEQAS IIA monoclonal protein identification scheme distribution 136 . N Latex FLC assays on the BNII and ProSpec (SMS. Diag. – BNII-SMS and SMS. Diag-ProSpec-SMS, respectively) showed similar λ sFLC assay precision to Freelite assays, but with a lower mean value. (Reproduced with permission from UK NEQAS).

39.4. College of American Pathologists scheme

The College of American Pathologists (CAP) has recently introduced a proficiency testing scheme for sFLCs. Three serum samples are distributed every 6 months, and currently over 250 participants are enrolled in the scheme. In contrast to The Binding Site and UK NEQAS schemes described above, the CAP sFLC scheme does not include proficiency testing for serum electrophoresis, which is tested separately.

39.5. Randox International Quality Assessment scheme

The Randox International Quality Assessment scheme (RIQAS) for Specific Proteins, incorporating FLCs, has been accredited by the UKAS since 2002 and is currently accredited to the ISO 17043 standard. Twelve liquid stable serum samples are distributed every 6 months with over 180 samples having been distributed to date. There are currently around 830 participants in the scheme with approximately 65 reporting results for FLCs.

39.6. German Institute for Standardisation scheme

The German Institute for Standardisation's Gesellschaft zur Förderung der Qualitätssicherung in Medizinischen Laboratorien scheme (abbreviated to INSTAND e.V.) provides a monoclonal protein scheme with over 760 participating laboratories reporting IFE results. Since 2007, sFLCs have been added and there are currently over 120 laboratories reporting sFLC results. Two plasma samples are distributed 4 times per year.

Test Questions

1. How do absolute sFLC values reported by N Latex FLC assays and Freelite assays compare?

Answers

1. EQA scheme results indicate that the assays do not compare well and are not interchangeable *(Section 39.3 and Chapter 8)*.

Index

A

C

I

W